FRAMES OF REFERENCE
for Pediatric Occupational Therapy

THIRD EDITION

PAULA KRAMER, PhD, OTR, FAOTA

Professor and Chair
Department of Occupational Therapy
College of Health Sciences
University of the Sciences in Philadelphia
Philadelphia, Pennsylvania

JIM HINOJOSA, PhD, OT, BCP, FAOTA

Professor
Department of Occupational Therapy
Steinhardt School of Culture, Education, and Human Development
New York University
New York, New York

Wolters Kluwer | Lippincott Williams & Wilkins
Health

Philadelphia • Baltimore • New York • London
Buenos Aires • Hong Kong • Sydney • Tokyo

Acquisitions Editor: Emily Lupash
Managing Editor: Linda G. Francis
Marketing Manager: Allison Noplock
Design Coordinator: Stephen Druding
Production Editor: Marian A. Bellus
Compositor: Laserwords Private Limited, Chennai, India

351 West Camden Street   530 Walnut Street
Baltimore, Maryland 21201-2436 USA   Philadelphia, Pennsylvania 19106 USA

Printed in China

Library of Congress Cataloging-in-Publication Data

Frames of reference for pediatric occupational therapy / [edited by] Paula Kramer, Jim Hinojosa. —3rd ed.
   p. ; cm.
  Includes bibliographical references and index.
  ISBN-13: 978-0-7817-6826-9
  ISBN-10: 0-7817-6826-8
  1. Occupational therapy for children. I. Kramer, Paula. II. Hinojosa, Jim.
  [DNLM: 1. Occupational Therapy—methods. 2. Child Development. 3. Child. 4. Disabled
Children—rehabilitation. 5. Infant. WS 368 F813 2009]
  RJ53.O25F73 2009
  615.8'515—dc22

                              2008046747

CCS0715

We dedicate this book to the children, families, and colleagues with whom we have worked who have changed our lives and perspectives. Ultimately, this book is dedicated to the children whose lives may be changed by this book.

CONTRIBUTORS

Kimberly A. Barthel, BMR, OTR
NDTA OT Instructor
Labyrinth Journeys
Victoria, British Columbia, Canada

Cheryl Ann Colangelo, MS, OTL
Occupational Therapist
North Salem Central School District
North Salem, New York;
Clinical instructor
Columbia University;
Instructor, Mercy College
Dobbs Ferry, New York

Craig Greber, BHMS (Ed), B Occ Thy
Senior Lecturer in Occupational Therapy
School of Health and Sport Sciences
Faculty of Science, Health and Education
University of the Sunshine Coast
Maroochydore DC, Australia

Kristine Haertl, PhD, OTR/L
Associate Professor
Department of Occupational Science and
    Occupational Therapy
The College of St. Catherine
St. Paul, Minnesota

Jim Hinojosa, PhD, OT, FAOTA
Professor
Department of Occupational Therapy
Steinhardt School Culture, Education, and
    Human Development
New York University
New York, New York

Margaret Kaplan, PhD, OTR/L
Associate Professor, Occupational Therapy
    Program
State University of New York
Downstate Medical Center
Brooklyn, New York

Jane Koomar, PhD, OTR/L, FAOTA
Executive Director
Occupational Therapy Associates;
Board President
Sensory Processing Institute for Research and
    Learning (SPIRAL) Foundation
Watertown, Massachusetts

Paula Kramer, PhD, OTR, FAOTA
Professor and Chair
Department of Occupational Therapy
College of Health Sciences
University of the Sciences
    in Philadelphia
Philadelphia, Pennsylvania

Shelly J. Lane, PhD, OTR/L, FAOTA
Professor and Chair
Department of Occupational Therapy;
Assistant Dean of Research
School of Allied Health Professions
Virginia Commonwealth University
Richmond, Virginia

Aimee J. Luebben, Ed.D., OTR, FAOTA
Professor of Occupational Therapy
University of Southern Indiana
Evansville, Indiana

Teresa A. May-Benson, ScD, OTR/L
Clinical Director
Occupational Therapy Associates-Watertown;
Research Director
Sensory Processing Institute for Research and
    Learning (SPIRAL) Foundation
Watertown, Massachusetts

Mary Muhlenhaupt, OTR, FAOTA
Clinical Research Coordinator
Child and Family Studies Research Programs
Thomas Jefferson University
Philadelphia, Pennsylvania;
Occupational Therapy Consultant
Phoenixville, Pennsylvania

Laurette Joan Olson, PhD, OTR
Associate Professor
Mercy College
Dobbs Ferry, New York;
Occupational Therapy Consultant
Mamaroneck Public Schools
Mamaroneck, New York

Karen Roston, MA OTR/L
Candidate for Doctorate of Professional Studies
New York University
New York, New York;
Senior Occupational Therapist
New York City Department of Education
New York, New York

**Charlotte Brasic Royeen, PhD,
OTR, FAOTA**
Dean of Edward and Margaret Doisy College of
    Health Sciences
Professor of Occupational Science and
    Occupational Therapy
Saint Louis University
St. Louis, Missouri

**Roseann C. Schaaf, PhD,
OTR/L, FAOTA**
Associate Professor and Vice Chairman
Department of Occupational Therapy
Thomas Jefferson University
Philadelphia, Pennsylvania

Sarah A. Schoen, PhD, OTR
Director of Applied Research
SPD Foundation
Greenwood Village, Colorado;
Assistant Professor, Rocky Mountain University
Clinical Instructor
University of Colorado at Denver and Health
    Sciences Center
Denver, Colorado

Mary Shea, MA, OTR, ATP
Kessler Institute for Rehabilitation
Clinical Manager, Occupational Therapy
West Orange, New Jersey

**Susanne Smith Roley, MS,
OTR/L, FAOTA**
Project Director, USC/WPS Comprehensive
    Program in Sensory Integration
USC Division of Occupational Science and
    Occupational Therapy
Los Angeles, California;
Coordinator of Education and Research,
    Pediatric Therapy Network
Torrance, California

**Colleen M. Schneck, ScD,
OTR/L, FAOTA**
Department Chair and Professor
Department of Occupational Therapy
Eastern Kentucky University
Richmond, Kentucky

Tien-Ni Wang, MA
Doctoral Candidate
Teaching Fellow
New York University
New York, New York

**Jenny Ziviani, PhD, MEd,
BA, BAppSc(OT)**
Associate Professor
Division of Occupational Therapy
The University of Queensland
Brisbane, Australia

The need for occupational therapy services has risen exponentially with the increase in adverse conditions affecting children's health including poverty, disease, complications from multiple births, and rates of disabilities due to autism. We as occupational therapists are challenged, therefore, to provide services to a wide range of children having specific pediatric conditions and their families in an ethical, professional, and efficacious manner. Paula Kramer and Jim Hinojosa's third edition of *Frames of Reference in Pediatric Occupational Therapy* discusses the legitimate tools of occupational therapy pediatric practice. I argue that this book is, in fact, an important and essential tool for any pediatric occupational therapy student or practitioner. It is one tool that will assist any of us, be it a student, new graduate, or someone like myself with a few decades of practice under her belt, to conceptualize and revise pediatric occupational therapy practice by current standards including new and emerging theory as well as international trends in use of professional language.

There are many aspects of this book that are simply stellar.

- It is easy to read.
- It takes complex concepts and presents them in an easy to understand manner.
- It is extremely comprehensive in terms of a variety of theoretical references.
- It reflects high academic and practice standards.
- It is very practical in that it reaffirms the need to use multiple frames of references in practice.

Personally, I really appreciate the emphasis the editors have placed upon critical reasoning and conscious use of self as two key elements of pediatric occupational therapy practice. For, regardless of our technology and sophisticated knowledge and understanding of the field, our application of such is only as good as our critical reasoning and our ability to use ourselves well in the treatment process.

Frames of Reference for Pediatric Occupational Therapy well reflects occupational therapy's longstanding and exceptional use of theory, and multiple theories, as legitimate tools of practice. For our practice must not only be evidence based, but must additionally be theoretically based or referenced. Over 20 years ago I had the good fortune to serve as the first and only occupational therapist serving as a research analyst in the Office of Special Education in the U.S. Department of Education. Part of my job was to oversee research grant competitions primarily involving those in special education. After having worked there for about 2 years and having seen the relatively "atheoretical" approach of most research in special education, and having had many a conversation about how occupational therapy approached working with children having similar characteristics as those being studied in the many research grants, the Division Director, Dr. Marty Kaufman, shared with me his observation that pediatric occupational therapy was a very theory-rich and theory-related profession, especially as compared to special education. It is high time to highlight and emphasis our rich theoretical foundations.

Thus, I take great pride in this book about pediatric occupational therapy practice that is so theory laden. If only all books in occupational therapy were of this bent! The theory driven approach of Kramer and Hinojosa takes us far beyond the technical, and firmly plants us in the realm of professional practice. Their scholarly leadership in taking us to this level is acknowledged and greatly appreciated.

So, take heart in the strong and vibrant theory-referenced approach to pediatric practice that this book conveys. It helps us all in occupational therapy to better serve humanity!

Charlotte Brasic Royeen
Glen Carbon, Illinois
June 14, 2008

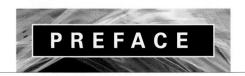
PREFACE

"Without theory, practice is but routine born of habit." Louis Pasteur

We strongly believe that practice needs to be based on theory. The frame of reference provides an effective vehicle for putting theoretical information into practice, a blueprint for the therapist. The question arises, why do a third edition? And the answer was clear to us, to include the changes and updates of both theory and practice and include new knowledge that is being used in practice.

We relied on feedback from users of the text and other expert reviewers, to reorganize and update the new edition. All of the chapters have been updated to reflect changes in theory and practice. The first section holds critical background information for current pediatric practice. The structure of the frame of reference has been put up front as that is the heart of the text. The second section contains the various frames of reference. This third edition supports the evolution of the profession to recognize the importance of occupation and all of the frames of reference have been revised to include the importance of occupation and participation in life. This includes several new frames of references, such as an original approach to teaching and learning, the Four Quadrant Model; an innovative frame of reference to enhance childhood occupations, SCOPE-IT; and a creative frame of reference to enhance social participation. A major thrust of this revision was the updating of material. Content was overhauled to reflect changes in the field. The final section presents important issues in applying frames of reference.

As with previous editions, this third edition is meant to be an effective tool for teaching pediatrics to entry-level students, however it can be equally effective for therapists who want to enhance the use of theory in their practice, and for those who are seeking new and updated approaches to interventions. The book continues to provide pediatric information organized through the structure of frames of reference.

For this edition, we used the language of the World Health Organization's International Classification of Functioning, Disability, and Health (ICF). Incorporation of ICF language broadens the appeal of the book. This language resulted in an emphasis on the importance of the child's ability to participate in meaningful activities of life (occupations). It is our hope that both new and experienced therapists will use this text to bring new approaches into their practice and update their knowledge of their favorite frames of reference. We hope that practice never becomes habit and is continually updated through the use of current theory.

Paula Kramer, PhD, OTR, FAOTA
Jim Hinojosa, PhD, OT, FAOTA

ACKNOWLEDGMENTS

We waited a long time, in the publishing world, to create this third edition. It was our goal that it should contain new knowledge and make a significant contribution to pediatric practice. We think this edition really achieves those goals. All the chapters which appear in previous editions have been updated and we have added new chapters that we believe are relevant to current practice. We hope this third edition will enrich the literature on pediatric occupational therapy.

There are many people to thank who helped us, directly or indirectly, to make this possible. First and foremost, we thank our parents as they are critical to our development and success. Our families have always been there for us, providing love, support and encouragement, especially David and Andrew Hunt, and Steven A. Smith. Dr. Anne Cronin Mosey has strongly influenced our thinking, organization, and professional development, and we gratefully recognize her contribution to the body of knowledge of occupational therapy.

A special thanks to all the authors who contributed to this book, and to their spouses, significant others, families and friends who were supportive to them and thus assisted them in producing such fine work. We are fortunate that they consider us to be their friends as well as their colleagues. Our colleagues at University of the Sciences in Philadelphia and New York University have always provided us with encouragement, support, and feedback throughout this project. We are very appreciative of the efforts of the entire team at Lippincott Williams & Wilkins who have been tremendous supporters of this book. We are grateful to our students for their questions and observations which have always stimulated our growth. Their feedback as students and therapists have continually contributed to our development and shown us that this book is valuable and well used.

The pictures in this book are critical to illustrating the text. Numerous families and colleagues contributed photos and we are very grateful that they have allowed their children to appear in this book. It makes the text much richer. We would like to specifically thank Karen Buckley, Yael Goverover, and Maria Mendoza and David Smith for their photographs. Two professional photographers were helpful to us, Daniel Hunt and Pam Sevenbergen.

Finally, we are indebted to our colleagues who continue to develop the art and science of pediatric occupational therapy.

CONTENTS

PART I: FOUNDATIONS OF PEDIATRIC PRACTICE   1

PART III: ISSUES WHEN APPLYING FRAMES OF REFERENCE   569

PART I

Foundations of Pediatric Practice

CHAPTER 1

Structure of the Frame of Reference

JIM HINOJOSA • PAULA KRAMER • AIMEE J. LUEBBEN

Healthcare professionals use theory to guide their practice. Theories are predictions of what will occur under certain circumstances. When people hear the word "theory," they tend to think of something that is complex, esoteric, difficult to understand, and completely impractical. A frame of reference uses pieces of one or more theories and makes them practical and useful. On the basis of one or more theories, a frame of reference is an accepted structure for organizing theoretical material and translating information into practice. The scaffolding of a frame of reference organizes theoretical material needed for problem identification and solution in occupational therapy service delivery.

Before learning about the usefulness of frames of reference, it is critical to have a basic understanding of theory. The purpose of a theory is to inform the theorist's intentions and the use of theory refers to how professionals actually put the theory into practice. Sometimes theory is not complex: people develop simple theories all the time.

When a person observes something and thinks that what he or she observed is repeated often in the world to create a pattern, he or she is developing a theory. For example, when we observe children playing on a slide in a playground, we might see that older children are more likely to go down the slide immediately and have fun. Younger children may get to the top of the steps of the slide and seem anxious and reluctant to come down without coaching or encouragement. Our theory might state that young children are fearful of going down a slide until they have repeated pleasurable experiences. This theory can be confirmed by observing other children in other playgrounds; this establishes validity through repeated observations (Figure 1.1).

In science, theories are based on the observation of phenomena. Scientists categorize what they have observed and then use that categorization to make predictions between objects or events. Theories are the formalized collection of concepts, definitions, and theoretical postulates, which predict relationships between behaviors and events in specified circumstances. A theory also has underlying assumptions.

Concepts, which provide the basis for categorization, are labels of phenomena that have specific, definable characteristics. Definitions (the specific, definable characteristics of concepts) are critically important to theory because they identify the shared characteristics of a concept, allowing people to determine which phenomena are included in the concept and which are not. Some of the concepts in this first example are older children, young children, height, slides, and anxiety. In this example, concepts have

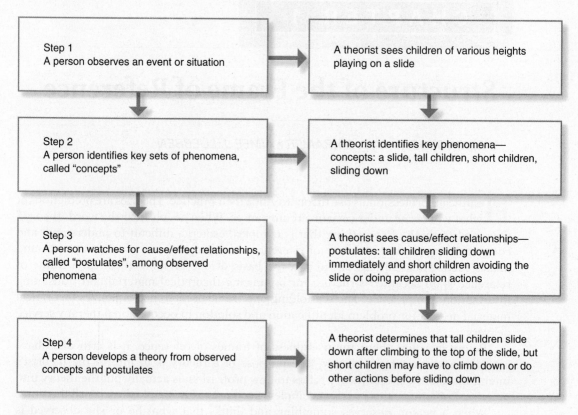

FIGURE 1.1 Establishing validity of a theory through repeated observations.

definitions based on our observations of the playground. Older children are physically larger and at least 2 ft tall. Younger children are smaller and shorter than 2 ft. Height is the size of a child in inches and feet. Slides are structures in the playground that are triangular in shape, with a means of going up on one side and a smooth surface on the diagonal side that allows a child to move down freely and smoothly. Anxiety is defined as behaviors including stopping at the top of the slide, crying, whining, or expressing fear. A theorist defines concepts in the way concepts are used, not necessarily using a dictionary definition or language that reflects common use. Once a theoretical concept is defined, the definition must be used consistently throughout the theory. If a new theory is developed or adapted, the theorist may modify the definition.

Theoretical postulates state the relationship between two or more concepts. Using the same example, one postulate maintains that younger children who hesitate at the top of a slide show anxiety (Figure 1.2). A second postulate holds that older children who go down the slide without stopping show no anxiety (Figure 1.3). A third postulate would be that the slide provokes anxiety in some children.

As explained earlier, a theory comprises concepts, definitions, and theoretical postulates. These concepts, definitions, and postulates define the parameters of the theory.

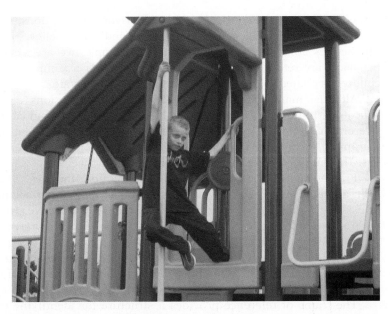

FIGURE 1.2 Child showing trepidation about a new motor act.

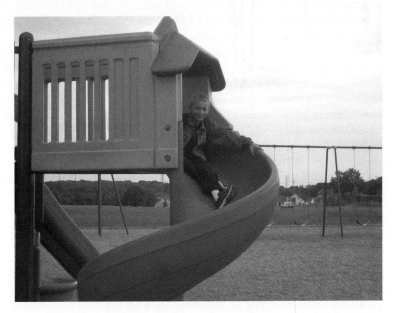

FIGURE 1.3 Normal child enjoying going down the slide.

A theory is developed consistent with underlying assumptions, in which the therapist believes. An assumption is something that an individual believes in and never questions. All theories contain assumptions. In our example, we are assuming that children's behaviors are reflective of emotional state. Another assumption is that the size of the children is related to their ability and to their feeling state.

Although many theories are shared by various professions (e.g., some psychologists, educators, physical therapists, and physicians use developmental theory), a frame of reference customizes theoretical information so that it can be used by occupational therapists. A frame of reference uses theoretical information to develop a theoretical base that guides evaluation and application to practice.

Frames of reference are based on one or more theories. The frame of reference is an accepted vehicle for organizing theoretical material in occupational therapy and translating it into practice through a functional perspective. In the pediatric arena, the frame of reference offers an outline of fundamental theoretical concepts relative to particular areas of function. The frame of reference serves as a guideline for assessing functional capacities in a client and offers a method for conceptualizing and initiating intervention. Frames of reference, therefore, enable the therapist to use theory in practice.

The frame of reference provides a structure for identifying relevant theories and then based on this information, outlines guidelines that occupational therapists use when assessing and providing intervention. This textbook comes from a perspective that all interventions begin with a thorough understanding of the child and family and their unique situation. For credibility of the profession, interventions must be theory based.

It is common for occupational therapy textbooks to focus on diagnostic categories (e.g., cerebral palsy, Down syndrome, etc.). Occupational therapists must learn about diagnostic categories. Diagnostic categories provide critical information needed to understand the child and his or her impairments and disabilities. Under discussions of treatment, diagnostic categories tend to be linked with specific strategies for intervention. The inherent premise, in this type of a textbook, is that a person chooses an intervention based on the diagnosis of the client. Although a diagnosis may provide insight into a child's disabilities, occupational therapists are concerned primarily with functional performance. Material organized around diagnostic categories does not always address the essential focus of the occupational therapy process. Occupational therapists are concerned with disabilities and impairments that may result from a diagnosis rather than the diagnosis itself. In addition, a child may exhibit several other needs not described in the diagnostic category but still fundamental to intervention planning.

Theories that serve as the basis for frames of reference address the strengths and limitations of the child and family. They do not focus solely on diagnosis, disability, or impairment. This book comprises articulated frames of reference that delineate the relationship between theory and practice. The frame of reference is designed first to highlight traditionally used theories, then to relate that information to function, and, finally, to organize that information for the purpose of intervention. The frame of reference essentially is a blueprint for evaluation and intervention.

The frame of reference is a method of organizing knowledge so that it could be used for planning and implementing intervention. The frame of reference consists of components: a theoretical base, function–dysfunction continua which includes indicators of function and dysfunction, a guide for evaluation, postulates regarding charge, and application to practice. The concept of indicators of function and dysfunction as defined by Mosey (1981, 1996) has been expanded to a section "Guide for Evaluation." Additionally, we have added another component, "Application to Practice" (Kramer & Hinojosa, 1999).

The purpose of the "Guide for Evaluation" section is to suggest methods and tools that may be used to evaluate a client's performance that would be compatible with a particular frame of reference. The "Application to Practice" component articulates for the occupational therapist how the frame of reference is used for treatment. This component is meant to clarify how a therapist moves in practice clinically from a theoretical perspective through the process of evaluation and the identification of specific problem areas to intervention.

Application to practice describes the media and modalities a therapist would employ for a particular frame of reference. This component also gives some specific examples of this application to the therapist. The context, including physical environment, in which this frame of reference may be used and the possible modifications to that environment are presented in this section. Including environment within application to practice allows a better understanding of the intervention process, giving more attention to the context of intervention.

The challenge to any therapist is the application of theoretical knowledge to practice. Moving from theory to practice is a complex process; it entails taking ideas that are abstract and bringing them to a level at which they can be used. When choosing a frame of reference, the occupational therapist looks at the child's needs, strengths, limitations, and environment. With a comprehensive understanding of all these issues, the therapist chooses the most appropriate approach for the child and within the context for service delivery. The frame of reference delineates the perspective of the occupational therapist when approaching the child.

These concepts are abstract and can be understood best through the use of examples. The examples presented are intended to clarify some of the ideas introduced. Our example frame of reference deals with facilitating reciprocal interaction with preschool children with autism. The frame of reference was written by Brunner, Gonzales, & Green-Taub (2003). This example is not intended to be a completely developed frame of reference but, rather, a brief example that exemplifies the various parts needed to understand the structure. The title of the frame of reference is "Facilitating Reciprocal Social Interaction in Preschool Children with Autism." The following section provides a descriptive overview of the characteristics of a theoretical base that provides the core thinking of the frame of reference. After the discussion of a theoretical base, the example is provided. This format is repeated throughout the rest of the chapter.

THEORETICAL BASE

Professional education provides occupational therapists with a broad knowledge base. One aspect of this educational process is the study of various theories. "A theory is concerned with how and under what circumstances those events happen and how they are related. The purpose of theory is to make predictions about the relationships between events or phenomena" (Mosey, 1981, p. 30). Theories provide therapists with ways of understanding the effects of their actions on the subsequent reactions of the child.

Generally, we talk about theory-based intervention in occupational therapy. If intervention is based on theory, a therapist is able to understand the relationship between the treatment and the subsequent reactions of the child. For example, if the theory states a relationship between tickling and laughter, when a child is tickled the therapist should then expect the child to laugh. If the child does not laugh, then the theory also should provide a means for the therapist to understand the lack of response. Most often, therapists do not use theories as a whole. Instead, they tend to select sections from various theories and organize these pieces of information together in a way that it will be meaningful to assist an individual. During this process, therapists are creating a new conceptualization of theoretical information, not new theories themselves (Hinojosa, Kramer, & Pratt, 1996). Intervention should be based on theoretical information because the therapist should be able to describe the postulated links between the intervention and the expected changes in the child.

Sometimes therapists have difficulty transforming theory from a classroom concept into practice. It is as if the theoretical knowledge is separated from practice. Sometimes therapists believe that practical knowledge constitutes a set of specific skills or techniques that are separate from theory. Both theoretical and practical levels of knowledge must be integrated. An organized, consistent treatment plan for the child flows from the clear understanding of the underlying theories. The underlying reasons for any intervention have to be clearly understood. The therapist's actions do not come from intuition but from a well-designed intervention based on thorough theoretical understanding. The frame of reference, therefore, provides cohesion between theory and intervention in a practical manner, with the theoretical base providing the framework for the actual intervention.

The theoretical base provides the foundation of the entire frame of reference. The theoretical base may draw from one or more theories. If more than one theory is used, the theories must be consistent internally or operating from the same basic premises (Mosey, 1981). A comprehensive frame of reference must contain theoretical information of both constant and dynamic theories. Constant theories, which are static theories, are concerned only with describing relationships between phenomena. These static theories do not describe a change process or how change occurs. For example, theories of anatomy describe the human body and the relationships of the various body parts to each other. Theories of anatomy are not concerned with explaining how the body develops or matures; therefore, these theories are considered constant. In pediatrics, some developmental theories are considered constant theories. These theories, which are constant, describe the specific stages and characteristics of the child within those stages, but not how a child moves from one stage to the next. Developmental theorists of the constant variety believe that development is stage specific and one set of skills has to be mastered before the individual moves onto the next set of skills. These theories rely on the natural development of children without an explanation of what should occur if development is delayed in any way.

To be useful in a frame of reference, constant theories are used in combination with dynamic theories. Dynamic theories are those that are concerned with change and describe the theoretical information the therapist will use to promote change in the individual. The types of dynamic theories primarily used in pediatric practice are developmental, acquisitional, and operational. Change occurs in many ways. Neurobiological theorists are concerned with the sequential changes that occur within the individual, with primary focus being on the progression in a specified pattern rather than stages, based on changes in the body, the central nervous system, and psychological growth. Acquisitional theories are based on learning and interaction with the environment, with change depending on the individual's ability to learn new skills or behaviors rather than on developmental stages or maturation. Operational theories are based on environmental changes that assist the individual to improve performance or function. These improvements in performance or function depend on environmental adaptations and are external to the individual (Hinojosa, Kramer, & Pratt, 1996).

When an occupational therapist works with an individual, the ultimate goal is to improve the person's ability to function; therefore, the theoretical base needs to have a dynamic theory to explain how this change in function will occur. Included in the theoretical base are assumptions, concepts, definitions, and postulates. Furthermore, the theoretical base states the relationship between all these elements. The elements of theoretical base follow in the Brunner, Gonzales, & Green-Taub (2003) example.

Theoretical Base for Facilitating Reciprocal Social Interaction in Preschool Children with Autism

Children with autism demonstrate difficulties engaging in social interactions with other individuals. This frame of reference addresses the need for facilitation of reciprocal social interaction skills in preschool children with autism during gross motor play. More precisely, it is intended for children between the ages of 3 and 5 who, though diagnosed with autism, demonstrate an understanding of cause and effect. For inclusion in the frame, a child's vision and hearing should be intact, and he or she must be able to walk independently. Additionally, the child must share the same language as the therapist and participants involved in gross motor play activities.

Autism has been defined in various ways. Kanner (1943) was the first to identify the disorder specifically. In his description, a child's extreme social isolation is an integral and salient feature of autism. It is generally defined in terms of four specific criteria: (1) an onset before the age of 30 months; (2) impaired social development; (3) impaired communicative development; and (4) "insistence on sameness," as shown by stereotyped play patterns, abnormal preoccupations, or resistance to change (American Psychiatric Association, 1994; Rutter, 1978). Children with autism frequently have behavioral and skill deficits that interfere with their ability to engage in appropriate play (Lantz, 2001; Lantz, Nelson, & Loftin, 2004). They tend to play alone and do not have interest in engaging in play with other children (Thomas & Smith, 2004).

"Reciprocal social interaction" is the physical and/or verbal exchange between two or more people that influences the successive behavior of each. This exchange involves a mutual passing back and forth, a response on the part of each individual to a cue emitted by the other (Dalton, 1961). A child's ability to establish relationships with people and inanimate objects requires initiating and responding behaviors from the child. This is affected by any impairment he or she may have in social interactions. "Initiating behaviors" are those social behaviors that are directed toward another individual to start an interaction. These behaviors have not been preceded by a behavior from another individual. Conversely, "responding behaviors" are those directed toward another individual which is in reaction to the behavior of that individual. Initiating and responding behaviors may be verbal or nonverbal. Verbal behaviors include vocalizations directed to another individual, excluding whining, screaming, or crying (Ragland, Kerr, & Strain, 1978).

With autism, a child's use of nonverbal behaviors to aid in social interaction is impaired. More specifically, the child demonstrates (1) inappropriate eye contact, which is considered to be the child's visual contact with the eyes of another person; (2) delayed or lack of a "social smile," which is a facial expression showing pleasure in response to a positive social situation (Agnes, 1999); and (3) a lack of body postures and gestures, such as waving, pointing, reaching, or orienting one's body toward an individual or object (Rapoport & Ismond, 1996). Children with autism also have difficulties with imitation skills. This interferes with their abilities to engage in reciprocal social interactions (Figure 1.4). Imitation occurs when a child produces similar behaviors that have been exhibited by another individual (Baer, Peterson, & Sherman, 1967).

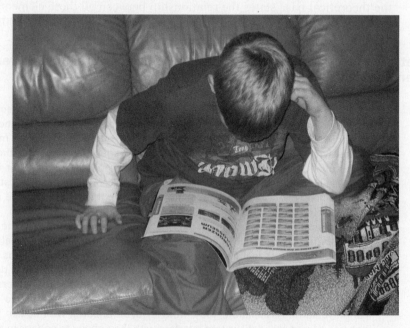

FIGURE 1.4 Child with autistic spectrum disorder focusing on a book with limited awareness of the external environment.

Social learning theory incorporates the concepts of modeling and reinforcement (both vicarious and direct external) to create an environment in which learning can take place (Bandura, 1977). "Modeling" is the process through which an individual forms an idea of how new behaviors are performed by observing others. This information is then stored in memory to direct an individual's actions in the future. Reinforcement is a learning process wherein the person gets feedback from the environment. A person's cognitive awareness is considered to be an integral part of this process. With "direct external reinforcement," persons adapt behaviors based on the consequences of one's own life experiences. "Vicarious reinforcement" occurs when the positive or negative consequences of a modeled action is observed.

According to Bandura's theory, individuals acquire new skills and behaviors in social situations through active engagement in the learning process. Learning takes place as a result of direct external reinforcement, when an individual continues those forms of successful behaviors that have positive effects and rejects those that have unfavorable outcomes during direct life experiences. Learning also takes place through modeling. An individual will pay greater attention to models that have engaging qualities and may not attend to models that lack these qualities. Additionally, a person will attend better to a model's behavior if that behavior is of interest to the person. Through the process of vicarious reinforcement, an individual will replicate the observed model's behaviors, which result in positive consequences or rewards, when in similar situations in the future. Conversely, an individual will not adopt those modeled behaviors which resulted in negative outcomes.

Although there are many definitions, there is no scholarly consensus regarding what specifically constitutes "play." Play is the primary occupation of children (Reilly, 1974). It is a complex set of behaviors characterized by a dynamic process that involves a particular attitude and action. Play involves exploration, experimentation, repetition of experience, and imitation of a child's surroundings (Takata, 1974). The interaction between the child and the environment that is controlled and motivated by the child with no limitation of the real world is also considered to be play (Bundy, 1991). There are also many different types of play, though this frame of reference uses "gross motor play" as a therapeutic modality. Motor play is crawling, running, jumping, climbing, throwing, kicking, and catching; chasing, wrestling, and engaging in other forms of rough and tumble play (Cook & Sinker, 1993).

Assumptions

Theorists develop theories with their own world view. These theories are consistent with the values and beliefs of the theorist. As discussed previously, assumptions are underlying theoretical ideas that are held to be true and are not questioned or tested in any way. In other words, assumptions are basic beliefs. All theories have assumptions. In a frame of reference, a theoretical base comprises several theories. Because each theory has assumptions, it is essential to understand the assumptions of each theory. If a frame of reference includes more than one theory, the theories must share similar assumptions for congruency. For example, psychoanalytic theories cannot be used with behavioral theories. If the theoretical base draws from several theories, then all the assumptions made must be accepted by all of those theories and the assumptions must not be in conflict with each other.

Assumptions from the example:

- Gross motor play increases alertness in some children whereas it decreases excess energy in other children.
- Interactional and self-occupying activities help focus a child's attention in a structured, self-controlled manner.
- Gross motor play facilitates the child's development in social interaction skills.

Concepts

Concepts are labels which describe phenomena that have been observed and have shared characteristics. The concept is a descriptor that the theorist uses to describe a specific set of phenomena. Theorists must define all concepts. Concepts are the fundamental building blocks of a theory. Theories are made up of many concepts. Theorists decide on the concepts (which is the label) that describe the set of phenomena. Therefore, different theorists may use different descriptors to describe the same set of phenomena. As occupational therapists put the theory into practice, they develop a frame of reference. The first step in developing a frame of reference is to start with a theoretical base. Sometimes this can be a complicated process if the therapist finds the same set of phenomena called "different things" (labeled as "different concepts") by different theorists. This may present a challenge, as the therapist must select the most appropriate concept label for the problem which the frame of reference will address. Once the therapist decides on the concept label, this label must be used consistently through the frame of reference. The individual reading the frame of reference must accept the concept label as selected by the developer of the frame of reference to describe that set of phenomena. Some concepts within a theory may be more important than others. The following are concepts identified in the example frame of reference.

Concepts from the example:

- Reciprocal social interactions
- Initiating behaviors
- Responding behaviors
- Reinforcement
- Modeling

Definitions

Definitions explain the meaning of important concepts. In the theoretical base, definitions are generally drawn from the theories that are used. Keep in mind that every concept in a theoretical base should be defined in terms of what it means to the particular frame of reference. The therapist must accept the definitions used by the developer of the theoretical base and is not free to assign his or her own definitions to any concepts in the frame of reference. It should be noted that frequently concepts and their definitions are identified together in the theoretical base and are not always in separate sections. Here are examples of specific definitions within the example frame of reference.

> Reciprocal social interactions: the physical and/or verbal exchange between two or more people that influences the successive behavior of each
>
> Initiating behaviors: those social behaviors that are directed toward another individual to start an interaction
>
> Responding behaviors: those directed toward another individual which is in reaction to the behavior of that individual; initiating and responding behaviors may be verbal or nonverbal
>
> Reinforcement: learning process wherein the person gets feedback from the environment
>
> Modeling: the process through which an individual forms an idea of how new behaviors are performed by observing others (Figure 1.5).

Theoretical Postulates

Theoretical postulates state the relationship between concepts. Within the theoretical base, all concepts are related in some way. Theoretical postulates describe the relationship between concepts. Within a theoretical base, the relationships between

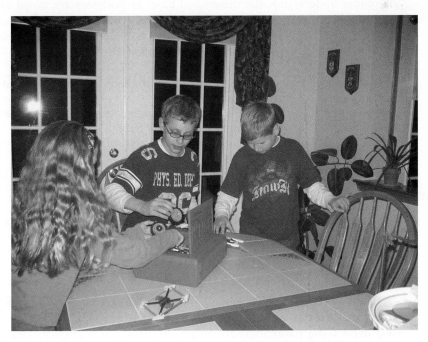

FIGURE 1.5 Children modeling interaction on a group task for a child with autistic spectrum disorder.

important concepts are made clear by postulates. Relationships between concepts may be quantitative or qualitative. Other types of relationships are temporal, spatial, causal, correlative, or hierarchical. Theoretical postulates are statements that describe connections between concepts. A clear understanding of these connections provides structure for the theory and an understanding of how concepts relate to each other in the theory. Theoretical postulates serve as the linking mechanism between concepts.

The theoretical base is constructed from concepts, definitions, and the theoretical postulates from several theories. When developing a theoretical base, the occupational therapist selects theoretical information (concepts, definitions, and theoretical postulates) to provide a foundation for the guideline for intervention. The process of developing the theoretical base involves selecting the appropriate theoretical information needed to address the clinical problem identified. The therapist skillfully selects theoretical information to write a theoretical base that is logical and comprehensive. A major aspect of this process is to select suitable theoretical postulates that clearly state the theoretical rationale in relationship to the problem being addressed.

One specific type of theoretical postulate is a hypothesis. The hypothesis states the theoretical postulate in a way that it can be measured and tested. A hypothesis includes operational definitions that allow variables to be observed and quantified. Most often, hypotheses are not explicitly written in the theoretical base but are implicit when the reader understands the theoretical base. Hypotheses are based on concepts of the dynamic theory, relating to stated postulates. Hypotheses can be tested within a frame of reference. The following are theoretical postulates that provide linking mechanisms between concepts in the example frame of reference:

- Children with autism frequently have behavioral and skill deficits that interfere with their ability to engage in appropriate play.
- A child's ability to establish relationships with people and inanimate objects requires initiating and responding behaviors from the child.
- Through the process of vicarious reinforcement, an individual will replicate the observed model's behaviors.

Organization of the Theoretical Base

When therapists begin to use a new frame of reference, they should be certain to understand the theoretical base and its component parts. The theoretical base sets the stage for the entire frame of reference. To move from theory to implementation of the frame of reference into practice, it is critical to understand the theoretical base, usually the most complex and abstract section in the frame of reference.

The theoretical base broadly delineates areas of concern in the frame of reference within the broader context of occupational therapy. The beginning of the theoretical base defines the parameters for using the frame of reference. This information may include the characteristics of children and their problems that this frame of reference addresses. Further, it might describe service delivery models where it is most likely to be used. The theoretical base identifies the various theories that provide the basis for the frame of reference, all underlying assumptions, and major concepts with definitions.

Within a theoretical base, there is an organizational structure, a design that describes how each of the parts fits together to form a whole. When learning a frame of reference, it is important to understand its design or the way in which it is organized. The way the theoretical base is organized should be reflected in all subsequent parts of the frame of reference. For example, if the theoretical base presents concepts in a particular sequence or progression, then that order should be reflected in all other parts of the frame of reference. This format enables the therapist to see the organizational design of the frame of reference and follow the same order in the application of the theoretical base to intervention. This again highlights the importance of the theoretical base. In the example frame of reference, a conceptual hierarchy is implied by the order of the concepts that are presented in the theoretical base (e.g., initiating behaviors occur before responding behaviors). When studying the theoretical base of a frame of reference, it may be helpful to keep the following questions in mind:

1. What are the assumptions?
2. What are the concepts?
3. What are the definitions of the concepts? Do the definitions provide meaning for the concepts?
4. What are the theoretical postulates? Are the relationships understandable?
5. How is the theoretical base organized?
6. What is the design of the theoretical base? Is the design understandable?

FUNCTION–DYSFUNCTION CONTINUA

This frame of reference section, function–dysfunction continua, clearly identifies those areas of function with which the frame of reference is concerned. After reading a theoretical base, a person should be able to identify the specific areas of performance important to an individual's skills and abilities. Performance related to skills and abilities are the areas the occupational therapist evaluates to determine whether the child is functional or dysfunctional. Concepts with corresponding definitions from the theoretical base identify what therapists consider to be functional. Likewise, concepts and definitions identify what represents dysfunction. Each function–dysfunction continuum covers one area of performance important to the particular frame of reference. A frame of reference generally has several function–dysfunction continua, which are labeled as such because human performance rarely can be classified as good or bad, able or disabled. The situation usually is not so clear-cut. Function is at one end of the spectrum and dysfunction is at the other, and human performance may fall at any point along this scale: Occasionally a frame of reference will have one function–dysfunction continuum.

Function _____ Dysfunction

The functional end of the continuum represents what the therapist expects the child to be able to do, whereas the dysfunctional end of the continuum represents disability:

Function _____ Dysfunction

Expected ability   Disability

Function–dysfunction continua come directly from the theoretical bases of the frames of reference and, therefore, are specific to those frames of reference. They cannot be taken out of context. In the case of the example frame of reference, there are two function–dysfunction continua: initiates behavior and responding behaviors (Tables 1.1 and 1.2).

Indicators of Function and Dysfunction

Underneath each function–dysfunction continuum are either lists of behaviors, physical signs, or some type of functional scale, such as a test score. These are called "indicators of function or dysfunction." When the frame of reference uses lists of behaviors or physical signs, there is one list of expected abilities at the functional end of the continuum. Another list (or the opposite of the "functional" list) identifies behaviors or physical signs that are considered areas of concern, which represent the dysfunctional end of the

TABLE 1.1 Indicators of Function and Dysfunction for Initiating Behaviors

Initiates Behaviors	*Does Not Initiate Behaviors*
FUNCTION: Able to put into action a social behavior directed at another person to start an interaction	DYSFUNCTION: Unable to put into action a social behavior directed at another person to start an interaction
Indicators of Function	**Indicators of Dysfunction**
Makes eye contact with another person to get his or her attention during gross motor play	Does not make eye contact with another individual during gross motor play
Positions self so that he or she is oriented toward another person to get his or her attention during gross motor play	Does not position himself or herself toward another individual or moves away from another individual during gross motor play
Gestures to an object or toward a person to indicate a desire to begin gross motor play	Ignores objects or people in a gross motor play situation
Verbalizes interest to begin gross motor play	Nonverbal and/or shows no interest in a gross motor play situation

TABLE 1.2 Indicators of Function–Dysfunction for Responding Behavior	
Responding Behaviors	*Does Not Demonstrate Responding Behaviors*
FUNCTION: Responds appropriately to another person in reaction to that person's behavior	*DYSFUNCTION*: Responds inappropriately or not at all to another person in reaction to that person's behavior
Indicators of Function	**Indicators of Dysfunction**
Makes eye contact when his or her name is called	Does not respond when his or her name is called
Makes eye contact when given verbal instruction	Does not make eye contact or does not respond to verbal directions
Socially smiles in response to a positive action exhibited by another person during gross motor play	Shows no facial response to a positive action from another person
Demonstrates imitative behaviors of another person during gross motor play	Does not demonstrate imitative behaviors during gross motor play
Verbally responds when asked a question during gross motor play	Will not respond verbally when asked a question during gross motor play

continuum. During the evaluation process, the therapist uses these lists of behavior and physical signs to identify strengths and areas of concern.

Sometimes a functional scale is used for evaluation. Some areas of human performance exhibit wide variations in expected or acceptable performance. For example, grasping an object involves many motoric steps. A child may have developed part of this and still be functional in relation to his or her age but may not have developed the whole sequence of grasping. This child, because he or she has not fully mastered grasping, still would not fall at the functional end of the continuum. In some frames of reference, a functional scale is used to identify expected or acceptable ranges of behaviors or performance rather than specified abilities. For example, a child's activity level could be considered dysfunctional if he or she was at the far end of either side of the continuum, either very active or extremely sedentary.

After the therapist performs an evaluation, he or she can then look at the results and check them against these descriptive lists or functional scales. The more behaviors or physical signs that the child exhibits indicative of dysfunction, the closer the child will be to the dysfunctional end of the continuum, showing that he or she needs intervention. Likewise, the fewer characteristics indicative of dysfunction that the child exhibits, the closer the child will be to the functional end of the scale.

Tables 1.1 and 1.2 are two function–dysfunction continua and the indicators of function and dysfunction from the example frame of reference.

GUIDE FOR EVALUATION

This section identifies how the therapist would approach the evaluation process within a particular frame of reference. The guide for evaluation may serve as an evaluation protocol in defining the areas of performance that the therapist should assess. The evaluation should relate to the indicators of function and dysfunction. Through the evaluation process, the therapist determines where the child falls on each function–dysfunction continuum. Is the child closer to function, or does he or she have so much difficulty with this area of performance that he or she has to be considered in need of intervention?

Specific assessment tools or a specified evaluation protocol may be identified. Most important, the guide for evaluation directs the therapist in the areas that he or she should be looking at to determine if the child needs intervention. This guide should include both standardized and nonstandardized assessments. Standardized assessments are preferable because they are based on psychometric integrity. In reality, there are not always standardized assessments that are consistent with the frame of reference. Each frame of reference has nonstandardized methods of evaluation. They may include a set of activities or tasks that provide necessary information. The occupational therapist uses tools, either standardized or nonstandardized, that will provide an appropriate baseline of performance and assist in developing a meaningful plan for intervention. Although it is often difficult to choose or devise evaluative tasks, the therapist should avoid falling back on "old favorites." Following the indicators of function–dysfunction, the therapist selects tasks to assess these specific behaviors. Assessments should not be chosen on the basis of the therapist's comfort level but on whether the therapist will obtain the necessary data needed for the intervention plan.

Because there is no one ideal assessment for the example frame of reference provided in this chapter, the therapist would have several options. One option might be to observe the child and determine the child's behaviors in play situations with other children. Another option might be to use a standardized play scale and see how the child's performance relates to data on the play of children without disabilities. If using the second option, the therapist has to recognize that these test data alone would not provide enough information to develop a plan for intervention, and another supplementary assessment, such as an observation of the child's interaction with others, would be necessary. Supplementing standardized assessment data provide information about the child in a broader context (as related to the play of children without disabilities), while still providing specific information about that child (through observation of the child in interactions with others). Using the indicators of function and dysfunction as the guide for evaluation, the therapist can determine whether the child can be considered functional or dysfunctional in terms of this specific frame of reference.

POSTULATES REGARDING CHANGE

There are two types of postulates, theoretical postulates and postulates regarding change. Theoretical postulates, found in the theoretical base of the frame of reference, state the relationship between two or more concepts. As indicated before, a dynamic theory, in the theoretical base, has theoretical postulates that explain the change process. The theoretical postulates provide the foundation for the development of the postulates regarding change. Postulates regarding change clarify the relationship between dynamic theory and the guidelines for how the therapist should intervene with the child. Postulates regarding change, like function–dysfunction continua, must relate back to the theoretical postulates in the theoretical base. There are both general and specific postulates regarding change. General postulates regarding change explain the context in which intervention will take place. The specific postulates regarding change describe the interaction between the therapist, the environment, and specific techniques that the therapist will use to bring about change. The specific postulates regarding change are always used in conjunction with the general postulates regarding change.

Postulates regarding change, which are critical for the occupational therapist, move the frame of reference closer to the more concrete level of practice and farther from the abstract level of theory. Think of the postulates regarding change as "if-then" or cause-effect statements, which state that if the therapist acts, then a resultant effect is more likely to occur. The statements are descriptive and guide the therapist's behavior and actions. As action-oriented statements, postulates regarding change convey to the therapist the type of environment that should be created to produce change or the type of technique needed to bring about change. The result can be a change in the child's performance, skills, behavior, or an enhancement of normal growth and development that has been impeded by dysfunction.

The general postulates regarding change encompass more than the physical environment of the intervention setting. These postulates that are general in nature involve the entire context: the emotional climate, the social interaction with the therapist and significant others, and various activities to which the child is exposed. It is important to note that therapists often do not actually create the change in the child, but they do create an environment that allows the change to take place (Mosey, 1981, 1986). The therapist may create an environment that should enhance normal growth and development by providing the child with specific activities that he or she has not engaged in previously.

Specific postulates regarding change relate to the use of a specific therapeutic technique. These specific postulates regarding change state the type of action the therapist should take to bring about an explicit response in the child. For example, if the therapist applies direct pressure to the insertion of a muscle, then the muscle should relax. Because a context that allows for change is important, it is rare that a frame of reference will have only postulates regarding change that describe the use of specific techniques. Most frames of reference include postulates regarding change that relate to the context and the therapist's direct actions.

Postulates regarding change are the turning points in the frame of reference. Postulates regarding change transform abstract material stated in the theoretical base into practical actions that need to be taken by the therapists to facilitate change in the child. Postulates regarding change give the therapist a mechanism for using the frame of reference to plan intervention, providing a theoretically sound protocol for the therapist to follow.

The following are sample postulates regarding change from the example frame of reference.

General Postulates regarding Change

> If a child is in an environment wherein he or she is provided with positive direct external reinforcement for the demonstration of reciprocal social interaction skills, then the child will be more likely to continue to repeat those forms of successful behaviors.
>
> If a child is in an environment that provides opportunities to interact with people and observe another individual's reciprocal social interactions (as well as the positive consequences of those interactions), then the child will be able to improve his or her reciprocal social interaction skills.
>
> If a child is in an environment wherein he or she observes models that have engaging qualities and are demonstrating behaviors that are of interest to the child, then the child will respond better and be more likely to imitate the modeled behaviors.

Specific Postulates regarding Change

> If a child participates in gross motor play and is provided with positive, direct external reinforcement for initiating social interactions with another individual, then the child will be more likely to initiate interactions (Figure 1.6).

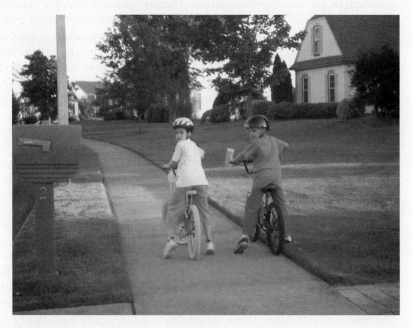

FIGURE 1.6 Children riding together in social play.

If a child participates in gross motor play and observes other individuals being positively reinforced for initiating social interactions, then the child will be more likely to demonstrate these initiating behaviors in the future.

If a child participates in gross motor play and is provided with positive direct external reinforcement for responding appropriately in a social situation, then the child will be more likely to duplicate this action.

If a child participates in gross motor play and observes other individuals being positively reinforced for responding appropriately in social situations, then the child will demonstrate similar responding behaviors in the future.

APPLICATION TO PRACTICE

Application to practice is guided by the postulates regarding change, which describe how an occupational therapist puts theory into action to facilitate change in the child. Some frames of reference require a more in-depth explanation of the key concepts used to promote functional performance. Other frames of reference require additional descriptions of the actions to be taken by the therapist. Certain frames of reference may require specific examples of the therapeutic process. Often it is difficult for even the most experienced therapist to make the move from the theoretical stage to practical application without additional explanation. This section eases that transition from theory to practice. In other words, this section is meant to provide added information for the therapist to put this frame of reference into practice effectively.

In the "Application to Practice" section, there is additional description of how to use the specific techniques and modalities according to the theory. This section identifies and delimits the appropriate intervention modalities for this frame of reference. Then the "Application to Practice" section clarifies how to use, provide intervention appropriately and efficiently, along with specific examples. Within this, inherently, therapists can see skills they may need to develop to use the frame of reference effectively.

For example, within the example frame of reference presented in this chapter, the therapist would provide gross motor play opportunities for the child, which allow for interactive experiences. Some examples of the gross motor activities employed in this frame of reference are climbing, running, jumping, throwing, catching, tumble play, and wrestling. Within these play sessions, the therapist will model appropriate behaviors and observe the child for signs of imitative behaviors. Direct external social reinforcement will be given to the child as reciprocal behaviors increase. As the child progresses and responds to physical and verbal cues, additional children will be added into the play session to allow for generalization of interactive skills.

This section is not meant to be a cookbook for application. Instead, application to practice is meant to provide clarification, where necessary, by:

- Stating the specific intervention modalities that the therapist needs to understand and be skillful in so that the frame of reference can be applied in practice.
- Describing specific techniques and strategies that the therapist employs to implement the frame of reference successfully.

• Describing how to combine theory with intervention.
• Bringing theory to a practical level and giving clear examples of implementation.

REFERENCES

Agnes, M. (Ed). (1999). *Webster's New World College Dictionary* (4th ed.). New York: Macmillan.

American Psychiatric Association. (1994). *Diagnostic and Statistical Manual of Mental Disorders: DSM-IV* (4th ed.). Washington, DC: American Psychiatric Association.

Baer, D. M., Peterson, R. F., & Shennan, J. A. (1967). The development of imitation by reinforcing behavioral similarity to a model. *Journal of the Experimental Analysis of Behavior*, *10*, 405–416.

Bandura, A. (1977). *Social Learning Theory*. Englewood Cliffs, NJ: Prentice-Hall.

Brunner, A., Gonzales, D. C., & Green-Taub, J. (2003). *Facilitating Reciprocal Social Interaction in Preschool Children with Autism*. New York University, Unpublished manuscript.

Bundy, A. C. (1991). Play theory and sensory integration. In A. G. Fisher, E. A. Murray, & A. C. Bundy (Eds). *Sensory Integration: Theory and Practice* (pp. 46–68). Philadelphia, PA: FA Davis Co.

Cook, J. L., & Sinker, M. (1993). Play and the growth of competence. In C. E. Schaefer (Ed). *The Therapeutic Powers of Play* (pp. 65–80). Northvale, NJ: Jason Aronson Inc.

Dalton, R. H. (1961). *Personality and Social Interaction*. Boston, MA: D. C. Heath & Company.

Hinojosa, J., Kramer, P., & Pratt, P. N. (1996). Theoretical foundations of practice: developmental principles, theories, and frames of reference. In J. Case-Smith, A. S. Allen, & P. N. Pratt (Eds). *Occupational Therapy for Children* (3rd ed., pp. 25–45). St. Louis, MO: CV Mosby.

Kanner, L. (1943). Autistic disturbances of affective contact. *Nervous Child*, *2*, 217–250.

Kramer, P. & Hinojosa, J. (1999). Structure of the frame of reference. In P. Kramer, & J. Hinojosa (Eds). *Frames of Reference for Pediatric Occupational Therapy* (2nd ed., pp. 83–118). Baltimore, MD: Lippincott Williams & Wilkins.

Lantz, J. (2001). Play time: An Examination of Play Intervention Strategies for Children with Autism Spectrum Disorders. *The Reporter*, *6*(3), 1–7,24.

Lantz, J. F., Nelson, J. M., & Loftin, R. L. (2004). Guiding Children with Autism in Play: Applying the Integrated Play Group Model in School Settings. *Teaching Exceptional Children*, *37*, 8–14.

Mosey, A. C. (1981). *Occupational Therapy: Configurations of a Profession*. New York: Raven Press.

Mosey, A. C. (1986). *Psychosocial Components of Occupational Therapy*. New York: Raven Press.

Mosey, A. C. (1996). *Applied Scientific Inquiry in the Health Professions: An Epistemological Orientation* (2nd ed.). Bethesda, MD: American Occupational Therapy Association.

Ragland, E. U., Kerr, M. M., & Strain, P. S. (1978). Behavior of withdrawn autistic children: Effects of peer social initiations. *Behavior Modification*, *2*(4), 565–578.

Rapoport, J. L. & Ismond, D. R. (1996). Developmental abnormalities in the first years of life. In J. L. Rapoport & D. R. Ismond (Eds). *DSM-V Training Guide for Diagnosis of Childhood Disorders* (pp. 85–92). New York: Brunner/Mazel Publishers.

Reilly, M. (Ed). (1974). *Play as Exploratory Learning*. Beverly Hills, CA: Sage Publications Inc.

Rutter, M. (Ed). (1978). *Autism: A Reappraisal of Concepts and Treatment*. New York: Plenum Press.

Takata, N. (1974). Play as a prescription. In M. Reilly (Ed). *Play as Exploratory Learning* (pp. 209–246). Beverly Hills, CA: Sage Publications Inc.

Thomas, N. & Smith, C. (2004). Developing Play Skills in Children with Autistic Spectrum Disorders. *Educational Psychology in Practice*, *20*(3): 195–206.

CHAPTER 2

Developmental Perspective: Fundamentals of Developmental Theory

PAULA KRAMER • JIM HINOJOSA

Occupational therapy intervention with a child is based on an understanding and appreciation of normal human development. Developmental theories have typically described patterns or sequences of development that are accepted as being characteristic for children. The most commonly used developmental theories are sequential in nature and tend to fall into three general categories: a linear progression, a pyramidal approach, and spheres of influence on the child.

TRADITIONAL DEVELOPMENTAL PERSPECTIVES

Those theorists who support the idea of linear progression believe that components of a process must occur before the skill as a whole is acquired or learned (e.g., Freud, 1966; Gesell & Amatruda, 1947; Kohlberg, 1969). This is similar to the links in a chain, wherein each link provides an important piece toward the strengths of the whole chain. Other theorists view progression as being more pyramidal in nature (Ayres, 1972, 1979; Erikson, 1963; Llorens, 1976; Piaget, 1963; Reilly, 1974). They believe that there must be a basic foundation from which skill development evolves. In this perspective, all blocks at the base of the pyramid must be strong and placed securely to provide support.

Those therapists who view development as linear have a perspective that it is made up of the components of a process and the resultant conditional responses. As the child develops, behavior represents a continual set of sequences. Other theories that support this perspective have been proposed by Pavlov & Anrep (1927); Skinner (1974), and Kaluger & Kaluger (1984). Behaviorism and learning theory are based on this theoretical perspective; however, currently these theories have become more complex and are not thought to be truly linear.

Those therapists who view development as pyramidal tend to be concerned with the development of each level of function to provide the foundation for higher level skills. Processes that take place at lower levels only provide the foundation on which processes that are more sophisticated may develop. Inherent in this view is the idea that skills are stage specific, that is, a skill that evolves in one stage forms a component part for the behaviors that take place at a later stage. These ideas have been proposed by Piaget (1963); Gagne (1970), and Maslow (1970). Currently, some theorists have less clearly defined pyramids but share the assumptions of the stage-specific theorists. Instead of stages, the theorists previously mentioned believe that development appears within spheres of influence sharing the assumption that higher level skills are based on lower level skills. This pyramidal view of development is thought to be a more contemporary perspective than the linear view of development.

Within the pediatric context, the linear and pyramidal processes qualify as developmental, even though each differs greatly in its perspective of what development actually means. Development may occur through learning and skill acquisition, or it may occur through maturation, wherein subsequent skills are created on the basis of preestablished foundations, or there can be a combination of learning and maturation. All these viewpoints involve an attempt to understand the patterns of progression. Each of these theoretical perspectives describes a particular pattern of progression in a child's development differently, yet each shares the generally accepted principles of human development (Daub, 1988).

NEW PERSPECTIVES ON CHILD DEVELOPMENT

The newer perspectives on child development tend to assume that there are wide varieties of spheres of influence that interact with the child to promote development. Humphry & Wakeford (2006) note that these different perspectives on development may be more consistent with an occupational therapy approach. There is the traditional approach that focuses on nature, referred to as the "sociobiological approach," (Lerner, 2002) which states that development is genetically inherent and is not changed by interaction with the others or the environment. There is the organismic approach (von Bertalanffy & Woodger, 1933; Humphry & Wakeford, 2006), based on systems theory, which purports that child is made up of subsystems and that the organism changes based on its interaction with the environment. This perspective puts forth that one cannot learn about one part of an organism separate from the whole organism. The child is viewed as active and as the source of the behavior. The child is the center of development and change in the child is self-directed based on the interaction the child has with the environment.

The metatheoretical stance emphasizes that the development of the child is based on both heredity and environment. This perspective incorporates the perspective that the nervous system is plastic and that there is a strong influence on context to promote change and development of the child (Lerner, 2002). This perspective is more consistent with the concept of nurturing as a way of promoting growth and change in the child. Currently, many theorists favor this perspective.

Another perspective, which emphasizes context, is the dynamic systems theory. This perspective views development as an open system, wherein genetic activity, neural activity, behavior, and environment (including physical, social, and cultural environment) dynamically interact to promote the child's development. There is a capacity for development throughout the life span. As these four systems interact, development

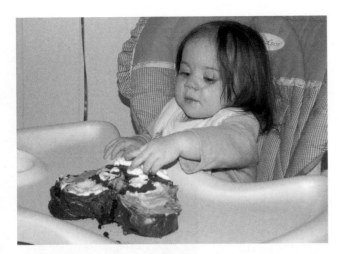

FIGURE 2.1 Child reaching for a first birthday cake.

occurs. There may be constraints on the interaction among these systems that influence development (Lerner, 2002). From this perspective, while we as therapists may think in terms of eye–hand coordination, the infant reaching out to grab an object may be operating on a purely sensory level (Figure 2.1). However, this may become more directed by internal genetic and neural activity, by the environmental response from parents and other children, or from the interaction with the toy itself.

Holistic Person-Context interaction theory (Magnusson & Stattin, 1998) views the child as part of a complex integrated and dynamic person–environment system. This theory states that it is not possible to understand the child's functioning without understanding his or her social system. The child and the environment develop as an integrated dynamic totality, with both being equal in importance. One cannot be studied without the other. This perspective draws on concepts used by family systems theorists (Haley, 1976; Minuchin, 1974), who view the developing child within the context of the family. Similarly, the child with an illness or developmental delay affects the entire family and its interactions.

Occupational therapists have begun to accept developmental theories that have a broader perspective and explore the external influences on the child. Occupational therapists value a different perspective on interaction rather than the traditional dynamic systems theory. It has been proposed that the child interacts with the environment resulting in change in the child and then the child has an impact on the surrounding environment, thus changing the environment as well. This is a constant interactive approach between the child and the environment, resulting in change in both (Davis & Polatajko, 2004).

Humphry & Wakeford (2006) take this one step further suggesting that there are reciprocal adaptations that occur between engagement with the objects and the influences between the engagement with the object and with the internal child factors (Figure 2.2). A limitation of all these developmental perspectives is the Western-based assumption that the environment is external to the child. Some Eastern philosophies view the environment as part of the individual as a whole (Iwama, 2006).

FIGURE 2.2 A child decorating a cookie.

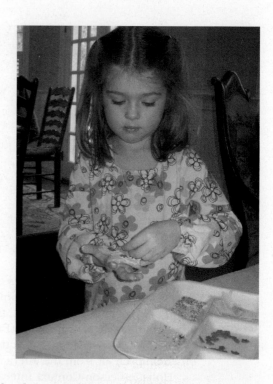

The introduction of a wider variety of developmental theories presents an interesting conundrum for occupational therapists. The newer theories are very consistent with the views of therapists regarding the importance of the environment, the plasticity of the neural system, the role of nurturing in development, and the criticality of involvement in meaningful activities to enhance growth. Yet, these same theories question the age-specific and stage-specific developmental theories that occupational therapists have used for many years. The traditional developmental theories are mainstays in our educational programs and prevalent in most of our developmental evaluation tools. Philosophically, therapists need to explore and understand the newer theories and determine how they can be used to support intervention. Additionally, if these newer theories are more consistent with our beliefs and assumptions about the environment, neural system, and meaningful occupations, then we should consider the need to develop evaluative tools that are more consistent with these perspectives, rather than relying on traditional age-specific and stage-specific theories and evaluations.

Newer Developmental Perspectives and Occupational Therapy

At this point in time, it would be important for occupational therapy to embrace the knowledge from all these developmental perspectives to the extent possible, thereby maintaining an understanding of age-specific and stage-specific development and incorporating an understanding of the vast additional perspectives on issues that can promote development. Regardless of which theories are used by the therapist, the goal is to facilitate movement of the child from one skill or behavior to another higher level skill or behavior.

These developmental theories provide a foundational knowledge for pediatric occupational therapy, but our perspective is broader and more unique than basic development. As occupational therapists, we concentrate more on how development translates into functional performance rather than the pure sequential nature of development. The developmental theories previously discussed do not provide us with enough information about skill acquisition or the mastery of activities of daily living. Our perspective of development centers on how the child performs meaningful occupations within the context of the developmental foundation (Coster, 1995).

Although occupational therapists learn about all aspects of development, our major concern is with the child's ability to translate development into action. Pediatric occupational therapists share a unique viewpoint in their concern for development of performance skills. Occupational therapists are concerned with children being able to function within their own environments to the best of their abilities. This viewpoint requires consideration of the many different factors that can influence a child's overall development. We are inherently concerned with the child's abilities and how human and nonhuman influences affect the development of these abilities. The child's abilities may be seen as a composite of various specific skills. To address the development of these skills, therapists concentrate on ascertaining the child's developmental level, which refers to a determination of each child's patterns and sequences of development and then on an evaluation of the level that has been attained. At the same time, therapists should also consider the myriad factors that are now believed to effect development.

A child does not develop in a vacuum. He or she is part of an ever-changing dynamic process because changes occur continuously in internal and external environments. A child's body and mind represent the internal environment and are greatly influenced by growth and maturation. Human and nonhuman objects are part of the external environment. These two worlds influence the child's development separately and together. The importance of each environment varies with each child's capabilities, the specific demands of a situation, the objects involved, and the performance required. Although a child is considered to have many separate areas that develop independently, motor, psychological, and social development all are interrelated and interdependent. In reality, although a child's motor development may be discussed in isolation, it cannot be considered independently of the child's whole life. Some variables that affect motor development also involve the neurophysiological status, the orthopaedic status, early sensory and cognitive experiences, and the family situation. The child who is unable to walk may have limited access to interaction with his peers and, therefore, may have difficulty with age-appropriate social development.

Rates of development vary from child to child, with no two children being exactly alike. There is a range of normalcy within progression and rates of development. For example, the accepted developmental sequence purports that a child creeps before walking. Usually, children spend several months mastering creeping, but some children progress very quickly through this stage and begin to attempt to walk soon after they have started to creep. One also needs to look at the environment, and how it can enhance or inhibit the progressive skills. When viewing normal development, however, it was always thought to be orderly, predictable, and sequential. However, one needs to explore the external factors of the environment, the interaction with care providers, the cultural climate, and physiological changes in the child. To be sure, there always is some degree of individuality with a child, with one aspect at times being more important than another is. For instance, at an earlier stage in life, motor performance may be more imperative than cognitive performance. Finally, development does not always occur at a consistent rate but rather in spurts that alternate with rest periods, at which time consolidation of skills takes place, much influenced by external factors. As a child begins to ambulate, he or she usually starts to ignore previous favored toys that required him or her to be sedentary. Instead, he or she now wants to explore his or her environment with newfound freedom.

Traditionally, once a child's pattern, sequence, and level of development are determined, an occupational therapist can address needs in two ways. First, the therapist can establish the performance skills a child has or can develop at his or her current level of function. The child who cannot walk or talk still may be able to participate actively in self-feeding. Second, based on a pattern or sequence of development, a therapist can determine a child's deficits and the possible influencing factors. On the basis of some hypotheses, a therapist uses knowledge about normal growth and development, anatomy, neurophysiology, and life tasks to develop an intervention plan that is sensitive to any sequela of disease or to any known data about the development of the particular systems in which a child has deficits.

With the advent of new theories of development, occupational therapists also have increased concern for other factors that may influence development. These include the environment, family life, cultural influences, nurturing, growth facilitating experiences, and other factors. Knowledge about the characteristic pattern of the development of a particular performance skill must be balanced by the particular child's direction, rate, and sequence of development, as well as the external factors of the environment and experiences that can influence the performance skill.

Perhaps the easiest area to understand is motor progression, which usually is presented in a format that identifies the sequence in which the child acquires the ability to move. This progression, like those of other systems, inherently includes the acceptance of two basic assumptions: (1) development has natural order and (2) development is sequential. Now, on top of this overlay the perspective that environment, stimulation, interaction, and the child's personal characteristics can affect and change the supposed natural order of development. Therefore, although there may be a general sequential order that each child seems to follow, it is not necessarily the only order to achieve basic skills. This order may be modified and changed by the external factors that interact with the child and the role of the individuals who are nurturing the child. Development, therefore, becomes a much more multidimensional process, with influences from many more sources than just a set of age-specific and stage-specific skills and behaviors. Some children develop faster in one area, some slower, and each child may not follow the exact sequence as variations may be promoted by external forces. The therapist has to consider not only the chronological age and developmental age but also the social and emotional age of the child. Experience tells us that no child's development is even across all of these areas, at any given time.

IS THERE REALLY A DEVELOPMENTAL FRAME OF REFERENCE?

Is there a developmental frame of reference? The developmental perspective, whether purely age-specific and stage-specific or influenced by a multitude of additional external forces, forms a foundational knowledge that is important to all pediatric occupational therapists. Most of the frames of reference presented in this text presume that the therapist has a firm knowledge of the developmental perspective and its impact on the skill acquisition of the child. However, there is no one specific developmental frame of reference presented here, but rather a compendium on recent perspectives of development. It is our viewpoint that there is no one specific developmental frame of reference for pediatric occupational therapy. We believe that what is commonly referred to as the "developmental frame of reference" is truly a frame of reference wherein the therapist uses various contemporary legitimate tools of the profession to facilitate the traditionally accepted sequence of normal development. This involves the clinical reasoning of the therapist, a manipulation of the environment, the use of teaching and learning theories, the provision of additional growth-enhancing experiences, and conscious use of self. In these situations, the therapist identifies the critical skills needed by the child within the generally accepted normal developmental sequence, and uses these tools and external factors to facilitate the development of those skills. The introduction and understanding of new perspectives on child development that are consistent with the assumptions and values of occupational therapy can be effectively used to enhance our interventions with children.

REFERENCES

Ayres, A. J. (1972). *Sensory Integration and Learning Disorders*. Los Angeles, CA: Western Psychological Services.

Ayres, A. J. (1979). *Sensory Integration and the Child*. Los Angeles, CA: Western Psychological Services.

Bertalanffy, L. V., & Woodger, J. H. (1933). *Modern theories of development: An introduction to theoretical biology*. London: Oxford University Press.

Coster, W. (1995). What is the unique occupational therapy perspective on development? In S. Cermack, A. Henderson, & S. Ray (Eds). *Proceedings of the Pediatric Occupational Therapy: Challenges for the Future in Education and Research. U.S. Department of Health and Human Services, the Maternal and Child Health*. Boston, MA: Boston University.

Daub, M. M. (1988). Occupational therapy—base in the human development process. In H. L. Hopkins, & H. D. Smith (Eds). *Willard and Spackman's Occupational Therapy* (7th ed., pp. 43–75). Philadelphia, PA: JB Lippincott Co.

Davis, J. A., & Polatakjko, H. J. (2004). Occupational development. In C. H. Christiansen, & E. A. Townsend (Eds.), *Introduction to occupation* (pp. 91–119). Upper Saddle River, NJ; Prentice Hall.

Erikson, E. H. (1963). *Childhood and Society* (2nd ed.). New York: Norton & Co.

Freud, S. (1966). *Standard Edition of the Complete Psychological Works of Sigmund Freud*. London: Hogarth Press.

Gagne, R. M. (1970). *The Conditions of Learning* (2nd ed.). New York: Holt, Rinehart, & Winston.

Haley, J. (1976). *Problem-Solving Therapy*. New York: Harper & Row.

Humphry, R., & Wakeford, L. (2006). An occupation-centered discussion of development and implications for practice. *American Journal of Occupational Therapy, 60*(3), 258–267.

Iwama, M. K. (2006). *The Kawa Model: Culturally Relevant Occupational Therapy*. Philadelphia, PA: Churchill Livingstone, Elsevier Science.

Kaluger, G., & Kaluger, M. F. (1984). *Human Development: The Span of Life* (3rd ed.). St Louis, MO: CV Mosby.

Kohlberg, L. (1969). Stage and sequence: The cognitive developmental approach to socialization. In D. Groslin (Ed.). *Handbook of Socialization Theory and Research* (pp. 347–480). Chicago, IL: Rand McNally.

Lerner, R. M. (2002). *Concepts and Theories of Human Development* (3rd ed.). Mahwah, NJ: L. Erlbaum Associates.

Llorens, L. A. (1976). *Application of Developmental Theory for Health and Rehabilitation*. Rockville, MD: American Occupational Therapy Association.

Magnusson, D., & Stattin, H. (1998). Person-context interaction theories. *Theoretical models of human development*, *1*, 685–759.

Maslow, A. H. (1970). *Motivation and Personality* (2nd ed.). New York: Harper & Row.

Minuchin, S. (1974). *Families and Family Therapy*. Cambridge, MA: Harvard University.

Mosey, A. C. (1968). Recapitulation of ontogenesis: A theory for practice of occupational therapy. *American Journal of Occupational Therapy*, *22*, 426–432.

Mosey, A. C. (1970). *Three Frames of Reference for Mental Health*. Thorofare, NJ: Charles B. Slack.

Pavlov, I. P., & Anrep, G. V. i. i. (1927). *Conditioned reflexes: An investigation of the physiological activity of the cerebral cortex*. London: Oxford University Press.

Piaget, J. (1963). *Psychology of Intelligence*. Paterson, NJ: Littlefield, Adams & Co.

Reilly, M. (1974). *Play as Exploratory Learning*. Beverly Hills, CA: Sage Publications Inc.

Skinner B. F (1974). *About Behaviorism*. New York: Vintage Books.

Travers, R. M. W. (1977). *Essentials of Learning*. New York: Macmillan.

CHAPTER 3

Domain of Concern of Occupational Therapy: Relevance to Pediatric Practice

AIMEE J. LUEBBEN • JIM HINOJOSA • PAULA KRAMER

A profession arises to address specific needs or concerns in society. The knowledge and services used in addressing societal needs become the discipline's domain of concern. In essence, a domain of concern defines the scope of practice, the breadth of a profession, and the expertise of practitioners. It is beyond the scope of this book to identify the entire domain of concern for the profession of occupational therapy. This chapter focuses, therefore, on the domain of pediatric practice.

Society rarely stays the same; as concerns in society change, a profession must respond accordingly. To remain viable and healthy, a profession needs to be dynamic, developing, and adapting to meet current needs and anticipate future concerns of society. As a discipline responds to the changing needs of society, the profession's domain of concern evolves.

Although a simple definition may serve the profession at the beginning, it is virtually impossible to use discrete terms when describing a domain of concern for a profession that has undergone ongoing evolution. Students and new practitioners may struggle with the complexity of this concept because they often seek a single, simple definition of their profession.

A profession must also adapt to changes in social priorities and in the ways that services are delivered. At various times, society has shown concern for a specific age-group or particular category of disability. This leads to an increased professional focus on those particular groups and may lead to specialized practice. This has been the case in occupational therapy in the United States. For example, pediatric occupational therapy practice has been influenced dramatically by societal changes. In the early 1970s, federal laws emphasized and supported the educational needs of special children and required occupational therapy as a related service. This idea was expanded during the 1980s when family-centered early intervention services for infants and toddlers became an area of concern and occupational therapy was identified as a primary service. During the 1990s, there was an increasing trend toward more community-based services and natural settings for intervention such as the home and school and assistive technology became a more important aspect of service provision. Federal legislation in the early 2000s has expanded the potential for school-based occupational therapists who have the education, training, and skills to provide leadership in the response-to-intervention movement which includes early intervention services that offer research-based intervention to individual children who do not qualify for special education but are in need of short-term assistance. Understanding what occupational therapy can offer is crucial; knowing the location of service delivery is also important. Currently, pediatric occupational therapists can be found in various settings including well-baby clinics, neonatal intensive care units, early intervention centers, preschools and Head Start programs, and school systems.

CLASSIFICATION SYSTEMS

A discipline needs a common language for many different reasons: to provide consistent communication among practitioners, to define a scope of practice both inside and outside the profession, to show evidence that intervention was effective, and to document services rendered for reimbursement sources. Over the years, the occupational therapy profession in the United States of America has adopted various classification systems that provide a common language.

A healthcare system–based classification system of uniform terminology (UT) is not a new idea. Occupational therapists working within the medical model have used what is now called the "International Classification of Diseases (ICD)" for years. The first edition of this system, the International List of Causes of Death (based on classification systems developed decades earlier) was adopted in 1893 by the International Statistical Institute. The World Health Organization (WHO), which assumed responsibility for the international classification, officially expanded the listing to include diseases, conditions, and injuries in 1948. Although the ICD-10 was adopted by WHO in 1994, many countries rely on an earlier version because of technology constraints. Because the ICD is the international standard diagnostic system used to classify diseases and other health conditions, the standard naming and measuring system allows coding, collection, storage, and analysis of morbidity and mortality statistics. The statistics can be compared at the individual, institutional, societal, and international levels (WHO, 2007).

The ICD, which allows for systematic naming and measuring across an etiological framework, is a member of the WHO family of classification systems. The system does not provide much information in terms of outcomes other than changes in mortality or morbidity rate by diagnosis. In 1980 WHO developed, for trial purposes, another classification system that was revised and subsequently published as the ICF (abbreviation used for the International Classification of Functioning, Disability, and Health). The ICF (WHO, 2001) is a biopsychosocial (a blending of medical and social models) framework of naming and measuring, designed to collect information about functioning, health, and well-being. Although initially designed for rehabilitation, this systematic standard framework for classification by functioning is designed to stand alone or work in conjunction with the ICD to provide international statistics about health outcomes.

A profession-developed classification system of UT based on functioning is not a new idea in occupational therapy. In the United States, the occupational therapy profession has been using a biopsychosocial framework to provide a uniform language, naming aspects of the profession's domain of concern, which predated the international classification system. In 1979, a document that came to be known as "Uniform Terminology" was approved by the American Occupational Therapy Association (AOTA) Representative Assembly to promote a uniformity of definition for practice within the profession (AOTA, 1979). To respond to the evolution of practice, AOTA then recognized the need to update the document on a regular basis to reflect current practice and to reemphasize the need for uniformity of definitions. In 1989, AOTA adopted the second edition of UT-II (AOTA, 1989), a revision that reflected current practice with a clarification of categories and refinement of definitions. A third edition (AOTA, 1994b) of UT-III refined common language and provided a needed expansion that included context and environments that influence performance. With an increase in UT complexity, AOTA (1994a) published a companion document to help occupational therapists apply the revised classification system to practice.

While UT was undergoing a fourth revision process, WHO published the ICF, which contains language very familiar to many occupational therapists. Rather than adopt the ICF, designed "to provide a unified and standard language and framework for the description of health and health-related states" (WHO, 2001, p. 3), AOTA (2002) replaced the UT document with the *Occupational Therapy Practice Framework: Domain and Process* (AOTA, 2002), commonly called the "Practice Framework."

The Practice Framework has increased the complexity of the domain of occupational therapy to a level some critics believe makes the classification system difficult to apply in practice. Nelson (2006) argued that in the Practice Framework, certain terms are no longer uniquely classified within one category, violating rules of logical definitions and classification. Gutman et al. (2007) maintained that terminology neither reflects the profession's domain nor spans clinical practice, that application may be difficult in fast-paced medical-model settings. Butts & Nelson (2007) demonstrated that practicing occupational therapists were not able to categorize terminology consistent with Practice Framework categories, indicating the Framework was not being used in the practice.

Table 3.1 provides a comparison of the UT-III, the Practice Framework, and the ICF. The table is arranged with the three classifications in the three main columns. The three main rows attempt to group similar aspects of the classifications. Although the three documents seem roughly similar, one-to-one comparison is not possible. In the main bottom row, all three classification systems include *contextual factors*, division categories with *context* in the name. The main top row of each classification contains *occupation-based life areas* (also called "activities and participation" in the ICF). UT-III and the ICF have some correspondence in the main middle row that provides *foundational body-level components*. To client factors (based on ICF body functions and structure), the Practice Framework adds other classification system categories (performance skills, performance patterns, and activity demands). See the bottom row of Table 3.1 for specifics.

International Classification of Functioning

This chapter uses the ICF, a worldwide taxonomy that provides a uniform language while offering assessment capabilities. The uniform language aspect is designed in stem-branch-leaf fashion: categories are mutually exclusive and lower-level order categories

TABLE 3.1 Comparison of Uniform Terminology III (AOTA, 1994b), the Practice Framework (AOTA, 2002), and the ICF (WHO, 2001)

	UT-III (AOTA, 1994b)	Practice Framework (AOTA, 2002)	ICF (WHO, 2001)
Life Areas (Occupations)	**Performance Areas** Activities of daily living; Work and productive activities; Play or leisure activities	**Areas of Occupation** Activities of daily living; Instrumental activities of daily living; Education; Work; Play; Leisure; Social participation	**Activities and Participation (Daily Life Area Domains)** Learning and applying knowledge; General tasks and demands; Communication; Mobility; Self-care; Domestic life; Interpersonal interactions and relationships; Major life areas; Community, social, and civic life
Foundational (Body-Level) Components	**Performance Components** Sensorimotor; Cognitive; Psychosocial	Client factors[a]; Performance skills[b]; Performance patterns[c]; Activity demands[d]	**Body Functions and Structures** Mental; Sensory; Voice and speech; Cardiovascular, hematological, immunological, and respiratory; Digestive, metabolic, and endocrine; Genitourinary and reproductive; Neuromusculoskeletal and movement-related; Skin and related structures
Contextual Factors	**Performance Context** Environment; Temporal aspects	**Context** Cultural; Physical; Social; Personal; Spiritual; Temporal; Virtual	**Contextual Factors** **Environmental Factors**: Products and technology; Natural environment and human-made changes to the environment; Support and relationships; Attitudes; Services, systems, and policies Personal factors

[a]Client factors (body functions and structures) correspond to ICF body functions and structures.

[b]Performance skills sections do not have direct correspondence to the ICF. The performance skill subparts, motor skills and process skills, have some similarities with ICF body functions. The performance skill subpart, Communication/interpersonal skills, has some similarity to two different ICF life areas: communication and interpersonal interactions and relationships.

[c]Performance patterns are mixed within the ICF. Habits are included in ICF personal factors (contextual factors), routines are within ICF general tasks and demands, and roles are not addressed explicitly with the ICF but are implicit in whether tasks or actions are considered activities (role of the self) or participation (roles beyond the self such as son, brother, pet owner).

[d]Activity demands correspond to ICF general tasks and demands and some contextual factors.

are subsumed under higher-order levels. The ICF allows occupational therapists to provide consistent communication with other disciplines and reimbursement sources, using terminology such as *activity, function, performance, functioning,* and *participation*—words that have been part of the occupational therapy lexicon for decades. A separate UT document that results in occupational therapists communicating among themselves may no longer be needed. Indeed, the viability of the profession may rest on the ability of occupational therapy to adapt the profession's language to the international standard naming and measuring system that allows coding, collection, storage, and analysis of statistics. For occupational therapists, using the ICF has an added benefit: This uniform language classification has an integrated coding system that allows measurement of baseline information for comparison with subsequent evaluation data. This universal classification and assessment tool provides a systematic method of building evidence to demonstrate the effectiveness of occupational therapy.

Although the ICF was divided into three rows in Table 3.1 to show similarities with UT-III and the Practice Framework, the international classification system has two parts—Part 1: Functioning and Disability and Part 2: Contextual Factors. Each part has two subdivisions. Part 1. Functioning and Disability comprises the subdivisions: (1) activities and participation and (2) body functions and structures. Part 2. Contextual Factors comprise the subdivisions: (1) environmental factors and (2) personal factors.

Occupation-Based Life Areas (Activities and Participation)

In the ICF, the activities and participation subdivision (of Part 1. Functioning and Disability) has nine daily life area domains: learning and applying knowledge, general tasks and demands, communication, mobility, self-care, domestic life, interpersonal interactions and relationships, major life areas, community and social and civic life. (Note: the term "domain," used as a subcomponent name in the ICF, is not equivalent to *domain of concern,* which is comparable to the scope of practice.)

To an occupational therapist, items within the nine ICF daily life domains are considered *occupations,* a core concept of the profession of occupational therapy. "Occupation, a collection of activities that people use to fill their time and give life meaning, is organized around roles or in terms of activities of daily living, work and productive activities or play/leisure" (Hinojosa & Kramer, 1997, p. 865). Occupations serve a multitude of purposes; people become involved in them for survival, necessity, pleasure, and for their personal meaning. Each individual's occupations comprise a unique combination of activities that are meaningful to that person. "Occupations are the ordinary and familiar things that people do every day" (Christiansen et al., 1995, p. 1015). People engage in occupations throughout their everyday lives to fulfill their time and give their lives meaning. An individual's unique occupations define that person. Depending on life situation and circumstances, the occupations that are important to the individual may change over time (Hinojosa & Kramer, 1997). Although the occupational therapy profession uses the term "occupation," the ICF uses the term "activities and participation" in nine daily *life areas,* also called "domains." This chapter works to integrate and unite occupational therapy terminology with ICF language. Therefore, the term "occupation-based life areas" is used in this chapter interchangeably with ICF *activities and participation*, ICF *life areas*, or ICF *domains*.

The flexibility of the ICF allows items within the activities and participation domains to be reclassified as an activity, defined as "the execution of task or action by an individual" or as participation, "involvement in a life situation" (WHO, 2001, p. 10). A simplified way of looking at activity versus participation is from a role standpoint. If a person does something in his or her "self" role, then that action is likely to be categorized as an activity. A person involved in a role beyond the self (e.g., functioning as a son, brother, student, or pet owner) is operating in participation mode. In other words, from an occupational therapy standpoint, occupations (tasks or actions) a person completes in the self-role would be classified as ICF *activities* and occupations (tasks and actions) an individual completes in other role are termed "ICF participation."

In addition to determining whether a part of a daily life domain is categorized as an activity or participation, qualifiers can be added to each. When qualifiers are used during the assessment process, the list of nine daily life area domains becomes a classification that allows quantitative measurement of baseline information to be compared with subsequent reevaluation data. For activities and participation, the two qualifiers are *performance* and *capacity*. In the ICF, performance is used the same way occupational therapists have used the term for years. Performance is what an individual is able to do in his or her current context (e.g., home, school) within society. For an individual, assessment of performance includes all equipment typically used in that environment. For example, if a person used eyeglasses to correct visual disabilities, the person would be assessed using his or her glasses. "Capacity" is a term used by the ICF to indicate a "naked person" assessment in a standard environment.

To assess capacity, the individual would be evaluated in a standard environment (e.g., a rehabilitation unit bathroom that is part of a simulated apartment) and as a naked person—with no equipment (not even eyeglasses) instead of in an environment that is authentic to the individual (e.g., home). Capacity assesses a person's true ability in a standard environment.

There are positive and negative aspects of the nine daily life domains in activities and participation. "Functioning," the positive aspect of activities and participation, is a term familiar to occupational therapists. A functioning person is able to live life effectively. The negative aspect of activities and participation has different terminology—there are activity *limitations* and participation *restrictions*.

The occupational therapy domain of practice includes various aspects of all nine daily life area domains of the ICF. For evaluation and intervention, therapists apply information from the learning and applying knowledge domain when they work on students' specific school functioning such as focusing attention, solving problems, and making decisions. Therapists use aspects of the general tasks and demands domain when working with a child on carrying out a daily routine, handling stress and other responsibilities, and operating alone or in a group. Although speech and language pathologists are responsible for many of the items in the communication domain, occupational therapists work with children on various communication domain aspects such as writing messages, using computers for writing, and comprehending body gestures. Mobility is a major domain for occupational therapists working with children.

The mobility domain includes changing and maintaining body positions, transferring from one surface to another, lifting and carrying objects, walking and moving, driving (e.g., bikes, four-wheelers, boats, cars, horse-drawn cart), and riding animals. The self-care domain is a primary area for pediatric occupational therapy. Aspects of this domain are expanded later in this chapter.

The domestic life domain includes acquiring goods and services, preparing meals, doing housework, and taking care of domestic animals. Pediatric therapists address this domain when they work with children on tasks involving making a bed, doing household chores, shopping, or taking responsibility for a pet. The interpersonal interactions and relationships domain is another area within the occupational therapy scope of practice. The focus is on this domain when therapists work with children on completing actions needed for basic and complex interactions with others (e.g., tolerance in relationships, interacting according to rules, and family relationships).

Another primary area for pediatric occupational therapists is the ICF domain, major life areas, which includes education (informal, preschool, school), vocational training, and higher education. Many pediatric therapists practice in natural settings such as school systems that include aspects of major life areas. Therapists may also address work and employment activities when they are working with older children or youth who are involved in transitions to employment or have remunerative employment such as paper routes, mowing lawns, or shoveling snow.

In the ICF, the community, social, and civic life domain includes community life, recreation and leisure, religion and spirituality, human rights, and political life and citizenship. This domain has an aspect that is a primary focus of pediatric occupational therapy—recreation and leisure—which includes play, sports, arts and culture, crafts, hobbies, and socializing. The emphasis of the remaining occupation-based life areas section of this chapter is on self-care as a whole domain and on the recreation and leisure section of the community, social, and civic life domain.

Self-Care

The self-care domain includes washing oneself, caring for body parts, toileting, dressing, eating, drinking, and looking after one's health (Figure 3.1). Depending on the individual situation of the children, the therapist may intervene either with the child, the care provider, or both to address aspects of the self-care domain. The ability to perform self-care activities independently is crucial to an individual's dignity. Therefore, this is a primary area of concern for pediatric occupational therapists and should not be overlooked in intervention.

Although it may be difficult for therapists to work with some self-care domain activities, it is critical that they do so because this may enable the child to become as independent as possible and to develop a positive sense of self. Although some frames of reference in this text do not address the self-care domain directly, it is understood that they are laying the foundation that allows the child to become independent in self-care.

Play, Recreation, and Leisure

The community, social, and civic life domain includes sections dealing with community life, recreation and leisure, religion and spirituality, human rights, and political life

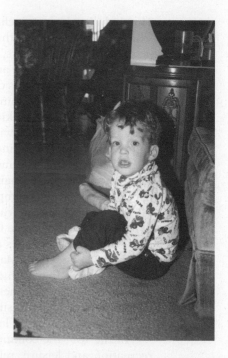

FIGURE 3.1 In the self-care domain, child taking off his socks.

and citizenship. The recreation and leisure section encompasses play (ranging from spontaneous, informal play to rule-based games such as cards), sports (e.g., soccer or bowling), arts and culture (e.g., reading for enjoyment, playing musical instruments, or going to the movie theater, art museum, art gallery), crafts (e.g., painting, sewing, scrapbooking), hobbies (e.g., collecting action figures, bugs, shells), and socializing (e.g., informal or casual gatherings, structured play dates).

Play, recreation, and leisure include those inherently gratifying activities in which a child chooses to engage. When used in therapy, play activities are selected for a child's amusement, enjoyment, or self-expression (Figure 3.2). Intrinsically, play, recreational, and leisure activities should be pleasurable, promoting the child's enjoyment or relaxation. Play, recreation, and leisure activities should encourage skill development through involvement with objects and interaction with others.

Play, recreation, and leisure activities are a natural part of a child's life, and the child without disabilities has many opportunities to engage in these activities. However, the child with disabilities may not have as many occasions to become involved. The primary exposure that the child has to play, recreation, and leisure activities may be in the context of a therapeutic experience. The expertise of the occupational therapist can be used to assist the child in playing as a means of self-expression and fun and as a means of assisting parents to strengthen their interaction with their child to provide a typical childhood experience (Hinojosa & Kramer, 1997).

For occupational therapists, play is a primary intervention when working with the pediatric population. Play activities are those things chosen by the child because they are amusing, enjoyable, relaxing, or self-expressive. Play often promotes skill development

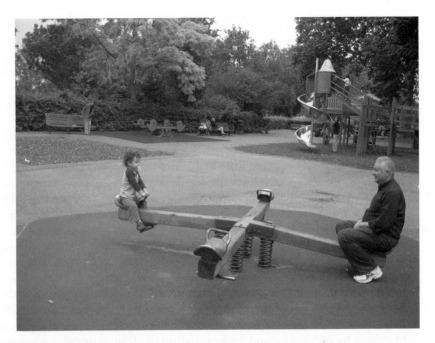

FIGURE 3.2 Child playing with his father on the seesaw.

and interaction with others. The occupational therapist uses play in two separate ways. First, the therapist tries to facilitate play exploration so that the child can try out various types of play and decide which ones he finds enjoyable. Second, the therapist uses play as a therapeutic modality to facilitate the functioning and development of the child. This aspect of play is addressed in Chapter 4.

Foundational Body-Level Components

In addition to the subdivision, activities and participation, Part 1. Functioning and Disability also contains the subdivision, body functions and structures. The body functions and structures subdivision has two sections: (1) body structures and (2) body functions. Aspects of the body structures section are related to the anatomical parts of the body (e.g., organs, limbs, and components). The eight chapters of body structure include structures of the nervous system; the eye, ear, and related structures; structures involved in voice and speech; structures of the cardiovascular, immunological, and respiratory systems; structures related to the digestive, metabolic, and endocrine systems; structures related to the genitourinary and reproductive systems; structures related to movement; and skin and related structures.

In the ICF, the physiological functions of the body systems are provided in the body functions, which include mental functions; sensory functions and pain; voice and speech functions; functions of the cardiovascular, hematological, immunological, and respiratory systems; functions of the digestive, metabolic, and endocrine systems;

genitourinary and reproductive functions; neuromusculoskeletal and movement-related functions; and functions of the skin and related structures. Body functions and body structures can be further coded as either positive or negative. The positive aspect is known as "functioning" (having functional integrity and having structural integrity for body functions and body structures, respectively). The negative aspect is called an "impairment," which has three qualifiers: extent (how much), nature (e.g., total absence, qualitative changes), and location (where).

There is a direct correspondence with the order of chapters in body structures (anatomy) section with the body functions (physiology). Additionally, there seems to be an overlap between the ICF body functions and structures components and ICD categories. The purposes of the two related classification systems, however, are not the same. Unlike the ICD that shows health conditions and service utilization, the body functions and structures component of the ICF is designed for the purpose of prevention or identification of a person's needs.

Separating body function and structure into foundational components allows the occupational therapist to understand the individual sections that make up the whole. By looking at the small sections, a therapist gains a better understanding of how the child processes information in these discrete areas. Through this specific examination of each discrete part, a more comprehensive understanding of the child's skills and deficits can be gained. A therapist's knowledge and understanding of the complex human organism increases by examining and understanding the foundational components of the human at the body level.

Foundational body-level components—body functions and structures—are closely interrelated, and each aspect embodies an area of the child's development. Understanding body-level functions and structures and their interrelation provides basic information about the child. From this point, the occupational therapist can develop appropriate interventions after considering the child's biological potential and developmental status.

Occupational therapists have expertise in three primary systems at the body function and structure level: (1) sensory functions and pain, (2) neuromusculoskeletal and movement-related functions, and (3) mental functions. Some occupational therapists may have specialized training to practice in areas that involve other foundational body-level components that are beyond the scope of this chapter.

Sensory Functions and Pain

In the ICF, the sensory functions and pain subcomponent comprise seeing functions (visual acuity, visual field functions, quality of vision, functions of the structures adjoining the eye such as nystagmus, and sensations associated with the eye and adjoining structures), hearing functions, vestibular functions, sensations associated with hearing and vestibular functions, additional sensory functions (taste, smell, proprioception, touch, temperature, vibration, pressure, and noxious stimuli), and pain. In this conceptualization, the critical concepts are the ability to take in sensory information and process this information.

Sensory functions are also based on the status of the central nervous system (CNS) and the child's neurophysiological responses. Sensory function responses are thought to develop from a generalized response to a more sophisticated discrete response to specific stimuli. The tactile system, for example, develops the ability to recognize internal as opposed to external sensation, such as interpreting light touch and pressure. The visual system likewise develops more sophisticated responses through recognition of pattern and color.

Understanding the sensory functions and pain subcomponent is critical to comprehending the sensory integration and Neuro-Developmental Treatment of references, and, to a lesser extent, the visual perception frame of reference. The occupational therapy student should be aware when reading each of these frames of reference that theoretical bases of each may conceptualize these subcomponents somewhat differently.

Neuromusculoskeletal and Movement-Related Functions

Neuromusculoskeletal and movement-related functions involve areas of development that underlie the motor aspects of behavior. This depends on the maturity of the CNS and the neurophysiological system. The neuromusculoskeletal and movement-related functions subcomponent includes functions of the joints and bones (mobility and stability of bones and joints), muscle functions (power, tone, and endurance), and movement functions (reflexes, involuntary movements, control and coordination of voluntary movements, involuntary movement functions such as tremor, gait patterns, and sensations related to muscles and movement functions such as muscle stiffness or spasm).

When these neuromusculoskeletal and movement-related functions are considered by pediatric occupational therapists, each is considered relative to the typical development of the child. It is not simply a case of whether the child has reflexes, for example, but at what level are the reflexes relative to the child's chronological and developmental age, and how they influence functioning. Most often these subcomponents are viewed relative to other motor behaviors and skills such as standing (Figure 3.3). This is particularly true in the Neuro-Developmental Treatment, biomechanical, and motor skill acquisition frames of reference.

Mental Functions

In the ICF, mental functions encompass two broad areas: global mental functions and specific mental functions. These broad areas allow the child to develop the cognitive and psychosocial abilities to handle life situations. Global mental functions include consciousness (state, continuity, and quality), orientation (time, place, person), intellectual (general cognitive functions and development across a life), global psychosocial (development of interpersonal skills needed to establish reciprocal meaningful social interactions), temperament and personality functions (extraversion, agreeableness, conscientiousness, psychic stability, openness to experience, optimism, confidence, trustworthiness), energy and drive (energy level, motivation, appetite, craving, impulse control), and sleep (amount, onset, maintenance, quality, functions involving the sleep cycle). An example of addressing global mental functions is an occupational therapist who is working with a child on alertness, functioning in groups with other children, curiosity, imagination and inquisitiveness, and confidence (Figure 3.4).

Specific mental functions include attention functions (sustaining, shifting, dividing, and sharing attention), memory (short-term, long-term, and retrieval), psychomotor

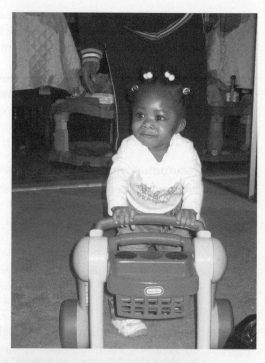

FIGURE 3.3 Child beginning to walk.

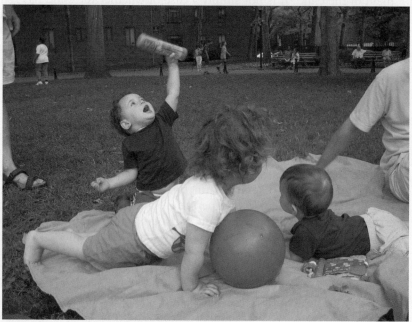

FIGURE 3.4 Children playing in a group encourages curiosity.

functions such as control (regulation of speed or response time such as moving and speaking slowly or excessive behavioral and cognitive activity) and quality (e.g., hand–eye coordination). Other specific mental functions are emotional functions (appropriateness, regulation, and range of emotion), perceptual functions (auditory, visual, olfactory, gustatory, tactile, and visuospatial perception), thought functions (pace, form, content, and control of thought). A therapist who is working with a child to improve perceptual skills in the area of form constancy or figure ground or to regulate emotions is addressing these foundational body-level subcomponents.

Additionally, specific mental functions also involve higher level cognitive functions of abstraction, organization and planning, time management, cognitive flexibility, insight, judgment, problem solving; mental functions of language (reception and expression of spoken, written and sign language); integrative language functions (organization of semantic and symbolic meaning, grammatical structure and ideas for the production of spoken and written language); calculative functions (simple and complex calculation); mental function of sequencing complex movements (commonly called "praxis" in the occupational therapy profession); and experience of self and time functions (experience of self, body image, experience to time). A therapist who addresses a child's organizational and time management skills or sequencing of movements (motor planning or praxis) is working on specific mental functions, a foundational body-level subcomponent.

These foundational body-level components appear to be directly related to the human occupation and coping frames of reference. However, the importance of foundational body-level components is much broader because it affects every area of the child's life. There is a complex interplay between and among the foundational body-level components, occupation-based life areas, and contextual factors.

Contextual Factors

Contextual factors are situations or factors that influence an individual's engagement in desired and/or required occupation-based life areas. In the ICF, Part 2. Contextual Factors has two subdivisions: (1) environmental factors and (2) personal factors. ICF environmental factors include the following categories: products and technology; natural environment and human-made changes to the environment; support and relationships; attitudes; and services, systems, and policies. While occupation-based life areas and foundational body-level components are internal to the child, environmental factors are external to the child. These external factors have an impact on the child's ability to engage in life areas. These factors may have a positive or negative effect. Positive environmental factors are called "facilitators" whereas negative factors are known as either "barriers" or "hindrances."

One category, products and technology, comprises both general products and technology as well as assistive products and technology. Products and technology include those for personal consumption (e.g., food, drugs); personal use in daily living; personal indoor and outdoor mobility; communication; education; employment; culture, recreation, and sport; and practice of religion and spirituality. Examples of products and technology are prescription medications, an adapted saddle for hippotherapy, a walker, pullover shirts for someone who cannot manipulate fasteners, a communication device, and a reacher.

This category also includes design, construction, and building products and technology of buildings for public use and private use, land development, and assets. Providing reasonable accommodations in the form of a ramp that allows a student who uses a wheelchair to enter a school and have an equal opportunity to engage in learning is one example of these types of products and technology. Another example is a community that develops an area of land for an accessible playground.

Another category is natural environment and human-made changes to the environment, which includes physical geography, population, flora and fauna, climate, natural events, human-caused events, light, time-related changes, sound, vibration, and air quality. Children with disabilities who live on an island accessed by a ferry, for example, may have a different level of access to occupational therapy services compared with those who live in a city with a therapy clinic down the street. A second example is an occupational therapist who may help children find fun activities for engagement inside buildings on days with a high pollen count.

Support and relationships is the third category of environmental factors. Included in support and relationships are immediate family; extended family; friends; acquaintances, peers, colleagues, neighbors, and community members; people in positions of authority; people in subordinate positions; personal care providers and personal assistants; strangers; domesticated animals, health professionals; and other professionals. The support and relationships category refers to all people and other living things with which the child interacts. This includes family members, peers, significant others, and pets (Figure 3.5).

The primary function of the family is to provide a supportive and nurturing environment for the child's development. The family shapes the child's ideological system and provides opportunities to develop interpersonal relationships (Turnbull, Summers, & Brotherson, 1986). A family consists of two or more persons who provide the environment in which the child develops and learns to become a member of society. Families usually include parents and children and may include other significant people. All family members' needs are recognized and supported in a well-functioning, healthy family.

Current American society has many different family configurations, including the immediate, extended, expanded, and single-parent households. The immediate (also called "nuclear") family consists of a couple who shares the responsibility of raising a child. The extended family is a group related through family ties or mutual consent that shares some part in child rearing. The expanded family is a complex combination of family configurations, involving a nuclear family, children, and significant others from previous relationships (Mosey, 1986). The configuration of this relationship among these different people is defined by the current and previous relationships. The single-parent household is one in which an adult assumes all the parental responsibilities.

The fourth category of environmental factors is attitudes, which includes individual attitudes of immediate family members; extended family members; friends; acquaintances, peers, colleagues, neighbors, and community members; people in positions of authority; people in subordinate positions; personal care providers and personal

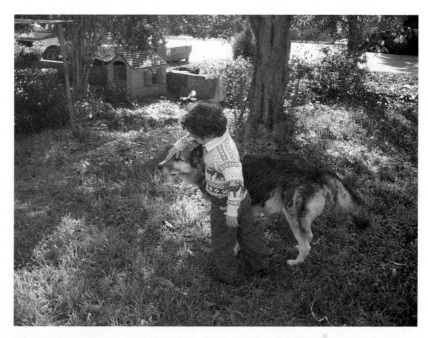

FIGURE 3.5 Child playing with his dog.

assistants; strangers; health professionals; and other professionals. Additionally the attitudes category includes societal attitudes and social norms, practices, and ideologies. Attitudes—which include customs, beliefs, behavior standards, and expectations—have an impact on the child's expectations of self and the parents' expectations of the child. Subsequently, cultural attitudes may reflect on the child's functioning. For example, in some cultures, it is acceptable for a child to use a bottle until he or she is ready to enter preschool, whereas in other cultures a child is weaned from the bottle once he or she becomes a toddler. This would impact on the child's exposure to a cup and his or her ability to drink from it. This is an example of a cultural attitude that affects functioning. Throughout life, attitudes influence what a person considers to be typical and what constitutes expected patterns of behavior. Within the process of intervention, the therapist needs to be aware of and sensitive to the cultural background and attitudes of each child encountered.

The fifth category is services, systems, and policies. Services may include benefits, programs, and operations; they are public, private, or voluntary by nature; and are established by individuals, groups, organizations, or governments. Systems, usually established by governmental entities, provide organizational control to organize and monitor services. Policies, which govern the systems, are the rules, regulations, standards established by various levels of government. A good example of services, systems, and policies in action and across time is the way in which pediatric occupational therapy has evolved and flourished since the 1970s because of changes in federal legislation in the United States.

Personal factors, the other part of Part 2. Contextual Factors, are not formally defined or classified by the ICF. Recognized as contributing to the outcome of various interventions, personal factors encompass any aspect of the particular background of an individual's life and living and include gender, race, age, fitness, lifestyle, habits, upbringing, coping styles, social background and so on. Personal factors also encompass the individualized aspects of a person an occupational therapist addresses during client-centered service provision.

The effects of personal factors on intervention are multifaceted. An individual's social background is a primary example of one aspect of personal factors a therapist must consider. Views on health and illness may be influenced by a child's cultural background, which is consistent with social background within personal factors. The ways in which people feel and act toward persons who have disabilities reflect cultural views or biases. This may be true of family members and therapists alike. The therapist should respond to cultural background identity. One way is to delineate how cultural background affects the selection of goals and the establishment of rapport (Levine, 1984). The perception of therapist and client may be "filtered through the screen of culture" (Hopkins & Tiffany, 1988, p. 108). For the pediatric occupational therapist, culture may outline the therapist–child–parent interaction. Consistent with the frame of reference, culture determines the choice of goals and the selection of legitimate tools and activities. "In every culture ... some activities are regarded as proper, some inappropriate, and other unacceptable for specific ages, social status, economic class, men or women, times of day, days of week, or seasons of the year" (Cynkin & Robinson, 1990, p. 10). Social background of the child also determines acceptable levels of functioning so that the therapist can decide on expected outcomes.

THE RELATIONSHIP OF THE OCCUPATIONAL THERAPY DOMAIN OF CONCERN TO INTERVENTION

The domain of concern of a profession defines the scope and focus of practice. The ICF, however, only provides an outline of the occupational therapy domain of concern. This classification system does not provide any in-depth information on the theoretical knowledge that underlies the practice of occupational therapy. By looking at the broad aspects of the ICF, therapists are able to identify occupation-based life areas, foundational body-level components, and contextual factors that require further assessment and possible attention. Once these areas, components, and factors have been identified, the therapist can choose a frame of reference that will address these specific concerns in more depth. Frames of reference address different aspects of practice. No one frame of reference addresses all aspects of practice fully. Some frames of reference focus more on occupation-based life areas (ICF activities and participation domains), some on foundational components at the body level, and some on contextual factors. Consequently, to treat all areas of concern with a particular child and family, the therapist may have to use more than one frame of reference.

Regardless of the specific frame of reference chosen when working with a particular child, pediatric occupational therapists draw from their expertise to view the child from various theoretical perspectives. This involves looking at a child relative to typical development and relative to that individual child's mastery of developmental milestones, which involves considering the child's chronological and developmental age.

Pediatric occupational therapists often begin by attending to the developmental aspects of the foundational body-level components that are important in determining the frame of reference used to guide intervention. This attention to foundational components is based on the therapist's understanding and appreciation for typical development. As defined by ICF, the body-level components (body functions and structures) are broad categories, sometimes too broad for dealing with an individual child. Because of the specific types of intervention, therapists need to divide these components into even smaller entities. When a therapist deals with a child who has grasp problems, for example, the categories of gross and fine coordination are not sufficient to understand and analyze these deficits. In this situation, the therapist needs to divide the child's functioning into even more discrete and specific aspects subcomponents.

Other times, therapists begin by focusing on the occupation-based life areas level—the activities and participation domains of the ICF. This requires looking at the overall functioning and determining areas in which the child is functioning well and areas in which the child may need assistance. To some, this is considered a more holistic or global view of the child's functioning. Additionally, some frames of reference concentrate on specific activities and participation domains more than others or to the exclusion of others. Again, therapists are concerned about the child's functioning within the ICF life areas, which are based in occupation, relative to his or her chronological and developmental levels. For example, the therapist may first determine how the child is performing in self-care and how that functioning relates to the child's chronological and developmental level and then explore which foundational body-level components may be contributing to any deficits in functioning. In this situation, the therapist again understands that functioning within the ICF life areas is not independent of foundational body-level components.

Finally, therapists may focus on contextual factors. When looking at the context, the therapist may first determine the demands on the child based on a particular environment or how a specific diagnosis, condition, or specific disability status may impact functioning overall. Once the therapist has determined the relationship of context to the child's functioning, then he or she can focus more specifically on occupation-based life areas or foundational body-level components. Pediatric occupational therapists are primarily concerned with the child's ability to function within his or her contexts. Therefore, it is acknowledged that foundational body-level components and contextual factors interact and have an impact on occupation-based life areas.

When occupational therapists use a specific frame of reference, they focus on certain aspects of the professional domain of concern. Although individual therapists may divide human functioning in different ways, what remains important is that the whole of what is considered to be human functioning still remains the same. More discrete and specific foundational body-level components, occupation-based life areas, or contextual factors serve a specific need for therapists' understanding of the children with whom they work. These arbitrary divisions of human functioning allow therapists to understand the parts of the whole to which children respond and then interact with their own environments. A therapist has a better perspective for analyzing the child's overall functioning by understanding the interplay of occupation-based life areas, foundational components, and contextual factors. This information gives the therapist a clear picture of how the child responds to situations and interacts with his or her environment.

Summary

All helping professions evolve and change to meet the needs of society. Within each of these professions, the profession's areas of expertise are considered their domain of concern. The domain of concern of occupational therapy encompasses foundational body-level components serving as the basis of occupation-based life areas. Foundational components and life areas are influenced strongly by contextual factors.

Life areas, the occupation-based activities and participation domains of the ICF, include learning and applying knowledge; general tasks and demands; communication; mobility; self-care; domestic life; interpersonal interactions and relationships; major life areas (such as education, work and employment, and economic life), and community, social, and civic life. Occupational therapists are always concerned with the functioning of their clients. The focus in pediatric occupational therapy is the child's functioning within various environments. The child's culture provides that setting for intervention and must be taken into account by the therapist.

In pediatric practice, the therapist is primarily concerned with three foundational body-level (ICF body functions and structures) components: mental function, sensory functions and pain, and neuromusculoskeletal and movement-related functions. Foundational body-level components are significant in the way in which the occupational therapist views intervention. Although these components are essential to intervention, the therapist should maintain the perspective of the total child.

REFERENCES

American Occupational Therapy Association. (1979). *Occupational Therapy Output Reporting System and Uniform Terminology System for Reporting Occupational Therapy Services*. Rockville, MD: American Occupational Therapy Association.

American Occupational Therapy Association. (1989). Uniform terminology for occupational therapy—second edition. *American Journal of Occupational Therapy, 43*, 808–814.

American Occupational Therapy Association. (1994a). Application of uniform terminology to practice. *American Journal of Occupational Therapy, 48*, 1055–1059.

American Occupational Therapy Association. (1994b). Uniform terminology for occupational therapy—third edition. *American Journal of Occupational Therapy, 48*, 1047–1054.

American Occupational Therapy Association. (2002). Occupational therapy practice framework: Domain and process. *American Journal of Occupational Therapy, 56*, 609–639.

Butts, D. S., & Nelson, D. L. (2007). Agreement between the *occupational therapy practice framework* classifications and occupational therapists classifications. *American Journal of Occupational Therapy, 61*, 512–518.

Christiansen, C., Clark, F., Kielhofner, G., Rogers, J., & Nelson, D. (1995). Position paper: Occupation. *American Journal of Occupational Therapy, 49*(10), 1015–1018.

Cynkin, S., & Robinson, A. M. (1990). *Occupational Therapy and Activities Health: Towards Health Through Activities*. Boston, MA: Little, Brown and Company.

Gutman, S. H., Mortera, M. H., Hinojosa, J., & Kramer, P. (2007). Revision of the occupational therapy practice framework. *American Journal of Occupational Therapy, 61*, 119–126.

Hinojosa, J., & Kramer, P. (1997). Statement: Fundamental concepts of occupational therapy: Occupation, purposeful activity, and function. *American Journal of Occupational Therapy, 51*, 864–866.

Hopkins, H. L., & Tiffany, E. G. (1988). Occupational therapy—a problem solving process. In H. L. Hopkins, & H. D. Smith (Eds). *Willard and Spackman's Occupational Therapy* (7th ed., pp. 102–111). Philadelphia, PA: JB Lippincott Co.

Levine, R. E. (1984). The cultural aspects of home care delivery. *American Journal of Occupational Therapy, 38*, 734–738.

Mosey, A. C. (1986). *Psychosocial Component of Occupational Therapy*. New York: Raven Press.

Nelson, D. L. (2006). Critiquing the logic of the *Domain* section of the occupational therapy practice framework: Domain and practice. *American Journal of Occupational Therapy, 61*, 511–523.

Turnbull, A. P., Summers, J. A., & Brotherson, M. J. (1986). Family life cycle: theoretical and empirical implications and future directions for families with mentally retarded members. In J. J. Gallagher, & P. M. Vietze (Eds). *Families of Handicapped Persons* (pp. 45–65). Baltimore, MD: Paul H. Brookes Publishing Co.

World Health Organization (WHO). (2001). *ICF: International Classification of Functioning, Disability and Health*. Geneva: WHO.

World Health Organization. (2007). *History of the Development of the ICD*. Retrieved July 19, 2007 from http://www.who.int/entity/classifications/icd/en/HistoryOfICD.pdf.

CHAPTER 4

Contemporary Legitimate Tools of Pediatric Occupational Therapy

PAULA KRAMER • AIMEE J. LUEBBEN • JIM HINOJOSA

Every health profession has a specific set of tools or instruments to use in bringing about change. These are referred to as the "profession's legitimate tools." Society accepts the professional as that person who is an expert in the use of these specific legitimate tools. These are tools in which all entry-level occupational therapists are competent. Competence comes from knowledge and skills, learned and practiced in school and in fieldwork, and from the scope of practice, defined by the profession, laws, and standard practice. Legitimate tools change over time because these tools are based on the knowledge of the profession, technological advances in society, and the needs and values of the profession and society. To bring about change in children, occupational therapists use various legitimate tools.

Most professions hold their legitimate tools in high regard. For some practitioners, legitimate tools are symbolic of the profession. Used daily as a means of interacting with clients, legitimate tools may be considered more tangible than the body of knowledge or domain of concern (Mosey, 1986). Many practitioners feel that the tools of their professions are unique, and, in some cases, this may be true. Although various professions often share legitimate tools, the uniqueness to each profession exists in the way the tools are used in the application of the frame of reference.

Each frame of reference addresses the process of change or the way in which the therapist promotes change in the client. Occupational therapy has various frames of reference that relate to many areas of practice. Legitimate tools are chosen by the therapist to match the particular frame of reference that he or she has determined to be appropriate for a particular client. Furthermore, specific legitimate tools are chosen based on their compatibility with the client's developmental level and the environment in which intervention is provided. Some legitimate tools are used by the profession as a whole but may be applied uniquely in pediatric occupational therapy. There have been extensive textbook discussions about the tools related to the profession and specific areas of practice (e.g., Bundy, Lane, & Murray, 2002; Christiansen, Baum, & Bass-Haugen, 2005; Crepeau, Cohn, & Schell, 2003; Mosey, 1986; Pendleton & Schultz-Krohn, 2006; Radomski & Latham, 2008). The ultimate goal in using legitimate tools is engaging an individual in occupations. All tools are always used as specified within the frame of reference.

This chapter presents an overview of selected legitimate tools for pediatric practice. Of these selected legitimate tools, two tools are core to the profession as they are used in all frames of reference. The two core tools are critical reasoning and conscious use of self. These core tools are implicit in all frames of reference and explicit in some. All other tools are optional and interchangeable and are consistent with the theoretical base of the specific frame of reference. These tools include activities, teaching and learning, nonhuman environment, and sensory stimulation with adaptive response and occupation. In addition to those presented here, other tools exist. Some are specialized and may be specific to one frame of reference. These tools may be discussed in the frame of reference. Some specialized tools require advanced education and training and, therefore, are beyond the scope of this book.

CRITICAL REASONING

Critical reasoning is the ability to understand and incorporate multiple concepts as well as views of culture, society, and the individual for effective problem solving. Clinical reasoning is a complex process used by occupational therapists to "plan, direct, perform and reflect on client care" (Schell, 2003, p. 131). The term "critical reasoning" is an amalgam of both concepts. Therapists continually need to do both: think and reason in order to effectively work with clients. To engage in effective practice, therapists have to consider a vast amount of information. They need to be able to determine what is important and what is not important at any given time based on priorities of the therapist and the client. Moreover, therapists need to be aware that these priorities can switch at any time. Simultaneously, the therapist also needs to identify problems and plan for intervention based on a frame of reference.

In choosing a frame of reference, a therapist has to have an awareness of the child, the presenting problems, and a wide variety of aspects surrounding and affecting the child. This takes into account the totality of the child including background and culture, the home and social environment, presenting problems, possible diagnosis and medical condition, and the context for intervention. On the basis of this information and possible additional information that may come from screening, observation, or discussions with other healthcare personnel, the therapist chooses a frame of reference. Once the frame of reference is chosen, the therapist continues with a comprehensive evaluation (Hinojosa, Kramer, & Crist, 2005). On the basis of results of the evaluation, the critical reasoning process becomes more intense as the therapist needs to consider a multitude of factors to develop a plan for intervention. First, the therapist explores whether this is the proper frame of reference to use with the child based on the problem areas that have been identified through the evaluation. If the therapist determines that this may not be the best frame of reference for the child, additional assessments may be needed from the perspective of another frame of reference. Once the therapist is comfortable that a particular frame of reference (or in some cases, multiple frames of reference) is the most effective way to approach intervention with the child, the therapist develops a plan for intervention. The development of the plan for intervention requires the therapist to reflect on all the various pieces of information about the child. This involves more than just planning for care and developing an intervention strategy. It requires being able to separate critical information from information that is of lesser importance at any given time.

CONSCIOUS USE OF SELF

Conscious use of self involves the occupational therapist's use of himself or herself as an agent to effect positive change within the therapeutic process. Although sometimes called "therapeutic use of self," the term "conscious use of self" is used here to indicate a phenomenon broader than "a practitioner's planned use of his or her personality, insights perceptions, and judgments as part of the therapeutic process" (AOTA, 2002, p. 628). Conscious use of self involves entering the child's world and relating to a child at his or her own level using emotional, developmental, physical, and sensory components.

Establishing a positive therapeutic relationship between the therapist and the child is an important result of the emotional component of conscious use of self. An important characteristic of this relationship is the therapist's ability to communicate, which includes developing rapport. Developing rapport involves making a child aware that the therapist cares and accepts the child at a current level of performance. In addition, developing rapport requires that therapists control their responses in a way that promotes children's ability to function or operate in their world.

In many cases, conscious use of self is expanded to interactions beyond the child to caregivers. Often the therapist includes parents, siblings, teachers, other classroom personnel, and other healthcare providers within the therapeutic relationship. To collaborate successfully, the therapist needs to interact with others in a positive manner and gauge the caregiver's understanding of the child. The therapist cannot dictate to caregivers, talk down to them, or be judgmental. This entails language, posture, gestures, and tone of voice that engages caregivers, ensuring that everyone can be an effective part in the therapeutic process. The conscious use of self in this sense therefore may mean that the therapist provides an appropriate role model for the family or classroom. The therapist's role with caregivers is flexible and needs to be open to change over time, depending on need.

Therapists can utilize conscious use of self with a developmental component. If the child is at a developmental level at which he or she spends most of his or her time on the floor, for example, then the therapist needs to work with the child on the floor. For the same child, objects and directions may have to be presented in a specific and concrete manner so that the child can understand them and respond. The conscious use of self in this example is the therapist's awareness of the child's level and the therapist's ability to adapt his or her posture and behavior to that level. Toys and therapeutic tools also need to be at the child's developmental level or slightly higher to stimulate the child's growth. The therapist has to have a clear understanding of the child's developmental level and skills to intervene at that same level or higher; otherwise, the intervention may be less than successful.

In the intervention process, therapists can also provide conscious use of self with a physical component. One example of the physical component is holding a toy to the side and above a child's head while encouraging reaching and opening an involved hand. Another physical example is the therapist who uses his or her body as a positioning device. For instance, a therapist in tailor sitting can use his or her legs to enhance an infant's tolerance to being positioned prone or add a dynamic balance element for a toddler seated in his or her lap. Some frames of reference make extensive utilization of the physical aspects of conscious use of self; for instance, handling and some of the neuromuscular facilitation techniques are used in the Neuro-Developmental Treatment frame of reference.

Some therapists incorporate a sensory component into conscious use of self. When working with infants, for example, a blonde therapist may choose to wear a black or navy shirt to provide a color contrast. For a child who is working on sensory processing issues, a therapist may select clothing to assist in the therapeutic session. For instance, a sweatshirt worn wrong side out provides extra softness and wool pants add a scratchy aspect in a therapeutic encounter. Therapists also can use scent (or the lack of scent) consciously. Wearing the same combination of soap, shampoo, and lotion can provide consistency in olfactory sensation for a child who is blind and using fragrant-free products may help a child who is hypersensitive to odors.

The skillful application of the conscious use of self develops with practice. A strong therapist builds a conscious use of self-repertoire that has various emotional, developmental, physical, and sensory components. Being an agent who effects positive therapeutic change is the reason why conscious use of self is a core contemporary legitimate tool of occupational therapy.

ACTIVITIES

Occupational therapists have always used activities as a therapeutic medium. Occupational therapists are concerned with a person's ability to engage in daily life occupations. Inherent in this concern is the ability to complete activities associated with and foundational to the various occupations. The goal of occupational therapy has always been to provide a person with the knowledge and skills to participate in the numerous activities that are part of daily life. Activities include the numerous things that people do as they live their lives (Hinojosa & Blount, 2004). Therapeutic use of activities is selecting the most appropriate activity for the client to create an environment within which the client can learn, develop skills, express feelings, and act on the environments toward a positive outcome.

Occupational therapists learn about the value and importance of activities as a core aspect of practice. The use of activities as a therapeutic tool requires that therapists understand the activities of people and the multiple factors that influence them. Some factors are age, culture, ethnicity, gender, physical environment, and personal preferences. An occupational therapist's knowledge and use of activity analysis and synthesis are basic to the use of activities as a therapeutic medium.

The way occupational therapists use activities as a therapeutic medium has changed over time. Currently, one way of looking at therapists' use of activities is to categorize them into purposeful activities and activities with therapist-defined purpose. Both these approaches require that the therapists be skilled in both activity analysis and synthesis.

Purposeful Activities

Purposeful activities are an inherent part of occupational therapy. "Purposeful activity refers to goal-directed behaviors or tasks … that the individual considers meaningful" (Hinojosa, Sabari, & Pedretti, 1993, p. 1081). An activity is purposeful when the *meaning* (purposefulness) of an activity is valued by the person performing the activity (Henderson et al., 1991). Everyday, as part of life, people perform purposeful activities. When people actively participate in purposeful activities, they focus on the task to be accomplished (Hinojosa, Sabari, & Pedretti, 1993). People focus on accomplishing a goal that may not be physical when engaged in purposeful activities. This requires a coordination of the persons' physical, emotional, and cognitive systems (Hinojosa & Blount, 2004).

Occupational therapists select purposeful activities for children from a wide range of activities. Pediatric occupational therapists select activities that are meaningful to the child. The activities should be developmentally appropriate and motivating to the child, meshing comfortably with the child's lifestyle and environment. Purposeful activities are those that have meaning to the child and that involve interaction with the human and nonhuman environments (King, 1978). Three common types of therapeutic activities are play, self-care, and learning activities.

Play

Play involves various purposeful activities that are fun. Erikson (1963) proposed the idea that play is the work of the child. Play is one category available among the tools of purposeful activity. Children learn through play. The various types of play include sensorimotor, constructional, imaginary, and group play. Sensorimotor play is characterized by the use of sensory stimulation with a motor component. Constructional play promotes pleasure through building and creating things. Imaginary play entails cognition combined with fantasy and creativity. Group play is an interactional process in which children work together with a relatively common theme. On the basis of developmental level, culture, and needs of the child, the pediatric occupational therapist uses and adapts the types of therapeutic experiences to the benefit of that child. Through the skilled therapeutic use of play as a tool, the therapist can enhance the child's enjoyment and success in therapy.

The ability to use play as purposeful activity requires specific knowledge and skills wherein therapy occurs around child-selected activities. Therapists construct therapeutic environments that allow the child to lead the direction of a therapy session. For example, a child might be working on increasing attention to task in socially appropriate situations. In advance of a therapy session, the therapist prepares the environment with several appropriate options based on the child's preferences and his or her stage of development. When the child enters the therapy environment, the therapist responds to the child's directives and at times becomes a playmate within the child's world. Each activity is personally meaningful for the child and leads to the achievement of a therapeutic goal.

Another classification of purposeful activities is the wide range of activities used to assist the child in development of self-care skills. Frequently, it is a challenge for therapists to engage a child in personally meaningful activities aimed at developing specific self-care skills. Therapists frequently use play such as dressing the doll or dressing up to develop the skills. Here again, it is the child's selection and participation in a fun activity that makes it a purposeful activity. As children mature, the motivation for attaining self-care skills may be self-motivated through peer pressure or parental concern. At this time, practice and repetition of specific activities themselves are purposeful.

Activities with a Therapist-Defined Purpose

Frequently, therapists will select activities because of their therapeutic value. The therapist presents the activity to the child because it has the greatest potential as a therapeutic medium. The therapist often does not consider whether the child finds the activity personally meaningful. The major criterion for selecting activity is that participation in that activity will lead to a projected outcome or address a specific deficit. At times, the child may even consider the activity unpleasant or boring. For example, if the child needs to learn to dress himself or herself, the therapist might select a frame of reference that requires practice and repetition. In this scenario, the therapist may have the child repeat putting on, taking off his or her shoes and socks, and tying his or her shoes. The child may not be interested in completing the activity without considerable encouragement and reinforcement by the therapist. To encourage participation, the therapist may use another more desired activity as a reward. At other times, the therapist might use other methods of manipulating the child's participation.

Activities that are defined and directed by a therapist are an important part of occupational therapy intervention with children because the intervention directly relates to the therapy goals. Therapists use their knowledge and skills about working with pediatric clientele to motivate children to participate in activities. Social interactions with the therapist or another child may facilitate participation. When the child engages in the therapist-directed activity, the therapist is focusing on the goals associated with the activity as an end product. In other words, participating in the activity is just a means to an end. While this may not be the desired practice at times, it is sometimes entirely necessary to achieve therapeutic goals. Often, the physical environment and the context are important elements to manipulate when presenting therapist-directed activities.

Activity Analysis

Activity analysis is the identification of the component parts of an activity (Buckley & Poole, 2004). Occupational therapists are continually fascinated by the parts that make up an activity. Even activities that seem simple because of their familiarity may actually be complex. The occupational therapist analyzes activities for use with client intervention. Through the use of this tool, the therapist identifies whether the child has the necessary skills to perform or complete the activity. Activity analysis also enables the therapist to teach the activity more successfully through a clear understanding of its component parts.

When working with children, activity analysis is a constant focus of the intervention process. The pediatric occupational therapist continually divides activities into smaller parts to determine which skills are necessary to complete the task or activity. This is just the first step in the intervention process. The next step involves observation of how the child reacts and interacts with the activity or its component tasks. The therapist then analyzes the activity and the child's participation in and reaction to it. This process provides the therapist with the information he or she needs to adapt, grade, or combine activities to make them effective in intervention (Hinojosa, Sabari, & Pedretti, 1993).

The complexity of the activity analysis process is illustrated in the simple activity of stacking blocks. The preliminary analysis entails gaining an understanding of the skills required for the child to stack blocks. The child needs to have beginning fine motor skills, the ability to grasp the blocks, and controlled release for stacking the blocks. Then, as the child begins to stack the blocks, the therapist observes the child's behavior and response to the blocks. The next step involves analyzing the child and activity in combination. The questions that follow are examples of what the therapist may ask to start this analysis:

1. Can the child pick up the blocks?
2. Can the child place the blocks neatly on the stack?
3. Does the child have difficulty letting go of or releasing the blocks?
4. Does the child exhibit other compensatory body movements when engaged in the task?
5. Is the child more interested in building the tower or knocking it down?
6. What is the level of the child's fine motor skills in this task?

The therapist answers these questions based on his or her preliminary analysis combined with the knowledge gained from observing the child perform the activity. The therapist needs to look at the answers to all these questions before he or she proceeds to know how to modify this activity to make it therapeutic for the child. Furthermore, the same activity may be different with another child because the reactions of the child and the answers to the previously stated questions would be different. Any activity becomes modified by the way a particular child interacts with the environment and how he or she performs the activity.

Activity Synthesis

The magician's sleight of hand is smooth and sinuous, creating an illusion which is not really there. The audience watches in awe, trying to reconcile the reality that they know exists, with what they think they are seeing. It seems so simple, and yet creating the illusion is so complex. In many ways, this is much like the activity synthesis created by the occupational therapy practitioner (Kramer & Hinojosa, 2004, p. 136).

Activity synthesis for an occupational therapist is changing or creating an activity so that it meets therapeutic goals and the child can participate in it. The specific frame of reference theoretical base guides the occupational therapist's synthesis of an activity.

Therapists begin to use activity synthesis when they consider how to adapt or modify an activity so that the child is able to participate in the activity. Activity synthesis begins with the therapist having completed a complete activity analysis. Therapists combine this knowledge about the activity with the specific child's situation and therapeutic goals. Important considerations are the child's personal goals, desires, capacities, and limitations. Fundamental to activity synthesis is a clear understanding of the child and the activities in which therapists expect the child to participate. At this point, the specific frame of reference guides the activity synthesis within the context of the frame of reference.

Before an activity can be synthesized, therapists must decide on the key elements that define the activity. For example, if someone is going to make chocolate chip cookies what must be part of making the cookies? The activity must have chocolate chips, dough, and a means of baking. Missing any one of these would not be making chocolate chip cookies. With this knowledge, therapists begin to think about how they can synthesize the activity to meet therapeutic goals by adaptation or changing the activity. Activity adaptation means elements of the activity are modified to meet the needs of the client and to facilitate positive change. Activities are adapted by modifying the child's position, the presentation of the materials, or the characteristics of the materials (e.g., shape, size, weight, or texture). Adaptation may also involve modifying the procedure or sequence of events for the activity, nature, and degree of interpersonal contact (Hinojosa, Sabari, & Pedretti, 1993).

Activity synthesis occurs within the parameters of the dynamic theory of the theoretical base. Therapists, guided by the dynamic theory, synthesize or adapt the activity so that the child can successfully complete it. Using synthesis, occupational therapists reconstruct activities taking into consideration the child's therapeutic goals, strengths, and limitations. Reconfiguration of the activities creates a situation wherein the child can engage in the activity with minimum fear of failure and probable success. The therapist continually adapts activities for the child. As discussed previously, an example of adaptation is the modification of stacking blocks. The therapist may use larger blocks, seat the child at a small table rather than on the floor, present one block at a time, or add Velcro to the blocks so that they may be attached more easily to each other. The possibilities of adaptation for this activity are endless, limited only by the therapist's creativity.

The frame of reference guiding the intervention will determine how the adaptation is made to the environment or the activity. Adaptations do not change the person (Kramer & Hinojosa, 2004). The child changes as a result of interacting in the controlled environment.

Occupational therapists' skills and abilities, understanding of the child, appreciation of the context, and their knowledge of the frame of reference are critical to activity synthesis. The use of a frame of reference guides the synthesis; the frame of reference outlines how therapists use, adapt, modify, or create activities (Kramer & Hinojosa, 2004).

Activity Groups

Activity groups are those that have a common goal that involves activities. As a tool, activity groups are used more often in some frames of reference than in others. In pediatric occupational therapy, therapists use activity groups as a tool to promote age-appropriate peer interaction in a therapeutic environment. Occupational therapists draw from their knowledge of child development, group dynamics, and a firm understanding of activities. Activity groups are used to develop play, task, social, and physical skills. The involvement of peers can be useful for facilitating motivation. The occupational therapist fosters group interaction in a safe and supportive environment. Activity groups may be set up in many different ways, where children work side by side on similar projects (a parallel group), when children work together on a common project (a cooperative group), and when children develop a project and implement it together (a cooperative group). There are various taxonomies for activity groups that are used in occupational therapy (e.g., Mosey, 1986).

THE NONHUMAN ENVIRONMENT

Life is contextual for everyone, including children. In fact, Humphrey & Wakeford (2006) advocate shifting to a contextual perspective to deliver pediatric occupational therapy services. Context includes both nonhuman and human environments, which are named, defined, and grouped slightly differently in three classification systems: the World Health Organization's International Classification of Functioning, Disability and Health (ICF); (WHO, 2001), the American Occupational Therapy Association's Practice Framework (AOTA, 2002), and Uniform Terminology III (AOTA, 1994). In this chapter, the term "nonhuman environment" is utilized in the manner of Mosey (1986), who used the tradition of Searles (1960). For a child, nonhuman environment includes all environmental aspects environment that are not human. Occupational therapists use the nonhuman environment as a legitimate tool of pediatric practice.

The nonhuman environment involves elements of space and time, comprises the natural environment and human-made changes in the environment, and includes products and technology. The nonhuman environment can be physical or virtual. The nonhuman environment may be different within the various spaces a child occupies and across time. For instance, a Midwestern little girl during a typical summer week may be at home, her grandparents' house, or Sunday school. In March, her weekly routine might also include school, Brownies, and soccer. The little girl's nonhuman environment includes natural environment (trees in the backyard and the state park she visits with her troop) and human-made changes in the environment (her home, school, a soccer field converted from prairie grass). She uses various products and technology; for example, she plays with toys, talks on a cell phone with her grandmother, watches her favorite television show, and uses a computer for homework. Some products act to ease transitions, from one stage of development to another or from one setting to the next. For example, a favorite teddy bear assisted this child's transition from a crib to a big girl bed, from her grandmother's spare bedroom, and to a hotel for a family vacation. The teddy bear also eased her transition during her daily routine. Although much of her context is physical, the girl's nonhuman environment may become virtual if she becomes absorbed in a book, movie, or computer game. From a temporal standpoint, the girl's nonhuman environment will vary as her abilities, interests, family situation—her overall life—changes across time.

Because using the nonhuman environment as a legitimate tool varies among occupational therapists, this section provides a focus on three commonly used kinds of nonhuman environment used by pediatric therapists. The three kinds of nonhuman environment are toys, pets, and technology.

Toys

Toys are particularly important learning tools in the nonhuman environment. Most toys are commercially designed, but toys can also be hand made or repurposed household objects. When repurposing household objects as toys, the therapist must consider human environment aspects including culture and gender. For example, graduated measuring cups found in many kitchen cabinets might be considered an occupation-based legitimate tool that could substitute for purchased nesting toys. In some cultures that have gender roles clearly delineated for children, however, it may be considered unacceptable for some male toddlers to play with kitchen utensils.

With toys, children can find basic stimulation, comfort, enjoyment and fun, and a sense of competency. Many commercial toys are available that provide basic stimulation. Some toys have been designed to stimulate single senses such as auditory, visual, vestibular, or tactile systems; other toys have multiple sensory components. There are commercially available baby toys that provide soothing sounds, vibrate, light up, and move; singly or in combination.

Children of all ages can find comfort in toys, both emotionally and physically. A favorite blanket, an animal toy, or a doll may become a companion for a child, providing continuity across different routines and across various developmental stages. A much loved doll, for instance, could go from the nursery to a dorm room.

Toys can create feelings of excitement, causing a child to lose track of time. In fact, using the word *toy* as a legitimate tool usually signifies a sense of enjoyment or fun from the child's standpoint. Without the aspect of enjoyment or fun, an object becomes a regular therapeutic tool.

Children develop a sense of competency from toys: they learn that they are able to do things. Toys can help children learn cause and effect and develop an initial understanding of task performance. The occupational therapist is skilled at using toys for intervention and at matching toys to the child. Toys may "grow" with the child, having different meanings at various ages and stages. For example, large brick-type blocks can be wrapped with towels and used as positioning devices early in life. The child may learn to throw blocks, then begin stacking the blocks, and at still another stage start building structures used in imaginary play.

Toys are used as legitimate tools in just about every frame of reference. Toys most often form the basis for play, a fundamental concept in an occupation-based frame of reference. Certain toys, a miniature piano for example, are designed to work on foundational skills such as fine motor coordination. Other toys, such as a swing set, may be designed for whole body movement and may have therapeutic parallels in equipment used for specific frames of reference such as sensory integration.

Therapists who use an acquisitional frame of reference sometimes use toys to provide practice and repetition to learn a specific skill; other times toys are provided as positive reinforcement or limited as negative reinforcement. Pediatric therapists who use a more biomechanical frame of reference can use toys as positioning devices. Across frames of reference, toys are often a universal learning tool in the nonhuman environment.

Pets

Pets are significant parts of the nonhuman environment for children of any age. A pet can help a young child move beyond the natural egocentrism of early childhood to relate to other living organisms. Older children can learn to take care of pets. Occupational therapists use pets as a nonhuman environmental legitimate tool for multiple purposes including a source of pleasure, companionship, a nurturing relationship, and a responsibility.

In some frames of reference, for example acquisitional, the pleasure of spending time with a pet could be used as a reward (positive reinforcement) for completing a task. For an occupation-based frame of reference, incorporating a pet into the environment during therapeutic intervention can provide companionship for a particularly difficult activity or a task a child considers not much fun. For instance, a little boy who would rather play videogames inside but is working on moving more quickly and safely in his outside physical environment could have the companionship of his dog as an intrepid sidekick on a daily hike. The occupational therapist could upgrade the difficulty of the hike by adding a leash and working on simple commands such as "stop" and "heel."

A pet can teach a child how to relate to other living beings, thus helping the child to develop a nurturing relationship that is respectful and caring. A therapist can work with the child to recognize a pet's nonverbal and verbal communication, by learning the meaning of a cat that circles and rubs against the legs, a dog with a wagging tail, a turtle retreated completely into a shell, purring versus loud meowing, and barking at various pitches and insistence levels. Looking for and assigning meaning to pet nonverbal and verbal cues can be generalized to interactions and relationships with persons.

With a pet, a child can learn responsibility and the importance of providing care to another living thing. Using an occupation-based frame of reference, for example, a pediatric therapist can recommend that a child have a chore of making certain that a pet has water. A younger child (or a child with physical disabilities) could take responsibility for checking to see if water is in the pet bowl and notifying a caregiver if the bowl is empty. As a child assumes more responsibilities, the therapist could work with the family to have the child complete additional steps of the task including washing the bowl with soap, rinsing the bowl squeaky clean, refilling the bowl with water, and setting the filled bowl into place.

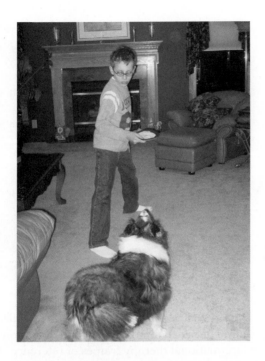

FIGURE 4.1 A child enjoys playing Frisbee with his pet.

Throughout life, pets can be a source of pleasure and companionship (Figure 4.1). The use of pets as a legitimate tool of the nonhuman environment is limited only by the imagination of the therapist.

Technology

Currently, technology, characterized as a kind of nonhuman environment, is pervasive in society. For children, technology has multiple purposes. Technology serves as an equalizer, maximizes potential, and creates a virtual environment.

Developed for persons with disabilities, assistive technology is designed to be an equalizer. Because of universal design, many products and features that were originally designed as separate assistive technology devices are now available to the general public in ordinary technology. Before recommending assistive technology, it is best to see if an intended function or feature is available in technology used by the general public. A primary example of incorporating stand-alone assistive technology products is the modern television. Since the mid-1990s, most televisions contain a caption-decoding microchip to allow closed captioning for people who are deaf (this feature is often used in noisy public spaces) and a device that allows a secondary auditory program (SAP), also called "video description," for persons who are blind. Often these features can be enabled after reading the product manual. Accessibility features (physical, auditory, visual, etc.) have been incorporated into many computer operating systems and word prediction, originally designed for persons with learning disabilities, has been built into cell phones or as autocorrect options in software applications.

FIGURE 4.2 A child playing a learning game on a computer.

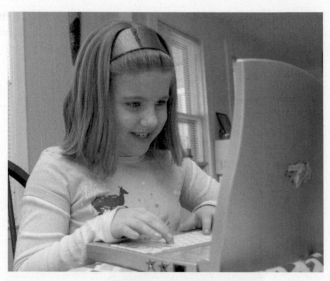

Technology also maximizes a child's potential (Figure 4.2). Previously called "adaptive equipment" (before federal legislation provided new language and definitions), assistive technology can be used in many occupational therapy frames of reference. Assistive technology can also play a role in other selected pediatric practice tools discussed in this chapter; however, this specialized type of technology is most often characterized as nonhuman environment.

Assistive technology devices are usually arranged in three general categories: speech generating devices (also called "augmentative communication systems"), mobility systems (which include wheelchairs and other devices), and electronic aids to daily living (EADL). Computer access, considered by many experts as a kind of EADL, is sometimes a fourth category. Devices within the assistive technology categories are available across a spectrum of levels from high tech to low tech.

For most people, the phrase "high tech" is synonymous with electronics-based devices. Electronic augmentative communication systems can assist children in functional communication and power mobility systems can help with functional mobility. Computers often provide assistance with educational activities and vocational exploration. Other high-tech EADL devices include page turners to read books and magazines, environmental control systems to manage lights and television, and robotic devices to help provide additional independence in activities of daily living. Because occupational therapists require specialized backgrounds to work with high-tech equipment (which is beyond the scope of this chapter), additional assistive technology information can be found in Cook & Hussey (2002) and Johnson, Beard, & Carpenter (2006).

At the other end of the spectrum, less expensive nonelectronic (low) technology continues to provide functional solutions for many children. Low-tech devices, under the guise of adaptive equipment, have been a primary staple in occupational therapists' practice repertoire for decades. Some children use picture boards for communication and others use walkers for mobility. Adaptive equipment catalogs are packed with low-tech equipment, primarily related to self-care. Catalogs have numerous pages of spoons and forks with built-up handles, nonspill drinking cups, and one-way straws to assist in feeding and eating; button hooks, elastic shoe laces, and long-handled shoe horns for dressing as well as various devices for grooming, oral hygiene, bathing and showering, and toileting. Many school-based, work-related, play, leisure, and recreational low-tech devices are also available.

Technology can create a virtual environment. For centuries, readers have experienced the virtual environments of books. Currently, technology makes available a wide variety of virtual environments in both scheduled format (e.g., televised cartoons) and on-demand (rented or purchased recordings of music, movies, and other entertainment). Gaming creates new worlds wherein children can interact in large social networks and competitions, using avatars and code names to represent themselves. Children can go to school online without leaving home. With assistive technology available, people in virtual worlds may not realize a child with severe disabilities is participating in the same activities as everybody else.

Pediatric occupational therapists may recommend technology to be used as a virtual environment to keep children safe. Used almost as an electronic pacifier, a virtual environment such as a favorite recorded movie can help ease plane trips, visits to the doctor's office, or even a long phone call at home. Therapists using a frame of reference with the word *acquisitional* sometimes use technology, especially technology that creates virtual environments, as rewards or positive reinforcement for completing specified tasks.

Using the nonhuman environment is essential to providing a contextual perspective in the delivery of pediatric occupational therapy services. Although toys, pets, and technology provided the focus for this section, there are unlimited ways occupational therapists use the nonhuman environment as a legitimate tool of pediatric practice.

TEACHING–LEARNING PROCESS

Occupational therapists, whether they consciously acknowledge the fact, use the teaching–learning process as a legitimate tool in just about every therapeutic encounter. Providing feedback to a child based on his or her performance is a prime example of the teaching–learning process in action. Pediatric therapists, even when they are not using the teaching–learning process directly with children, often engage in the teaching process as part of caregiver education. Caregiver education has become increasingly important to ensure follow through from specific therapy sessions and provide overall continuity of care.

Although both teaching and learning involve doing, the agent is different for each component of the process. In its most fundamental form, the therapist engages in the teaching component and the child is involved in the learning component. Teaching usually consists of giving instruction and providing demonstration, but often teaching is expanded to designing opportunities for active learning. Designing active learning opportunities involves creating contexts that are conducive for learning and planning therapeutic activities, which allow exploration and discovery and then the practice of new performance skills. Learning, which results in a relatively permanent positive change in performance, is the outcome of teaching–learning process.

Because the teaching–learning process has a grounding in behavioral approaches, teaching and learning are most often associated with frames of reference that include the word *acquisitional* in the theoretical base or title. Any other frame of reference, however, that uses terminology such as *trial* and *error, shaping, modeling, repetition, practice,* and *discovery* is using the teaching–learning process as a contemporary legitimate tool to effect positive change in occupational performance.

SENSORY STIMULATION WITH AN ADAPTIVE RESPONSE

Many of the activities used in occupational therapy involve the use of sensory stimulation as a tool. Blocks that are soft and fuzzy are often chosen by the therapist because of their tactile properties in addition to their use as a building tool. Therapists often use different tactile materials with children to determine how the child will respond and to provoke a specific adaptive response. Adaptive responses are responses that change over time based on the child's exposure to and integration of sensory input. The therapist needs to observe and understand the child's ability to process sensory information in order to effectively use this as a tool in treatment. Sensory stimuli are not limited to the tactile realm but may also include visual, auditory, gustatory, and olfactory stimulation to produce a response (Figure 4.3). Stimulation applied by the therapist, such as massage and positioning in a way to allow for improved engagement in a task, is also part of the sensory stimulation tool. Gross and fine motor activities may also include aspects of sensory stimulation to bring about a very specific adaptive response. Examples of this might include using a jumping activity to effect a neuromuscular response of increasing

FIGURE 4.3 Play involving multiple senses.

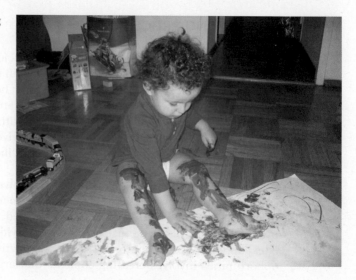

muscle tone, or using a grip adaptor on a pencil to revise a child's prehensile pattern when writing.

Therapists create environments that use sensory stimulation to provoke adaptive responses. Manipulating elements of the environments can elicit specific responses in children. Some therapists may use visual, auditory, olfactory and/or components and/or room to either stimulate or inhibit the adaptive responses of the child. Therapists skillfully match the environment of the treatment setting to obtain specific types of adaptive responses.

OCCUPATION

Occupation is used by therapists in intervention as a means to reach goals and as an outcome of successful intervention that children can engage in meaningful occupation. In this chapter, occupation will only be explored as a contemporary legitimate tool of the profession, as a means to reach a goal. One of the major ways that pediatric occupational therapists use occupation as a tool is through play. In order for play to be an occupation, it must be meaningful to the child. Ideally, the child should choose the particular play activity. All too often the therapist, not the child, chooses toys and play activities that fit the needs of the child and the goals of intervention. Another type of occupation that is often used in intervention is self-care. However, the specific play or self-care activity used in intervention must be meaningful to the child in order to be classified as an occupation (Hinojosa & Kramer, 1997). There are wide varieties of occupations that can be used in therapy; however, it is incumbent on the therapist to ensure that the specific activity chosen is meaningful to the child, and not just meaningful to the therapist as a way to achieve therapeutic goals.

Occupational therapy practitioners need to keep an individual's occupations in the forefront of their thoughts when using any legitimate tool. Interventions are always directed toward improving a child's ability to function within his or her occupations and in the roles as family member, sibling, player, or student. However, within the context of using any frame of reference, it is important to address the overall occupations of the child and to focus on the occupations of the particular child (Hinojosa & Kramer, 1997).

 Summary

This chapter has outlined the current major legitimate tools for pediatric occupational therapy. Other legitimate tools exist that have not been presented here but they are specific to one frame of reference and may be highly specialized. These specialized tools often require advanced education and training. The tools of the profession can change over time, just as practice changes over time. Because these tools are used within a frame of reference to create an environment for change, each frame of reference has tools that are more relevant and acceptable to it than to others. Within each frame of reference, the change process is outlined, delimiting the tools that are viable.

REFERENCES

American Occupational Therapy Association. (1994). Uniform terminology for occupational therapy—third edition. *American Journal of Occupational Therapy, 48,* 1047–1054.

American Occupational Therapy Association. (2002). Occupational therapy practice framework: Domain and process. *American Journal of Occupational Therapy, 56,* 609–639.

Buckley, K., & Poole, S. (2004). Activity analysis. In J. Hinojosa, & M. -L. Blount (Eds). *The Texture of Life* (2nd ed., pp. 69–114). Bethesda, MD: American Occupational Therapy Association.

Bundy, A. C., Lane, S. J., & Murray, E. A. (Eds). (2002). *Sensory Integration: Theory and Practice* (2nd ed.). Philadelphia, PA: FA Davis Co.

Christiansen, C. H., Baum, C. B., & Bass-Haugen, J. (Eds). (2005). *Occupational Therapy: Enabling Function and Well-Being* (3rd ed.). Thorofare, NJ: Slack Inc.

Cook, A. M., & Hussey, S. M. (2002). *Assistive Technologies: Principles and Practice* (2nd ed.). St. Louis, MO: Mosby.

Crepeau, E. B., Cohn, E. S., & Schell, B. A. (Eds). (2003). *Willard and Spackman's Occupational Therapy* (10th ed.). Philadelphia, PA: Lippincott Williams & Wilkins.

Erikson, E. H. (1963). *Childhood and Society* (2nd ed.). New York: Norton.

Henderson, A., Cermak, S., Coster, W., & Murray, E. (1991). The issue is: Occupational science is multidimensional. *American Journal of Occupational Therapy, 45,* 370–372.

Hinojosa, J., & Blount, M. -L. (2004). Purposeful activities within the context of occupational therapy. In J. Hinojosa, & M. -L. Blount (Eds). *The Texture of Life* (2nd ed., pp. 1–16). Bethesda, MD: American Occupational Therapy Association.

Hinojosa, J., & Kramer, P. (1997). Statement: Fundamental concepts of occupational therapy: Occupation, purposeful activity, and function. *American Journal of Occupational Therapy, 51,* 864–866.

Hinojosa, J., Kramer, P., & Crist, P. (2005). Evaluation: where do we begin? In J. Hinojosa, P. Kramer, & P. Crist (Eds). *Evaluation: Obtaining and Interpreting Data* (2nd ed., pp. 1–17). Bethesda, MD: American Occupational Therapy Association.

Hinojosa, J., Sabari, J., & Pedretti, L. (1993). Position paper: Purposeful activity. *American Journal of Occupational Therapy, 47,* 1081–1082.

Humphrey, R., & Wakeford, L. (2006). An occupation-centered discussion of development and implications for practice. *American Journal of Occupational Therapy, 60,* 258–267.

Johnson, L., Beard, L., & Carpenter, L. B. (2006). *Assistive Technology: Access for all Students.* Upper Saddle River, NJ: Pearson Prentice Hall.

King, L. J. (1978). Towards a science of adaptive responses. *American Journal of Occupational Therapy, 7,* 429–437.

Kramer, P., & Hinojosa, J. (2004). Activity synthesis as a means to occupation. In J. Hinojosa, & M. -L. Blount (Eds). *The Texture of Life* (2nd ed., pp. 136–158). Bethesda, MD: American Occupational Therapy Association.

Mosey, A. C. (1986). *Psychosocial Components of Occupational Therapy.* New York: Raven Press.

Pendleton, H. M., & Schultz-Krohn, W. (Eds). (2006). *Pedretti's Occupational Therapy* (6th ed.). St. Louis, MO: Mosby, Elsevier Science.

Radomski, M. V., & Latham, C. A. T. (Eds). (2008). *Occupational Therapy for Physical Dysfunction* (6th ed.). Philadelphia, PA: Lippincott Williams & Wilkins.

Schell, B. A. B. (2003). Clinical reasoning: the basis of practice. In E. B. Crepeau, E. S. Cohen, & B. A. B Schell (Eds). *Willard and Spackman's Occupational Therapy* (10th ed., pp. 131–139). Philadelphia, PA: Lippincott Williams & Wilkins.

Searles, H. F. (1960). *The Non-Human Environment.* New York: International Universities Press.

World Health Organization(WHO). (2001). *ICF: International Classification of Functioning, Disability and Health.* Geneva: WHO.

CHAPTER 5

The Perspective of Context as Related to Frame of Reference

MARY MUHLENHAUPT

Descriptions of pediatric occupational therapy practice in the 1950s (Gleve, 1954; Swartout & Swartout, 1954) represent programs located primarily in hospitals, specialized clinics, and medical units. During that era, services were provided for children with permanent physical limitation or prolonged periods of restricted activity and convalescence because of illness. Occupational therapists implemented interventions that created opportunities for socialization, restored function, and promoted psychological adjustment to altered physical capacities and limitations in activity because of illness or disease. In the following years, occupational therapy developed in specialized schools and treatment centers for youth with mental retardation (Bower, 1961; Curzon, 1962), and then in public schools, with services provided for children with perceptual motor difficulties (Erhardt, 1971).

A major shift in pediatric occupational therapy was facilitated in the mid-1970s when Public Law 94–142, the Education for All Handicapped Children Act (Federal Register, 1977) was enacted (Note: this law is the predecessor to the current Individuals with Disabilities Education Improvement Act of 2004). For the first time in the United States, federal regulation mandated access to public schools, affording all children (aged 3 to 21, as consistent with individual state law), regardless of their abilities, the right to equal educational opportunities in the public education system. As school districts enrolled students with differing abilities, occupational therapists were among various support personnel whose expertise was designed to assist students with disabilities to benefit from special education (Federal Register, 1977; Turnbull & Turnbull, 1978). Subsequent amendments to this federal education legislation changed the eligibility age ranges in all states to include children with disabilities, from birth to 21 years of age (Federal Register, 1986). Under federal provisions for early intervention, states began implementing programs that emphasize supporting families to help their young children (from birth to 3 years of age) develop and learn within the environments and situations that represent natural learning opportunities for all early childhood development (Hanft, 1988; Campbell, Bellamy, & Bishop, 1988).

In the 21st century, pediatric occupational therapy encompasses prevention, developmental, remediation, and enrichment interventions. The central focus of contemporary occupational therapy practice is to enable individuals to participate in everyday occupations as an essential pursuit that influences their health and well-being (Law, 2002). Through childhood occupations, children interact with people and environments, learn and practice skills, develop physical and psychosocial competence, explore interests, and master roles that enable them to transition to adulthood (Case-Smith, Richardson, & Schultz-Krohn, 2005; Law et al., 2006). The unique and essential focus of pediatric occupational therapy practice extends from its goal to engage children in everyday activities through which they gain experience and practice, learn, develop, and realize their potential.

Contemporary occupational therapy practice arenas for children include medically based settings such as neonatal intensive care units, pediatric acute care and rehabilitation units, intermediate and long-term healthcare facilities, and hospital-based outpatient clinics. Independently managed private practices offer office-based as well as itinerant services within the community. In addition to public and private schools and preschools, occupational therapists provide services in families' homes, child care settings, or in other community-based settings, such as the library's weekly parent–child music group or a summer day camp program. These latter practice settings call for therapists to integrate occupational therapy perspectives into the everyday activities, routines, and situations which already exist in those settings, so that all children can grow, learn, and play together. Table 5.1 summarizes features that distinguish contemporary pediatric service settings.

New knowledge and shifting paradigms within and beyond our discipline, medical advances that cure as well as protect children from illness and disability, the development and use of technology, and changing fiscal and governmental factors are some of the influences that have driven the transformation in pediatric occupational therapy throughout the last 55 years. Numerous other changing variables, such as population demographics, family structures, lifestyles, and roles of children and youth in society have shaped practice as well. All these factors represent only some aspects of the *context* in which pediatric occupational therapy services have developed and continue to evolve.

WHAT IS CONTEXT?

The American Heritage College Dictionary (2007) defines context as "the circumstances in which an event occurs, a setting" (p. 309). In reference to language, context is defined as "the part of text or statement which surrounds a particular word or passage and determines its meaning" (American Heritage College Dictionary, 2007, p. 309), implying a shaping or controlling influence. We derive a particular understanding from a remark as it is heard within a speech, yet the same comment may convey an entirely different sense when considered in isolation, or as part of another discourse. Context contributes significance and has bearing on the entities it encompasses. It originates from the Latin word, contextus, which means a joining together.

The International Classification of Functioning, Disability and Health framework (World Health Organization, 2001) includes context, composed of both personal and environmental factors, as an integral dimension of the health of individuals

TABLE 5.1 Distinguishing Features of Pediatric Service Settings

	Hospital	School System	Home Based	Private Practice	Child Care Center
Governance	Healthcare, managed care organization, and Board of Trustees	State Education department, local Board of Education, and building administration	Family culture and norms	Independent corporation, partnership, or individual owner	Corporation, partnership, individual owner, or sponsoring agency
Funding	Public, private funds, endowment, and charities	State and federal government, local taxpayers	Third-party payment, medical insurance, federal and state funding, out-of-pocket	Third-party payment, private insurance, and out-of-pocket	Medical insurance, federal/state subsidies, early intervention programs, and out-of-pocket
Focus of care	Treating acute or chronic disease/dysfunction/conditions	Student's participation and progression within the education curriculum, preparation for higher education, employment, independent living	Family system and child as part of the family	Specific to agency's mission	Nurturance, health and safety, developmental progression
Peer relations/supervision	Therapy department with director and hierarchical supervision by medical and administrative staff	Principal is administrator of multidisciplined staff. Therapist as employee or contractor	Employee or agency contractor traveling to homes on itinerant basis. Supervision from building administration and home agency personnel	Therapist functions solo or with group of related professionals	Therapist as contractor into child care center. Administrative supervision from building administration and home agency personnel
Intervention setting	Simulated environment structured around dispensing care as a priority	Multiple school-based and community-based environments (least restrictive settings), as determined by educational team	Natural home and family settings and activities	Simulated settings in center-based practice, may include home-based and community-based setting	Caregiver-child/children in settings that simulate home and preschool environments
Provider/consumer relations	Brief, intermittent contact, episodic care in 1:1 relationship	Therapist works with system, programs, education staff, students and parents, short-term to long-term contacts	Therapist in 1:1 relationship with family/child, short-term to long-term contacts	Therapist in 1:1 relationship with family/child, short-term to long-term contacts	Therapist in direct relationship with child care provider and may include direct relationship with child; short-term to long-term contacts

and of populations. In occupational therapy, context is described as a "variety of interrelated conditions within and surrounding the client that influence performance" (American Occupational Therapy Association, 2002). Cultural, physical, social, spiritual, virtual, and temporal contexts are considered in the occupational therapy process. The child development field recognizes that multiple and complex contexts, described as "unique combinations of genetic and environmental circumstances" (p. 8), influence children's capacities, what they do, and how they grow, learn, and mature (Berk, 2006).

Context is related to that which it surrounds; therefore, specific contextual features that are relevant vary according to individual points of interest. For example, when we consider the options within the after-school activity program in a large city school district, broad concerns such as the system's current strategic goals and operating budget, as well as space allocation, the numbers, interests and capabilities of students, along with the resources of personnel who implement the program, are some of the variables that influence the content that is offered. In a more narrowly focused circumstance, our attention is different. Consider a situation in which the occupational therapist attends to the play behavior of a 3-year-old boy during outdoor recess period in his preschool. The availability of toys at his home and in school, his family's views on play, the attributes of the recess area, his teacher's role in encouraging or allowing certain play schemes, and the influence of his playmates are some of the features that influence what he pursues during the recess period. Even the boy's interests and motivations related to his motor or cognitive skills have a bearing on his behavior. While distinct and contrasting contextual factors are important in these two scenarios, a common denominator across each is that in addition to the personal attributes that individuals bring to any situation, both human and nonhuman elements in the immediate and more remote environments impact capacities and expectations and enable or constrain outcomes.

This chapter describes and highlights how context is relevant in occupational therapy for children. Contextual influences impact the ways in which occupational therapy services are distinguished and utilized within a practice setting, and in addition, affect the scope of the therapist's contribution to the programs offered. Contextual features also shape a child's participation and performance. Knowing about all of these variables is important when occupational therapists define their roles and responsibilities and consider a frame of reference to guide their service in any situation. Furthermore, the perspective of context helps occupational therapists to understand and interpret what the child is doing and whether the behavior serves or interferes with his or her function. Consequently, the occupational therapy process requires that the therapist consider contextual variables within the child and within his or her surrounding environments when evaluating, planning and implementing intervention, determining progress toward outcomes, and discontinuing service. Occupational therapists need to learn about and use the specific context of the service system as well as the context that influences an individual child to design and provide individualized assistance and support that are valid and reasonable in the situations, settings, and routines that are most familiar to that child.

LOCUS OF PEDIATRIC PRACTICE — HEALTH AND EDUCATION

Healthcare and education represent two broad *systems* in which pediatric occupational therapy services are delivered currently. Systems concepts help us understand both the context and the complexities of the healthcare and education institutions. Mosby's Dictionary of Medicine, Nursing, and Health Professions (2006) defines systems theory related to healthcare as "a holistic medical concept in which the human patient is viewed as an integrated complex of open systems rather than as semi-independent parts. The health care approach in this theory requires the incorporation of family, community and cultural factors as influences to be considered in the diagnosis and treatment of the patient" (p. 1814).

Bertalanffy (1968) described the open system as a complex of interacting elements that is characterized by (1) relationships within its internal environment and (2) relationships between the system and external environments. An open system is defined by its relationships and a view that does not see the system through these relationships as inaccurate. Interdependence between the system and external environment is an important concept. The open system receives and responds to information generated from interactions (1) within itself (subsystems) and (2) with the external environment. Each exchange provides feedback to which both the system and the external environment respond. Therefore, the environment has the potential to influence the system and changes in the system have the potential to influence both the system and the environment. One cannot understand the system by separating it from its environment or by breaking it into component parts because, by doing this, the relationships that give the system its identity and attributes no longer exist. This chapter reflects these concepts of connectedness and relationships in the occupational therapy process and the therapist's selection of frame of reference in pediatric practice.

INFLUENCES THAT SHAPE HEALTH AND EDUCATION CONTEXTS

Multiple factors inside and outside of health and education shape these systems (Table 5.2) and help define consumer access, as well as the variety, quality, and cost of occupational therapy and other services provided. Unique philosophies, values, tools, and practices distinguish each system. Other influential features extend from the level of society at large to the individual communities in which programs are located. As examples, substance abuse, malnutrition, and social issues that include homelessness, violence, and poverty affect neighborhoods and their populations. These concerns impact the needs of families and their children and affect their ability to seek and receive services. Providers' professional and personal perspectives represent another dimension of the context that characterizes each system and its programs (Hall, 2005). The following sections raise several specific issues that influence contemporary health and education systems and are important for occupational therapists to consider.

Current views of disability support the inclusion of all persons in society (Villa & Thousand, 2002; Smith, 2007). The American Occupational Therapy Association (AOTA,

TABLE 5.2	Categories of Factors Influencing Health and Education Systems
Policy	Governmental—federal, state, and local; accreditation bodies; health organization/health plans
Environmental	Political and social climates; science and research, technology; philosophical beliefs, history and current knowledge in medicine and education; social perspectives
Population characteristics	Regional and community demographics—age, gender, and culture
Fiscal and materiel resources	Within systems/agencies/programs
Individual characteristics	Healthcare and education beliefs/interests; financial resources; personal health practices and behavior; personal attributes/capacities

2004) and other associations (Council for Exceptional Children, 2003; TASH, 2000a,b) that promote the rights of individuals with disabilities have adopted positions in support of inclusive practices for all children in home, school, and community settings. Client-centered perspectives in health care (Hanna & Rodger, 2002; Schauer et al., 2007) and the self-determination movement support consumer-focused care and the rights of all persons to define and choose their preferred lifestyles and the activities they pursue (Erwin & Brown, 2003; Poulsen, Rodger, & Ziviani, 2006; Shapiro, 1993). Family-centered approaches recognize the strengths of families and support them in active decision making regarding their children's care (Committee on Hospital Care, 2003). Recent perspectives also suggest a shifting paradigm in pediatric rehabilitation, moving away from an emphasis on biomedical approaches in favor of more functionally oriented outcomes and interventions that promote children's participation in society (Binks et al., 2007; Rosenbaum & Stewart, 2007). All these points mean that providers who work with children with disabilities need to hold high expectations for their clients' participation in home, school, and community-based activities, along with typically developing children. They need to anticipate and facilitate involvement by families and children in making choices about the goals, activities, and opportunities that are meaningful to them.

In its latest national poll, the U.S. population continues to reflect increasing diversity in its cultural composition (US Bureau of the Census, 2000). A family's cultural beliefs are connected to their interpretation of child health, causes of disability, and preferred plan of care (Mandell & Novak, 2005). When people of diverse cultures access medicine and healthcare in the United States, language barriers, divergent beliefs, and contrary treatment approaches may challenge both providers and recipients and lead to clashes that interfere with the care process (Fadiman, 1997; Barry, 2002). From a Western viewpoint of medicine and healthcare in the early 2000s, how does a local hospital reach out to the community and what types of programs are offered when the surrounding population represents Hmong immigrants who value spiritual intervention in dealing with their children's illnesses and disabilities? During recent years, greater attention has been directed to the need for physicians and healthcare personnel, educators, child care providers, and others working with children and their families to respect multiple different cultural, ethnic, and linguistic heritages (Hanson, 2004). Lynch (2004) describes cross-cultural competence as "the ability to think, feel, and act in ways that acknowledge, respect, and build on ethnic, [socio-] cultural, and linguistic diversity" (p. 43). The provision of culturally competent care has been associated with positive healthcare outcomes (Callister, 2005; Clay, 2007). As a result, occupational therapists can expect that contemporary health and education systems include initiatives (McPhatter & Ganaway, 2003; Mutha & Karliner, 2006; Martin, 2007) designed to facilitate communication and interactions among individuals from diverse backgrounds. These efforts prompt service providers to adopt ways of thinking and behaving that enhance their relationships with families and enable them to accept varying perspectives that families bring with them.

Telemedicine and the relatively new terms, e-health and e-learning, describe healthcare and education practices which are supported by the Internet, wireless, and other related technologies. These tools and processes provide alternate channels for communication and instruction, improved access to information and other strategies that streamline and enhance multiple aspects of service provision. In relation to children, their environments and activities—computers, arcade games, and virtual toys—along with learning, recreational, and social opportunities available through the Internet are a part of many home, school, and community activities in which children engage. The virtual environments afforded by these electronic media are becoming more important in children's lives, presenting beneficial as well as potentially unfavorable influences (Ziviani & Rodger, 2006) and ultimately contributing to the landscape of health and education systems.

Principles of accessible design and assistive technology solutions, combined with digital age technology, contribute to the development of universal curriculum, teaching methods and materials that are more easily accessed by all students, regardless of whether special learning needs are present (Rose & Meyer, 2002). Recent scientific and technological advances offer robotics as a tool to promote children's development (Michaud et al., 2007) and "smart" wheelchairs using mobile robot technology to enable independence (Simpson, 2005). Continued applications of universal design, ubiquitous computing, or *ubicomp*, as well as pervasive and intuitive technologies have the potential to increase children's participation in valued and meaningful activities and to alter service delivery. As an example, CareLog and Abaris, prototype automated capture devices, offer new strategies for professionals and consumers. These mobile computer-aided applications are designed to assist caregivers and providers as they implement and assess interventions to promote participation at home and in the classroom for children with autism (Kientz et al., 2007).

Both healthcare and education systems espouse evidence-based approaches within the programs and services they provide. Dr. David L. Sackett et al. describe evidence-based medicine as the "integration of best research evidence with clinical expertise and patient values" (Sackett et al., 2000, p. 1). Sackett's work has influenced the development of evidence-based approaches in rehabilitation (Law, 2007). Occupational therapists practice evidence-based approaches within their evaluation, planning, and implementation processes (Lee & Miller, 2003; Tickle-Degnen, 2000). The No Child Left

Behind Act of 2001 (NCLB, 2002) requires that federally funded education programs be grounded in scientifically based research. IDEA 2004 provisions require the use of instructional strategies that are supported by scientifically based research. The federal regulations also stipulate that related services (including occupational therapy) be "based on peer-reviewed research to the extent practicable" (Federal Register, 2006, p. 46788). Supporters of evidence-based practice in education see incorporating scientific research as a "means for improving education and developing a knowledge-base for what works" (Beghetto, 2003, p. 4).

The emphasis on evidence-based approaches in medicine, healthcare, and education creates a context in which informed decision making and accountability are essential elements in practice by all providers in these systems. Occupational therapists need to present families and other adults involved with a child's program with unbiased information about the potential benefits and limitations of a range of intervention options, or acknowledge uncertainty when the implications of specific strategies are unknown. Data-based decision-making practices are increasingly emphasized in children's services (Chen et al., 2004; Bayona et al., 2006; Reid et al., 2006). Therapists need to work with other team members to design and implement measurement systems so that once intervention begins, data about the child's participation in targeted settings and activities is routinely collected. This data is reviewed, and based on trends in the child's behavior the course of intervention is continued, adjusted, or replaced. As a result, practice decisions are informed by evidence that is relevant for the individual child.

ORGANIZING PARADIGMS IN PEDIATRIC HEALTH AND EDUCATION SYSTEMS

Capra (1996) defines a social paradigm as "a constellation of concepts, values, perceptions, and practices shared by a community, which forms a particular vision of reality that is the basis of the way the community organizes itself" (p. 6). The curative model, the palliative model, and the ecological model described in this chapter represent distinct social paradigms that can be identified in children's healthcare and education systems (Table 5.3). In addition to influencing how programs and services are utilized within the system, these different paradigms have some bearing on expected roles and relationships for providers in these systems. Any one of the paradigms is not associated exclusively with either healthcare or education systems. It is also important to recognize that contextual dimensions (both human and nonhuman) that influence any "community" may support or limit particular elements of these models in that system. Therefore, any of the paradigms may not be reflected in its entirety in a practice setting within either the healthcare or education system.

CURATIVE MODEL PARADIGM

The curative paradigm is embodied in the medical model in which the person and his or her attributes are the center of attention and are considered to be the base

TABLE 5.3 Three Social Paradigms in Healthcare and Education Systems		
	Curative Model Paradigm	*Palliative Model Paradigm*	*Ecological Model Paradigm*
Goal	Cure	Improve function and reduce symptomatology/dysfunction	Achieve performance and function across relevant/desired environments
Method	Treat the diagnosis	Address person and environment: reduce undesired and enhance desired traits/components	Create options for child's relationships with others and increase participation across environments
Cause of the problem	Physical and biological phenomena	Multiple variables within human organism, environment, or both	Multiple variables in person–environment dimensions and dynamics
Model of thinking	Reductionistic; analysis of data	Incorporating mind–body connection and synthesis of data	Holistic; mind–body–environment interaction and interrelations
Assessment based upon	Pathophysiology, scientifically based data, professional expertise	Pathophysiology, scientifically based data, professional expertise, and child/family/caregiver perspective and subjective views	Scientifically based data, professional expertise, child/family/professional/other relevant person's views of environment dimensions and dynamics
Relevance of human organism	A host for disease/dysfunction, compliance with treatment plan	Source for valuable information needed to supplement clinical findings and plan treatment	Child/family/caregiver capable of making choices and of influencing development
Intervention based upon	Professional's expertise and discretion, individual's medical history and physical diagnosis, and knowledge of clinical/hard science	Client-determined goals related to their life and diagnosis, in cooperation with professionals	Client-determined goals, consensual decision making, family is a peer on team
Service delivery	Subspecialties provided by multiple providers, each with focused perspective; unit of care provider–patient dyad	Providers with diverse expertise, well-developed communication skills; unit of care provider focused on person and environment	Collaborative and consultative relationships with family and each other; providers with well-developed interpersonal skills; unit of care provider focused on person within immediate and broad environments
Team process	Multidisciplinary	Interdisciplinary	Interdisciplinary/transdisciplinary
Intervention success measured by	Cure is achieved; dysfunction/symptomatology is eliminated/reversed	Patient/family perspectives combined with scientific data regarding symptom abatement/relief	Sufficiency of environmental options to enable family/child to function across desired situations/communities

upon which function depends. Mosby's dictionary defines the medical model as "the traditional approach to the diagnosis and treatment of illness . . . focuses on the defect, or dysfunction, within the patient, using a problem-solving approach. The medical history, physical examination, and diagnostic tests provide the basis for the identification and treatment of a specific illness. The medical model is thus focused on the physical and biologic aspects of specific diseases and conditions . . . ." (Mosby, 2006, p. 1167). The belief that an individual's function and operational behavior depend on the integrity of its underlying parts is a central concept in medical model approaches. This approach views person and environment as separate, predominated healthcare during the 20th century (Stewart & Law, 2003).

Personal factors within the human system represent the valued context in this model. The external context—factors in the environments surrounding the person—is not central to understanding function or treating conditions that impact performance. The curative model of medical care is focused on alleviating symptomatology as its goal (Fox, 1997). Component systems within the individual, which are believed to contribute to the expression of observed behaviors, are analyzed. Diagnostic testing is used to identify and define dysfunction and symptomatology within components. Once determined, pathology is treated. Psychosocial aspects are addressed separately from the condition. The medical cure model views the selection of a treatment approach as a scientific question, best answered by the professional using objective, scientifically based data (Fox, 1997).

Teamwork in the medical model is based on principles of multidisciplinary function which recognize various providers whose work with a client is generally accomplished separately from each other throughout most stages of their care (McCallin, 2001). Individual team members, each seen as specialists with their own discipline's particular expertise and perspective toward defined aspects of human function, evaluate, plan, and implement their own intervention. Information about the different treatment programs and their results is shared through written reports and team meetings. As the model has ultimate respect for scientific and biomedical knowledge, the physician assumes a commanding position as the authority in the care process.

PALLIATIVE CARE PARADIGM

Palliative treatment is defined as "therapy designed to relieve or reduce intensity of uncomfortable symptoms but not to produce a cure" (Mosby, 2006, p. 1381). A "management" intent is embraced, rather than a goal to cure the identified deviation or dysfunction that resides within the individual or "fix the problem." Palliative approaches focus on preserving and enabling the individual's function and enhancing quality of life despite the static or progressive disease or biopsychosocial differences that he or she experiences. A mind–body connection in relation to disease and illness is acknowledged in this model. Value is placed on understanding the client's perceptions and knowing his or her preferences related to outcomes and to choice of intervention options.

Both personal and environmental contexts are important concerns for evaluation in this paradigm. Diagnostic tests and procedures that focus on the individual are implemented. In addition, information from the client, family, and other important caregivers regarding a subjective assessment of the individual's goals and current status contributes to evaluation data. Other environmental factors including cultural, social, and ethical points are legitimate concerns within the evaluation process. The client and his or her family or caregivers are also a part of the decision-making courses in this model.

Analysis of information, intervention planning, and implementation are accomplished through a team process with interdisciplinary components (McCallin, 2001). Members of distinct professions may or may not share roles and responsibilities as they complete evaluations in the data-gathering phase. However, as an essential element, they work together to review evaluation findings and then develop intervention recommendations. Interdisciplinary team function requires that each individual member recognizes cross-discipline perspectives when using discipline-specific information to contemplate optimal intervention in a given situation. Team communication and collaboration enables the client, his or her significant caretakers, and service providers to consider numerous variables as targets of intervention and then, work together as a group to develop a unified program plan. Once team decisions are made regarding the recommended program, interventions are implemented by members of the disciplines that are specified. Treatment methods include remediation, adaptation, support, and other intervention strategies to help the individual and his or her caretakers deal with differences and improve conditions.

The palliative care paradigm includes views that may be considered in opposition to the curative paradigm just discussed. As explained, cure of pathology is not a goal in this model. Therapists using palliative care approaches adopt a more "generalist view" incorporating diverse perspectives as they participate in a care process that deals with both physical and social aspects of the human system along with influences from relevant environments. When compared to the curative paradigm, different possibilities are evident during evaluation, planning, and intervention phases because this model solicits information from additional sources beyond those on which the curative care model depends. In this model, the provider's manner may be considered "more caring" or communicative as the person receiving service is asked to contribute information to the evaluation and treatment planning processes.

A recognized specialty in England, pediatric palliative care is practiced in the United States for children with serious or life-threatening conditions (Browning & Solomon, 2005; Meier & Beresford, 2007). Programs that emphasize a child's capacities rather than limitations, and those that seek to build on the assets of child and environment, also referred to as "strengths-based approaches" (Blundo, 2001), represent this model. Their views are compatible with the interest of palliative care in bringing affirmation to the individual's life (Perron & Schonwetter, 2001).

ECOLOGICAL MODEL PARADIGM

The ecological paradigm draws from the social model of disability (Oliver, 2004) in which societal aspects of everyday life are recognized as significant influences when addressing an individual's function and performance. An acceptance that human development occurs in relation to a context is critical in the ecological perspective. Human ecology is defined as "the study of interrelations between individuals and their environments, as well as among individuals within an environment" (Mosby, 2006, p. 904). In this perspective, interactions with people and relationships within and across environments and settings are identified and valued among the diverse influences that contribute to growth and maturation. Culture and society are included as important influences on the developing child. This model appreciates that various environmental variables may be more significant in projecting health outcomes than are the characteristics of the individual (Stewart & Law, 2003), and reflects the belief that disability can be reduced when social and physical aspects of the environment are included as targets of intervention (Stark et al., 2007).

Opportunities for team planning are an integral part of this perspective, with team-work approaches reflecting components of the interdisciplinary or transdisciplinary processes. Members of the transdisciplinary team work across disciplines functioning together as a unit (McCallin, 2001), and not as a group of individuals representing and promoting distinct professions. Collaborative efforts, shared roles, and mutual responsibilities are characteristic throughout evaluation, planning, and program implementation. Communication skills and interpersonal relations are important as individuals with varied backgrounds share their expertise related to the child. Profession-specific language and concepts are translated to be understood by those without a similar professional background.

Services based on this model focus on child–environment interaction as a means to effect change and measure progress. The creation of options that enable the child to engage and participate in his or her environments are valued intervention objectives. Many inclusive settings and programs that support services and interventions in "natural settings" espouse principles based on ecological perspectives. The primary service provider model used in special education programs (Rainforth, 2002) is another example that represents features of the ecological paradigm.

CONSIDERING CONTEXT WHEN PLANNING OCCUPATIONAL THERAPY SERVICE

When shifting from a large-scale view and looking more narrowly at occupational therapy services for children, systems views and knowledge about context present various considerations that impact upon how the occupational therapy process is conceptualized, planned, and implemented for consumers served in either health or education systems. In addition to the larger context of the health or education system, which has already been discussed in this chapter, the context of the child for whom the occupational therapy program is developed requires consideration.

Children grow, develop, and change with the influence of intrinsic variables as well as those from immediate and extended environments. Bronfenbrenner's bioecological perspectives provide a framework from which to understand the relationship of these contexts on the developmental process. A person's biological, cognitive, emotional, and behavioral characteristics are at the core of this model (Bronfenbrenner & Morris, 2006).

Human development is explained through episodes of both stability and change in the biopsychological characteristics of the individual together with reciprocal relationships between the individual and his or her environments over time (Bronfenbrenner, 2005a). These interactions, occurring on a regular basis, are referred to as "proximal processes" and are seen as the *"primary engines of development"* (p. 6). Over the course of a child's life, these processes become increasingly more complex. Parent–infant daily bottle-feeding experiences, attending an older sibling's basketball games, outdoor play with neighborhood peers, and completing a group project during a classroom work period are some examples of situations and opportunities in which proximal processes abound. Recognizing the value and impact of these everyday occurrences, the occupational therapist intervenes in the context of the daily activities, routines, and experiences in which a child engages to influence his or her growth and development.

The child's environment is a context with multiple layers, each a system that provides either direct or indirect influence on his or her growth and performance over the life span. The most proximal, the *microsystem*, is defined as "a pattern of activities, roles and interpersonal relations experienced by the developing person in a given face-to-face setting with particular physical and material features and containing other persons with distinctive characteristics of temperament, personality, and systems of belief" (Bronfenbrenner, 2005b, p. 148). The family and home environment represents an early microsystem for infants. The infant who attends a community child care setting for part of the week experiences two different microsystems. As children grow, the number of microsystems present in their lives increases. School, home, church, and the club soccer league are examples for a particular teenager. The activities, experiences, relationships, and even the distinct characteristics of persons in each of these settings are recognized as important influences on the child's development.

Moving away from the child's immediate context, Bronfenbrenner identifies several dimensions that can influence proximal processes and thereby impact development. Connections and relationships between a child's microsystems (e.g., home and school partnerships between parents and teachers) make up the *mesosystem*. Links between settings in which the child's surrounding adults engage (parent's workplace and parent's graduate education program or parent's workplace and home) define the *exosystem*. At the broadest level, the *macrosystem* includes cultural belief systems, societal patterns of behavior, and resources.

In summary, the bioecological perspective posits that a child's development results from the influence of multiple circumstances and attributes within the child together with regularly occurring relationships and interactions between the child and the world in which he or she exists. This model acknowledges the central contribution of the family and their distinct attributes. Contextual dimensions that surround the child and family unit influence the important persons and circumstances within a child's everyday experience and consequently, have relevance on how the child grows and matures.

The Family

For the purpose of this book, the primary function of the family is to provide a supportive and nurturing environment for the child's development. The family is a child's first context for development and in terms of power and breadth of influence, the family surpasses other contexts which support a child's growth and development (Berk, 2006). Families are characterized by various features including membership (single or dual parent family, inclusion of extended family members, siblings, and pets), size, ethnicity, socioeconomic status, traditions, and lifestyle preferences. Diverse combinations of beliefs, resources, and interests contribute to the nature of each family. Consistent with its culture, the family system shapes the child's ideological system and provides opportunities to develop interpersonal relationships (Parke, 2004; Seligman & Darling, 2007). As a social system, patterns of connectedness, relationships, and interdependence are essential to the family's function. Subsystems within families—parent–parent, parent–child, parent–sibling, and family–extended family—add to the dynamics and complexities of the family unit (Figure 5.1). Change introduced into one subsystem influences other subsystems and the system as a whole. As discussed previously, the relationships and opportunities within the family are significant influences on the child's development (see the discussion earlier in this section).

Although the entry-level therapist should have a strong knowledge base related to occupational therapy, he or she may not have as much information about family operations and interactions. It is beyond the scope of this text to cover in-depth material related to working with families; however, the issues that follow are important whenever any frame of reference is applied in the context of the family. Occupational therapists need to learn about the ways in which each family functions and appreciate the normal

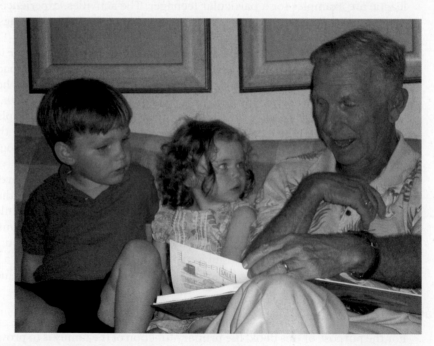

FIGURE 5.1 A grandfather reading to his grandchildren.

conflicts that are inherent in child rearing. To work effectively with families, therapists need to understand that the parenting process is not always a positive experience. While in a well-functioning family, the needs of all family members are recognized and supported, conflict naturally occurs even in the most capable families. In addition to understanding family dynamics, the therapist has to recognize the potential influence that he or she may have on the family. To provide the most effective intervention, the therapist must work together with family members, being careful not to impose his or her values or concerns onto the family.

Working with families requires that therapists acquire specific knowledge and skills for effective communication and interpersonal relations. Families value reciprocal communication with their children's healthcare providers (Chambers & Childress, 2005; Hanna & Rodger, 2002). When asked, many place a high priority on receiving information and making informed decisions about options that are available (Nolan, Orlando, & Liptak, 2007). To be responsive, the therapist must approach the family as a partner in this endeavor. Each family has its own needs and concerns. Therapists need to take time to listen to parents' perspectives, interests, and priorities throughout all phases of the occupational therapy process. A family or caregiver's ability and willingness to contribute information may vary over the course of their involvement in programs and services that support their child's development. They should have multiple opportunities to communicate with the professionals who are involved in their child's life. These interactions should be nonjudgmental to meet the needs of all participants. Through a relationship based on mutual trust, issues related to the child and family are discussed openly. This collaboration can provide the therapist with a clear perspective of the real-life demands faced by the family and child, and help the therapist learn about how the child's special needs impact on the family and their ability to nurture and support their child.

Effective occupational therapy intervention requires that the therapist be sensitive to the child's unique environment, including family and culture. When a therapist conducts an evaluation or plans intervention without regard to the important people in the child's environment, the evaluation is incomplete and subsequent intervention recommendations may not be appropriate. It is vital that the child's culture and family be considered in the application of any frame of reference (Figure 5.2). The human environment is not specifically mentioned in the theoretical bases of all frames of reference. For example, the Neuro-Developmental Treatment frame of reference does not address family issues. Nonetheless, it is important for the therapist to consider this domain when completing an evaluation, designing, and implementing a comprehensive intervention plan, and therapists who use the Neuro-Developmental Treatment frame of reference usually consider family support and education when implementing intervention. They recognize that their interventions will be less effective if they cannot be reinforced on a frequent basis during the family's routine activity. Some frames of reference include the family and the human environment as aspects of their theoretical bases. These frames of reference go so far as to involve family members or caregivers directly or indicate their influence in the application to practice. Examples of this are found in the frame of reference to enhance childhood occupation: SCOPE-IT and the frame of reference to enhance social participation.

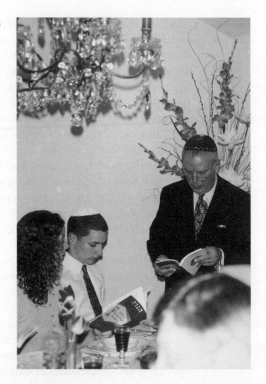

FIGURE 5.2 Observance of a cultural tradition within a family.

When providing ongoing occupational therapy services to a child, the therapist is usually in contact with the parents, although the extent of this interaction generally is determined by the setting and service delivery model. In any situation, opportunities that are available for interaction can also be affected by the willingness of the therapist and parent or teacher to collaborate. An occupational therapist should make an effort to develop open and sustained communication with the adults who are the child's primary caregivers, discussing goals and the types of interventions that may be implemented and responding to questions that arise. For example, in school system practice, while the teacher is often the therapist's primary contact on a day-to-day basis, therapists make efforts to reach out to parents through phone, e-mail contact, written notes, or face-to-face meetings. Therapists solicit information from families and along with other team members. They provide families with regular progress monitoring reports about the child's participation in the curriculum. Parents are also included in discussions and decisions regarding any changes in their child's program.

Therapists need to be aware of how some families see the position of authority that is implied by the role of therapist, and they must be careful not to abuse that power. As the center of concern for the child, the family has the real power in the therapist–family relationship. Family members can facilitate or sabotage the intervention process. Therapists have to be concerned with the expectations and responsibilities that they impose on families. Depending on the frame of reference chosen, therapists must be realistic about the role that the family plays in the intervention process. Furthermore, they need to recognize that family members are not experts in the use of the profession's legitimate tools.

An occupational therapist must be willing to accept that he or she does not have all the answers and seek more information from family members or other resources when needed. Intervention plans may require an adjustment or change in the frame of reference to meet a family's goals. When interventions do not work, the therapist must examine several areas. Reasons for failure may be the choice of the frame of reference, the cultural influence that impacts on the demands of the particular intervention, unrealistic expectations by either the therapist or the family, or the "fit" between the personalities of the therapist and family members.

Many professionals are sometimes apprehensive about working directly with parents and other family members. Often, family issues are overwhelming. The therapist may not feel adequately prepared to deal with family reactions or may feel uncomfortable with a parent's distress, anger, or frustration. Ironically, parental feelings of elation over achievements may also be overwhelming to the therapist. Recognition of these feelings may make it easier for the therapist to understand this range of emotions and contribute to his or her ability to develop working relationships with families. Experience in working with families and sensitivity to the parenting process can also help.

SOCIAL PARADIGMS AND OCCUPATIONAL THERAPY PRACTICE

Occupational therapy professional training is influenced by social paradigms as they exist within the sponsoring educational institution. Coursework may be aligned with a perspective that is representative of any of the views discussed in this chapter and subsequent learning is assimilated with students' own personal values, beliefs, and ways of thinking. Clinical or field-based training further contributes to students' experience, understanding, and points of view. Entry-level therapists bring these influences into the practice setting, integrating their perspectives with those of the system (Table 5.2) as they apply the occupational therapy process to benefit consumers served. The consistency between the model that characterizes the setting, perspective of the therapist, and the chosen frame of reference is important and may contribute to the success of the intervention and the understanding of the occupational therapy process by family members, administrators, and other professionals in the program. In the following sections, the different practice approaches and types of interventions used by the therapists who are grounded in a curative, palliative, and ecological model are discussed.

Pediatric Occupational Therapy from a Curative Paradigm

Occupational therapists who practice in a curative medical model focus on the individual child. Environmental elements that may influence performance are not a primary target for consideration. Evaluation approaches and assessments emphasize child attributes—performance skills and the underlying cognitive, perceptual, sensory, and neuromuscular processes that contribute to observed behavior. Through the process, differences or deviations from typically developed capacities and functions are identified. Intervention is designed to change or correct dysfunction that has been identified through the evaluation. Although the therapist may not believe that he or she can "cure" the problem, the anticipation is that performance will be vastly improved by reducing pathology or dysfunction in the underlying components. Therapists using a medical curative model tend to select frames of reference based on neurophysiology and neuropsychology or on neuromotor and other theories explaining causal relationships between component parts within the human organism. These frames of reference stress the identification and remediation of pathology or dysfunction in any of the sensorimotor components that contribute to the child's task performance. The curative perspective and frames of reference that represent this view may be applied more successfully within settings that are medically oriented or in instances of acute problems or other conditions that are likely to be resolved (e.g., recovery following a broken arm or rehabilitation for a child with Guillain-Barré syndrome).

Along with other discipline-specific professionals, the occupational therapist is the "expert provider." Intervention that is indicated is delivered primarily through direct interaction with the child, either in a dyad between child and discipline-specific provider or in some instances, through a small group of several children that is led by the professional. To support programs that address this priority, usually space and equipment are needed for child-centered evaluation and intervention procedures. For example, a spacious environment with a supply of various sized positioning aids and an obstacle-free area for the therapist to use when handling the child in various movement planes is well suited for therapy based on the Neuro-Developmental Treatment frame of reference. Locations for curative model interventions are chosen solely with the intervention in mind because treatment does not focus on environmental circumstances related to the child's performance.

The agency that espouses this paradigm expects discipline-specific approaches from providers who represent distinct programs, with each generally maintaining an interest and expertise in a targeted domain of child function and behavior. In larger agencies, groups of therapists constitute the "therapy department." Separate physical therapy, occupational therapy and speech therapy divisions may be differentiated. The departmentalized arrangement provides the occupational therapist with direction and supervision concerning care. There is ample opportunity for therapists to interact and collaborate with others who "speak the same language" and share similar interests. An occupational therapist working with a child who poses a treatment challenge may involve another department colleague to review the case and treatment regimen so that additional or revised intervention strategies may be considered. This type of interaction may be facilitated by a department in-service structure reminiscent of "medical rounds" occurring in traditional hospital environments. The peer support provided through these exchanges is particularly valuable to an entry-level therapist. The collaborative opportunity is also rewarding for the therapist who enjoys a mentoring relationship with other colleagues. Conferences and continuing education events are frequently scheduled in-house for staff members' participation. As a result of these offerings, department members often acquire a similar knowledge base about interventions relevant to the population served by the agency.

This model is illustrated in a hospital's developmental clinic. Evaluations target specific domains of child performance and are completed independently by professionals, each in a specialized environment (e.g., the individual provider's office, examination or "testing" room). The occupational therapist focuses on the child's neurological, orthopedic, muscular, cognitive and sensory-perceptual systems, as well as performance skills and patterns that contribute to occupational performance. Each therapist identifies pathology and then develops a plan of care that reflects the profession's intervention approach to remediate the dysfunction. Selection of the frame of reference that guides the process is determined by the individual therapist and his or her perspective relative to the diagnosis. A team meeting, led by the physiatrist, provides an opportunity for all to report their findings and recommendations. The physiatrist develops prescriptive referrals for follow-up services, authorizing a specific plan of care to each discipline. Professionals representing the prescribed disciplines then implement their intervention, sharing progress reviews through summary reports that are sent to the physiatrist and copied for the child's central file.

Pediatric Occupational Therapy from a Palliative Paradigm

The child along with human and nonhuman features of his or her surrounding environments are significant contexts for the occupational therapist whose practice reflects the palliative perspective. The evaluation process includes procedures that assess the child's performance skills and patterns. Data gathering also focuses on learning about the priorities and concerns of the family or caretakers and other important adults, such as the classroom teacher. Knowing how they view the child's strengths and needs, and what they perceive as important and meaningful for the child to accomplish, are essential information that contributes to program planning. As the child is able to contribute, his or her perspectives are solicited as well. The need to collect this information requires that the therapist incorporate interview procedures and be skilled at asking relevant questions and facilitating dialogue and discussion. Evaluating performance in areas of occupation, understanding what the child wants and needs to do, and learning about the environments in which participation is expected are important concerns. The occupational therapist may evaluate the child's self-feeding skills once breakfast is served in the hospital unit, or by visiting and observing in the school cafeteria during the scheduled lunch period. When this type of contextual opportunity is not available, simulated environments (e.g., a room that has been renovated into a small apartment) may be available or may be temporarily constructed by the therapist to evaluate performance areas.

The occupational therapist and other evaluators may complete their own processes in isolation, each summarizing the findings in a separate written report. The evaluation may also be a combined responsibility of persons from different disciplines. As an example, the occupational, physical, and speech therapists may each evaluate different aspects of the child's performance, with perspectives from all three therapists integrated into one report. During a meeting, each professional presents his or her evaluation results for review and discussion by all team members. It is important to recognize that in this model of interdisciplinary function, intervention priorities and recommendations are not determined until the team members, including the family, meet together and reach consensus.

Palliative approaches focus on the client and his or her family as the unit of care (Perron & Schonwetter, 2001). Interventions may be directed toward the caregivers or teachers, offering support and specific strategies that they implement in their ongoing interactions with the child. Service may also be provided directly by the therapist to the child, either individually or in group situations. Because the environment is valued as a context that influences behavior, the settings, activities, and routines that represent the child's everyday experiences are a focus as well. The occupational therapist looks for and identifies opportunities already available in the child's environment that support participation and reinforces their benefit to others who are concerned with the child's development. The therapist also implements modification or change to address environmental variables that constrain participation.

Home and community visits to the settings in which children grow, learn, and develop may serve as the primary venue for service delivery. Elements of practice may also require that routine service settings occasionally be adjusted or temporarily replaced to provide the milieu that is designed for specific procedures (e.g., a specialized location may be required for the fabrication of hand splints and adapted grips on pen, pencil, scissors, rulers, and other tools to support function in the child with whose current motor skills limit participation in classroom tasks).

Therapists choose various frames of reference that emphasize operational theories, such as the biomechanical frame of reference for positioning children for functioning. Intervention strategies may include developmental, remedial, and compensatory approaches. Methods that are compatible with the child's everyday context and can be embedded into available routines are preferred over the use of unusual, contrived, or separate strategies. As a result, multiple opportunities become available to enable the child throughout his or her everyday experiences. For example, with the aid of a slant board placed on a particular student's desk, he is able to hold his pencil and write for the duration of each classroom lesson period, affording him increased opportunities to practice penmanship skills. When therapist-implemented activity is indicated, consideration is given to how the involvement occurs so that it fits within the naturally occurring context. When specialized procedures that do not integrate into the routines and activities in the child's usual settings are required, they are provided in separate locations.

Programs that support this model encourage interdisciplinary teamwork and collaboration across disciplines. Separate, discipline-specific offices may be located in close proximity or designated work spaces may include accommodations that are shared by multiple disciplines. Social workers or psychologists are often involved, working closely with families, therapists, and other personnel throughout the care process. The occupational therapist or any other team member may function in the role of case manager and assume responsibility for leading the team to complete the evaluation, and then develop and monitor the intervention plan. Providers weekly schedules may include regular periods reserved for phone contact or face-to-face meetings with families and other team members.

Pediatric Occupational Therapy from an Ecological Paradigm

Occupational therapy practice reflecting the ecological paradigm addresses the child, family, caregivers, and other persons who are important in his or her life, along with multiple variables in the environments surrounding the child. Relationships between the child and the circumstances and conditions in his or her natural environments are relevant and valued concerns for the therapist. This therapist learns about the human and nonhuman environmental variables which may support or limit a child's function and participation. Programming seeks to optimize relationships and interactions between the child and the adults who provide support, and between the child and peers. Further, improving relationships between the child and the activities he or she pursues, materials used, and the settings and situations experienced is a goal. The successful outcome of this program planning is the child's engagement in everyday routines that provide the most advantageous opportunities for learning. These enduring experiences are valued as significant contexts for a child's development.

Evaluation includes procedures that are contextualized within the typical activities that the child experiences, reflecting functional or curriculum-based assessment (Rubin & Laurent, 2004) and "authentic assessment" practices (Neisworth & Bagnato, 2004). Using these strategies, the therapist goes beyond identifying and quantifying a child's differences in relation to standards that represent accomplishments of same-aged peers. This assessment reveals what the child is currently able to do within a valued and relevant context, despite developmental challenges. Environmental scans and analyses of activities and materials contribute information about the surroundings in which the child's participation is expected. Data about the relationships the child has with persons, activities, materials, and other environmental features is also gathered. Through interviews therapists learn about parent, caregiver, and teacher concerns. The occupational therapist needs to rely on strong interpersonal skills and be able to ask questions and listen to know about their perspectives and experiences. While this process may require additional time at the start, once completed, available data leads the team to plan appropriate and individualized interventions that are compatible within the typical types of situations in which children learn (Meisels, 2001).

Team cooperation is characteristic throughout service provision, beginning with the evaluation phase. More than one discipline may be represented by evaluators who are simultaneously present with caregivers to observe the child in settings and situations which he or she routinely experiences, such as the community-based child care center. Observation during a period of caregiver–child interaction, or group free-play may be combined with other interactions between child and evaluators. The evaluators work together with parents and other caregivers to review and discuss the child's participation and performance from different perspectives, and then identify the child's strengths and needs. Together they define relevant outcomes that are focused on enabling the child's participation in the routines and situations that are typical within the settings that are the child's early learning environments. The occupational therapist works closely with families and members of other disciplines to reach consensus regarding program priorities and an appropriate intervention plan. This may mean that a particular area of concern identified by the occupational therapist is not accepted by the team for immediate attention. For example, the developing self-dressing needs of a 3-year-old boy may be weighed with less urgency as the team plans and implements a cohesive approach to facilitate oral communication in the preschool classroom. Multiple areas of expertise may be combined into one summary report that documents evaluation findings and programming recommendations.

Frames of reference that emphasize person–environment interaction and relations are applicable in settings that reflect the ecological paradigm. Specific examples include the SCOPE-IT and the frame of reference to enhance social participation. These frames of reference involve aspects of the immediate and extended environments that are relevant for the child. Intervention is provided through functional activities that are already available, or readily incorporated into existing routines, integrating occupational therapy perspectives within the child's context. This affords multiple opportunities for the child's engagement, exploration, practice, and skill development. Because participation and development is influenced by family and important adults in the child's life—caregivers, teachers or other persons who regularly interact with the child, including his or her peers—intervention is designed to help them learn about ways they can positively influence the child's development through their interactions.

The occupational therapist identifies adaptations and modifications that promote the child's participation in the activities and situations that ordinarily exist and serve as natural learning opportunities. Strategies that are easily embedded into the everyday routines and experiences that are typical for the child are emphasized over the provision of separate, episodic procedures by therapists or others in contrived situations or specialized environments. This may mean that the therapist highlights and reinforces desirable strategies and approaches that already are present within the child's environment (such as specific visual cues provided by the classroom teacher to prepare a student for an upcoming transition to a new activity) so that their use continues. The therapist's intervention may include instruction or training to help classroom staff learn new strategies and prompts they can use to support and facilitate a student's participation throughout the customary school routines. For example, the specific presentation or placement of materials for the child in the classroom, use of modified tools, or altered sequences of activities may be recommended to the teacher and assistant in the classroom. When interventions need to be delivered by the occupational therapist, this option is generally implemented as a time-limited service (Ziviani & Muhlenhaupt, 2006). As the model emphasizes social contexts and relationships, activities may be structured for implementation in homogenous or heterogeneous groupings with other children.

Continued interest in including children with disabilities into all areas of community life has brought attention to the environmental discrepancies that exist for many children and families accessing new situations (Stewart & Law, 2003; Ziviani & Muhlenhaupt, 2006). An ecological perspective provides a framework that places relevance on those discrepancies and their relation to the child's participation in meaningful activities and as an influence on his or her development. Occupational therapists apply this approach in early intervention services with infants and toddlers and it is particularly suited to support inclusive education programs for students of all ages.

APPLYING FRAMES OF REFERENCE IN CONTEXT

Occupational therapists understand that context is so influential that it is impossible to interpret the child's behavior without understanding the unique contextual cues that support or limit his or her task performance (Dunn, 2007). When systems processes and influences are understood, an analysis can be made of the relationships between (1) a system's attributes, (2) a therapist's expertise and thinking approach, and, subsequently, (3) the ways in which an occupational therapy program may be designed and applied for a specific child. Then, therapists need to carefully select and apply frames of reference in practice. Throughout the occupational therapy process, therapists must consider the congruity between their own views along with those that characterize the settings in which their service is provided. They need to devise ways to incorporate the chosen frame of reference with the setting's social paradigm to provide interventions within the system's context. These considerations help the therapist to effectively integrate principles of occupational therapy evaluation, program planning, implementation, and outcome assessment for relevant and meaningful pediatric services.

FAMILY AND PROFESSIONAL RELATIONSHIPS IN THE CONTEXT OF HEALTH AND EDUCATION SYSTEMS

Children who receive occupational therapy services have contact with various other professionals who address their health and medical needs and who administer or implement programs to support their growth and development. As discussed earlier, these professionals have distinct beliefs, values, and attitudes. In addition, each brings a preconceived view of his or her own role, as well as the roles and responsibilities of other professionals involved. Consequently, despite a common interest in helping the child to grow, develop, and participate in relevant activities and environments, each lends a different viewpoint to the situation and his or her unique perspectives generate individual concerns and goals for the child. However, pediatric occupational therapists and other child developmental specialists can take advantage of various processes so that they do not operate in isolation. The occupational therapist needs to regard family, caretakers, and other professionals as equals on the team. A reciprocal relationship enables the therapist to learn about important perspectives that are particularly relevant within the occupational therapy process for children. The collaborative partnership between families and pediatric professionals is one of the foundations for effective services for children (Keen, 2007; Lynch & Hanson, 2004).

Multiple partnerships, communication, cooperation, and teamwork strategies are advocated among disciplines and across programs to support for the needs of families and their children. The Individuals with Disabilities Education Improvement Act (Federal Register, 2006) requires teamwork to plan and implement individualized programs that meet the unique educational needs of children with disabilities. Further, therapists working with children in either hospital or community-based programs identify benefits from various collaborative practices with members of other disciplines (Malone & McPherson, 2004). Interaction among professionals requires mutual respect and support as well as an understanding of different roles and goals (Giangreco, 2000; Hall, 2005; Rainforth, 2002). To achieve this rapport, professionals must communicate with each other and be willing to learn from one another. They must recognize and solve problems that arise when professionals from multiple disciplines interact and, ultimately, participate effectively in teams. Occupational therapists can draw from their educational background concerning psychosocial functioning to understand the workings of the team and become an important contributing member. Coursework related to facilitating the group process is also useful.

Many entry-level occupational therapists initially feel insecure about working as a full-fledged team member. It takes skills to collaborate effectively with other professionals. All occupational therapists in pediatric practice need to become confident in their own roles so that they participate successfully with other professionals who work with children. To do so, they must understand their profession, the structure of pediatric frames of reference, and how they may fit within different systems that serve the needs of children. Then, they need to carefully select and apply frames of reference in practice and teach other team members about occupational therapy perspectives. With experience, sensitivity, and self-examination of their own interactions, they rapidly acquire the skills needed to be an effective team member.

The following issues are important points to consider when using any frame of reference in the context of a professional team:

- Team members include the family and as appropriate, the child, and all have equal status and should work toward facilitating positive change for the child and his or her family.
- Occupational therapists should be concerned about whether they are speaking the same language as other team members. Each frame of reference has its own jargon, which should be translated for mutual understanding by all who participate in the team, including family members and the child, as appropriate.
- Any one team member can sabotage team function and, therefore, negatively affect the intervention process.
- Occupational therapists cannot see themselves as being all things to all children. They need to understand the important contributions that can be made by other professionals and discuss these openly with other team members.
- Occupational therapists must be aware of the strengths and limitations of their profession and accept that they do not have all the answers. They must be willing to examine their plans and adjust or even make a change in the frame of reference, and modify their interventions to meet unified team goals for the child and his or her family.

Once interventions are implemented, occupational therapists need to ensure that the child's performance is assessed. If the desired change in targeted behavior is not evident, therapists must ask questions. Is the planned intervention being used? Does the child have enough opportunities to participate in the intervention? Is the intensity of the intervention sufficient? Various issues need to be explored without looking for blame. This requires communication with other team members and may require a review of the specific intervention. Additional collaboration may be required to redefine the team's approach or another frame of reference may be used by the occupational therapist. Therapists should keep in mind that the overriding concern is how best to meet the needs of the child and his or her family.

 ## Summary

The influences and attributes that distinguish healthcare or education systems, along with several agency-centered and community-focused variables (from inside and outside of the agency) contribute to how an individual agency structures its programs and delivers services to families and their children. Ultimately, this mix has implications for all phases of the occupational therapy process—from initial referral, throughout evaluation, to the selection of an appropriate frame of reference, program implementation, progress monitoring, discharge planning, and discontinuation of services. To continue to meet the needs of consumers and offer relevant and valued service in ever-changing healthcare and education systems, occupational therapists need to continually think about how they apply the profession's values, beliefs, standards, practices, and research base in their provision of services.

Occupational therapy services are also influenced by human interpretation of values, beliefs, and needs. To that extent, intervention becomes subjective because feelings color the definition of these systems. Collaboration among occupational therapists, family members, and other professionals is essential to provide the most appropriate support for children and families in any service system. The occupational therapist must be aware, however, that although the therapist's perspectives and expertise are important, the values and beliefs of the child and his or her family take precedence. A collaborative relationship is one in which a foundation of cooperation is established to support effective working relationships, family concerns are a priority, issues are discussed openly, and decisions are made mutually.

REFERENCES

(2007). *American Heritage® College Dictionary of the English Language* (4th ed.). Boston, MA: Houghton Mifflin Company.

American Occupational Therapy Association (2002). Occupational therapy practice framework: Domain and process. *American Journal of Occupational Therapy, 56*, 609–639.

American Occupational Therapy Association. (2004). Occupational therapy's commitment to nondiscrimination and inclusion. *American Journal of Occupational Therapy, 58*, 668.

Barry, B. (2002). Trends and issues in serving culturally diverse families of children with disabilities. *Journal of Special Education, 36*(3), 131–138.

Bayona, C., McDougall, J., Tucker, M., & Nichols, M. (2006). School-based occupational therapy for children with fine motor difficulties: Evaluating functional outcomes and fidelity of services. *Physical and Occupational Therapy in Pediatrics, 26*(3), 89–110.

Beghetto, R. (2003). *Scientifically Based Research. ERIC Digest 167—April 2003.* http://eric.uoregon.edu/publications/digests/digest167.html. Retrieved October 31, 2007.

Berk, L. E. (2006). *Child Development* (7th ed.). Boston, MA: Allyn & Bacon.

Bertalanffy, L. (1968). *General System Theory: Foundations, Development, Applications*. New York: George Braziller.

Binks, J. A., Barden, W. S., Burke, T. A., & Young, N. L. (2007). What do we really know about the transition to adult-centered health care? A focus on cerebral palsy and spina bifida. *Archives of Physical Medicine and Rehabilitation, 88*(8), 1064–1073.

Blundo, R. (2001). Learning strengths-based practice: Challenging out personal and professional frames. *Families in Society: The Journal of Contemporary Human Services, 82*, 296–304.

Bower, L. (1961). The occupational therapist's role with mentally retarded children. *American Journal of Occupational Therapy, 15*, 61–62.

Bronfenbrenner, U. (2005a). The bioecological theory of human development. In U. Bronfenbrenner (Ed). *Making Human Beings Human: Bioecological Perspectives on Human Development* (pp. 3–15). Thousand Oaks, CA: Sage Publications Inc.

Bronfenbrenner, U. (2005b). Ecological systems theory. In U. Bronfenbrenner (Ed). *Making Human Beings Human: Bioecological Perspectives on Human Development* (pp. 106–173). Thousand Oaks, CA: Sage Publications Inc.

Bronfenbrenner, U., & Morris, P. (2006). The bioecological model of human development. In W. Damon, & R. Lerner (Eds). *Handbook of Child Psychology, Vol. 1: Models of Human Development* (6th ed., pp. 793–828). Hoboken, NJ: John Wiley and Sons.

Browning, D., & Solomon, M. (2005). The initiative for pediatric palliative care: An interdisciplinary educational approach for healthcare professionals. *Journal of Pediatric Nursing, 20*, 326–324.

Callister, L. (2005). What has the literature taught us about culturally competent care of women and children. *MCN, American Journal of Maternal Child Nursing, 30*, 380–388.

Campbell, P., Bellamy, G., & Bishop, K. (1988). Statewide intervention systems: An overview of the new federal program for infants and toddlers with handicaps. *The Journal of Special Education, 22*, 25–40.

Capra, F. (1996). *The Web of Life: A New Scientific Understanding of Living Systems*. New York: Double-day.

Case-Smith, J., Richardson, P., & Schultz-Krohn, W. (2005). An overview of occupational therapy for children. In J. Case-Smith (Ed). *Occupational therapy for children* (5th ed., pp. 2–31). St. Louis, MO: Mosby.

Chambers, C., & Childress, A. (2005). Fostering family-professional collaboration through person-centered IEP meetings: The "true directions" model. *Young Exceptional Children, 8*, 20–28.

Chen, C., Heinemann, A., Bode, R., & Granger, C. (2004). Impact of pediatric rehabilitation services on children's functional outcomes. *American Journal of Occupational Therapy, 58*(1), 44–53.

Clay, D. (2007). Culturally competent interventions in schools for children with physical health problems. *Psychology in the Schools, 44*(4), 389–396.

Committee on Hospital Care. (2003). Family-centered care and the pediatrician's role. *Pediatrics, 112*, 691–696.

Council for Exceptional Children. (2003). Appendix 4. CEC professional policies. In. *What Every Special Educator Must Know: Ethics, Standards and Guidelines for Special Educators* (pp. 151–196). Arlington, VA: Council for Exceptional Children.

Curzon, W. (1962). Training of mentally handicapped children in day training centres. *Developmental Medicine and Child Neurology, 4*, 537–542.

Dunn, W. (2007). Ecology of human performance model. In S. Dunbar (Ed). *Occupational Therapy Models for Intervention with Children and Families* (pp. 127–155). Thorofare, NJ: Slack Inc.

Erhardt, R. (1971). The occupational therapist as a school consultant for perceptual-motor programming. *American Journal of Occupational Therapy, 25*, 411–414.

Erwin, E., & Brown, F. (2003). From theory to practice: A contextual framework for understanding self-determination in early childhood environments. *Infants and Young Children, 16*(1), 77–87.

Fadiman, A. (1997). *The Spirit Catches You and Then You Fall Down*. New York: Farrar, Struas and Giroux.

Federal Register. (1977). *The Education for all Handicapped Children Act of 1975*, P.L. 94–142, Vol. 42, No. 163, August 23, 1977.

Federal Register. (1986). *The Education for all Handicapped Children Act Amendments of 1986*, P.L. 99–457, #20, USC § 1401, October 8, 1986.

Federal Register. (2006). *The Individuals with Disabilities Education Improvement Act of 2004*, P.L. 108-446, Vol. 71, No. 156, August 14, 2006.

Fox, E. (1997). Predominance of the curative model of medical care. *Journal of the American Medical Association, 278*(9), 761–763.

Giangreco, M. (2000). Related services research for students with low-incidence disabilities: Implications for speech-language pathologists in inclusive classrooms. *Language, Speech and Hearing Services in the Schools, 31*(3), 230–239.

Gleve, G. M. (1954). Occupational therapy in children's hospitals and pediatric services. In H. Willard, & C. Spackman (Eds). *Willard and Spackman's Occupational Therapy* (2nd ed., pp. 138–167). Philadelphia, PA: JB Lippincott Co.

Hall, P. (2005). Interprofessional teamwork: Professional cultures as barriers. *Journal of Interprofessional Care, 19*(Suppl 1), 188–196.

Hanft, B. (1988). The changing environment of early intervention services: Implications for practice. *American Journal of Occupational Therapy, 42*, 724–731.

Hanna, K., & Rodger, S. (2002). Towards family-centred practice in paediatric occupational therapy: A review of the literature on parent-therapist collaboration. *Australian Occupational Therapy Journal, 49*, 14–24.

Hanson, M. (2004). Ethics, cultural, and language diversity in service settings. In E. Lynch, & M. Hanson (Eds). *Developing Cross-Cultural Competence: A Guide for Working with Children and Their Families* (pp. 3–118). Baltimore, MD: Paul H. Brookes Publishing Co.

Keen, D. (2007). Parents, families, and partnerships: Issues and considerations. *International Journal of Disability, Development and Education, 54*(3), 339–349.

Kientz, J., Haynes, G., Westeyn, T., & Starner, T. (2007). Pervasive computing and autism: Assisting caregivers of children with special needs. *Pervasive Computing, 6*, 28–35.

Law, M. (2002). Participation in the occupations of everyday life. *American Journal of Occupational Therapy, 56*, 640–649.

Law, M. (2007). *Evidence-Based Rehabilitation* (2nd ed.). Thorofare, NJ: Slack Inc.

Law, M., Petrenschik, T., Ziviani, J., & King, G. (2006). Participation of children in school and community. In S. Rodger, & J. Ziviani (Eds). *Occupational Therapy with Children: Understanding Children's Occupations and Enabling Participation* (pp. 67–90). London: Blackwell Science.

Lee, C., & Miller, L. (2003). Evidence-based practice forum: The process of evidence-based clinical decision-making in occupational therapy. *American Journal of Occupational Therapy, 57*, 473–477.

Lynch, E. (2004). Developing cross-cultural competence. In E. Lynch, & M. Hanson (Eds). *Developing Cross-Cultural Competence: A Guide for Working with Children and Their Families* (pp. 41–75). Baltimore, MD: Paul H. Brookes Publishing Co.

Lynch, E., & Hanson, M. (2004). Steps in the right direction: implications for service providers. In E. Lynch, & M. Hanson (Eds). *Developing Cross-Cultural Competence: A Guide for Working with Children and Their Families* (pp. 449–466). Baltimore, MD: Paul H. Brookes Publishing Co.

Malone, M., & McPherson, J. (2004). Community and hospital-based early intervention team members' attitudes and perceptions about teamwork. *International Journal of Disability, Development and Education, 51*(1), 99–116.

Mandell, D., & Novak, M. (2005). The role of culture in families' treatment decisions for children with autism spectrum disorders. *Mental Retardation and Developmental Disabilities Research Reviews, 11*(2), 110–115.

Martin, J. (2007). Community conversations with parents to improve perinatal care. *Zero to Three, 27*(5), 30–38.

McCallin, A. (2001). Interdisciplinary practice—a matter of teamwork: An integrated literature review. *Journal of Clinical Nursing, 10*(4), 419–428.

McPhatter, A., & Ganaway, T. (2003). Beyond the rhetoric: Strategies for implementing culturally effective practice with children, families, and communities. *Child Welfare, 82*(2), 103–124.

Meier, D., & Beresford, L. (2007). Pediatric palliative care offers opportunities for collaboration. *Journal of Palliative Medicine, 10*(2), 284–289.

Meisels, S. (2001). Fusing assessment and intervention: Changing parents' and provider's views of young children. *Zero to Three, 21*(4), 4–10.

Michaud, F., Salter, T., Duquette, A., & Laplante, J. (2007). Perspectives on mobile robots as tools for child development and pediatric rehabilitation. *Assistive Technology, 19*(1), 21–36.

(2006). *Mosby's Dictionary of Medicine, Nursing and Health Professions* (7th ed.). St. Louis, MO: Mosby, Elsevier Science.

Mutha, S., & Karliner, L. (2006). Improving cultural competence: Organizational strategies for clinical care. *Journal of Clinical Outcomes Management, 13*(1), 47–51.

Neisworth, J., & Bagnato, S. (2004). The mismeasure of young children: The authentic assessment alternative. *Infants and Young Children, 17*, 198–212.

NCLB. No Child Left Behind Act of 2001, Public Law 107-110, 115 Stat. 1425. (2002). Retrieved October 31, 2007 from http://www.ed.gov/policy/elsec/leg/esea02/index.html.

Nolan, K., Orlando, M., & Liptak, G. (2007). Care coordination services for children with special health care needs: Are we family-centered yet? *Families, Systems and Health, 25*(3), 293–306.

Oliver, M. (2004). If I had a hammer: the social model in action. In J. Swain, S. French, C. Barnes, & C. Thomas (Eds). *Disabling barriers—enabling environments* (2nd ed., pp. 7–12). Thousand Oaks, CA: Sage Publications Inc.

Parke, R. (2004). Development in the family. *Annual Review of Psychology, 55*, 365–399.

Perron, V., & Schonwetter, R. (2001). Hospice and palliative care programs. *Primary Care: Clinics in Office Practice, 28*(2), 427–440.

Poulsen, A., Rodger, S., & Ziviani, J. (2006). Understanding children's motivation from a self-determination theoretical perspective: Implications for practice. *Australian Occupational Therapy Journal, 53*, 78–86.

Rainforth, B. (2002). Perspectives. The primary therapist model: Addressing challenges to practice in special education. *Physical and Occupational Therapy in Pediatrics, 22*(2), 29–51.

Reid, D., Chiu, T., Sinclair, G., & Wehrmann, S. (2006). Outcomes of an occupational therapy school-based consultation service for students with fine motor difficulties. *Canadian Journal of Occupational Therapy, 73*(4), 215–224.

Rose, D., & Meyer, A. (2002). *Teaching Every Student in the Digital Age: Universal Design for Learning.* Alexandria, VA: Association for Supervision & Curriculum Development.

Rosenbaum, P., & Stewart, D. (2007). Perspectives on transitions: Rethinking services for children and youth with developmental disabilities. *Archives of Physical Medicine and Rehabilitation, 88*(8), 1080–1082.

Rubin, E., & Laurent, A. (2004). Implementing a curriculum-based assessment to prioritize learning objectives in Asperger syndrome and high-functioning autism. *Topics in Language Disorders, 24*, 298–315.

Sackett, D., Straus, S., Richardson, W., & Rosenberg, W. (2000). *Evidence-Based Medicine: How to Practice and Teach EBM* (2nd ed.). New York: Churchill Livingstone.

Schauer, C., Everett, A., del Vecchio, P., & Anderson, L. (2007). Promoting the value and practice of shared decision-making in mental health care. *Journal of Psychiatric Rehabilitation, 31*(1), 54–61.

Seligman, M., & Darling, R. B. (2007). *Ordinary Families, Special Children: A Systems Approach to Childhood Disability* (3rd ed.). New York: Guilford Press.

Shapiro, J. P. (1993). *No Pity.* New York: Random House.

Simpson, R. (2005). Smart wheelchairs: A literature review. *Journal of Rehabilitation Research and Development, 42*, 423–436.

Smith, P. (2007). Have we made any progress? Including students with intellectual disabilities in regular education classrooms. *Intellectual and Developmental Disabilities, 45*(5), 297–309.

Stark, S., Hollingsworth, H., Morgan, K., & Gray, D. (2007). Development of a measure of receptivity of the physical environment. *Disability and Rehabilitation, 29*(2), 123–137.

Stewart, P., & Law, M. (2003). The environment: paradigms and practice in health, occupational therapy, and inquiry. In L. Letts, P. Rigby, & D. Stewart (Eds). *Using Environments to Enable Occupational Performance* (pp. 3–115). Thorofare, NJ: Slack Inc.

Swartout, G., & Swartout, R. (1954). Pediatric occupational therapy—a reappraisal. *Journal of Pediatrics, 44*(1), 112–115.

TASH. (2000a). *Resolution on Life in the Community.* Washington, DC.

TASH. (2000b). *Resolution on Quality Inclusive Education.* Washington, DC.

Tickle-Degnen, L. (2000). Gathering current research evidence to enhance clinical reasoning. *American Journal of Occupational Therapy, 54*, 102–105.

Turnbull, R., & Turnbull, A. (1978). *Free Appropriate Public Education: Law and Implementation.* Denver, CO: Love Publishing.

US Bureau of the Census. (2000). *Profile of General Demographic Characteristics: 2000.* Retrieved December 31, 2007 from http://censtats.census.gov/data/US/01000.pdf.

Villa, R., & Thousand, J. (2002). Inclusion: welcoming, valuing, and supporting the diverse learning needs of all students in shared general education environments. In W. Cohen, L. Nadel, & M. Madnick (Eds). *Down Syndrome: Visions for the 21st Century* (pp. 339–356). New York: Wiley-Liss.

World Health Organization (WHO). (2001). *International Classification of Functioning, Disability and Health*. Geneva: WHO.

Ziviani, J., & Muhlenhaupt, M. (2006). Student participation in the classroom. In S. Rodger, & J. Ziviani (Eds). *Occupational Therapy with Children: Understanding Children's Occupations and Enabling Participation* (pp. 241–260). London: Blackwell Science.

Ziviani, J., & Rodger, S. (2006). Environmental influences on children's participation. In S. Rodger, & J. Ziviani (Eds). *Occupational Therapy with Children: Understanding Children's Occupations and Enabling Participation* (pp. 41–66). London: Blackwell Science.

PART II

Frames of Reference

CHAPTER 6

A Frame of Reference for Sensory Integration

ROSEANN C. SCHAAF • SARAH A. SCHOEN • SUSANNE SMITH ROLEY • SHELLY J. LANE • JANE KOOMAR • TERESA A. MAY-BENSON

OVERVIEW

The sensory integration frame of reference was developed by A. Jean Ayres (Ayres, 1972a, 1979, 1989), an occupational therapist with postdoctoral training in education psychology and neuroscience. Ayres developed the theory of sensory integration to explain behaviors she observed in children with learning problems—behaviors that were not adequately explained by existing perceptual motor theories. The theory of sensory integration postulates that adequate processing and integration of sensory information is an important foundation for adaptive behavior. This idea is illustrated in Figure 6.1—the senses, integration of their inputs, and their end products (Ayres, 2005).

In this model Ayres shows how the interactions between the sensory systems—the auditory, vestibular, proprioceptive, tactile, and visual systems—provide integrated information that contributes to increasingly complex behaviors or "end products" and learning. For example, the vestibular and proprioceptive systems contribute to the ability to develop adequate posture, balance, muscle tone, gravitational security, and movement of the eyes in coordination with head and body movements. These, in turn, interact with the tactile system to provide an important foundation for adequate body awareness, coordination of the two sides of the body, and praxis. Together these sensory motor skills form the foundation for eye–hand coordination, visual perceptual skills, and engagement in purposefully activity. In combination with the auditory system, the sensory systems contribute to speech and language development and provide an important foundation for behaviors needed for learning such as maintaining an appropriate level of activity and emotional stability as well as the ability to concentrate or organize behavior for paying attention in the classroom. Although this frame of reference has been updated and expanded upon as the theory of sensory integration has evolved, the basic premise that the sensory systems and the integration of their inputs are important contributors to learning and behavior remains the key postulates in the theory of sensory integration.

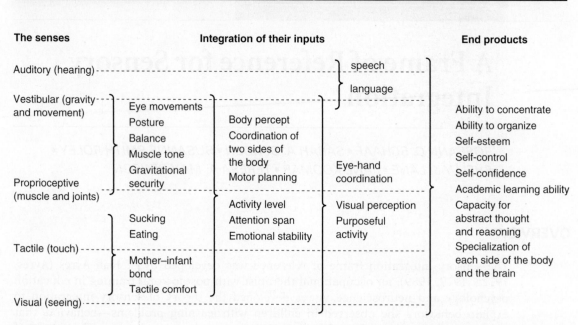

Sensory integrative processes

The senses	Integration of their inputs	End products

FIGURE 6.1 From Sensory Integration and the Child: Understanding Hidden Sensory Challenges. Copyright © 2005 by Western Psychological Services. (Reprinted by permission of the publisher, Western Psychological Services, 12031 Wilshire Boulevard, Los Angeles, California, 90025, USA [www.wpspublish.com]). Not to be reprinted in whole or in part for any additional purpose without the expressed, written permission of the publisher. All rights reserved.

THEORETICAL BASE

The theory of sensory integration combines concepts from human development, neuroscience, psychology, and occupational therapy into a holistic framework for viewing behavior and learning. Ayres defined sensory integration as "The neurological process that organizes sensations from one's body and from the environment and makes it possible to use the body effectively in the environment" (Ayres, 1989, p. 22). Ayres appreciated the multifaceted nature of the sensory integrative process and regarded it as a brain behavior process (Figure 6.2). Accordingly, there are seven basic theoretical postulates that form the foundation for the sensory integration frame of reference.

1. Sensory information provides an important foundation for learning and behavior (Figure 6.3).
2. Sensory integration is a developmental process.
3. Successful integration and organization of sensory information results in and is further developed by adaptive responses.
4. The "just right challenge" provides the milieu for sensory integration to occur.

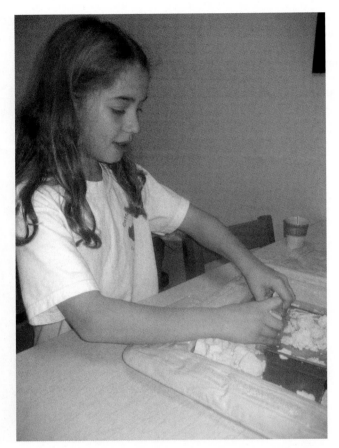

FIGURE 6.2   Children learn through exploration with their senses.

5. Children have an innate drive to seek meaningful experiences from their environment.
6. As a result of neuroplasticity, enriched experiences effect change in the nervous system.
7. Sensory integration is a foundation for physical and social engagement and participation in daily life activities and routines.

Each theoretical postulate will be elaborated on in the subsequent paragraphs.

Sensory Information Provides an Important Foundation for Learning and Behavior

The unique contribution of the sensory integration theory is its focus on the sensory systems as information sources. Sensory integration theory considers all of the sensory systems as important contributors to behavior and learning, but in particular emphasizes the "body-related" senses—tactile, vestibular, and proprioceptive sensations. According to the theory of sensory integration, these body-related senses provide the reference point relative to the environment, critical to all learning and behavior. For example, in order to move one's body effectively to accomplish a task, sensory

FIGURE 6.3 The sensory integration frame of reference focuses on the tactile, vestibular, and proprioceptive sensations to create "body maps" that are used to guide movement and motor planning.

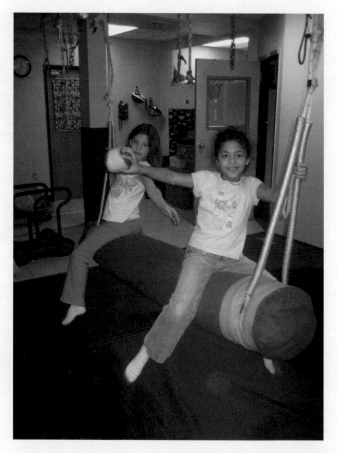

integration theory posits that the brain must receive and integrate proprioceptive, tactile, and vestibular information about the position and location of the body. Current sensory information is checked against the existing "body sensory map" developed from previous sensory and motor experiences to continually update the brain's knowledge about the body. This information is used to plan and execute movements. Knowledge and feedback from successful movement experiences provide increasingly complex perceptions and enhance the individual's ability to act and interact effectively in response to environmental demands. The senses, their receptor end points in the nervous system, and their posited contributions to development and learning are described in Table 6.1.

Sensory Integration is a Developmental Process

Sensory integration is based on an understanding that development unfolds in a sequence, and is influenced by the experiences one has during development (Ayres, 2005). Ayres states: "(the) environment acts upon the innate tendencies ... and molds and modifies them" (Ayres, 1972a, page 6). Nowhere is this more evident than during

TABLE 6.1 The Sensory Systems

Receptors	Sensation Detected	Features and Functions	Organization	Primary Central Projection	Cortical Projections	Links to Sensory Integration Theory
Somatosensory pathway: DCML						
Muscle spindle Golgi tendon organ Meissner's corpuscle Merkel receptor Pacinian corpuscle Ruffini ending Hair receptor	Proprioception, vibration Movement of touch on skin	Transmit information related to object/surface size, form, and texture Convey spatial and temporal aspects of touch Input is fast and direct	Precise somatotopic organization throughout Little convergence Few relays Processing of information takes place at each synapse	Ventral posterior lateral nucleus of thalamus Reticular formation	Primary and secondary somatic cortex Areas 5 and 7 of parietal lobe	Activity in anterolateral pathways can be decreased by simultaneous activation in low-threshold mechanoreceptors that feed DCML Projections from anterolateral pathways to reticular formation important for emotional and arousal aspects of touch
Somatosensory pathway: anterolateral (spinothalamic, spinoreticular, and spinomesencephalic)						
Free nerve endings	Pain, crude touch, temperature, tickle, neutral warmth, itch	Signal to CNS that body tissue is at risk of damage Transmission has both fast and slow aspects	Somatotopic, but less specific More convergence	Ventral posterior lateral, intralaminar, and medial nuclei of the thalamus Reticular formation Periaqueductal gray Tectum Hypothalamus	Primary and secondary somatosensory cortex Other thalamic nuclei	Projections from intralaminar thalamic nuclei are reflected broadly in cortex; also linked to behavioral arousal Integration of discriminative inputs leads to perception of self, and interpretation of tactile environment; lays foundation for praxis and organization of behavior
Somatosensory pathway: trigeminothalamic						
	Discriminative touch and proprioception from face and mouth Pain, temperature, and nondiscriminative touch		Somatotopic	Principal sensory nucleus of the trigeminal nerve Spinal nucleus of the trigeminal nerve Trigeminal nuclei project to ventral posterior medial nucleus of thalamus	Primary somatosensory cortex	

(continued)

TABLE 6.1 (Continued)

Receptors	Sensation Detected	Features and Functions	Organization	Primary Central Projection	Cortical Projections	Links to Sensory Integration Theory
Vestibular pathway: vestibular						
Hair cells in the utricial and saccule Hair cells in the semicircular canals	Linear and angular movement of the head	Position and movement of the head in space Maintenance of balance and equilibrium Coordination of the head and eyes; gaze stabilization during movement Detection of speed and direction of movement Maintain muscle tone	Otolith organs: hair cells oriented either toward or away from striola, within utricle (horizontal) and saccule (vertical); orientation results in ability to transmit information about linear movement in all directions Semicircular canals: hair cells embedded in cupula Hair cells in both structbreakures are tonically active; displacement either increases or decreases activity, information CNS of movement	Vestibular nuclei Cerebellum	Area 3a (region near face representation in SII), 2v of the cortex Posterior parietal (Area 5)	Vestibular nuclei are important integrative centers, receiving input from cerebellum, visual and somatosensory pathways, as well as ipsilateral and contralateral vestibular information Cortical region 3a also receives proprioceptive and visual information; linked to perception of body orientation in extra personal space Critical in maintenance of upright, antigravity posture Working with visual system, determines movement of self in space and detects movement of self vs. objects
Vestibular pathway: audition						
Hair cells in the organ of corti, within the cochlea	Sound detection and localization	Combination of different sound wave frequencies and intensities gives sound the qualities we recognize Response to sound is function of fact that basilar membrane is wider and more flexible at apex Perception requires simultaneous action of many cortical regions	Tonotopic Amplitude tuning curve	Ventral and dorsal cochlear nuclei Ventral nucleus bilateral projections to superior olive, onto to inferior colliculus Dorsal nucleus to inferior coliculus Multiple parallel pathways project from nuclei	MGN to auditory cortex	Superior colliculus projections role in for integration of visual and auditory information Sound interpretation results in auditory map of space and development of sense of location Interpretation of spoken words assists in understanding emotional meaning of communication Considered "higher level" sensory processing system within sensory integrative theory base; very complex cortical representation and interpretation

Vestibular pathway: visual

| Rods and cones in the retina | Cones: day vision, and color
Rods: night vision | Identify objects, position in space, movement through space, color, shape
Contrast and movement detection | Much integration within layers of retina
Receptors project to bipolar cells; these project to ganglion cells
Ganglion cells form optic tract
Cones: little convergence onto ganglion cells, resulting in high degree of spatial resolution; found primarily in central retina
Rods: significant convergence, high light sensitivity, low resolution; absent from central retina, found in periphery
Substantial interaction between receptor cells and other retinal cells prior to transmission to CNS
Detailed organization of information carried throughout this system (retinotopic) | Most ganglion cells project to the lateral geniculate nucleus of the thalamus; primary processing center and gateway to cortex
Optic tract fibers also project to hypothalamus, pretectum, superior colliculus | Primary visual cortex
Primary visual cortex projects to extrastriate regions, dorsal and ventral streams
Response to new visual stimuli
Lateral geniculate is primary processing center; receives streams of information
Lateral geniculate also receives input from reticular formation, thus regulating alertness and attention; this links modulates visual input | Dorsal stream: analyzes visual motion and responsible for visual control of action; navigation through space
Ventral stream involved with perception of visual world and object and face recognition (shape and color)
Hypothalamic projections have role in synchronizing biological rhythms (i.e., wake/sleep)
Tectal projections responsible for directing eye and head movements that bring image into central retina for optimal resolution; thus role in orienting eyes and head in Considered "higher level" sensory processing system within sensory integrative theory base; very complex cortical representation and interpretation and beyond |

CNS, central nervous system; DCML, dorsal column–medial lemniscal; MGN, medial geniculate nucleus.

early development as the infant first experiences touch from the caregiver and responds with a visual regard and a smile! These early sensory experiences and simple motor responses of the infant, combined with the caring and nurturing responses of the caregiver, result in a process of neuronal processing and integration that will lay the foundation for higher level sensory motor activity, emotional regulation, and social skills. Accordingly, therapy that utilizes a sensory integration frame of reference follows a developmental approach, starting at the child's current developmental level and then progressing to more complex, higher level actions and interactions.

Successful Integration and Organization of Sensory Information Results in and is Further Developed by Adaptive Responses

The individual's ability to make adaptive responses to constantly changing sensory environments is a pivotal consideration in the sensory integration frame of reference. Ayres (1972a) defined an adaptive response as an "appropriate action in which the individual responds successfully to some environmental demand" (p. 22). Ayres elaborated this concept calling it "organism-environmental interactions" (p. 22). She stated that the action of the environment upon the organism, and the reaction of that organism upon the environment, is the essence of a sensory integrative response (Ayres, 1972a). Therefore, when encountering a new situation, the individual draws upon previous understanding of one's abilities and competences and modifies them accordingly to organize new behavior and meet the current demand. Successfully meeting ongoing challenges, in other words, making these adaptive responses, provides increased motivation and skill to engage in further complex, challenging activities (Figure 6.4). For example, during play in a safe environment, a child discovers new ways to play with objects and people, and thus, exhibits adaptive responses. Subsequently, these adaptive responses create the foundation for further, more complex play actions and interactions. The sensory integrative process, therefore, facilitates successful responses to environmental demands resulting in adaptive responses. Further, increasingly complex adaptive responses are both an indicator of ongoing sensory integration and an outcome of sensory integration.

The "Just Right Challenge" Provides the Milieu for Sensory Integration to Occur

The term "just right challenge" refers to the activity that has the capacity to build new skills and abilities while adjusting for the current level of function of the child. Learning occurs when a child meets and successfully accomplishes a challenge. During intervention guided by sensory integration theory, the "just right challenge" is facilitated by the therapist and provides the milieu where learning occurs. Creating the "just right" sensory and motor challenges engages the child, and invites participation and success. Ongoing clinical reasoning allows the therapist to accurately assess the child's abilities and the environmental context; anticipate the child's needs, developmental level, and interests; grade the sensory and motor difficulty of the activity; and create the context that engenders motivation, spontaneous play, and successful performance. These concepts will be discussed in greater detail in the section "Application to Practice."

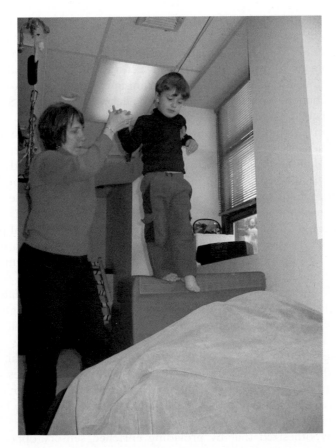

FIGURE 6.4 The therapist sets us an achievable challenge so the child is motivated to try activities that may be beyond the current skill level.

Children Have an Innate Drive to Seek Meaningful Experiences from Their Environment

Ayres believed that children have an innate drive to explore, interact with, and master their environments. Therapy based on the sensory integration frame of reference provides an environment whereby the child's innate/inherent motivation to participate and gain mastery is stimulated. By crafting intervention that provides the just right challenge, the therapist provides the context and affordances that ignite the child's desire, that is, "innate drive" to act and interact with the people and objects in the environment.

Sensory Integration Promotes Neuroplasticity

Neuroplasticity, defined as the nervous system's ability to change in response to environmental input and demands, is one of the key theoretical concepts of the sensory integration frame of reference. Ayres built her theory on research showing that the nervous system is shaped by environmental and sensory inputs (Ayres, 1979). New findings and knowledge demonstrate that the nervous system is even more plastic, complex, and integrated than Ayres and others believed at the time and thus, the principles on which the theory of sensory integration were built are still held in high regard in the scientific community (Jacobs & Schneider, 2001; Kraemer, 2001). More recent research on the mechanisms of neuroplasticity demonstrates that structural, molecular, and cellular changes in neural functions are possible, and that meaningful sensory motor activities are mediators of these changes (Greenough, Black, & Wallace, 1987; Kandel, Swartz, & Jessell, 1995; Kempermann & Gage, 1999; Merzenich et al., 1984).

The theory of sensory integration is built on this principle of neuroplasticity and proposes that optimal sensory experiences that invite action and active participation influence the growth and development of the nervous system and, subsequently, behavior. To act and interact in the world, the individual must filter and organize countless bits of information entering the brain and respond to the changing environment. Studies of environmental enrichment in both animals and humans support this concept and show that rich, meaningful sensory motor experiences promote neuronal processing. For example, classic studies of primates show that there is an increase in the cortical representation of fingers when they are provided enriched opportunities for manual tactile exploration (Jenkins et al., 1990 as cited in Kandel, Schwartz, & Jessell, 1995). Similarly, classic enriched environment studies, from the Greenough laboratory (Volkmar & Greenough, 1972; West & Greenough, 1972; Floeter & Greenough, 1979), show that enhanced sensory motor opportunities result in increased synaptic density and efficiency.

Contemporary research continues to validate these findings. Brown et al. (2003), for example, showed that rodents involved in active sensory motor activities such as running in a wheel cage demonstrate better ability to learn maze tasks. Further, changes in the hippocampus area of the brain in these same animals were potentially linked to this enhanced learning and memory.

Similarly, Ayres hypothesized that by providing enriched sensory opportunities processed at the level of the brain stem, and stimulating the child's motivation via the limbic system with the "just right" sensory and motor challenges, change will occur both neurologically as well as behaviorally as the child makes higher level adaptive responses and is more willing to tackle challenges in everyday life (Smith Roley, 2006).

Sensory Integration is a Foundation for Participation

Ayres (1979) believed that sensory integration provides an important foundation for engagement in meaningful, health-promoting activities that support participation in life. As such, occupational therapy using a sensory integration frame of reference is designed to improve sensory processing and integration as a basis for enhancing successful participation in daily occupations (Parham & Mailloux, 2001; Spitzer & Smith Roley, 2001). Sensory integration considers the dynamic interactions between the individual's abilities/disabilities and the environment as illustrated in Figure 6.5 (Spitzer & Smith Roley, 2001). This figure shows the interaction between sensory integration and occupation, illustrating how the basic processes of sensory modulation and sensory discrimination interact to support praxis, postural/ocular/oral control, and

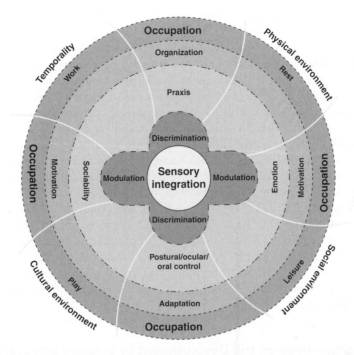

FIGURE 6.5 The dynamic process of sensory integration. The relationship of sensory integration to engagement in daily occupations can be likened to a rolling wheel. In this case, sensory integration is the hub. The spokes are sensory modulation, supporting practice skills and postural, ocular, and oral control. These spokes link to a rim of adaptation, motivation, and organization. The wheel supports the tire of occupations—work, play, leisure, and rest. This wheel spins in an occupational context of the physical, social, and cultural environment. The wheel (in its entirety and in its parts) and the environment are in constant interaction, exerting forces on each other. In the case of the sensory integrative wheel, the degree of flexibility and interaction with the occupational context may be much greater than that of a literal wheel rolling through physical space. (Reprinted by permission of the publisher, Smith Roley, S. Blanche, E. I., & Schaaf, R. C. [2001]. *Understanding the nature of sensory integration with diverse populations*. Austin, TX: PRO-ED, Inc.)

emotional and social development, which subsequently form the basis for organized behavior, motivation to act and interact in the environment, and adaptation to environmental demands. These, in turn, support occupational engagement in multiple areas such as work, play, leisure, and rest within the social, physical, and cultural contexts.

Sensory integration deficits disrupt the child's and family's ability to participate in daily routines such as mealtimes, grooming, bedtime routines, social activities such as family gatherings and shopping trips, and community activities such as school and organized sports. During self-care routines, slow, imprecise, and poorly regulated responses to sensations make dressing, eating, and grooming habits difficult for a child. For example, a child with tactile sensitivity will avoid manipulating things with his or her hands; a child with poor tactile discrimination is likely to have difficulty with manipulative hand skills needed for grooming (e.g., difficulty negotiating fasteners on clothing, difficulty grading the amount of muscle activity needed to squeeze a tube of toothpaste, or difficulty using utensils to eat neatly). While participating at school, children with sensory integrative dysfunction may be distracted by the intensity and multiple types of sensory stimuli in areas such as the classroom, playground, and lunchroom and have trouble paying attention and participating appropriately with the other children. The child with poor somatosensory feedback in the hands may have difficulty with handwriting, whereas the child with poor vestibular-mediated postural control will have difficulty maintaining a seated posture. In addition, social participation, which involves navigation of a vastly complex world of sensory and motor demands, is often difficult for children with sensory integration problems. Children who have difficulty perceiving, tolerating, and integrating sensations also have difficulty negotiating the unpredictable and changing stimuli associated with social activities (Smith Roley, 2006). These children tend to fall out of step with their peers and demonstrate inappropriate or immature behavior. Participation issues are discussed in more detail in the section entitled "Outcomes of Adequate Sensory Integration."

Historical Perspectives on the Development of Sensory Integration Theory

Ayres' work originally focused on children and adults with autism and developmental and neuromotor delays, and in the 1970s established a new role for occupational therapists in the treatment of children with learning disabilities. By the 1970s, Ayres created a series of standardized assessments and structured clinical observations, designed innovative therapeutic equipment, and conducted numerous research studies to validate her theories and interventions.

Beginning in the 1960s, Ayres created a series of assessments designed to evaluate sensory and motor processes including tactile perception and discrimination, visual perception, motor planning, vestibular processing, and bilateral motor skills culminating in the *Southern California Sensory Integration Tests* (SCSIT), a series of 17 norm-referenced standardized tests designed to identify sensory integration dysfunction (Ayres, 1972b). The use of standardized measures that identified deficits, patterns of dysfunction identified through factor analyses and the way in which it guided intervention, marked significant advances in evidence-based practice for occupational therapy. Ayres revised the SCSIT and published the new series of 17 tests as the *Sensory Integration and Praxis Tests* (SIPT, Ayres, 1989). These new tests, while maintaining a focus on the tactile, vestibular, visual, and proprioceptive systems, bilateral motor coordination, and visual motor skills, expanded the measures of praxis.

Ayres' intervention differed from interventions of her day in that prior interventions were adult directed and prescribed therapeutic activities designed to ameliorate a motor problem. In contrast, Ayres' sensory integrative approach offered a specially constructed and malleable therapeutic environment in which the child physically participated in activities with the therapist in the context of play. These activities were designed to provide vestibular, tactile, and proprioceptive opportunities that were fun, satisfying, and led to increased problem-solving abilities and motor skills.

Patterns of Sensory Integration Dysfunction

Ayres conducted numerous factor analyses using the SCSIT and later the SIPT that validated sensory integration theory (Ayres, 1972c, 1977, 1989). These factors identified patterns of sensory integrative disorders that are heterogeneous and involve multisensory systems (Parham & Mailloux, 2005). Although the factors differ slightly in various analyses, there is consistency across research findings that include difficulties with sensory modulation, sensory discrimination and perception, vestibular processing, and dyspraxia (Parham & Mailloux, 2005). Several factor analyses showed high factor loadings between tactile defensiveness and hyperactivity and distractibility (Ayres, 1972c), and thus Ayres (1979) defined "tactile defensiveness" as "a tendency to react negatively and emotionally to touch sensations" (pg. 107).

Ayres conducted one cluster analysis that identified four dysfunctional groups: low-average bilateral integration and sequencing deficits, visual and somatodyspraxia, dyspraxia on verbal command, and generalized sensory integrative dysfunction; and two typical groups, low-average and high-average sensory integration and praxis (Ayres, 1989). Mulligan (1998) conducted a confirmatory cluster analysis that revealed patterns consistent with the findings of Ayres. A recent cluster analysis by May-Benson (2005) supported the patterns identified by Ayres and Mulligan and also suggested an additional subgroup of children with praxis problems who demonstrate difficulties with ideation.

Ayres' factor studies were criticized as a result of the small sample sizes and the varying number of tests administered (Cummins, 1991; Hoehn & Baumeister, 1994). Subsequently, Mulligan (1998) conducted a confirmatory factor analysis using 10,000 SIPT data sets to examine the constructs proposed by Ayres. Mulligan's (1998) results suggested a four-factor model: visual perceptual deficit, bilateral integration and sequencing deficit, dyspraxia, and somatosensory processing deficit. Each of these factors was highly correlated in a factor called "generalized sensory integrative dysfunction" (Mulligan, 1998) and later, "sensory integration dysfunction" (Ayres, 2003).

Ayres identified unusual responsiveness in other sensory systems such as gravitational insecurity (a fear response to movement against gravity), auditory hypersensitivity, and visual distractibility (Ayres, 2005). In earlier works, Ayres noted that children with autism often exhibited behaviors that suggested poor modulation of sensory information and began to formulate a new subtype of sensory integrative dysfunction that involved dysfunction in sensory modulation (Ayres, 1979; Ayres & Tickle, 1980). Specifically, Ayres' early work identified two types of problems with sensory modulation—a dysfunction in sensory registration (sometimes referred to as "under-responsiveness") and sensory over-responsiveness. This factor was elaborated on and expanded in the 1990s by Royeen and Lane (1991), Dunn (1999a), and Miller et al. (2007) and is described in further detail in the subsequent text.

In summary, Ayres' work and that of her colleagues resulted in the identification of types of sensory integration deficits that were based on (1) factor and cluster analyses using data from the SCSIT and later the SIPT, (2) intelligence quotient (IQ) and other assessment data, and (3) clinical observations of behaviors associated with sensory processing problems. These include the following:

1. Sensory modulation dysfunction is an atypical response (over-responsiveness, under-responsiveness, or excessive seeking or avoiding) to sensory experiences or situations.
2. Somatodyspraxia includes poor ability to plan and execute novel motor actions associated with signs of poor perception of touch and poor body scheme/body awareness (Ayres, 1972b, 1985, 1989, 2005).
3. Bilateral integration and sequencing deficit is defined as poor ability to coordinate both sides of the body and atypical postural and ocular mechanisms associated with signs of inefficient processing and perception of movement and body position (Ayres, 1972b, 1985, 1989, 2005).
4. Somatosensory processing deficits are poor discrimination of tactile and proprioceptive information.
5. Vestibular processing deficit includes poor awareness and tolerance of gravity and movement through space.
6. Visuodyspraxia includes poor visual perception and visual motor integration.[1]

The function–dysfunction continua associated with each of these cluster groups are described in detail in the section entitled "Function–Dysfunction Continua for the Sensory Integration Frame of Reference."

KEY SENSORY INTEGRATIVE ABILITIES

The abilities supported by sensory integration are consistent with the patterns of function and dysfunction identified through research. They include sensory modulation, sensory discrimination (primarily tactile, vestibular, and proprioceptive as well as auditory, visual, taste, and smell), postural-ocular control, praxis, and bilateral integration and sequencing.

Sensory Modulation

The ability to modulate sensation contributes to the capability to sustain engagement despite variability in the intensity of sensations from the body or environment, and contributes to emotional stability, behavior, arousal, activity level, and attention. *Sensory modulation* refers to an individual's ability to respond adaptively to sensation over a broad range of intensity and duration (Lane, 2002; Smith Roley, 2006). Sensory modulation provides the foundation to perform adaptively in day-to-day occupations. Adequate sensory modulation supports the ability to maintain an optimal level of arousal, attention, and activity to meet the demands and expectations of the environment and task; it requires grading one's response to the degree, nature, or intensity of the sensory information (Miller et al., 2007) (Figure 6.6).

---

[1]This group is related to the form and space perception cluster Ayres identified in her early studies.

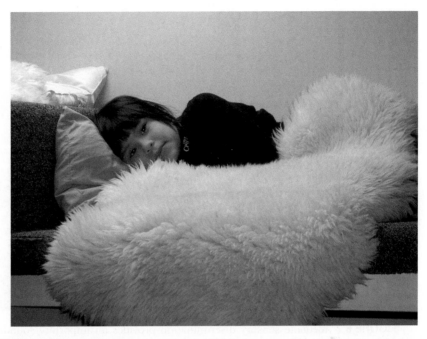

FIGURE 6.6 Children with adequate sensory modulation are able to tolerate various sensations offered in the environment.

Sensory Discrimination

Sensory discrimination refers to the individual's ability to interpret and differentiate between the spatial and temporal qualities of sensory information—or the "where is it," "what is it," and "when did it occur" response. The ability to discriminate sensory information allows the development of perceptions of events and self in action and contributes to skill development, learning, social interactions, and play that especially involves fine, discrete responses such as object manipulation. Each sensory system has discriminative functions that contribute to the individual's knowledge of sensory input and preparation for a response. *Somatosensory discrimination* refers to the ability to discriminate touch and proprioceptive stimuli. Tactile discrimination provides information about the spatial and temporal qualities of the environment by perceiving the qualities of information from skin receptors. *Proprioceptive discrimination* provides an understanding of the body's (muscles, joints, and tendons) position and the load or tension on muscles and joints. Together tactile and proprioceptive information provide important information that helps the child develop a "body awareness" or "body scheme," which in turn provides the foundation for efficient motor planning (praxis) (Figure 6.7). *Discrimination of vestibular* stimuli allows the individual to know where the head is in relation to the rest of the body and in relation to the environment at large by providing information about the position of the head relative to gravity, and the speed and direction of body movements. Vestibular discrimination works with somatosensory discrimination and

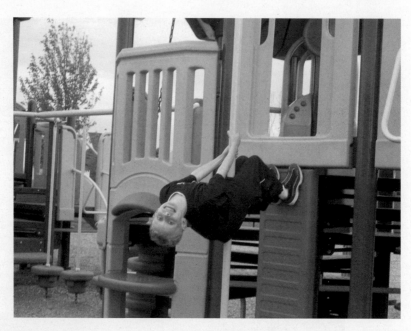

FIGURE 6.7 Adequate sensory discrimination provides an important foundation for successful actions in the environment.

contributes to postural control, balance, and equilibrium. *Discrimination of visual stimuli* provides the foundation for being able to visually discern the position and location of objects. There are many kinds of visual discrimination such as visual figure ground perception, visual rotation, and visual motor abilities. Visual discrimination interfaces with vestibular, proprioceptive, and auditory information to coordinate eye and head movements and to provide a map of the three-dimensional world relative to the body's position in space. *Auditory discrimination* allows us to differentiate sounds used in speech so that we can detect the location of sounds and difference between a "p" and a "t" in such words as "sheep" versus "sheet." Auditory discrimination is essential for understanding spoken language, following directions, and learning to read or write.

Postural-Ocular Control

Postural-ocular control involves activating and coordinating muscles in response to the position of the body relative to gravity and sustaining functional positions during transitions and while moving. Postural responses are required for any action needed during physical engagement. Postural control emerges as the individual develops activation and coactivation of muscle groups that support movement. Postural control is dependent not only on adequate muscle tone, coactivation of muscles, and ability to activate muscle synergies but also on adequate ability to integrate sensory information from the vestibular, proprioceptive, visual, and tactile systems. These systems contribute to our ability to maintain upright and antigravity postures as well as to move efficiently through the environment. For example, antigravity postures such as prone extension and supine flexion develop to support the infant's ability to raise his or her head against gravity and initiate movement. These provide the basis for more complex postural mechanisms that allow the child to move in and out of a midline position and maintain balance and equilibrium. Balance and equilibrium are components of postural control that are modulated by the vestibular, proprioceptive, and visual systems. Daily activities require coordinating the position of the body relative to gravity by organizing not only upright postures but also the coordination of the two sides of the body. These repetitive daily actions that are part of postural-ocular control and bilateral integration and sequencing are reliant on accurate sensory information to be executed well. Once learned, these movements do not require praxis (Figure 6.8).

Praxis

Praxis is the ability to conceive of, plan, and organize a sequence of goal-directed motor actions. Praxis enables us to adapt and react quickly to novel environmental

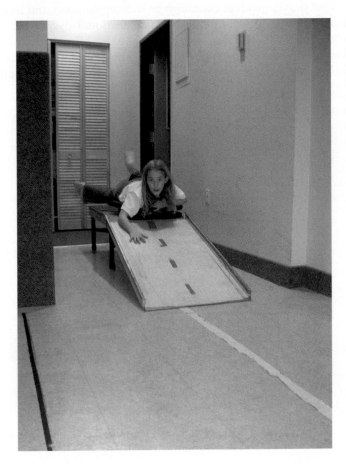

FIGURE 6.8 Adequate postural control provides an important foundation for movement. Here, prone extension posture is facilitated using a scooter board activity. The vestibular stimuli obtained while riding down the scooter further facilitates prone extension.

demands in a meaningful and efficient manner. When engaged in learning a new skill or problem solving a complex action or task, a great deal of praxis is required (once a skill is learned, less praxis is required). As day-to-day engagement in the physical world requires constant adaptations to novel situations and no action is ever performed exactly the same way twice, praxis is probably required to varying degrees in every action we make. Praxis is developed through meaningful and successful motor interactions with the world (Figure 6.9). Repetition of successful actions encodes the action in a motor engram or "neural map" in our nervous system. We draw upon this "library" of motor engrams when faced with novel situations to plan and organize a response. The more successful experiences we have, the more motor engrams are available for use to build new motor plans easily and effortlessly. Well-established engrams allow us to access feedforward processes for automatic and highly skillful actions. Feedforward refers to information from the senses that facilitate activation of the motor control system prior to use in an action. These motor engrams are therefore the building block of praxis, particularly motor planning, and contribute to formation of body scheme and body awareness.

Ayres (1985) felt that praxis involves cognition as well as planning and motor skills and, accordingly, labeled three aspects of dyspraxia: ideational dyspraxia, difficulty planning, and poor execution. What this means is that the term "praxis," as used in sensory integration, is not interchangeable with the phrase "motor planning." Motor planning, the bridge between ideation and execution, is that ability to organize and plan a

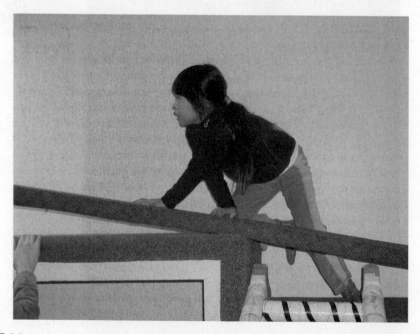

FIGURE 6.9 Praxis is developed through meaningful and successful motor interactions with the world.

motor action. It is related to and depends on the ability to sequence movements or tasks. Motor planning is believed to be largely dependent on tactile proprioceptive sensory inputs, although visual perceptual and visual spatial skills are also often associated with this area of function. Most often, problems in motor planning are reflected in difficulties in planning body movements. Daily life activities, such as dressing, bathing, or organizing one's books and papers for school, that should be automatic often take a great deal of attention and effort and still may not be done well when difficulties with motor planning exist. Visual perception and visual spatial skills interact intimately with motor planning abilities, and specialized problems in visual perceptual motor planning may be seen in completing two-dimensional and three-dimensional planning such as with constructional praxis (e.g., building with blocks) and visual motor praxis (e.g., drawing or writing). These specialized problems related to visual perception will be discussed separately in more detail below. Motor planning is only one aspect of praxis and the others will be discussed in the section "Sensory Integration: Current Updates."

Bilateral Integration and Sequencing

Bilateral integration and sequencing is the ability to use two parts of the body together for motor activities, and is another feature of praxis. Bilateral coordination and sequencing of actions is built on the immediate perception of the body's position or movement in space and the ability to use the two sides of the body together. These skills used in common daily activities such as clapping, riding a bike, or opening a container are dependent on adequate vestibular-proprioceptive processing. They also rely on lateralized sensory and motor skills including slightly faster and better hearing from the right ear (in right handers), right-left discrimination, crossing the body's midline, and establishment of hand preferences for tool use. Bilateral coordination skills serve as the foundation for the development of bimanual skills used in managing fasteners on clothes such as shoe tying and unilateral skills such as writing and throwing.

Related to bilateral integration and sequencing is postural control and bilateral coordination. Postural control forms the foundation for fluid, controlled movement and is essential when performing projected action sequences, that is, a sequence of motor acts put together to accomplish a goal in future time and space such as running to catch or kick a ball or coordinating the position and time to kick a soccer goal or make a basket.

SENSORY INTEGRATION: CURRENT UPDATES

Ayres indicated that the theory of sensory integration is constantly evolving and is informed and modified as new research is generated (Ayres, 1972a). Ayres, herself, advanced the theory on the basis of literature reviews and research and it continues to be refined primarily based on the work of occupational therapists and supporting evidence emerging in neuroscience and psychophysiology (Bundy, Lane, & Murray,

2002; Schneider, 2005; Smith Roley, Blanche, & Schaaf, 2001; Stein, 2007). The theory of sensory integration will continue to change shape and form, be affirmed or transformed, as new knowledge from basic and clinical sciences is added.

Current research refines the understanding of sensory integration function and dysfunction. The patterns identified through research fall into categories broadly classified as deficits in sensory modulation, sensory discrimination, postural, bilateral integration and sequencing, and dyspraxia (Bundy, Lane, & Murray, 2002; Miller et al., 2007). These categories are not mutually exclusive; for example, a modulation deficit may be seen with deficits of discrimination and/or praxis. Praxis deficits are typically seen in combination with deficits in sensory discrimination. Postural, bilateral integration, and sequencing problems are often seen in combination with vestibular-proprioceptive–based problems and, sometimes, somatodyspraxia. As new knowledge is generated, various researchers and theorists have suggested new ways of organizing the categories and subtypes of sensory integrative dysfunction. For example, Bundy, Lane, & Murray (2002) and Miller et al., (2007) propose revised versions of Ayres' original model of sensory integrative dysfunction as is discussed below.

Updates in Sensory Modulation

Ayres originally introduced tactile defensiveness as a disorder of sensory modulation, explaining it as an imbalance in protective versus discriminative functions (Ayres, 1965). Since that time Knickerbocker (1980), Royeen and Lane (1991), Dunn (1999b), and Miller et al. (2007) elaborated on Ayres' original conceptualization about sensory modulation.

Sensory modulation takes place as the central nervous system regulates the neural messages about sensory stimuli. It is defined as one's ability to respond adaptively to sensation over a broad range of intensity and duration (Lane, 2002; Smith Roley, 2006). When it works, sensory modulation contributes to adequate arousal level and attention and thus, facilitates engagement in day-to-day occupation. A disorder in sensory modulation is reflected in behavior that does not match the demands and expectations of the environment and task; it is the result of difficulty in grading of the behavioral response to the degree, nature, or intensity of the sensory information (Miller et al., 2007). Disorders of modulation can involve over-responsiveness or under-responsiveness to sensation from the internal or external environment; some investigators also define "sensory seeking" as a deficit in sensory modulation, different from over-responsiveness and under-responsiveness (Miller et al., 2007) and still others include sensory avoiding (Dunn, 1999b). Problems with modulation may occur in any sensory system, but are best documented in the tactile system (Ayres, 1972a, 1979; Bar-Shalita et al., 2005; Schneider, 2006). While deficits in modulation may occur in single sensory systems, they may also be seen in multiple systems simultaneously. Clinical observations suggest that an individual can be over-responsive in one sensory system while at the same time under-responsive in another. Further, it is possible that responsiveness within a sensory system can fluctuate, such that an individual can be over-responsive at one time point, and/or typically under-responsive at another time point.

Another type of sensory modulation dysfunction, gravitational insecurity, was originally identified by Ayres and later elaborated on by May-Benson & Koomar (2007).

These later investigators recently published a measure to assess gravitational insecurity in children. Preliminary data shows that even children with very mild gravitational insecurity were able to be discriminated from typical peers. Children with gravitational insecurity were found to be fearful when their feet were not touching the ground or were on a raised or unstable surface, when their head changed position out of upright, or when they moved unexpectedly through space (especially backwards). In addition, they found that gravitational security improves as the child ages (May-Benson & Koomar, 2007).

To evaluate sensory modulation, Dunn (1999a) created an assessment tool, The Sensory Profile, that allowed parents, caregivers, and teachers to rate a child's responses to sensory activities. Dunn also developed a model to describe the cluster groups that emerged from factor analysis of her data from the sensory profile (Dunn, 1999b). Dunn's work proposed that children with sensory modulation deficits not only demonstrate over-responsivity and/or under-responsivity to sensation but also display sensory behaviors in four characteristic patterns—sensory sensitivity, sensory avoiding, sensory registration, or sensory seeking. The child's behavioral presentation depends on whether he or she acts in accordance with the proposed sensory threshold or attempts to compensate for the threshold. Dunn's model of sensory modulation is illustrated in Figure 6.10. In this model, a child who has a low threshold for sensation may either show sensory sensitivity or sensory avoiding behaviors, whereas a child with a high threshold for sensation may show either low registration or sensory seeking behaviors.

Using data from physiological studies that examine autonomic nervous system activity during sensory stimuli, Miller et al. (2007) also developed a model of sensory modulation proposing that there are only three subtypes of sensory modulation dysfunction: over-responsivity, under-responsivity, and seeking/craving. Miller et al. (2007) outline their thinking in a proposed nosology of sensory processing disorders

	Sensory sensitivity	
	Low threshold	High threshold
Behavioral		
	Increased sensitivity	Decreased sensitivity
Behavioral response in accordance with sensitivity level	**Hyper responsive behaviors** (i.e., highly active and reactive)	**Hypo responsive behaviors** (i.e., lethargy, passivity) "Low registration"
Behavioral response to compensate for sensory sensitivity	**Sensory avoider**	**Sensory seeker**

FIGURE 6.10 Dunn's model of sensory processing. According to Dunn, children with problems in sensory modulation fall into four categories based on their sensitivity to sensation and their behavioral response to it. Reprinted by permission of the publisher. *Sensory Profile.* Copyright © 1999 by Harcourt Assessment, Inc. Reproduced with permission. All rights reserved.

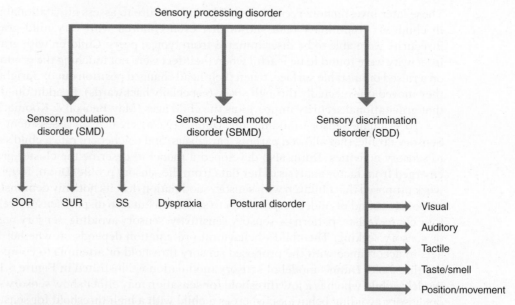

FIGURE 6.11 Proposed nosology of sensory processing disorders. Reprinted by permission of the publisher. *SOR*, sensory over-responsivity; *SUR*, sensory under-responsivity; *SS*, sensory seeking. (From Miller, L. J., Anzalone, M. E., Lane, S. J., Cermak, S. A., & Osten, E. T. [2007]. Concept evolution in sensory integration: A proposed nosology for diagnosis. *American Journal of Occupational Therapy, 61*[2], 135–140.)

as depicted in Figure 6.11. This group of investigators proposes that the term "sensory integration dysfunction" be renamed "sensory processing disorder" and that it include three disorders: sensory modulation disorder, sensory-based motor disorder, and sensory discrimination disorder. It should be noted that this nosology is under development and requires further research to validate the proposed subtypes, and thus, there is no consensus in the field. Within this nosology, Miller et al. (2007) defined the three subtypes of sensory modulation dysfunction as described below.

Sensory over-responsivity is defined as responses to sensation that are quicker in onset, and stronger in intensity than would be expected for most children that may be met behaviorally by withdrawal and avoidance of the sensation(s), or by more aggressive outbursts designed to allow escape from the sensation (Dunn, 1999b; Miller et al., 2007). *Sensory under-responsivity* is defined as a disregard or passive response to sensory stimuli; responses are less intense or slower in onset than those typically expected. The individual finds it difficult to get engaged, feels lethargic, and self-absorbed, and seems unaware of sensation, thus lacking an inner drive for exploration. Others describe children with under-responsivity as having sensory registration deficits in that they do not appear to register (notice/acknowledge) the sensation present in their environment (Smith Roley, 2006). *Sensory seeking/craving* is defined as an intense, insatiable desire for sensory input; available input appears to be less than what is needed for the individual to feel satiated; individuals energetically engage in actions geared to adding more intense sensation, constantly moving, touching, watching moving objects, and/or seeking loud sounds or unusual olfactory or gustatory experiences (Miller, James, & Schaaf, 2007). Miller provides some psychophysiological evidence to support her theoretical conceptualization of the sensory modulation subtype (McIntosh, Miller, & Hagerman, 1999; Miller, James, & Schaaf, 2007) that show children who are over-responsive demonstrate greater electrodermal activity (sympathetic nervous system activation of a "fight or flight response") during exposure to sensory stimuli than children who respond to sensation in a typical manner (McIntosh, Miller, & Hagerman, 1999).

To guide treatment of sensory modulation dysfunction, Miller et al. (2002) propose an ecological model of sensory modulation that includes external factors of culture, environment, relationships, and task that influence basic intrinsic emotions, sensory processing, and attention in children. Miller et al. (2002) suggest that children with sensory modulation dysfunction process stimuli differently than typically developing children and children with other clinical disorders such as fragile X syndrome or attention deficit with hyperactivity disorder, and she provides psychophysiological data to support her conceptualization (Miller et al., 2001). Miller's work has further elaborated on the subtype of sensory modulation; however, further research is needed to evaluate the nosology as it relates to the theoretical conceptualizations presented by Ayres (1972a) or Bundy, Lane, & Murray (2002). Nevertheless, as a result of the efforts of Miller et al., two diagnostic classification references now include children with sensory processing disorders: the Diagnostic Classification of Mental Health and Developmental Disorders of Infancy and Early Childhood, Revised (known at the "DC:0-3 R") (Zero to Three, 2005) and the Diagnostic Manual for Infancy and Early Childhood of the (Interdisciplinary Council on Developmental and Learning Disorders ICDL, 2005).

Updates on Sensory Discrimination

The discrimination of sensory information involves the ability to identify and interpret the qualities of the sensory experience. For example, somatosensory discrimination informs the individual about the size, weight, texture, location, and color. In contrast to simply registering (being aware of) and tolerating the information, as in sensory modulation, the sensory discrimination process occurs when the individual interprets the qualities of the experience, integrates them with past memories or associates them with past experiences, and formulates perceptions about the object, event, or person. The complexity of this discrimination process can be seen in the multiple aspects of even a single sensory system such as touch. Touch from a friend includes the pressure, texture, size, duration, location, and temperature. These various qualities are discriminated, integrated, and associated with previous experiences of touch from that friend as well as from other friends.

The sensory integration frame of reference focuses on sensory discrimination in the somatosensory system as relates to the development of body scheme and body awareness, and in the vestibular and proprioceptive systems as they contribute to postural-ocular control and timing and sequencing of body movements. Visual discrimination is also highlighted as discrimination of form, space, and contrast as it provides the foundation for the development of visual perceptual and visual motor skills. Integrating discrete sensory information forms a basis for understanding and interpreting environmental cues and using this information to act and interact with the environment, as originally proposed by Ayres (1972a) has been further validated in animal studies (Stein, 2007). For example, during the daily activity of brushing our teeth, oral tactile sensation is associated with all other sensory features of this experience: the position of the body relative to gravity; the force of the proprioceptors required to maintain stability and mobility patterns; the visual input from the immediate environment and spatial surround; the auditory information from ambient sounds and speech sounds; smells and tastes if appropriate, and whatever the state of the inside of the body, such as hungry or full, and the result is successful completion of the activity. In contrast to this ability to glean crucial information from the multisensory environment, the child with sensory discrimination deficits is unable to extract appropriate meaning from the sensory stimuli received. These children often demonstrate poor body awareness, poor visual perceptual skills, and difficulty with fine, coordinated movements that rely on sensory feedback from their muscles and joints for efficient execution.

Updates on Praxis

Adaptive interaction with the world requires the ability to accurately perceive sensations from the environment and to make an appropriate motor response. Within a sensory integration frame of reference, the ability to conceptualize, plan, and execute intentional and meaningful motor actions in response to these environmental demands is referred to as "praxis" (Ayres, 1985). Praxis is conceptualized as more than just motor coordination or motor movement. It is a neurocognitive process of identifying and planning out how to make an effective goal-directed motor response to a specific situation. Ayres (1979) stated that "Praxis is the ability of the brain to conceive of, organize, and carry out a sequence of unfamiliar actions" (p.183). Thus, as a process, praxis consists of several subprocesses or abilities including ideation (the ability to conceptualize and intentional motor action), motor planning (the ability to organize one's actions), sequencing (the ability to order one's actions in an appropriate way), execution (the ability to coordinate and produce a controlled, precise, and refined motor response), and feedback (the ability to perceive, recognize, and act on the results of one's actions).

The concept of "praxis" within sensory integration is unique as it specifies these subprocesses and conceptualizes the entire motor process from the initiation of an intention to act through adaptation of an action in response to feedback in the particular situation of making a meaningful adaptive response. In addition, the sensory integration frame of reference specifies that disorders in praxis have a sensory basis. Praxis requires sensory and motor memories of previous actions that can be retrieved when a new action plan is needed. Accurate sensory perceptions help the individual create an accurate plan of action (Figure 6.12).

Children who have praxis problems are often identified as having dyspraxia. They may appear clumsy or awkward in their movements and have difficulty playing with

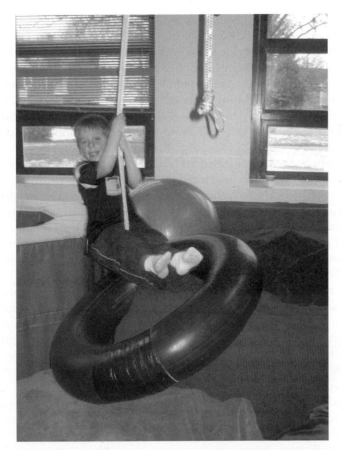

FIGURE 6.12 Praxis is a neurocognitive process of identifying and planning out how to make an effective goal-directed motor response to a specific situation.

toys or engaging in school and home daily living activities. Children with dyspraxia may have difficulty conceptualizing an idea for an activity, creating a plan for the activity, or generalizing or transferring learned motor plans to new situations. Children with dyspraxia frequently work much harder and exert more effort than typically developing children to learn a skill such as riding a bicycle or tying their shoes. Children with dyspraxia may not be that fluent in his or her movements and have difficulty with unexpected changes in situations that require a larger repertoire of potential solutions, such as overcoming an obstacle in the path or a difference in the grade of the riding surface. A child with dyspraxia may demonstrate a deficit in any or all of the various subcomponents of the praxis process (Ayres, 1972a, 1979, 1985).

To assist understanding of motor performance problems and to facilitate intervention, researchers have attempted to identify various subgroups of children with praxis problems. Ayres drew heavily on knowledge obtained from the adult apraxia literature when developing her theories about childhood developmental dyspraxia. Her initial cluster and factor analyses led her to identify two types of motor performance problems in children: somatodyspraxia (often referred to as "dyspraxia" or as "developmental dyspraxia") and vestibular-based bilateral coordination and sequencing deficits (Ayres, 1965, 1966, 1969, 1971). Somatodyspraxia has its foundation in somatosensory (e.g., primarily tactile but also proprioceptive) discrimination deficits, which interfere with the development of body scheme and body awareness. Somatodyspraxia was frequently found in conjunction with visual spatial deficits suggesting an important role of visual perception in praxis functioning. This subtype of dyspraxia is characterized by poor motor planning and difficulties learning and organizing motor actions. Specialized problems in oral-motor planning may also been seen, which may impact articulation or eating skills.

Bilateral integration and sequencing deficits have their foundation in poor vestibular-proprioceptive discrimination, which interferes with the ability to coordinate, sequence, and execute motor actions quickly and efficiently. Problems are found especially in those actions that require coordination of two parts of the body. Problems with timing and sequencing movement through space, such as throwing and catching a ball or running across a sports field may also be seen. In particular, postural-ocular problems, which also have their basis in poor vestibular-proprioceptive processing, are often seen in conjunction with bilateral integration and sequencing problems (Ayres, 1985).

At this time it is not clear whether bilateral integration and sequencing is an aspect of praxis or a separate type of sensory integrative dysfunction.[2] In an attempt to clarify this issue, Miller et al. (2007) suggested a category called "sensory-based motor disorders" with a subcategory of postural and ocular disorders (Figure 6.11). They noted that postural disorder, including poor stability in the trunk, poor righting and equilibrium reactions, poor trunk rotation, and poor oculomotor control, involves vestibular, proprioceptive, and visual motor problems. They suggested that postural and ocular disorders could be seen with or without dyspraxia. When seen as an aspect of dyspraxia, these investigators suggested that difficulty with bilateral integration and rhythmicity were observed.

While Ayres initially conceptualized these two problems as unique deficits, she later questioned whether they reflected different aspects of some unifying practic function (Ayres, Mailloux, & Wendler, 1987). More recent work by (Mulligan, 1996, 1998, 2000, 2002) and Lai et al. (1996) has supported this perspective and they suggested that there is an underlying construct of dyspraxia, which may subserve the various subgroups of children. It is possible that somatodyspraxia and bilateral integration and sequencing deficits reflect various aspects of practic functioning based on differing sensory inputs (e.g., tactile/somatosensory inputs vs. vestibular-proprioceptive inputs). Clinically, it is important to distinguish these. One way to distinguish them is to examine whether the praxis issues are related to problem-solving novel or non-habitual actions, or difficulties with bilateral coordination during learned repetitive

---

[2]While there is some evidence that bilateral integration and sequencing is a subtype of praxis (with praxis as a common underlying function with several subtypes of dysfunction, including somatodyspraxia or motor planning problems, ideational dyspraxia, and bilateral integration and sequencing deficits) rather than a separate subtype of sensory integrative dysfunction this issue is not clear at this time (May-Benson, *personal conversation*, January 3, 2008). Others feel that bilateral integration and sequencing is a separate subtype of sensory integrative dysfunction that often includes poor vestibular processing, postural, and bilateral integration difficulties, oftentimes in association with sequencing difficulties (Smith-Roley, *personal conversation*, January 3, 2008).

actions. Visuopraxis, constructional praxis, and praxis on verbal command may reflect additional aspects of practic behavior in response to visual and auditory inputs. Reeves and Cermak (2002) proposed that dyspraxia in children with sensory integration problems may be conceptualized as a unitary function with various levels or types of dysfunction. They identified two types of praxis problems, somatodyspraxia and bilateral integration and sequencing deficits, and suggested that somatodyspraxia reflects the more severe problem, a conclusion supported by a Rasche analysis of the SIPT subtests by Lai et al. (1996). They also recognized a generalized practic dysfunction in which the child demonstrates problems in both of the above-mentioned areas. More recently, May-Benson (2005) suggested a deficit in ideation that may fall somewhere between these two problems in terms of severity of motor dysfunction.

The relationship between motor performance and sensory systems, as proposed in the sensory integration frame of reference, has also been confirmed by researchers in other fields as well. For example, poor visual spatial skills have been associated with decreased motor performance (Rosblad, 2002). Poor kinesthetic skills (which are frequently referred to as "decreased proprioceptive processing") have been found to be related to poor motor performance (Dewey, 2002). Similarly, subgroups of children with poor balance (probably reflecting decreased vestibular processing) and decreased coordination (Conrad, Cermak, & Drake, 1983) have been identified. Other than work by Ayres et al., the relationship between motor performance and somatosensory/tactile function has not been examined. Like Ayres, however, in addition, to differences in performance on motor tasks, these researchers also found that children in their various subgroups frequently had differential performance on nonmotor academic, language, visual perceptual, and visual motor tasks. This suggests that the different subgroups of children may differ not only on motor performance but also on other aspects of performance. While research on children with motor performance problems outside of the sensory integration frame of reference has not demonstrated consistent subgroups of children, it is encouraging that similar groupings of motor performance problems emerge across disciplines (Dewey, 2002).

Within the sensory integration frame of reference, the most recent advancement in the understanding of praxis has been in the subcomponent of ideation. While this component of praxis has been discussed and deficits identified in the adult literature, this is an area of praxis that has not received much attention in the pediatric literature. Ayres (1985) originally specified that ideation involved conceptualizing a goal for an action and some idea of how to achieve that goal. Thus, in regard to the praxis process, an idea is not just the final goal, but some sense of the larger steps needed to achieve that goal. For instance, a child on a playground looks around and sees other children going down a slide, and then decides to go down the slide herself. However, since she is playing on the other side of the playground, she needs to develop some idea about the steps needed to achieve that goal—she must cross the playground to go over to the slide, climb the slide, and then go down the slide. The conceptualization of ideation was recently expanded on by May-Benson (2005), who presented a model for ideation. In this model, ideas for motor actions may originate from perception of objects in the environment or from previously performed and internalized motor schemas. The ability to recognize object and environmental affordances, the qualities or properties of an object which inform one about possible actions, (Gibson, 1979) was identified as a critical element in a child's ability to generate ideas for motor actions.

May-Benson & Cermak (2007) developed a standardized assessment of ideational abilities. Studies conducted using this assessment in conjunction with other measures of behavior/attention, motor performance, and language further illuminate our understanding of ideational problems in children with dyspraxia. May-Benson (2005) found that children with ideational problems do not have an absence of motor ideas, rather they have a paucity of ideas. For instance, when asked what they could do with common items, such as a length of cord or hula-a-hoop, they demonstrate a limited range and variety of motor ideas and actions. In addition, approximately one half of the children with dyspraxia examined demonstrated below average ideational abilities suggesting that decreased ideation is a more common practic problem than previously thought. Motor, behavioral/attention, and language characteristics of children with ideational deficits were further examined (May-Benson, 2005). She found that children with the worst ideational problems did not have the most severe motor planning problems, cognition, or language skills. Like Ayres' factor and cluster studies, May-Benson's (2005) cluster analysis of children with dyspraxia with and without ideational problems and typical peers found a subgroup that demonstrated generalized dysfunction, a subgroup with very poor motor planning/motor skills and adequate ideation, two typical groups, and a group with very poor ideation and moderate problems in motor planning/motor skills. She further found that the subgroup with the worst ideational abilities had above average IQ and language skills, which is contrary to popular belief that only cognitively impaired or the most motorically impaired children demonstrate ideational deficits.

In conclusion, "praxis" is the term used to describe difficulties with ideation, planning, and execution components of praxis. Bilateral integration and sequencing difficulties may also be viewed as a type of dyspraxia but more research is needed to determine if the sensory and motor disorders associated with this subtype of sensory integrative dysfunction are more like a dyspraxia or a separate dysfunction.

OUTCOMES OF ADEQUATE SENSORY INTEGRATION

The overall outcome of adequate sensory integration is successful participation in life activities in the home, school, community, and other environments, or to enhance successful participation in daily occupations. To achieve this outcome, the sensory integration frame of reference focuses on sensory motor areas that provide the foundation for successful participation including: (1) the ability to modulate, discriminate, and integrate sensory information from the body and from the environment; (2) self-regulation to regulate and maintain an arousal level, and/or an activity level needed to appropriately attend and focus on the task or activity; (3) maintaining postural control including muscle tone, strength and balance, ocular control, and bilateral coordination and laterality; (4) adequate praxis; (5) organizing behavior needed for developmentally appropriate tasks and activities; and, (6) development of self-esteem and self-efficacy. These outcomes build on each other and provide the foundation to support the child's participation in

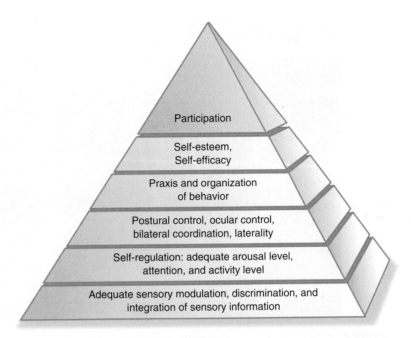

FIGURE 6.13 Outcomes of the sensory integrative process.

self-care, play, social activities, and academic tasks that are developmentally appropriate as exemplified in Figure 6.13.

Modulation, Discrimination, and Integration of Sensory Information

This is the most primary and basic aspect of the sensory integration process and involves the capacity to grade responses to sensory stimuli (sensory modulation) as appropriate for the situation at hand, discriminate the qualities of sensation (sensory discrimination), and give meaning to information from two or more senses simultaneously (sensory integration). These provide an important foundation for higher level behaviors as depicted in Figure 6.13.

Self-Regulation

Self-regulation is the ability to regulate and maintain an arousal level, activity level, and attention/focus as appropriate for the demands of the task or activity (Figure 6.14). It also includes the ability to modulate mood, self-calm, delay gratification, and tolerate transitions in activities (DeGangi, 2000). Self-regulation is a by-product of good sensory modulation, discrimination, and integration and is closely linked to arousal regulation, activity level, and attention. Self-regulation, in the sensory integration frame of reference, refers to the ability to achieve an appropriate arousal state needed for participation in everyday activities in response to sensory experiences (Schaaf & Smith Roley, 2006).

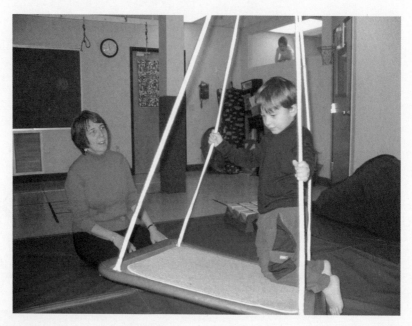

FIGURE 6.14 Self-regulation is the ability to achieve an appropriate arousal state needed for participation in everyday activities in response to sensory experiences.

Self-regulation is dependent on one's ability to modulate responses to sensory input and influences arousal regulation, mood, activity level, and attention or ability to focus. Arousal regulation reflects the functioning of the autonomic nervous system, which regulates the child's state of readiness to respond. Behaviorally it is characterized by the child's ability to respond in an appropriate manner to the intensity and duration of environmental stimuli. When over-responsivity, under-responsivity, or sensory seeking behaviors occur, there is greater likelihood of poor arousal regulation. For example, if the child is over-responsive he or she may shut down and therefore appear "under-aroused." Another over-responsive child may present with a heightened state of arousal to all experiences resulting from a basic fear of the threatening stimuli. Sensory seeking behaviors can also lead to overarousal as the stimuli the child may seek is not "organizing" but rather is "disorganizing" resulting in a difficulty to calm and focus on tasks and activities. Accordingly, adequate self-regulation and an optimal arousal level impact on activity level and ability to attend to activities needed for participation in daily life activities.

Postural Control and Bilateral Motor Coordination

Postural control and bilateral motor coordination includes the ability to utilize and maintain antigravity postures (prone extension, supine flexion, upright sitting, etc.); coordinate eye and head movements; use the two sides of the body together in a coordinated way; and develop unilateral dominance for skilled tasks. These foundational abilities reflect adequate vestibular and proprioceptive processing and provide the basis for higher level skills.

Praxis

Praxis is the ability to create, plan, and execute adaptive motor actions to meet the ongoing changes and challenges in the environment. It is dependent on adequate reception, discrimination, and integration of sensory information and the ability to regulate responses to these stimuli (self-regulation). Praxis allows us to plan and sequence actions that are essential for the effortless and automatic ability to participate in daily life tasks and activities. It is also an important component of sensory integrative process by generating an ongoing repertoire of learned actions that are available for dealing with unexpected changes in situations or the need for novel solutions. Thus, it provides a foundation for successful participation in daily occupations.

Praxis and the organization of behavior are outcomes of sensory integration that are closely related. The ability to create, plan, and execute adaptive motor actions, and to organize oneself in time and space to complete these acts is essential for the completion of complex daily tasks and participation in life activities. Praxis and organization of behavior depend on adequate reception, discrimination and integration of sensory information, and ability to regulate responses to these stimuli (self-regulation). Collectively, these abilities allow us to plan and sequence multiple temporal spatial interactions in the present and future and thus are important components of the sensory integrative process as they provide an important foundation for successful participation.

Organize Behavior Needed for Developmentally Appropriate Tasks and Activities

The ability to organize behavior relative to time and space is essential to the completion of complex and developmentally appropriate daily tasks and activities. Along with praxis, organization of behavior allows us to sequence multiple temporal spatial interactions in the present and future. This ability to organize motor actions is closely related to the ability to organize daily occupations.

Self-Esteem

Self-esteem refers to the child's self-concept and confidence. In psychology, self-esteem reflects a person's overall self-appraisal of his or her own worth. Self-esteem encompasses both beliefs (e.g., "I am competent/incompetent") and emotions (e.g., triumph/despair and pride/shame). Behavior may reflect self-esteem (e.g., assertiveness/timorousness and confidence/caution) and is often manifested by the child's willingness to take on new challenges and to feel good about his/her accomplishment of a task. Self-esteem can apply specifically to a particular dimension (e.g., "I am good at soccer and feel proud of my math homework") or to a global feeling (e.g., "I believe I am a good person and feel proud of myself in general"). Children with dysfunction in sensory integration are particularly vulnerable to problems in self-esteem as a result of repeated experiences of failure in daily life activities such as play, social participation, and academics. Even the ability to appropriately modulate reactions to sensory stimuli can impact on the children's development of self-esteem as they often incorporate the feedback they get from others about their behavior suggesting that they are "bad," "lazy," or "not good at anything."

Participation in Self-Care, Leisure, and Academic and Social Activities

Participation in self-care, leisure, and academic and social activities is the final outcome of the sensory integration process. Participation in these activities involves the ability to produce a suitable adaptive response to the dynamic and multiple demands of everyday life (environmental mastery). This environmental mastery depends on adequate modulation, discrimination, and integration of all sensory systems, the ability to regulate and modulate responses to sensory information, praxis, and the organization of one's behavior. Together they form the foundation for participation in the occupations of daily life. Among the key challenges for children with dysfunction in sensory integration include participation in play and school activities.

Play

Play is the occupation of children. Play requires interaction between the individual and the environment (Neumann, 1971). For play skills to develop, there needs to be an intrinsic motivation to play, the ability to share control with a play companion, and the ability to engage in fantasy and pretend. Like academic functioning, play is one of the broad-based occupational performance outcomes of sensory integration. It builds on the foundational components of sensory integration. Play requires ideation, planning, sequencing, and execution of motor actions as well as the ability to modulate, discriminate, and integrate sensory information (Figure 6.15).

Academic Skill

Academic skill refers to the child's ability to participate in the learning process and includes abilities such as maintaining attention/focus on school tasks, using appropriate motor skills and motor planning to execute the many tasks associated with school performance such as handwriting, maintaining appropriate sitting posture, or negotiating objects in one's desk. Accordingly, adequate academic skills are partly dependent on the foundational skills and abilities of the sensory integration process (Figure 6.16).

Social Participation

Social participation refers to the child's ability to engage and interact meaningfully with peers and family. It is unique to each child because social participation is intimately related to a family's culture, priorities, and community. Successful social participation can be described as a child's ability to conform to cultural norms in the contexts of daily life (Cohn & Miller, 2000). Social participation can range from being able to play successfully with a sibling or peer to being able to go to the grocery store, attend a family Thanksgiving celebration, or go to church regularly. Most important in achieving

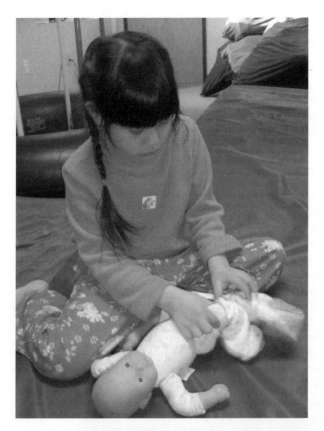

FIGURE 6.15 Play is an outcome of adequate sensory integration—it requires ideation, planning, sequencing, and execution of motor actions as well as the ability to modulate, discriminate, and integrate sensory information.

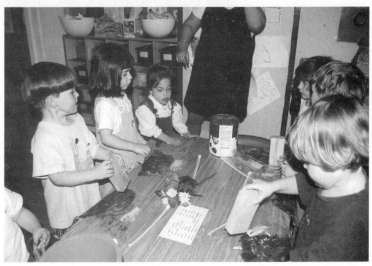

FIGURE 6.16 The foundational skills of sensory integration provides a basis for the learning behaviors needed for successful participation in academic activities.

appropriate social participation is the ability to self-regulate and to utilize praxis to create and enact plans for social participation.

Daily Occupations

Participation in daily occupations is the ultimate end product of sensory integration. It reflects the ability to perform all of the daily tasks and activities of childhood. Clearly these skills are age dependent. They reflect the child's ability to complete activities of daily living, to have successful relationships, to perform academic tasks, and to play with peers.

Populations for Whom This Frame of Reference is Used

The sensory integration frame of reference was originally applied to children and adults with developmental delays and behavior that were not accounted for by neuro-motor dysfunction (Ayres, 1986; Ayres & Tickle, 1980). In the 1970s, Ayres' research funding directed her to investigate children with learning disabilities who presented with sensory and motor challenges that were not attributed to damage in the central nervous system (Ayres, 1976), and it is still useful for these children currently. Although it was never intended to explain the neuromotor or cognitive disorders evident in populations with cerebral palsy or Down syndrome, commonly individuals with these and other disorders exhibit sensory integration deficits making this an important adjunct to other therapeutic interventions (Smith Roley, Blanche, & Schaaf, 2001; Schaaf & Smith Roley, 2006; Schaaf & Miller, 2005). The sensory integration frame of reference has been applied to various populations including infants born at risk and/or with regulatory disorders (DeGangi, 2000); children with autistic spectrum disorders (Parham & Mailloux, 2001; Mailloux & Smith Roley, 2001), fragile X syndrome (Hickman cited in Smith Roley, Blanche, & Schaaf, 2001), and attention deficit hyperactivity disorder (ADHD) (Ognibene, 2002; Yochman, Parush, & Ornoy, 2004); children with cerebral palsy and other motor disorders (Blanche, 2002; Blanche, Botticelli, & Hallway, 1995); children experiencing trauma and attachment disorders (May-Benson & Koomar, 2007); and children from environmentally deprived situations (Cermack, 2001).

In particular, children with autism spectrum disorders (ASDs), present with a significant prevalence (80% to 90%) of sensory processing problems (Kientz & Dunn, 1997; Tomcheck & Dunn, 2007; Rogers & Ozonoff, 2005). Poor sensory processing, especially sensory modulation dysfunction, is believed to contribute to the maladaptive behavioral profile of these children and impact on their ability to participate in social, school, and home activities (Anzalone & Williamson, 2000; Schaaf et al., 2002). Children with ASD often demonstrate extreme aversion to sensory stimuli; avoidance of noisy situations; and fearfulness of typical activities that involve touch, sounds, and movement. Alternatively they may display excessive seeking of sensory stimuli with unusual preoccupation with smells or visual stimuli and overengagement in activities that involve touch, sounds, or movement (Huebner, 2001; Kientz & Dunn, 1997; Mailloux, 2001; Mailloux & Smith Roley, 2001). Self-reports from individuals with ASD confirm these findings and are particularly potent in terms of describing the impact of sensory dysfunction on participation in daily life activities (Grandin, 1995; O'Neill & Jones, 1997; Parham & Mailloux,

1995; Williams, 1992). These descriptive self-reports portray how over-responsiveness, under-responsiveness, or intense seeking of the typical sensations of daily life pervade behavior and limit their ability to participate fully in society.

POSTULATES OF THE SENSORY INTEGRATION THEORETICAL BASE

The evolving theoretical base of sensory integration includes 10 basic postulates. Each postulate supports the theoretical base which states that it is critical that the therapist promotes growth and development toward the outcomes of the sensory integration process.

1. An optimal state of arousal is a prerequisite for adaptive responses to occur.
2. Sensory integration occurs during adaptive responses.
3. Multiple sensory systems may be needed to facilitate an optimal state of arousal.
4. Adaptive responses must be directed toward the child's current developmental level.
5. Activities that reflect the "just right challenge" produce growth and development.
6. Problems with sensory modulation, or in the foundational abilities, contribute to deficits in the end product abilities.
7. The child needs to be self-directed, with therapist guidance, for sensory integration to occur.
8. Adaptive responses are elicited through activities that facilitate sensory modulation, discrimination, and integration, resulting in improved postural control, praxis/bilateral integration, and participation.
9. Intervention is directed to underlying deficits in sensory modulation, discrimination and integration, and/or foundational abilities, and not toward training in specific skills or behaviors.
10. As the child achieves increasingly complex adaptive responses in therapy, changes will be evident in the outcome abilities such as self-regulation, self-esteem, social participation, academic performance, and participation in daily life routines and activities.

FUNCTION–DYSFUNCTION CONTINUA FOR THE SENSORY INTEGRATION FRAME OF REFERENCE

The theoretical base of a frame of reference delineates those problems with which the frame of reference is concerned. The skills and abilities outlined in the theoretical base serve as a guide for the therapist's evaluation during which a determination is made regarding whether the child is functional or dysfunctional relative to this frame of reference. The concepts outlined in the sensory integration frame of reference are defined so that the clinician can identify areas of performance that need to be assessed. Behaviors are examined within the context of the function–dysfunction continua to determine the need for intervention. A cluster of behaviors is necessary to be identified as requiring intervention using a sensory integrative approach.

The function–dysfunction continua included in this chapter are the culmination of Ayres' factor and cluster analyses (Ayres, 1972b, 1977, 1986) and Mulligan's (1998) cluster groups from her recent confirmatory factor analysis study. These include the following:

- Atypical responses (i.e., unusual over-, under-, or fluctuating responsivity) to the sensory aspect of materials, activities, or situations (sensory modulation disorder)
- Poor ability to conceptualize, plan, and execute motor actions associated with signs of poor perception of touch and body position (somatodyspraxia)
- Poor ability to coordinate both sides of the body, and atypical postural and ocular mechanisms associated with signs of inefficient processing and perception of movement and body position (bilateral integration and sequencing deficit)
- Poor visual perception and visual motor integration (constructional and visuodyspraxia)

Sensory Modulation Abilities

Sensory modulation describes the way in which an individual responds to sensory stimuli in the environment. When functional, sensory modulation means that an individual is able to respond in a manner, which is appropriate to the degree, nature, and intensity of the sensory information experienced. However, difficulty can be encountered when the individual does not respond appropriately to the incoming stimuli and is unable to adapt the response to every changing circumstance in daily life. Proposed are three subtypes of sensory modulation disorder: over-responsivity, under-responsivity, and sensory seeking (Miller et al., 2007; Miller, James, & Schaaf et al., 2007).

Sensory Over-Responsivity

Sensory over-responsivity is characterized by an excessive or exaggerated response to sensory stimuli that are not perceived as threatening, harmful, or noxious by typically developing children (Table 6.2). This term subsumes sensory defensiveness, gravitational insecurity, and aversive responses to input. The fight, flight, or freeze reactions manifested by individuals who are over-responsive can produce anxiety, hyperactivity, and inattention. Over-responsivity can occur in one sensory system (i.e., tactile defensiveness) or in multiple sensory systems.

For children with sensory over-responsivity standing on-line may be problematic because of the "threat" of being touched from behind. Other areas that may be problematic are entering a crowded room because of the possibility of being bumped by others or by being overwhelmed by noise. Additionally, meeting others in a social situation where a hug is expected may be problematic if someone else is initiating the hug. Generally over-responsiveness is most evident when someone else is in control of the sensation. Because unknown environments present unknown sensory challenges, transition to a new environment may be particularly stressful and may be met with strong behavioral reactions. Further, there may be a cumulative effect of sensation, such that a very strong reaction may be observed to be seemingly innocuous sensation simply because of the "buildup" of sensation throughout the day.

TABLE 6.2 **Indicators of Function and Dysfunction in Sensory Modulation: Sensory Over-Responsivity**

Typical Responsivity	*Sensory Over-Responsivity*
FUNCTION: Typical response to sensory stimuli	*DYSFUNCTION*: Excessive or exaggerated response to sensory stimuli
Indicators of Function	**Indicators of Dysfunction**

Touch
    Comforted by touch
    Explores all types of play materials with hands
    Wears all types of textured clothing
    Participates willingly in daily living activities with tactile components
	Bothered by tactile aspects of daily living activities
	Bothered by specific types of clothing
	Bothered by specific textured materials

Auditory
    Not bothered by sounds that occur in daily activities
    Attends gatherings of all sizes
    Participates in community social activities
	Distressed by environmental noises (vacuum cleaner, blender, siren, and toilet flush)
	Avoids gatherings such as birthday parties, malls, parades, restaurants, and church services

Visual
    Comfortable in lighted areas
    Enjoys a variety of colors and patterns
	Bothered by brightly colored or patterned materials
	Bothered by visually cluttered environments

Proprioception
    Comfortable with activities that require graded force and coordinated use of muscles
    Freely engages in sustained muscle activation or traction to joints
	Avoids climbing activities
	Dislikes hanging from jungle gym

Vestibular
    Enjoys movement in all planes of space and in various directions (up/down, back/forth, and rotary)
    Engages in climbing in activities
	Avoids playground swings, slides, or jungle gym
	Avoids climbing activities

Smell Not bothered by typical daily smells across environments	Bothered by food smells as well as smell of household or hygiene products Avoids some environments because of smells

Taste
    Eats a variety of textured foods
    Enjoys a range of spicy to bland foods
	Avoids lumpy, slimy, or soft foods
	Avoids spicy or salty foods
	Avoids mixed consistencies

Historically tactile defensiveness was the first form of sensory over-responsivity defined (Ayres, 1979), but defensiveness was also identified in the olfactory and auditory systems (Knickerbocker, 1980). As noted earlier, over-responsivity has been documented in single sensory systems (e.g., tactile defensiveness) (Ayres, 1979) and across several sensory systems (i.e., sensory defensiveness).

Sensory Under-Responsivity

Sensory under-responsivity describes children who exhibit less response to sensory information than the situation demands, taking longer time to react or requiring a higher intensity/longer duration of sensory messages before they are moved to action (Table 6.3). They often appear apathetic or lethargic and can be misunderstood as being lazy, unmotivated, or self-absorbed.

Children with under-responsivity may exhibit passive behavior. Children who do not detect, register, or notice sensation in the environment do not have a drive to interact or to engage in occupation. Unfortunately because of their uncommonly "good" behavior, these individuals are often overlooked; they do not have behavior problems in school or at home and they do not act out in new environments or during times of transition. As a result, under-responsivity may go unnoticed.

Sensory Seeking

Sensory seeking describes children who actively look for or crave sensory stimulation and seem to have an almost insatiable desire for sensory input (Table 6.4). Often, these children are in constant movement and may engage in unsafe behaviors to satisfy their need for sensory input. They can be seen as extreme risk takers, whose sensory needs interfere with attention. Sensory seeking children are overly active, constantly moving, touching, watching moving objects, and/or seeking loud sounds or intense olfactory or gustatory experiences. They may engage in risky behaviors such as climbing and jumping from playground equipment that is not designed for this activity as well as excessive spinning, mouthing of objects, touching things, or making noises.

All three subtypes can interfere with one's ability to engage in social interactions and to participate in home and school routines.

Sensory Discrimination

Ayres (1972a) proposed that the ability to motor plan movements was dependent on the development of an internal representation of the body. This unconscious knowledge of the body was theorized to be the result of somatosensory information coming from the skin, joints, and muscles. Thus, when information from the somatosensory system is inaccurate or imprecise, there will be a deficit in the child's ability to develop and utilize motor memories to guide future planned movements (Table 6.5).

TABLE 6.3 Indicators of Function and Dysfunction in Sensory Modulation: Sensory Under-Responsivity

Typical Responsivity	Sensory Under-Responsivity
FUNCTION: Exhibits typical response to sensory stimuli **Indicators of Function**	*DYSFUNCTION*: Exhibits less response to sensory information than the situation demands **Indicators of Dysfunction**

Touch
    Acknowledges touch
    Notices texture of all types of play materials on hands
    Shows appropriate reaction to being wet, cold, hot, or dirty
	Does not notice when touched
	Does not respond to pain, such as bumping, falling, cuts, or bruises
	Does not notice dirt, wet
	Does not notice something too hot or too cold
	Does not notice drooling or food on face

Auditory
    Responds to name when called
    Acknowledges unexpected sounds such as fire drills, hall bells, and so on
    Able to follow verbal directions given once
    Attends gatherings and is a participating member in community social activities
	Does not respond when name is called
	Does not respond to verbal directions given only once
	Does not respond to unexpected loud sounds
	Tends to be quiet, passive, or withdraw in social situations

Visual
    Responds to visual stimuli; enjoys various colors and patterns
    Attends to visual cues at home, school, and in the community
	Does not notice activity in a busy environment
	Does not notice the visual reminders in the classroom or on the blackboard
	Misses the visual cues in the environment (home, school, and community)

Proprioception Appropriately grades force and power in use of tools	Performs movements in a slow and plodding fashion May have a weak grasp
Vestibular Actively engages in movement and climbing activities	Gives little indication of like or dislike of movement
Smell Notices strong or noxious smells	Does not notice strong or noxious odors

Taste
    Eats when hungry
    Notices very spicy, hot, or sour foods
	Does not seek food when hungry
	Able to tolerate extremely spicy foods—more than cultural norm

TABLE 6.4 Indicators of Function and Dysfunction in Sensory Modulation: Sensory Seeking

Typical Responsivity	*Sensory Seeking*
FUNCTION: Exhibits typical response to sensory stimuli	*DYSFUNCTION*: Actively looks for or craves sensory stimulation
Indicators of Function	**Indicators of Dysfunction**
Touch	
Enjoys touch, hugs, and typical family expressions of affection	Touches people to the point of irritating them
Explores all types of play materials with hands	Overly affectionate
Participates willingly in daily living activities with tactile components	Engages in pinching, biting, and scratching
	Seeks out touching, feeling, or vibrating objects
Auditory	
Able to modulate volume of voice	Speaks in a loud voice
Engages in reciprocal conversations	Make noises for the sake of making noise
Alerts appropriately to varied sounds	Likes loud volume of the TV, radio, and so on
Not bothered by sounds that occur in daily activities	Difficulty taking turns when talking
Attends gatherings of all sizes	
Participates in community social activities	
Visual	
Comfortable in lighted areas	Excessive preference for fast changing images on the TV or movies
Enjoys a variety of colors and patterns	Excessive watching of flickering or blinking lights
Not disoriented by extraneous visual stimuli in the environment	Watches spinning objects
Proprioception	
Moves in a smooth and fluid manner	Always bumping, crashing, or falling on purpose
	Falls out of chair
	Fidgets, wiggling, and restless throughout the day
Vestibular	
Enjoys movement in all planes of space	Engages in excessive amounts of movement; cannot sit still
Engages in climbing in activities	Tends to be a daredevil, engages in movement with no regard for safety
Challenged by new motor activities	Twirling/spinning throughout the day
Calmed following movement activities	
Smell	
Responds appropriately to typical daily smells	Eats only foods with strong flavors
	Smells people/objects
	Smells toys/objects during play
Taste	
Eats a variety of textured foods	Licking, sucking, and chewing nonfood items
Enjoys a range of spicy to bland foods	Always putting things in mouth
Uses food appropriately to regulate energy and arousal	Prefers crunchy, chewy, or hard foods to the exclusion of other textures

TABLE 6.5 Indicators of Function and Dysfunction in Sensory Discrimination

Discriminates Sensory Input	*Difficulty Discriminating Sensory Input*
FUNCTION: Ability to develop and use motor memories to guide planned movements **Indicators of Function**	*DYSFUNCTION*: Deficits in ability to develop and use motor memories to guide planned movements **Indicators of Dysfunction**

Touch/proprioception
   Able to identify object in hand without looking
   Able to localize touch on body
   Able to identify shape drawn on the back of the hand
   Awareness of position and body parts
	Has trouble performing fine motor tasks without looking
	Has trouble identifying an object in hand without looking
	Cannot discriminate shape drawn on hand
	Does not know where touched without looking
	Has difficulty maneuvering through space without bumping into objects

Visual
   Able to track objects
   Able to localize and follow a moving target
   Able to maintain stable vision with eyes moving or head moving
	Difficulty keeping track of place on a page
	Difficulty following a moving object with eyes
	Difficulty copying from the blackboard

Proprioception
   Able to use graded force, timing, and distance appropriately in play and daily activities
   Able to detect body position in relationship to gravity
   Awareness of body position and weight of body part
   Able to maintain posture at table for class and home activities
   Strength and endurance for indoor and outdoor activities with peers
   Moves in a smooth and fluid manner
	Difficulty balancing without using vision to assist
	Cannot judge timing and distance in ball play
	Cannot use appropriate pressure with writing implements
	Cannot judge appropriate force for daily activities
	Poor extension against gravity
	Decreased core stability
	Poor balance
	Lack of postural background movements
	Delayed standing and walking balance
	Fatigues easily
	Low endurance
	Feels loose or floppy
	Poor posture during table top activities

Vestibular
   Ability to sit still comfortably
   Ability to move through space without tripping and falling
   Established coordinated use of the two sides of the body and both hands
   Coordinates the two sides of the body especially for tool use with the preferred hand coordinated with the nonpreferred hand use for assist
	Has difficulty maintaining good posture and leans, fidgets, or sits on feet or legs
	Falls over easily
	Poor oculomotor control while moving
	Poor body spatial awareness
	Poorly coordinated use of the two sides of the body, as in jumping, skipping, hopping, catching, or throwing a ball
	Right-left confusion
	Delayed or lack of hand dominance
	Poor lateralization of hand function
	Avoidance of crossing midline
	Does not spontaneously use one hand to assist the dominant hand
	Difficulty sequencing tasks

Dyspraxia

Praxis is the ability to make adaptive motor responses to the environment. When praxis is functioning well, an individual is able to effortlessly and automatically adapt to and successfully meet challenges and changes in the environment. A dysfunction in this process is referred to as "dyspraxia," an overarching term that refers to problems in the overall praxis process.

Somatodyspraxia is described as a deficit in learning new motor skills, planning new motor actions, and generalizing motor plans. The ability to motor plan is key to somatopraxis and central to the child's ability to make adaptive responses (Table 6.6). New motor skills are learned easily without much conscious attention. When motor planning abilities are not working well, the child struggles to complete new or complex motor tasks. Learning new skills is an arduous process that is difficult and takes a great deal of time and effort. Frequently, the child must consciously think about and plan out every motor action as if it was a brand new skill.

Somatodyspraxia is the most common form of dyspraxia seen in children with sensory integrative disorder and is closely related to deficits in somatosensory processing. Some children (i.e., some children with cerebral palsy or nonverbal learning disabilities) have motor planning problems that are not tied to somatosensory problem. These types of motor planning problems are not considered to be a problem in sensory integration.

TABLE 6.6 Indicators of Function and Dysfunction in Somatodyspraxia

Learns New Motor Skills	*Deficit in Learning Motor Skills*
FUNCTION: Completes new or complex motor tasks	*DYSFUNCTION*: Struggles to complete new or complex motor tasks
Indicators of Function	**Indicators of Dysfunction**

Ideation
  Ability to recognize and act appropriately on the affordances of objects or the environment
  Ability to generate multiple ideas of play with new pieces of equipment
	Difficulty conceptualizing a goal for action
	Difficulty knowing what actions are appropriate to use with a given object
	Often uses objects in inappropriate ways (e.g., stands on a therapy ball)

Motor planning
  Able to easily learn new motor tasks in school and after school activities
  Adapts easily to changes and uses a range of motor strategies
	Clumsy
	Difficulty learning new motor tasks
	Cannot ride a bicycle
	Difficulty developing a movement strategy for accomplishment of a goal

Execution Uses smooth, fluid, controlled movements	Movements may be stiff or rigid Movements may be ballistic with difficulty working within midrange positions

It is important to ascertain that there is a sensory component to the motor planning problem before determining that it is somatodyspraxia.

Children with somatodyspraxia have difficulties with body boundaries and therefore frequently invade others space. They are clumsy, frequently tripping and falling and avoid or may have difficulty participating in sports. Performing activities of daily living such as brushing teeth, dressing, or eating are difficult for them. Unintentionally, they may break toys and push or shove others. They are disorganized, often losing things like toys, books, mittens, and shoes. In addition, they have difficulty using tools like writing utensils, scissors, fork, and knife.

Children with somatodyspraxia have specific difficulties in oral motor praxis, which may result in poor articulation, difficulty in chewing, or inability to learn how to whistle. Because many children with somatodyspraxia are aware of how hard they work to complete tasks that are easy for others and how often they fail, self-esteem problems are common with these children. Because they are unable to follow other children's plan, these children often have a strong need to be in control of play and daily life routines. This inflexibility can impact on interpersonal skills with peers and make transitions or schedule changes throughout the day difficult. Because these children are frequently so ineffective in their control over the environment, they often have an external locus of control; they may attribute a failure to complete a task to someone else or the environment. Children with somatodyspraxia frequently do not anticipate the end result of their actions and therefore may appear impulsive and frequently may put themselves in unsafe or at-risk situations.

Ideation

Ideation is the conceptualization of a goal and some idea of the steps necessary to achieve that goal. Children who have difficulty with ideation do not recognize play opportunities with novel toys so they tend to act on all toys with a limited set of behaviors such as lining up, throwing, swinging, or breaking. They tend to use limited, very familiar, and often scripted play themes such as re-enacting a book or movie which other children may not wish to participate in. Frequently, they lack the ability to represent objects and so they may be very concrete in their thinking (e.g., a stick is a stick and not a bat). Children with ideational problems often do not engage in much independent active play. They often are unable to play independently and require a parent or more skilled peer to structure their play. They are easily frustrated and may demonstrate acting out behaviors as a result. They may not take motor risks. Children with ideational problems are typically talkers and not doers. They frequently have very good language skills and will talk to avoid having to actually do a task. Some children with ideational problems may have relatively good motor skills and do well in structured sports but not be able to participate well with peers in free play.

Motor Planning (Organization of Motor Actions)

Motor planning is the ability to automatically organize a motor act so that it can be performed or implemented. This involves the internal process of organizing one's motor actions, without consciously planning out the action.

Execution (Production of the Motor Movement — More Related to Motor Control Than Praxis)

Finally, execution involves the implementation or production of motor movements. This requires motor control for accurate implementation of the action that has been planned. In execution, motor control is more critical than praxis.

Bilateral Integration and Sequencing Dysfunction

Bilateral integration and sequencing dysfunction include deficits coordinating two sides of the body effectively and difficulty sequencing. When working well, bilateral integration is readily observable in children's ability to smoothly and skillfully complete developmental activities that require the use of the two sides of the body together in a coordinated fashion such as jumping, hopping, skipping, riding a bike, or using two hands together to accomplish a task such as cutting with scissors (Table 6.7). Problems in bilateral integration and sequencing skills are usually seen in conjunction with vestibular-proprioceptive problems. Because they share a vestibular basis, difficulties in postural-ocular control are also often seen with bilateral integration and sequencing dysfunction problems. Difficulties in bilateral integration and sequencing are characterized by difficulties with lateralization skills, establishment of hand dominance, and difficulties with crossing the midline. Problems with skilled coordination of actions that require smooth and efficient timing and spatial accuracy are often seen in these children and manifested in sports activities. Sequencing of motor actions tends to be particularly difficult; therefore, completing multistep activities may be hard even when the child is able to easily complete the component parts individually. In addition, postural and oculomotor difficulties, which often accompany bilateral integration and sequencing problems may further compromise a child's ability to perform skillful actions. Difficulties in these areas may also be associated with poor visual motor skills and poor oral motor skills.

In general, bilateral integration and sequencing dysfunction problems are functionally milder than somatodyspraxia. Children with bilateral integration and sequencing dysfunction problems typically have relatively good ideation and motor planning skills, but have difficulty with anticipatory actions, refined timing, and spatial coordination of movements. They tend to have particular difficulties with actions and activities that require integration of vision and movement. Projected action sequence problems (i.e., a sequence of motor acts put together to accomplish a goal in future time and space such as running to catch or kick a ball or coordinating the position and timing to kick a soccer goal or make a basket) are also particularly characteristic of children with bilateral integration and sequencing dysfunction.

Children with bilateral integration have difficulty coordinating two parts of the body for bimanual tasks such as holding paper to write or using a knife and fork. They may have difficulty with activities involving timing and movement through space such as running across a field to catch or kick a ball. Difficulty coordinating eye–hand activities such as throwing or catching a ball are common. They have difficulties with bilateral tasks such as hopscotch, riding a bike, jumping jacks, or pumping a swing, coordinating a sequence of movements, crossing the midline, and knowing right from left. Often they

TABLE 6.7 **Indicators of Function and Dysfunction in Bilateral Integration and Sequencing**

Bilateral Integration and Sequencing	Difficulty with Bilateral Integration and Sequencing
FUNCTION: Ability to use two sides of the body in a coordinated fashion **Indicators of Function**	*DYSFUNCTION*: Difficulty using two sides of the body in a coordinated fashion **Indicators of Dysfunction**

Vestibular
    Holds head in midline when needed
    Coordinates body position with head movements and *vice versa*
    Moves in and out of midline during transitional movements gracefully
    Maintains a symmetrical upright posture during sustained sitting and standing
    Regains a vertically aligned posture automatically when moving through space and equilibriums is disrupted
    Stabilizes eyes during head movement
    Established hand preference for tool use
    Uses nonpreferred hand as a functional assist
	Poor extension against gravity
	Poor balance, righting, and equilibrium responses
	Poor coordination of head, neck, and eyes
	Difficulty sitting or standing up straight while holding still
	Difficulty balancing without using vision to assist
	Jumps around when trying to balance rather than holding still
	Holds body in asymmetrical postures when moving
	Poorly coordinated use of the two sides of the body, that is, jumping, skipping, hopping, catching, or throwing a ball
	Right-left confusion
	Delayed or lack of hand preference
	Avoidance of crossing midline
	Does not spontaneously use one hand to assist the preferred hand during needed tasks
	Difficulty sequencing tasks

Proprioception
    Able to grade force, timing, and distance in play and daily activities
    Uses the correct amount of strength during activities, corrected for weight, size, and distance
    Able to detect relative body position in relationship to other body parts
    Awareness of body position and weight of body part
    Strength and endurance for indoor and outdoor activities with peers
    Moves in a smooth and fluid manner, grading movements as appropriate for the task
	Cannot judge how to position the body to ensure proper timing and distance during ball play
	Cannot use appropriate pressure using writing implements
	Cannot judge appropriate muscle force for daily activities
	Difficulty maintaining appropriate posture for static or dynamic activities
	Does not adjust body position relative to movement of other body parts
	Poor adjustment of body posture when balancing, for example, fixing shoulders and holding them in high guard or holding the leg out straight
	Fatigues easily
	Low endurance
	Feels loose or floppy

(continued)

TABLE 6.7 (Continued)	
Bilateral Integration and Sequencing	*Difficulty with Bilateral Integration and Sequencing*
Coordination of two parts of the body and sequencing of body movements	
Can complete multiple step activities, that is, sports, karate, and exercise routines	Decreased core stability
Able to complete bimanual activities	Poorly coordinated use of the two sides of the body, that is, jumping, skipping, hopping, catching, or throwing a ball, and tying shoes
Able to demonstrate good timing through activities such as eye–hand coordination and throwing/catching ball skills	Difficulty with anticipatory, feedforward movements, and actions
Able to play various sports games	Difficulty completing tasks with several steps and hands working together
	Difficulty peddling a bike
	Difficulty learning exercise routines or dance steps
	Difficulty with bimanual tasks like tying shoes, holding paper, and writing
Ocular motor	
Symmetrical use of the eyes for all tasks	Difficulty organizing visual gaze
Stabilizes eyes during head movement to sustain a stable visual field	Disorganized or uncomfortable while moving or needs to go very slowly
Able to stabilize the head during eye movements for tracking and locating objects	Poor ability to track or locate objects, especially those that are moving
Coordinates actions with visual gaze	Does not look at what they are doing
Can watch moving objects and track across different planes and spatial distances	Loses track of object visually as they move near to far
Can shift gaze between horizontal and vertical planes and between near and far	Loss of balance during head movements especially when looking at something besides where they are going
Oral motor	
Can make various verbal and nonverbal sounds such as humming or saying words	Difficulty with articulation
Can move tongue in all directions, up, down, side-to-side including managing food inside all areas of the mouth	Difficulty with sucking, chewing, or swallowing sequences
Clear articulated speech	Difficulty blowing bubbles or a whistle
	Sloppy eater

tend to remain in an upright posture as they have difficulty moving the head out of upright to go over, under, and through planes of movement. Frequently children with bilateral integration and sequencing dysfunction have related difficulties with postural and oculomotor control. They may have difficulty staying in their seat or copying from a blackboard.

These children are often overlooked because overtly observable problems may not manifest until later in school when sequencing and organizational demands increase. They may appear to be good at sports in early years as they often are good at running about, but have problems in later years when increased timing and precision are needed.

Poor Visual Perception and Visual Motor Integration (Visuodyspraxia)

Visual perception is critical to many of the abilities described earlier and is a common deficit addressed by the sensory integration frame of reference. Vision is particularly relevant to our ability to maintain upright postures, to learn about objects, and to provide us with information about the position of our body in space. Visual perceptual abilities are an important component of many cognitive skills that relate to success in school, finding one's way in the environment, and performing simple dressing tasks such as finding one's clothes in a drawer or the closet. Visual motor skills include the ability to use vision to direct hand and body movements (Table 6.8). Visual motor skills

TABLE 6.8 Indicators of Function and Dysfunction in Visual Perception and Visual Motor Skills

Visual Perception and Visual Motor Skills	*Poor Visual Perception and Visual Motor Skills*
FUNCTION: Ability to use vision to direct hand and body movements **Indicators of Function**	*DYSFUNCTION*: Inability to use vision to direct hand and body movements **Indicators of Dysfunction**

Visual form and space perception
   Shape constancy
   Able to match shapes regardless of orientation in space, size, or color
	Difficulty matching objects by spatial orientation

Figure ground perception
   Able to find an object hidden in a distracting background
   Able to find matching clothes
	Trouble finding objects in distracting background

Visual motor integration
   Copy by imitation
   Copy with model present
   Copy from memory (i.e., shapes, letter, numbers, etc.)
	Unable to accurately copy drawings, handwriting difficulties

Visual spatial abilities
   Visual control of movement through space
   Guides movement of the limbs; support balance
	Unable to negotiate movement in the environment without bumping into objects or falling
	Unable to judge speed of moving objects, as in crossing the street or in the playground

are dependent on adequate visual tracking, coordination of eye–head movements, and coordination of eye–hand movements. Adequate visual motor skills are an important component of successful participation in academic activities, as well as sports and play activities.

GUIDE TO EVALUATION

Typically, the reason for referral to occupational therapy for an evaluation is based on the child's difficulties in participating in everyday skills and activities rather than a specific diagnosis. When the child's health and participation is hindered as a result of sensory-related concerns, an occupational therapy evaluation using a sensory integrative frame of reference is indicated. The therapist selects assessments that identify the contribution of the sensory systems to the difficulties that hinder a client's ability to meet desired expectations in one or more areas including participation in activities of daily living, education, play, sleep, and leisure activities at home and in the community; social participation; and performance skills and patterns, including habits and routines (Smith Roley, 2006).

Therapists can use several methods of assessment to identify the child's area of strength and need, including formal assessments, parent questionnaires about the child's developmental history and sensory-related behaviors, an occupational profile (Schaaf & Smith Roley, 2006), and structured and unstructured observation (Windsor, Smith Roley, & Szklut, 2001). Each piece of data helps to clarify and focus the therapist's clinical reasoning and direct intervention (Blanche, 2006).

Table 6.9 provides a clinical reasoning framework that guides the therapist through the assessment process. It also contains some resources for assessment. The therapist begins with the presenting problems and the reasons the child and his or her family is referred to occupational therapy. These include issues that are related to participation in daily activities such as difficulty learning activities in the classroom or difficulty completing self-care activities such as donning clothing or organizing behavior during daily morning routine. These issues become both the reasons for referral and the outcome goals for intervention (Schaaf & Smith Roley, 2006).

The therapist collects the assessment data to inform his or her clinical reasoning about how the child processes sensory information from one or more sensory channels, how this information is integrated, and the way in which this information is used during ongoing development. The following section explains the key components of the evaluation process in this frame of reference.

Record Review

Familiarity with the client is an important part of the assessment process. The therapist verifies and reviews the subject's historical information including medical, educational, and therapeutic reports, developmental history, and an occupational profile. These tools help the therapist determine if the child's difficulties have a sensory basis, and

TABLE 6.9 Clinical Reasoning Guidelines and Suggested Resources for Occupational Therapy

Steps for Clinical Reasoning during the Assessment Phase	*Suggested Strategies*	*Suggested Resources*
Identify the strengths of the child and family	Observe the environment Talk with the family Observe the child Observe child–family interactions Review the child's history	Background Information and Occupational History Profile (Smith Roley & Schaaf, 2006)
Identify the occupational dilemmas	Define and describe current concerns and how these relate to performance of daily activities	Background Information and Occupational History Profile (Schaaf & Smith Roley, 2006)
Determine if occupational dilemmas may be related to sensory motor deficits	Use indicators of function/dysfunction to guide your clinical judgment	(Ayres, 1972, 1979, 1989, 2006) (Schaaf & Smith Roley, 2006) (May-Benson & Koomar, 2007) (Parham & Mailloux, 2005)
Choose appropriate assessments to evaluate sensory and motor areas	Conduct formal and informal assessments of sensory and motor skills and abilities	SIPT (Ayres, 2003) *Sensory Processing Measure* (Parham et al., 2007; Miller-Kuhaneck et al., 2007) Sensory Profile (Dunn, 1999a) Clinical Observations of Sensory Integration (Blanche, 2002)
Summarize data and determine its relationship to clients occupational dilemmas	List behaviors and possible underlying sensory or motor mechanisms	Blanche (2006)
Develop goals for intervention	On the basis of occupational dilemmas and proposed sensory motor basis, develop goals that are consistent with assessment findings and parents/teachers identified needs	Mailloux (2006)

SIPT, Sensory Integration and Praxis Tests.

accordingly, to conduct specific assessments to determine the specific type and range of the sensory-based deficits.

Identifying Patterns of Dysfunction

The therapist uses clinical reasoning to determine the best assessments to guide intervention taking into consideration time, cost, information obtained from a developmental history, and the intellectual level and attention span of the child. In this case, the therapist is guided by his or her understanding of the theoretical principles of sensory integration and the evidence to support intervention, combined with other assessments of sensory and motor skills.

The SIPT, a comprehensive assessment of sensory integration, is considered the "gold standard" for evaluating sensory integration and praxis (Ayres, 1989; Windsor, Smith Roley, & Szklut, 2001). It consists of 17 standardized, computer-scored tests designed to measure visual and tactile perception and discrimination, visual motor skills, bilateral integration and sequencing, praxis and vestibular-proprioceptive functions. Specifically, the SIPT provides a template for evaluating several aspects of praxis including construction, imitation, facial gestures, sequencing, visual spatial planning, and following unfamiliar verbal directions. It also includes tests of sensory motor skills such as standing and walking balance. The SIPT subtests are listed in Table 6.10. While the therapist is administering the test items, the therapist observes the child, evaluating the complexity of interactions with objects and people, and adaptability to change during the session. It is important during these observations to see what the child can do without prompts or instruction, using his or her own praxis abilities. This is frequently used in conjunction with specific clinical observations (Blanche, 2002).

The SIPT is standardized on children aged 4 to 8 years, 11 months. Standard scores are generated and graphed using Z-score standard deviations with the mean of zero (Figure 6.17). SIPT test scores are used in combination with a history, sensory questionnaires (Dunn, 1999b; Parham et al., 2007; Miller-Kuhanek et al., 2007), and clinical observations of sensory and motor skills (Blanche, 2002) to identify specific areas for intervention. Although the SIPT provides a useful evaluation of sensory integration and praxis, it is not appropriate for all clients.

TABLE 6.10 Sensory Integration and Praxis Tests (SIPT, Ayres, 1989) Subtest

Space visualization
Figure ground
Standing and walking balance
Design copying
Motor accuracy
Postrotary nystagmus test
Postural praxis
Constructional praxis
Oral praxis
Praxis on verbal command
Sequencing praxis
Bilateral motor coordination
Manual form perception
Kinesthesia
Graphesthesia
Finger identification
Localization of tactile stimuli

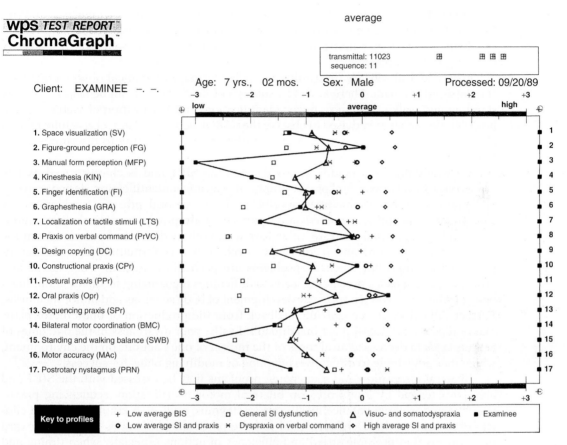

FIGURE 6.17 Sensory Integration and Praxis Tests (SIPT) graph of test scores.

Supplemental clinical observations are an integral part of the evaluation process. Initially recommended by Ayres and updated by Blanche (2002), these structured observations target behaviors related to response to sensation, muscle tone, righting reactions, postural stability, postural control, bilateral coordination, visual pursuits, organization of behavior, and projected actions sequences. Postrotary nystagmus (the reflexive response of the eyes after rotation) is a test of vestibular functioning that is part of the SIPT.

Sensory modulation deficits are best identified using observation in combination with parent/teacher/self-report scales such as the *Sensory Processing Measure* (Parham et al., 2007; Miller-Kuhaneck et al., 2007) and *Sensory Profile* (Dunn, 1999a). The sensory over-responsivity scales offer a unique contribution to the identification of sensory modulation dysfunction by specifically measuring sensory over-responsivity across all seven sensory domains and by combining an examiner-administered performance measure and a subjective, caregiver (for children), or self-report (for adults) measure. The scales provide a method to assess individuals in a standard manner across a diverse age range (3 years through adults) and across severity (subtle to overt behaviors). With further study, these scales may be able to contribute to evidence-based decisions related to whether a particular individual exhibits clinical signs of sensory over-responsivity (Schoen et al., in press).

Assessment of sensory discrimination is based more on clinical observations than standardized test data. There are a few subtests of the SIPT that can be helpful, such as standing and walking balance, finger identification, and localization of tactile stimuli; however, therapists are advised to observe the child in activities that will give information about his or her responses to sensory stimulation and the ability to discriminate this information.

Somatodyspraxia is readily assessed using the SIPT and is characterized by low scores on postural praxis, oral praxis, graphesthesia, finger identification, design copying, and motor accuracy. Sometimes specific problems in oral praxis, visual motor, or constructional planning are noted along with somatodyspraxia. In clinical observations, these children may demonstrate difficulties with both feedback (information from the senses after an action) and feedforward mechanisms, (information from the senses prior to an action) but feedback problems are particularly evident. Poor tactile and proprioceptive sensory processing leads to difficulties recognizing feedback about one's body movements, which impact the development of body schemas and motor memories. Further difficulties in recognizing feedback from the production of one's motor plans makes repeating successful actions difficult. Lastly, poor awareness of the outcomes of actions leads to decreased awareness of the impact of one's actions on the environment, which may contribute to difficulties adapting or modifying plans for success.

Bilateral integration and sequencing problems may be assessed with the SIPT and are characterized by low scores on bilateral motor coordination, sequencing praxis, standing and walking balance, postrotary nystagmus, and often graphesthesia. In clinical observations, these children tend to have particular difficulties with feedforward mechanisms that promote speed and efficiency of actions especially when timing and spatial demands are present.

Visual perception and visual motor integration are viewed as end products or outcomes of the sensory integration process. Subtests from the SIPT that are useful in identifying this area of dysfunction are space visualization, figure ground, and design copying. Additionally, there are many other assessments on the market that can provide information on this area (see Chapter 11).

Because some therapists do not have access to the SIPT, or their service delivery model does not allow the use of this tool, therapists must use other tools to evaluate the potential for sensory integrative dysfunction. While such tools are not as precise as the SIPT, they can provide valuable information. Therapists should consider the use of other tests which identify the behaviors and characteristics associated with sensory processing deficits.

Communication with Parents, Care Providers, and Teachers

The assessment process with children almost always involves communication, consultation, and collaboration with parents and other important people in the child's life such as extended family members, care providers, teachers, and other service providers. Establishing goals should be conducted in collaboration with parents, and may involve other individuals as well. Goals will be discussed and expressed in ways that relate to the results of the assessment, as well as the priorities and concerns of the family and others. During each key component of the assessment, the therapist uses reflective questions to gather needed information and frame the child's strengths and needs:

- What are the child's areas of competency and strength with the key daily life activities encountered?
- Do I understand the family's priorities for their child?
- Do the parents seem comfortable with the intervention plan?
- What can I do to meet the needs of the child as well as of family members?
- What is the best way to collaborate with the child's parents and share my observations?
- Do I need to spend more time talking to parents, provide more written materials, or suggest other audio, video, or print resources?

This information is used in combination with standardized assessment findings and clinical observations to develop a comprehensive intervention plan for the child.

POSTULATES REGARDING CHANGE

The postulates regarding change of this frame of reference describe the therapeutic environment that is necessary to facilitate change. The process of intervention is fundamentally based on the following 11 general postulates regarding change.

1. If the therapist provides a therapeutic environment with enticing equipment, the child will be more likely to engage in activities.
2. If the therapist provides a physically safe environment that allows for challenges to the child, then the therapist's attention can be directed toward facilitating the child's abilities.
3. If the therapist provides sensory opportunities in at least two of the three sensory systems (tactile, vestibular, and proprioceptive), then therapy will be more likely to support the child's development of self-regulation, sensory awareness, and/or awareness of movement in space.
4. If the therapist helps the child attain and maintain appropriate levels of alertness and affective state, then the child will be more likely to sustain engagement in therapeutic activities.
5. If the therapist utilizes an achievable challenge to sensory modulation, discrimination, and/or integration, then the child will achieve enhanced development in that area of challenge.
6. If the therapist provides challenges to the child's ability to conceptualize and plan novel motor tasks, then the child will be more likely to develop praxis and the ability to organize his/her behavior in time and space.

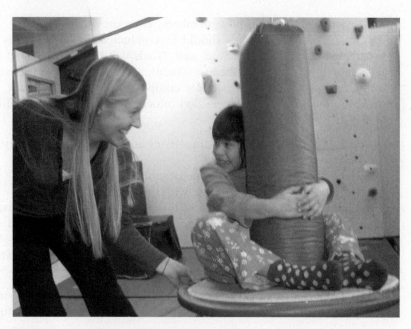

FIGURE 6.18 The sensory integration frame of reference uses child-directed, active sensory motor experiences at the just right challenge to facilitate adaptive responses. In this case, the child is using active flexion to remain on the swing while challenging balance and eye–hand coordination.

7. If the therapist collaborates with the child in the choice of activity allowing some degree of "child direction," then the child will be more likely to achieve an adaptive response (Figure 6.18).

8. If the therapist increases the complexity of the challenge so that the child needs to exert some degree of effort, then the child will be more likely to master the challenge and move to a higher level adaptive response.

9. If the therapist presents or facilitates challenges in which the child is successful in any of the following areas: sensory modulation, discrimination, postural/ocular/oral control, or praxis, then the child will be more likely to develop skills in the challenged area.

10. If the therapist creates an environment that supports play, then the child will be more fully engaged and will have more intrinsic motivation to engage in the therapeutic activities.

11. If the therapist establishes a positive therapeutic rapport with the child, there will be a greater likelihood of the child participating fully in the intervention.

Specific Postulates Regarding Change for Sensory Modulation Disorder

If there are deficits in sensory modulation, it is important to bring modulation within normal levels prior to addressing other areas of dysfunction. There are five postulates regarding change related to sensory system modulation.

1. If a child is over-responsive, under-responsive, or seeking sensory stimuli, then intervention must be directed initially toward facilitating an appropriate adaptive response to those sensory stimuli which are producing the maladaptive response.
2. If opportunities are provided for appropriate sensory responses to one sensory system, then the child will be more likely to show adaptive responses in the other sensory systems.
3. If the child's sensory modulation is brought to an optimal level, the child will be better able to address problems in foundational abilities and outcomes.
4. If the child's family, significant others, and teachers understand the child's sensory modulation issues, they will be more likely to structure daily life activities and routines to support an optimal level of arousal.
5. If the therapist supports the child's engagement in play activities that encourage modulation of sensations, then the child will be more likely to develop the ability to self-regulate their sensory responsivity.

There are five additional postulates regarding change related to sensory discrimination as it relates to sensory modulation.

1. If the child has opportunities to develop tactile, proprioceptive, and vestibular discrimination, he or she will be more likely to develop precise body awareness needed for skill development.
2. If the therapist provides opportunities for increased feedback regarding position and relation of body to environment, the child will be more likely to perceive the orientation and position of objects to one another.
3. If the therapist provides opportunities for the development of tactile discrimination skills, the child will be more likely to engage in manual use of the hands in skilled activities.
4. If the child is guided to develop visual pursuits during intervention, then he or she will be more likely to be successful in classroom-related visual activities.
5. If the therapist provides opportunities for visual discrimination activities (figure ground activities and visual spatial perception activities), then the child will be more likely to develop and utilize these skills for play and learning.

Postulates Regarding Change Related to Dyspraxia

It is important when treating praxis problems to address all areas of practic function. There are four postulates regarding change related to dyspraxia in general. Each subtype of dyspraxia also has specific postulates to address problems in that area.

1. If the child develops improved praxis, then he or she will more likely be successful in achieving skills.
2. If the therapist provides the "just right challenge" and the child produces effective adaptive responses, these successful experiences will develop motor memories which will serve as foundations for new actions.

3. If the therapist provides opportunities for the sensory-rich activities (tactile, proprioceptive, and/or vestibular) needed to enhance body awareness combined with practice opportunities at the just right level, praxis abilities will develop.
4. If the therapist provides sensory opportunities, which are at a meaningful intensity level with appropriate frequency and duration to promote sensory discrimination, praxis will develop.

There are four specific postulates regarding change related to somatodyspraxia.

1. If the child engages in activities rich in somatosensory input, he or she will be more likely to develop an improved body schema.
2. If the therapist provides an environment where the child must navigate the body through unusual size and shaped spaces out of an upright position, and must move in varying planes of space, he or she will develop improved body awareness and planning in space abilities.
3. If the therapist asks questions and guides the child in discovering and problem solving instead of directing, he or she will be more likely to develop the ability to self-generate motor plans.
4. If the therapist balances varying and increasing activity demands with the opportunity to repeat and adequately master the task, the child will develop improved motor planning.

The following four specific postulates regarding change relate to problems with ideational in somatodyspraxia.

1. If the therapist bridges the child's current experience with examples of similar previous experiences, he or she will develop improved ideation.
2. If the therapist provides the child with familiar mental images to describe the child's actions, he or she will be more likely to develop increased representational abilities and improved ideation.
3. If the therapist encourages the child to imitate and expand creatively on what the therapist is doing during the therapy session, then he or she will be more likely to develop ideation abilities.
4. If the child is guided to explore and develop an increased awareness of object affordances, he or she will be able to expand his or her repertoire of ideas for possible actions with the objects.

Specific Postulates Regarding Change for Bilateral Integration and Sequencing Deficits

There are four specific postulates regarding change related to bilateral integration and sequencing deficits.

1. If the child is provided with vestibular-proprioceptive experiences emphasizing balance, antigravity control, core stability, endurance, and crossing midline, he or she will be more likely to develop hand dominance and perform age-appropriate activities involving coordinated use of the two sides of the body.

2. If the child engages in movement activities that provide opportunities for visual motor challenges, he or she will develop improved timing and spatial skills.

3. If the child is actively engaged in the process of creating, setting up, participating in, and cleaning up an activity, then he or she will develop an internal sense of sequencing and self-organization.

4. If the child participates in multistep motor sequences (gross, fine, or oral), then he or she will be more likely to perform motor sequences more efficiently during daily life at home and at school.

Visual Perception and Visual Motor Integration

There is one postulate regarding change related to visual perception.

1. If the therapist integrates visual perceptual and/or visual motor tasks into therapy activities, the child will be more likely to generalize these skills to daily life activities at home and at school.

APPLICATION TO PRACTICE

Occupational therapy using a sensory integration frame of reference is a dynamic, process-oriented intervention. It does not follow a specific or prearranged set of therapeutic activities. As with most frames of reference used with children, intervention includes both direct therapy sessions for the child as well as family education and support. Some of the unique principles of intervention in the sensory integration frame of reference are the concepts of the just right challenge and the adaptive response. These concepts are defined in the theoretical base. Additionally, to use this frame of reference effectively, the child is an active participant in therapy sessions and intervention is child directed to a degree.

Setting Goals for Intervention

Once the assessment data has been gathered, the therapist utilizes this information to create goals and plan intervention. When considered and constructed carefully, goals convey significant components of the therapeutic process. Goal setting and the ongoing review process with the family offer many opportunities for therapists to identify specific areas for intervention, communicate their role with other members of the team, and monitor the effectiveness of the chosen intervention strategies. The most obvious purpose of creating goals is to guide intervention and to ensure that it has been successful. The outcome identified in a goal represents an agreed-upon target behavior and a way to measure progress toward that behavior. In the process of establishing goals, the therapist has the opportunity to reflect upon the intermediary steps that need to occur for a goal to be accomplished. Often called "objectives," "benchmarks," or "short-term goals," these intermediary steps can help to identify the functions, components, steps, or foundation skills that need attention in order for broader goals to be achieved (Mailloux, 2006).

To begin the process of setting goals, the presenting problem, underlying problem, and desired functional outcome must be identified. The presenting problem is the issue that brings the individual to occupational therapy. For example, a common presenting problem for school-age children is poor handwriting. The underlying problem is determined or at least hypothesized through the evaluation process, as well as through ongoing observations of the individual. In the sensory integration frame of reference, a presenting problem, such as poor handwriting, may be the result of an underlying problem in somatosensory processing and praxis. In addition, poor handwriting may be related to muscle weakness and poor motor control. Difficulties with visual perception may also play a role. The desired functional outcome is directly related to the presenting problem and is the same regardless of the underlying problem. However, the intervention is aimed at reaching the desired functional outcome utilizing strategies that address the underlying problem. Table 6.11 presents a sample format for goals in the sensory integration frame of reference, including the presenting problem, the underlying problem, and the desired functional outcome (Mailloux, 2006). This format is useful as it articulates the proposed underlying sensory basis of the child's participation difficulties, and guides the therapist in the appropriate choice of intervention targets (in this case, a focus on improved vestibular processing and improved postural and ocular control). The outcome measure of successful intervention will be not only improved vestibular processing and postural/ocular control but also, importantly, improved ability to copy assignments from the blackboard. Thus, the proposed method of goal identification and charting provides a system for tracking and monitoring progress in occupationally relevant outcomes.

Considerations for Intervention

The sensory integration frame of reference is most frequently utilized by occupational therapists as part of a total program of occupational therapy. The intervention is unique in that it addresses the underlying sensory motor substrates of dysfunction rather than just the functional difficulties itself. When sensory integration principles are used as part of occupational therapy, the therapist maintains the profession's focus on enhancing independence in life skills and utilizes the principles of sensory integration within the context of the professional domain to achieve these goals. Therapy is intended to be part

---

TABLE 6.11 Example of Targets for Educationally Related Goals

Presenting Problem	Hypothesized Underlying Problem	Desired Functional Outcome
Difficulty in copying from the blackboard	Inefficient processing of vestibular sensory input which affects the ability to extend the neck and to keep the head up; to coordinate head and eye movements; and to use bilateral hand movements	Adequate ability to copy assignments from the blackboard

of a comprehensive intervention program and as a supplement to, not a substitute for, formal classroom instruction. Therapy is not prescriptive, but rather it is individualized to meet the specific needs of each child and family (Bundy & Koomar, 2002).

This frame of reference provides opportunities for engagement in sensory motor activities rich in tactile, vestibular, and proprioceptive sensations. The therapeutic environment is designed to tap into the child's inner drive to play. The therapist uses keen observation skills to observe and interpret the child's behaviors and interests and then creates a playful environment in which the child actively pursues achievable challenges (Schaaf & Smith Roley, 2006; Bundy, Lane, & Murray, 2002). For example, a sensory integration frame of reference for a child with over-responsiveness to tactile and vestibular stimuli might include enticing opportunities for sensory-rich play that modulates sensory responsiveness while providing achievable challenges to experience sensory activities. This might include activities like climbing up a small platform, grabbing onto a trapeze bar, swinging, and then landing in a matted pit full of colorful balls. Thus, the intervention is child directed and therapist guided, using challenging and fun activities designed to modulate responsiveness to sensation, stimulate sensory and motor systems, and facilitate integration of higher level of sensory, motor, cognitive, and perceptual skills (see Schaaf & Smith Roley, 2006).

The therapist creates playful activities that challenge the child's skills and uses astute observation of the child's ability to process and utilize sensory information during these playful activities. This is a critical skill for therapists using this frame of reference. The therapist observes the child's responses during the activity and increases or decreases the sensory and motor demands to create a challenging and therapeutic environment. The previous stated postulates regarding change guide the intervention.

Play is consistently described as an intrinsic aspect of intervention focusing on sensory integration. Play marks activities as being "fun" or pleasurable. As a result the child wants to participate in therapy because play promises that no matter how challenging therapy will be, it will also be fun. The child experiences joy despite effort and work, which supports the child's continued and necessary active participation. These play experiences maintain motivation and facilitate praxis. Additionally this allows the child to develop play skills and to encourage participation in play. The therapist–child relationship is a critical component of a sensory integration frame of reference. This therapeutic relationship must be strong to support the child to engage in challenging activities.

Finally, to ensure that the therapeutic process is in keeping with the goals and needs of the family and the school personnel as well as meeting the overall goal of improving participation in home, school, and community activities, it is essential for the therapist to communicate with parents and other people important to the child's continued development, such as teachers. Time must be available to have scheduled meetings with parents and teachers of children receiving occupational therapy using a sensory integration frame of reference. The initial meeting should focus on results of the evaluation and delineating goals and objectives of intervention as discussed previously. Goals must explicitly relate to improved participation in daily life activities across multiple contexts. In addition, ongoing exchanges should be conducted throughout the course of therapy. These meetings should be directed toward helping individuals understand the role of the sensory systems and praxis affecting the child's performance and participation at home, school, and in the community.

The Physical Environment of Intervention

The physical environment needs to have adequate space to allow for the flow of vigorous activity. The arrangement of the equipment and materials needs to be flexible enough to allow for rapid changes in configuration during an intervention session. There should be several ceiling hooks with adequate spacing to suspend hanging equipment. The hooks should be set up in such as way that rotational devices can be attached to the ceiling support, allowing for 360 degrees of rotation. Bungee cords should be available for use with the hanging suspended equipment. There should also be a quiet space such as a tent, adjacent room, or partially enclosed area.

As with all therapeutic interventions, safety must be maintained at all times in the therapy environment. This is ensured though the use of mats, cushions, and pillows that are used to pad the floor underneath all suspended equipment. Equipment should be adjustable to the size of the child. All equipment must be routinely checked for safety. Therapists should take great care in self-monitoring their own safe use of equipment.

The following are examples of ensuring safety within the therapeutic environment. The therapist may adjust the height, distance, or location of equipment to prevent the child from bumping into hard surfaces, a wall, or a person. The therapist may move mats or pillows to where the child might fall or bump. The therapist may stay close and be ready to move or stabilize the child or equipment. Whenever the child is in an inverted position, the therapist watches the neck position and must be ready to stabilize or position the neck to insure that the child does not fall on his or her head/neck or put excessive pressure on the neck. The therapist may stop moving equipment if a child is starting to get off in midflight or to keep equipment from bumping into the child. The therapist may position his/her body to block the child from a potentially unsafe action such as jumping off a bolster onto a hard surface.

Equipment

The following is a list of items that are highly recommended for an occupational therapy clinic that uses this frame of reference.

- Bouncing equipment
- Rubber strips or ropes for pulling
- Therapy balls
- Platform swing
- Platform glider
- Frog swing
- Scooter board and ramp
- Flexion disc
- Bolster swing
- Tire swing

- Weighted objects such as balls or bean bags in various sizes
- Inner tubes
- Spandex fabric
- Crash pillows
- Ball pit
- Vibrating toys or massagers
- Various tactile materials
- Visual targets
- Climbing equipment
- Barrel
- Props to support engagement in play (dress up clothes, sports equipment dolls, and puppets)
- Materials for practicing daily living skills (school tools, clothing, hygiene, and other home-related objects)

Therapeutic Interventions Related to Modulation

Once the treatment environment and milieu is in place, intervention can be initiated. The therapist provides the child with various sensory opportunities, with the intent of providing at least two of the following three types of sensation: tactile, vestibular, and proprioceptive. These sensations are provided beyond the normal presentation of sensation that a child experiences in daily life and are graded to a greater or lesser intensity depending on the needs of the child. Sensation may be central to the goal of the activity such as drawing designs in shaving cream or may be more incidental to the goal such as placing some textured materials in the child's path while engaged in another activity. The therapist emphasizes the use of additional sensory feedback to compensate for and enrich those sensory systems that have been identified to be of concern.

Sensory activities can be facilitating, inhibiting, or regulatory/modulating depending on the quality, intensity, and duration of the stimuli. Refer to Table 6.1 for a description of the various qualities of sensory stimuli in each sensory system.

The therapist provides light touch, textures, shapes, or deep touch pressure. This may be by directly touching the child's skin or through play activities with tactile media such as shaving cream or play dough, in a ball pit, in a cloth tunnel, in a Lycra or net swing, or with textured toys.

When treating a child with tactile over-responsivity or defensiveness, the therapist would use increased pressure touch (tactile input with moderate pressure such as a hug or heavy pillow placed on the child's back) and increased proprioceptive aspects of the activity to help the child manage and adapt to tactile stimuli during activities. The therapist encourages the child to choose the types of tactile media that he or she desires and that feel good. Allowing the child to self-initiate and self-administer the input may make the activity less aversive. Textures may be introduced in a graded manner, starting with less bothersome textures, usually in combination with deep pressure, proprioceptive, and/or vestibular activities. Vestibular stimulation is often needed before, during, and after tactile play to help the child stay calm and organized.

Children who demonstrated high arousal can be treated with the use of heavy work activities, such as movement against weight or resistance. The therapist can use deep touch pressure, with activities such as hugging, a massage, or squeezing between objects, which may be calming for some children. Decreasing light touch can also help decrease arousal. Reducing other sensory stimuli such as visual clutter, bright lights, and simultaneous auditory stimuli also tend to have a modulating effect on the processing of light touch.

The use of light or intermittent touch tends to be alerting. This can be provided through activities that utilize objects which provide light, intermittent touch such as playing dress up with a feather scarf, or by playing in a large ball pit that is filled with textured objects rather than small hard balls (Figure 6.19).

The therapist provides opportunities for the child to obtain linear, orbital, rotary stimulation, or a combination of these, during activities in which the head and body are moving through space. The therapist often uses suspended equipment such as swings, but may also create activities in which the child moves through space without suspension such as using a scooter board on an inclined ramp or jumping up and down on a trampoline.

FIGURE 6.19 Dress-up activities can facilitate discriminative and light touch to and improve arousal and discrimination.

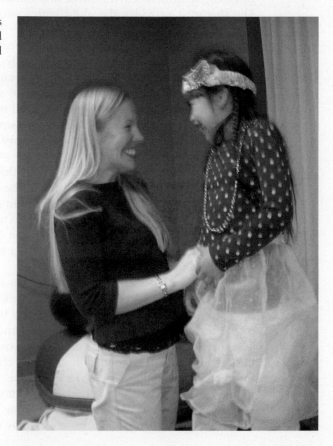

For children with low arousal in the vestibular system, the therapist would use fast, irregular (stop/start), and rotational movement, as these tend to be alerting. For children with high arousal in the vestibular system, the therapist would use slow, linear, and rhythmical movement as such movements tend to be calming. Increasing proprioceptive input or visual input during vestibular activities can help to modulate vestibular stimuli. Care should be taken in the use of visual stimuli because sometimes visual stimuli is disorganizing.

Children with gravitational insecurity require increased vertical movement and gradually moving the head and body in varied planes of space and against gravity during playful activities. These demands are graded slowly. It is helpful to initially allow the child to choose equipment that is on or close to the floor so that his or her feet remain in contact with the floor surface. The therapist needs to help the child feel safe. The therapist might encourage the child to practice falling onto soft pillows and mats. Proprioception can also be used to help the child modulate the "fear" response to movement.

The therapist provides experiences in which muscle tension, load, and stretch sensations (heavy work) are the dominant sensation. Heavy work is provided through active engagement of the child in movement activities that provide resistance or weight, which is greater than that experienced by the child during typical everyday activities. Such work activates the proprioceptive system by increasing the load on the muscles, requiring greater contraction of more muscle fibers and producing greater tension on the tendons. Heavy work can be incorporated through activities that require antigravity postures (such as a prone position in a net swing), weight bearing (such as climbing up an inclined ramp in quadruped), or increasing the weight that the child must negotiate during daily activities (such as using a backpack filled with books in it to walk from the classroom to the lunch room). Adding heavy work to activities can help decrease arousal and over-responsivity to sensory input. Common examples include having the child pull, push, or carry heavy/weighted objects/equipment; hang onto equipment or the therapist's hands; stretch; bear weight through the arms; extend or flex body against gravity (i.e., neck extension in prone).

A therapist can use proprioceptive input to influence arousal level. Increasing proprioceptive input tends to help facilitate optimal arousal (both calmness and alertness). Using activities that are constantly changing in their proprioceptive demands facilitate increased arousal. An example of such an activity might be alternating between pushing and pulling activities. Activities that require sustained muscle activity against gravity, such as using a rope to pull up a ramp while on a scooter board, are more likely to decrease arousal level.

When the therapist provides more than two types of sensory input (tactile, vestibular, or proprioceptive) then the child is more likely to develop self-regulation, sensory awareness, and an awareness of movement in space. The addition of such stimulation to motor activities in particular can facilitate body awareness. This can include using activities such as effort against gravity or moving with resistance from weight to increase proprioceptive feedback and awareness of one's body parts.

To improve somatodyspraxia, it is helpful to use proprioceptive activities to increase unconscious and conscious awareness of body position and body movement. This may be accomplished through practice with motor activities, use of a mirror while performing activities, and having the therapist and child talk through an activity to motor plan various novel activities.

Modulation of sensory stimuli is an important component of obtaining and maintaining optimal arousal level. Optimal arousal enables the child to participate in the activities with appropriate alertness, attention, comfort, and activity level. An optimal arousal level is necessary for the child to access environmental and sensory opportunities. For children with sensory modulation problems, specific sensory experiences might trigger overarousal. The child will have difficulty maintaining or regaining self-regulation during the activities and thus the role of the therapist is to (1) recognize the signs of overarousal, (2) try to modify the environment or the activities to decrease the likelihood of an overaroused response, and (3) utilize strategies to help the child maintain or regain self-regulation in the face of potentially disorganizing sensory activities. The therapist may challenge a child to expand his or her ability to maintain an optimal level of arousal in a more or less stimulating environment or with other challenging activities.

Therapeutic Interventions Related to Sensory Discrimination

Sensory discrimination is the natural next step after sensory modulation. Many of the techniques used for intervention in sensory modulation also apply to sensory discrimination. To help a child develop appropriate tactile discrimination, the child may discriminate size, shape, texture, location, and quality of a variety of tactile stimuli to various areas of the body with and without vision. For example, the child explores, feels, and identifies key aspects of objects without vision such as finding toys hidden in a bin of rice, guessing objects without seeing them, and finding a particular object in a container with other objects.

Tactile stimulation that forms the basis for somatodyspraxia includes providing the child with opportunities to encountering rich and varied stimuli to the skin, such as textured materials, while the child is performing motor actions. This helps to increase tactile feedback and awareness of one's body parts. Specific examples include stepping on, crawling over, hanging on, or moving through textured items such as fabrics, sheets, shaving cream, and so on. Rubbing textured items on the body before or during motor activities also helps to increase tactile awareness of one's body.

Therapeutic Interventions Related to Bilateral Integration and Sequencing

Children who are experiencing deficits in bilateral integration and sequencing require the therapist infuse vestibular input into activities involving increasing complexity of bilateral coordination and the timing of body movements. Common activities include targeting objects while in motion or coordinating one's body movements in time to achieve specified outcomes.

During playful activities, the child is encouraged to build postural tone against gravity through vestibular input. In dynamic movement activities, the child is required to stabilize his or her body, balance himself or herself, protect himself or herself from

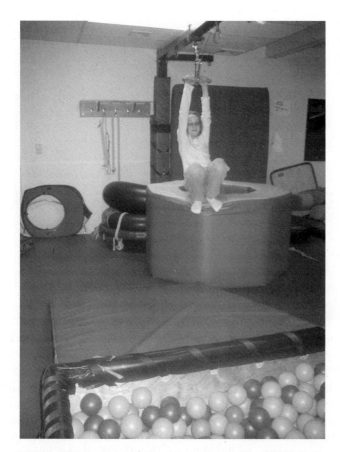

FIGURE 6.20 The therapist creates a playful environment in which the child actively pursues achievable challenges.

falling, and cocontract trunk and limbs during static and dynamic activities. Depending on whether the child has more difficulty when holding still, or when moving through space, the therapist provides activities that will gradually increase postural demands (Figure 6.20).

To develop postural, visual motor, visual perceptual skills, and bilateral integration, the therapist will provide various opportunities that are challenging to the child. This includes activities that will promote postural responses while in motion, the use of visual feedback while moving, and the use of two hands together. These activities are devised to be fun for the child so that the child will concentrate on the activity and responding, rather than thinking about using both hand together or maintaining his or her balance while in motion. These activities will promote postural, ocular, and bilateral motor development.

Therapeutic Interventions Related to Promoting Praxis

To encourage the ability to create ideas for planning and executing new and unfamiliar motor activities within the context of play, the therapist supports and guides the child's

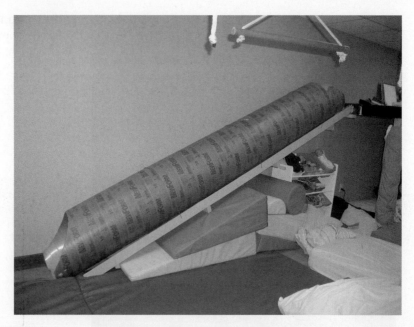

FIGURE 6.21 The environment contains equipment that is flexible in its use and can be used in varied ways and evokes creative problem solving in the child.

self-organization of behavior during play activities. This is accomplished by assuring that child-directed activities are a good match for the child's developing skills and abilities (the just right challenge) and covertly adjusts the environmental demands to ensure that the activity is successful (scaffolds the environment) (Figure 6.21). The therapist tailors or changes the activity in response to the child, so that the challenge presented to the child is not too difficult or too easy. The therapist presents or supports activities in which the child can be successful in response to sensory, motor, cognitive, or social challenge. The therapist allows the child to experience success in doing part or all of an activity. This promotes the development of self-esteem and self-confidence. Ultimately, involvement in such activities will facilitate self-regulation to provide positive and appropriate sensory and motor feedback utilized to develop body awareness and praxis.

The therapist treats the child as an active collaborator in the therapy process. The therapist provides structure and support for adaptive responses while allowing the child to be actively in control as much as possible in the choice of activities. This assists the child in developing ideational praxis. The therapist does not predetermine activities independently of the child.

SAMPLE INTERVENTION SESSION

The key components presented above represent a sophisticated blend of clinical reasoning embedded in the occupational therapy process and the theoretical principles of the sensory integration frame of reference. The intervention process is fluid and dynamic, as the therapist constantly evaluates and reevaluates the child's strengths, needs, and skills required for participation in life activities. An example of a typical session is shown in Table 6.12.

During treatment, goals and progress are recorded by noting observable changes in the child's ability to participate in sensory-based activities, regulate arousal level, increase repertoire of sensory motor skills, and improved ability to participate independently in daily life activities (see Schaaf & Nightlinger, 2007). In addition to direct intervention

TABLE 6.12 A Typical Treatment Session Using this Frame of Reference for a Child with Sensory Integrative Disorder (Schaaf & Miller, 2005)

Activity	Purpose	Example	Comments
Warm up	To ensure that the child is comfortable and relaxed for play	Greeting and playful interactions: "Hi did you come to play with X today?" What would you like to play with today?[a]	Favorite game is tossing bean bags at a large stuffed bear in attempt to knock it over
Active sensory motor play with a focus on multi-sensory input	To decrease sensory sensitivities and increase praxis	Swinging on space bag and crashing into large pillows and bolsters Space bag is set low to ground to offset any fear that the child might have and to encourage independence during this activity	Therapist sets up an environment with the child's needs in mind and then observes child, following the child's cues, to select activity[b]
Active sensory motor play with a focus on praxis	To decrease sensory sensitivities, improve awareness of body, and increase praxis	Therapist helps the child create a "bridge" (two triangular climbing devices with a flat bolster suspended between them) The child climbs up ladder (with assistance), climbs onto bolster, and then the child dumps into large "crash pad" (pillows)[c]	Therapist vigilantly observes the child's reactions and actions, encouraging the child as needed but allowing for as much self-direction and independence as possible[d]
Snack with a focus on socialization	To decrease oral sensitivities, expand food repertoire, and enhance socialization	The child brings a snack to share with another child; the child sets up snack, invites other child, and participates in snack	Mother packs food and beverage that the child enjoys in addition to one or two foods that the child is not familiar with or usually avoids

Therapy is contextualized in sensory-rich play and taps into the child's inner drive for competence (Ayres, 1979). The therapist artfully and skillfully creates enticing, achievable challenges for the child to promote the ability to process and integrate sensory information, and observes adaptive responses to these challenges (Schaaf & Nightlinger, 2007).

[a]If no response: I have your favorite game ready, do you want to play?

[b]Upgrade—add tactile and motor planning component (count to 3 and "crash" into pillows).

[c]If child is not willing to climb up to bridge, therapist downgrades by lowering ladder.

[d]Therapist uses playful language (singing) or pretend play (climbing into spaceship).

with the child, the therapist interacts and collaborates with parents, teachers, and others who are involved with the child to (1) help them understand and reframe the child's behavior from a sensory perspective, (2) adapt the environment to the needs of the child, (3) create needed sensory and motor experiences throughout the day in natural environments, and (4) assure that therapy is helping the child become more functional in daily life activities (Schaaf & Smith Roley, 2006).

The sensory integration frame of reference is a complex, multifaceted treatment approach that requires dynamic clinical reasoning based on the theoretical base. The following two case studies describe the clinical reasoning for assessment and intervention with children who have different types of sensory processing disorders. These case studies represent useful models of best practice that will assist therapists in learning and applying this frame of reference.

Michael's Case Study

Michael is a 2-year-old only child of a married couple, who are very devoted to him and to his progress. They also hold very positive beliefs about his ability to change, and develop increasingly more competent skills with therapy. Although they live in a relatively small two-bedroom home, they expressed a willingness to do whatever was recommended by his team of professionals to help him at home. Although on the autism spectrum, Michael clearly has a bond with his parents and prefers to have them with him. During unstructured time, Michael prefers to run around the room making only fleeting eye contact. Sometimes he will hide behind his parents, or, when he seems stressed, he looks quickly to them to reference them. He frequently flicks his mother's hair as a method of self-soothing. Michael has a few words and he will use his own signs to communicate such as tapping a toy to indicate his desire to have help with operating it such as tapping a square music cube to have the adult press the side to start the music. Michael's parents are a strong support for him and are an important part of his intervention process.

Shortly before Michael was referred for an occupational therapy assessment, he was diagnosed as having pervasive developmental disorder-not otherwise specified (PDD-NOS) and began receiving early intervention services. His parents were concerned about his difficulty going to sleep and waking up periodically throughout the night and resultant lack of sleep. Additionally, he had a limited repertoire of foods, which was believed to be due in part to reflux. They were also concerned with the frequency and intensity with which he seeks sensory input. They suspect that his excessive sensory seeking may be an attempt to help regulate his state of arousal. They are also concerned about his limited language skills and lack of willingness to use his hands to play with toys, other than using objects to "bonk" or hit against his arm or another surface. His lack of interest in playing with other children or any ability to engage in simple games such as peek-a-boo or hide and seek, or any form of imaginative play was also a concern. Overall, they feel that his strong need to try and regulate himself using sensory input interferes with his ability to focus on tasks and develop skills. These behaviors limit Michael's occupational performance.

Evaluation: Process and Results

Michael's parents completed a sensory history and spoke with a therapist by phone for an initial intake screening. The therapist wanted to determine if the presenting problems and difficulties with occupational performance might be related to sensory motor deficits. On the basis of these data, it seemed that there were sensory motor concerns that may benefit from further assessment and then participation in occupational therapy using a sensory integrative frame of reference. For example, the parents reported that his responses to auditory stimuli were variable—at times he was highly sensitive to sounds and at other times he appeared not to hear sounds at all. The same sound could be both bothersome and ignored. He was also reported to be easily overstimulated by visual stimuli including most of the available television programs for children. He was also reported to be particular about the types of textures he would allow in his mouth and touching his skin. He had difficulty with playground equipment and only liked to go on equipment which could have under his full control, such as climbing apparatus. As an infant, Michael was reported to have difficulty nursing and to be a poor sleeper. He had a short crawling phase and was an early walker.

The first step for the therapist was to determine what would be the appropriate assessments to use to evaluate sensory and motor areas. Owing to his parent's observations of Michael in his home environment and the therapist's ability to read earlier reports from his early intervention program, it was determined that an observational assessment of his responses to sensation, play, and engagement in daily life activities would be best suited to his needs as Michael would not be able to participate in standardized testing. During the evaluation, Michael showed a high state of arousal as noted by either a constant state of movement, either running around the room or "bonking" with an object, or hiding behind his mother. It was quickly noted that Michael had significant difficulty modulating sensory information. He became easily overstimulated by any background auditory stimulation as well as visual, tactile, and vestibular input in the environment. Observations of his behavior also revealed a variable response to vestibular sensations with an inconsistent desire to swing in infant swings that appeared to be related to the speed of the swing and how quickly he was pushed after getting into the swing. His parents indicated that he loved rough house play with Dad and that it was his favorite activity. He showed signs of poor proprioceptive awareness and motor planning challenges as he had difficulty trying to climb over low bolsters to reach his Dad. Also, when trying to imitate pushing the side of a music cube to turn the music back on, he did not use the appropriate amount of force. During a typical day, Michael would usually "bonk" objects for a minimum of 4 to 5 hours and seek hair twirling for 1 to 2 hours. If his mother allowed him to twirl her hair as long as he wanted, he would typically twirl it for 45 minutes at a time. He enjoyed his baths and often his parents found that he would give more visual engagement to a new toy when introduced in the bathtub. He could be taken out in a stroller, but could not walk outside with an adult as he would not hold hands and did not have any safety awareness for moving about a playground or taking a walk on a sidewalk.

The therapist's impression was that during the observation, Michael was very overwhelmed by a new environment, and the examiner and the novel opportunities for exploration that were offered to him. From the results of the sensory history, it appeared that Michael demonstrated sensory over-responsiveness/defensiveness to light touch, as he would pull quickly away when this was applied. In response to auditory and visual stimuli, Michael would appear to tune out when entering a room with many other children. This was interpreted as an indication of overload and an attempt to withdraw or shutdown from the auditory and visual input. Although this may be primarily a modulation problem, there is often an underlying discrimination problem for children. This may include poor discrimination regarding the location of the auditory input, and potentially visual spatial problems along with difficulty using ocular skills to locate objects visually. These problems may increase stress and heighten arousal. In addition, he was unwilling to explore any of the tactile bins offered to him, including those holding corn, rice, bean, or cornstarch. He also was unwilling to try any food or candy offered to him and often scrunched up his nose to indicate that he found the smell of the food unpleasant. His parents commented that he did not seem to like any sweets. It appears that his deficits in occupational performance are strongly related to his underlying sensory integration.

The evaluation also revealed that he had very limited postrotary nystagmus following 20 seconds of rotation and a great deal of difficulty organizing this type of input. He responded by looking dazed and overwhelmed and he did not wish to repeat the experience, evidencing that he was not able to organize vestibular input well. He exhibited difficulty with ocular control, low muscle tone, postural stability, and righting and equilibrium reactions. When seated in a swing with support, such as sitting in a "buddy boat" swing or inside an inner tube on a square platform swing, he was unable to sustain an upright position while in the swing and was leaning heavily into the swing. Although he could walk and run, he could not yet climb and hence avoided all ladders and stairs. He had great difficulty with motor planning, and needed to be helped in and out of swings and onto other pieces of equipment. He did not readily see the affordances in the room and, therefore, ran around rather than engaging independently in the opportunities the room presented.

The evaluation also revealed that Michael was able to engage in only limited interaction. He enjoyed up and down bouncing movement in the spandex hammock, where he could be fully supported while receiving deep touch pressure from the Lycra material (stretchy fabric), and could bang his leg to indicate he wanted more swinging. He was not able to indicate a desire for repeated movement or engagement with other activities. Further, Michael declined the use of crayons or other markers and he was not able to play with toys designed for 8- to 12-month babies with simple push operation. He was able to pick up Cheerios with his fingers and bring those to his mouth. He was unwilling to attempt to blow any infant whistles.

Overall, the evaluation indicated that Michael has sensory modulation difficulties. It appears that the modulation of all types of incoming sensations increases his arousal and keeps him in a constant state of flight or agitation. This makes it difficult for him to fall asleep and stay asleep or to feel safe enough to allow separation from primary caregivers. In addition, this high state of arousal may contribute to his sustained reflux and his constant need for self-soothing sensations from his "bonking," a largely proprioceptive and visual activity, and from twisting his mother's hair, a tactile and proprioceptive activity. The evaluation also found that he has difficulty discriminating proprioceptive and vestibular input, and most likely tactile stimulation, although this could not be adequately assessed at this time given his unwillingness to explore tactile materials. These difficulties do not allow him to have adequate body awareness for beginning play skills or motor planning of his own actions, which are necessary for successfully engaging in interactive play. Games such as peek-a-boo and hide and seek rely on a strong sense of object permanence as well as a strong internal sense of body scheme. In addition, his difficulty with postural and ocular skills does not allow him to sustain the initial phase of interactive activities. This affected his eye gaze and shared attention that allows for initiation of a play activity, his coordinated oral activities such as blowing bubbles, his eye–hand coordination activities such as using crayons or markers, and his total body movements such as climbing in and out of unfamiliar pieces of equipment at or near floor level.

Goals for Intervention

The immediate focus for Michael's occupational therapy intervention was in three main areas: sensory modulation to help regulate arousal level, sensory discrimination as a basis for body awareness and praxis, and postural and ocular control.

In terms of sensory modulation, it was critical to help Michael improve his ability to modulate sensation so that he could regulate his arousal level and stay organized in new and familiar environments. This became the first goal for intervention. In addition, since Michael had only rudimentary abilities to self-regulate, it was essential to help him through giving the parents and his caregivers' ways to help him to regulate. This included helping him learn that he could seek caregivers to provide him with activities that were regulating for him.

The second goal was to improve sensory discrimination of auditory, visual, gustatory, tactile, proprioceptive, and vestibular input as a basis for improved body awareness and praxis needed for participation in developmentally appropriate and meaningful activities. Specifically, the therapist wanted Michael to participate in play activities with his parents. This involved clear interpretation of sensory stimuli, knowledge of his body, and the ability to innately plan out movements (motor planning) to participate in the play activities.

The third goal was to develop ocular, postural, and oral skills to support his ability to use his eyes to gain needed information for play and interactions; postural skills to support his movement during play and oral motor skills to provide a foundation for language/speaking.

Lastly, Michael needed to use his self-regulation, praxis, postural, ocular, and oral skills to initiate and sustain simple plans for social and emotional engagement with parents, caregivers, and peers. In this way, Michael will lay the foundation for skill acquisition of language, cognitive, and motor abilities.

The Intervention Plan

In Michael's case, there is interplay between sensory modulation and sensory discrimination. Both areas need to be addressed. First, to help him attain and sustain a regulated state, it was necessary to work on sensory modulation and self-regulation simultaneously. In addition, sensory discrimination and postural, ocular, oral skills will allow him a greater ability to modulate incoming sensations, so both problem areas are addressed in tandem. Michael's intervention plan included individual therapy at a private occupational therapy clinic twice per week. The clinic setting offered the specialized equipment that Michael needed to begin to modulate and discriminate sensory information. Some clinical interventions included methods used to accomplish this included slow rocking in the platform swing and buddy boat as well as through deep squishes between two large foam-filled pillows, (Figure 6.22) and by singing rhythmical children's songs such as "Row-Row-Row Your Boat." Coupling songs with movement allowed Michael to begin to have a sense of predictability over the beginning and end of the movement. Michael's parent or nanny was present during all clinic treatment sessions in order to assist in helping to regulate him as well as to learn new ways to mutually regulate (Table 6.13).

FIGURE 6.22 Total body pressure touch (provided by large inflatables) and proprioception (provided by resistance to body [prone against gravity] and arms) can help to modulate tactile over-responsivity.

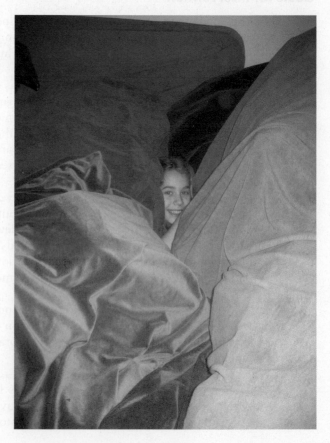

TABLE 6.13 Example of a Treatment Session for Michael

Activity	Purpose	Example	Comments
Warm up	To ensure that the child is comfortable; Sensory processing of vestibular stimuli to increase vestibular discrimination and improve body awareness needed for play and praxis	Slow gentle swings in the buddy boat with full support and frequent stops to allow for processing of the vestibular input; the therapist sings different songs for different directions of movement to start to give some way to differentiate the different ways his head and body were moving in space	Michael will make fleeting eye contact and at times move his body to indicate that he would like the swing to move again. He also seems to enjoy the songs the therapist sings as he would bonk more if the songs were discontinued
Active sensory motor play with a focus on praxis	To decrease sensory sensitivities, improve awareness of body, and increase praxis as a basis for appropriate play and interactions	After an initial period of 20 mins of organizing vestibular and proprioceptive input, a large tactile bin was put into the buddy boat swing for Michael to engage with while swinging; scoops were present to allow him to try and scoop and dump the beans	Therapist models the activity and also has a peer demonstrate the actions encouraging Michael's self-exploration as well as modeling of the other child's actions needed
Fine motor exploration	To increase ability to use toys; to allow for independent play activities rather than only self-stimulation	Michael is shown how to use the music cube and is assisted in pressing on the sides indicating different instruments with hand over hand motions	The therapist assists and then waits to allow time for Michael to take her hand or make a verbal indication of his desire to have another instrument played. She is careful to not allow him to be frustrated but rather to immediately respond to any indication of his desire to create sounds with the cube

Since vision was a strong sensory channel for him, the speech and language therapist assisted the parents in developing many ways to help Michael communicate using visual cues including creating computer games to facilitate problem solving. For example, they created a "Where's Daddy" video where his father would hide and Michael could use the mouse to click on different spots in the video image of the room to find his father. They also would create videos of places he would visit and ones including his friends, therapists, and teachers. These computer videos were very motivating for him before manipulation of three-dimensional toys.

Progress

Over the next several months, Michael began to show progress in his ability to modulate sensory stimuli and develop mutual regulation. In occupational therapy, he would stay on swings for longer periods of time, increasing from several minutes to 5 to 10 minutes as long as the therapist used frequent stops and starts combined with proprioceptive input to his legs as she used pulling of his legs to help change the movement of the swing. He was able to go to his parents and show them what he needed. For example, he might pull them to a large therapy ball to request bouncing to help with self-regulation. As his vestibular processing improved, Michael began to seek more challenging movements and postures. He and his Dad made up a game of having him slung over his Dad's back and hung upside down. Initially during this game, Michael hung freely, but over time, he would push up on his Dad's back, engaging his extensor muscles to look around while upside down demonstrating improved antigravity postural control. Later he began to enjoy side-to-side movement and greatly enjoyed when his Dad would hang him upside physically and swing him side to side as he twisted. Michael responded with improved postural and righting responses. These activities provided strong input to both Michael's semicircular canals as well as his gravity receptors while also providing strong proprioceptive input. In the home, toys were added, such as cans of different weights (filled with the original canned goods) on his low shelves in his room for him to take on and off and provide needed proprioceptive input in the context of an activity. A tactile bin of rice and beans with hidden toys in it was also added to work on tactile discrimination and manipulative hand skills.

Initially, during the clinic-based therapy, the "warm-up" phase took up most of the session. This was because the goal of self-regulation and modulation of sensory input was the focus. In addition, it was critical that a sense of physical and emotional safety be established for Michael before any other effective work could be done. This phase involved the use of a pillow for deep pressure input (Figure 6.23), controlled swinging in one of the suspended swings with adequate time in between swings to allow him to process the input.

As Michael was better able to process sensory input, he was able to tolerate higher and faster side-to-side movements in swings and we began to work on posture and strength. For example, we used a platform swing with a tube inside and the buddy boat. He began to sign "more" and make direct eye contact with his therapist to indicate he wanted more of this swinging when the swing stopped suggesting that his posture,

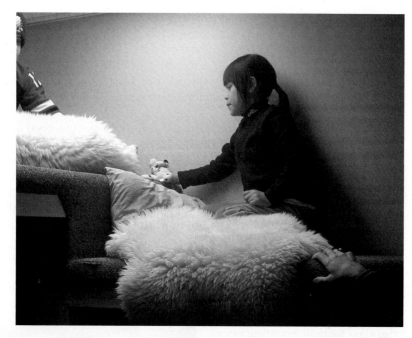

FIGURE 6.23 Tactile discrimination activities help build the differential awareness needed for movement and coordination.

oculomotor control, and interaction skills were improving. His sensory modulation also began to improve. Initially, it took 30 seconds or so for him to appear to fully register the input and then indicate he wanted more. As he was better able to organize this input, he would very rapidly indicate he wanted more as soon as the swing was stopped. The therapist used singing to help give a beginning and end to each period of swinging so that he could come to predict the changes in movement as well. At first, Michael was silent during treatment, but as he began to better process vestibular input he began to make vocalizations similar to a young infant who is experimenting with sound production.

Initially, Michael did not want to play in the ball pool or inside any tunnels or club houses. This is not unusual for a child who does not have a good sense of his own body and needs to use visual, auditory, and tactile contact to maintain his connection with others to help him know his whereabouts. In addition, the postural control needed to move oneself into and out of the ball pool was initially too challenging for him. But eventually, Michael could go into the ball pool with a therapist or caregiver and enjoy it. The therapist enhanced the experience of the sensation of tactile and proprioceptive input by playing a pulling game where he extended his arms to be pulled out of the pool again and again. At this time, his sleep also began to improve. It appeared that his improved self-regulation, sensory modulation, and increased knowledge of where he was in space resulted in a lower resting state of arousal, making falling asleep easier.

Eventually, Michael was able to use his postural muscles to move himself around in the swings, rather than being completely dependent. First he began to sit up, then moved into prone on elbows, then he moved into kneel standing and later standing while the swing continued to move. The day he moved to stand on his own while the swing was moving at a good pace, joy spread over his face—he knew this was an amazing accomplishment without any need for external praise, the ultimate in sensory integration intervention.

Michael's sensory discrimination also improved as evidenced in his improved body awareness, postural skills, and praxis. He began to propel swings independently. He could lie over the frog swing (a swing on a bungee cord with a large strap for the child to lie prone across) on his belly and propel the swing with his feet. Over time, he also began to hold on to a hula-a-hoop or the therapist's hands to be propelled. As he gained greater mastery of moving himself on a swing in the clinic, he began to do the same at home in his doorway swing. He also began to do simple oral motor plans such as blowing soap bubbles. Simultaneously, he began to say words, and could now say "swing, more, stop, again" sometimes combining two words such as "more swing" (Figure 6.24).

Despite the many gains that had occurred, his sensitivities to sound could still be acute, which he could now show us by covering his hands with his ears and crying out.

FIGURE 6.24 Providing activities that allow for head movement in various planes facilitates the vestibular systems and thus provides information about body and head position needed for posture and balance.

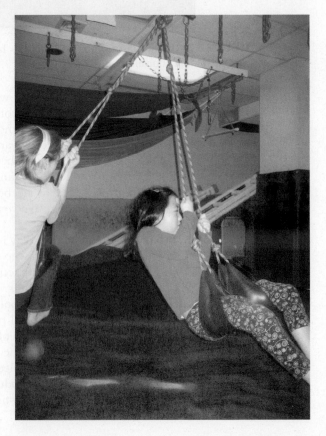

In some ways, it appeared that he had increased in his sensitivity in this area. But it was felt that initially he was so sensitive that he would move into overload and shutdown and his system would block out the sounds. Now, his apparent greater sensitivity was seen as progress, as he was able to stay with the incoming sensation without becoming overloaded and communicate to us that it was too much. Headphones, playing classical music, were introduced at this point which he was initially reluctant to try, but after several sessions where his mother held them lightly over his ears while he listened, he wanted the headphones and the organizing Mozart music. When the headphones went on, any self-stimulatory behavior would tend to stop immediately. His preschool made sure to have headphones available in the free play area for him to use during school to block out sounds.

Michael began to motor plan and sequence during activities, for instance pushing himself prone on the buddy boat swing, then running up and down a ramp, and then repeating this sequence. He started to copy other children's play for brief periods of time, especially if they were doing a climbing activity. He could now manipulate toys such as putting large coins in a bank and turn the handles on a busy box to gain access to the toy. But most importantly, he seemed to become increasingly relaxed and to smile more, at times grinning as he engaged in activities.

At 3.5 years, Michael was able to enter an integrated preschool program. Although very tired at the end of each half day, he was delighted to be there and would often point to the photos of his friends at school and the activities offered there on his computer at home. Initially he was not able to sit at circle time initially. After engaging in sensory strategies with his aide, such as bouncing prior to circle time and sitting in a chair that sits flat on the floor with a back support, he began to attend and participate in circle time. At home, Michael was able to go on family walks without running at all times and could sit at restaurants as well. These two activities were not stated goals at the beginning of the intervention; however, it became apparent that these would enhance the family's ability to engage in favorite occupations.

Through the use of the sensory integration frame of reference for intervention with Michael, he has been able to demonstrate improved self-regulation and modulation. He demonstrates an increased sense of body awareness, which was a necessary foundation for improved praxis. Most importantly, because of these gains, Michael has been able to interact more appropriately with his parents and peers. He has been able to enter an integrated preschool and has begun to engage in developmentally appropriate activities. The gains that Michael has made during this intervention have supported his involvement in positive functional occupational performance, at home, in school, and in his community.

Sophie's Case Study

Sophie is 7 years old and is the second child of a married couple, Tony and Maria, originally from Guatemala. Her older sister is 2 years older. They have a loving extended family that includes two sets of grandparents, aunts, uncles and cousins, and several routine caregivers who are very engaged with Sophie and her brother. Her parents are most focused on Sophie gaining in her academic skills, as the parents and older brother are very successful in their cognitive pursuits. There is a history of coordination problems in the family, so there is not a high value placed on physical activities. The family enjoys nature and taking walks but does not engage in biking, skiing, skating, or any individual or team sports.

Sophie was referred for an occupational therapy assessment by her speech and language therapist. The therapist identified verbal apraxia and suspects other sensory and motor delays that might benefit from occupational therapy intervention. The parent's primary concern was about Sophie's ability to sit and eat dinner with the family. They reported that Sophie had great difficulty sitting through meals and using utensils. They also reported that she had great difficulty getting dressed in the morning even when they laid out her clothes for her ahead of time. They also noted that although Sophie was a very warm and friendly child, she was not forming friendships in school where other children would invite her for a play date or to a birthday party. They commented that the other children in class seemed fond of her but that she seemed more like a pet to them rather than a peer.

The occupational therapist at her school previously completed an assessment focusing primarily on fine motor skills. She noticed some sensory issues and developed a sensory diet to help Sophie access classroom instruction. The speech pathologist felt that an occupational therapy assessment done outside of the school using the SIPT would be a good complement to the school assessments in helping the team to design a thorough Individual Educational Plan (IEP). Currently her IEP includes small group instruction for difficulties in reading and in mathematics.

Evaluation: Process and Results

During the evaluation, it was critical to determine if Sophie's problems in occupational performance related to sensory motor deficits. Her parents completed a sensory history and participated in a phone intake process with the occupational therapist conducting the assessment. There were many reports of sensory motor issues. Although Sophie was not reported to be overly sensitive to incoming sensations, she was reported to have difficulty coordinating her body and moving her body through space. Her parents noted that sometimes Sophie looks at her hands as though her hands were unfamiliar tools and their sense was that she did not have very good body awareness. They commented that when she took a bath, she would only wash herself with very large general motions, not seeming to be able to really scrub her arm and leg in its entirety, even though she appeared to be trying to do her best. In addition, Sophie was reported to have a low frustration tolerance with frequent comments that she could not do many age-appropriate activities and needed help. These behaviors are common for a child with dyspraxia and thus, it was recommended that Sophie obtain a complete assessment of sensory integration and praxis using the SIPT.

When Sophie came to the clinic, the SIPT was administered along with clinical observations and free play observations in the therapy rooms. It was also deemed important to observe Sophie both at school and at home.

When observing Sophie in her home environment, she did not seem to easily find things to play with. Her parents report that she is content to watch videos and do rough house play with her brother. These were two activities she was observed to initiate. When shown age-appropriate puzzles, construction tasks, or fine motor activities that were present in her playroom, she declined engagement. Her mother commented that she did not engage in those activities unless her brother or one of her parents did them with her. Her mother stated that those activities were not her preferred activities. However, her family did find that when given scraps of paper and a glue stick she greatly enjoyed making a collage.

While observing her during eating, it was noted that Sophie initially got in and out of her chair frequently and picked up all the food on her plate with her fingers. During one of her times up and out of the chair and moving around the kitchen, the examiner took her to the playroom and bounced her on a therapy ball that she had brought with her and gave Sophie sensory input to her hands using a bin of rice to search for objects. The examiner had learned from the school occupational therapist that tactile preparatory activities could be helpful to Sophie's engagement with fine motor activities. After this input, Sophie was able to return to the table and sit for 10 minutes and when handed her fork was able to use it to spear her food seven or eight times before putting it down and reverting to use of her fingers. This observation suggested that Sophie was neither processing tactile input well, and therefore was not aware of her hands, nor using them to explore and interact with her environment. In addition, the observed response to vestibular input suggested that Sophie required movement stimulation to help increase her attention and focus on activities. The therapist suspected that the movement input not only improved her awareness of her body and therefore her ability to move smoothly but also increased her arousal level to improve attention and focus.

When the evaluating therapist observed Sophie in the classroom, she noted that Sophie would often stop and observe the actions of the other children as they moved about the classroom, cafeteria, and playground at recess. The therapist reasoned that Sophie seemed to have difficulty both watching and then initiating an action. For example, it was quite difficult for her to both watch the children play and move her body so that she could socialize with them. Therefore, Sophie mostly engaged in her own independent play or simple watched the other children.

Building on her experience with Sophie during the home observation, the therapist reasoned that enhancing vestibular and tactile opportunities for Sophie may provide her with the sensory input needed to initiate purposeful movement and interactions. The therapist tried placing a Move n' Sit cushion in her chair to increase vestibular and tactile input. This seemed to be quite useful and organizing for her. Sophie was able to imitate the other children during a coloring activity suggesting that the input served to increase her arousal level and provide better body awareness needed for her to combine "watching and doing" during coloring. The therapist also provided a small bin with tactile materials (textured objects) prior to handwriting. Play in the tactile bin prior to handwriting activities seemed to increase Sophie's interest in picking up a pencil and trying to write, although the formation of letters was very laborious for her. It appeared that each letter must be planned out and was not automatically written, as one would expect of a second grader. Her teacher commented that she seemed to do the best when she had visual models and that she also loved art class and seemed to have some nice innate art abilities.

In addition to the observation data gathering in the home and classroom, the therapist completed the SIPT. During the evaluation, Sophie frequently asked the examiner how she was doing. She often requested that items be repeated, indicating that she was not feeling comfortable with being able to competently complete the test items. Sophie needed frequent breaks to complete all of the SIPT, but was always amenable to returning to the table tasks once a movement break was given.

The analysis of Sophie's SIPT revealed that Sophie has dyspraxia. Her scores on all of the SIPT were below −1.0 SD (design copying −2.2 SD, constructional praxis −2.4 SD, sequencing praxis −1.8 SD, praxis on verbal command −2.0 SD, postural praxis −2.7 SD, oral praxis −2.1 SD, and bilateral motor coordination −1.6 SD). In addition, Sophie's test scores indicated significant somatosensory delays. She received a score of −1.1 SD on kinesthesia, and there were many clinical observations (Blanche, 2002) that supported poor proprioceptive awareness. These included great difficulty doing thumb to finger touching especially with eyes closed, and segmented and jerky performance when completing slow controlled movements. Her scores on manual form perception −2.5 SD, finger identification −1.4 SD, and graphesthesia −1.4 SD all indicated tactile discrimination difficulties. In addition, she appeared to have some difficulty processing vestibular input. Although her score on postrotary nystagmus was −0.7 SD, she appeared to crave rotary movement. Other vestibular-related observations were poor prone extension, poor standing balance, especially with eyes closed, and poor ocular control, especially when following objects across midline.

In addition, Sophie had difficulty with space visualization −1.7 SD, but scored adequately on figure ground −0.3 SD. These findings suggest that Sophie has some difficulty with visual spatial skills, but relative strength in figure ground. This was consistent with her teacher's comments that learning through her visual system seemed to be a strength for Sophie. Although it seems paradoxical that Sophie used her visual system as a learning strength when her space visualization score was significantly low, children with poor body awareness, and especially poor vestibular processing, tend to also demonstrate poor visual spatial skills even when the visual system is a strong learning channel. The difficulty in spatial perception stems from poor awareness of self and objects in space, and this further underscores the need for Sophie to develop better body and spatial awareness.

Another finding was that Sophie was unable to sustain the supine flexion position against gravity for more than 1 or 2 seconds. At age 7, a child should be able to sustain supine flexion for at least 10 seconds (Blanche, 2002). On further assessment, it was noted that Sophie continued to have some head lag in pull to sit. This also supported the observation of poor antigravity flexion. Using typical development as a reference point, the therapist reasoned that this is a position where the infant explores his or her hands and brings hands, toes, and objects to their mouth. It appeared that this developmental stage of body exploration that assists the child in creating needed patterns for body scheme had most likely been largely absent for Sophie and contributed further to her poor body awareness and poor use of hands to explore and learn.

In the clinic, Sophie stood and stared at the equipment (whereas most children will actively explore and play on the enticing sensory motor equipment of a typical sensory integration clinic). When invited to explore the Jump 'n' Play, she asked what to do with it. When encouraged to explore it, she got inside and stood in the middle and said, "I do not want to play jail." The affordance of jumping on the inner tube and holding onto the metal bars while standing on the outside of the structure needed to be modeled for Sophie, suggesting that she was unable to develop and execute new motor plans for play and interaction.

When alone in a clinic room, Sophie would stay engaged with each activity the therapist helped her to initiate for at least several minutes, but if another child entered the room, she would immediately stop and stare at the other child. This behavior was very consistent with the behavior observed in her school. Sophie had great difficulty "watching and doing" simultaneously, for example trying to throw and catch. She could catch a large ball, but did not adjust the size of her hands to catch a smaller ball. She lost her balance while trying to kick a ball to the therapist. She was not able to pump a swing, gallop, or skip. She also was observed to have an immature fisted grasp on her pencil and she was not yet able to effectively cut more than a short straight line with scissors.

It was the impression of the therapist that Sophie demonstrated somatosensory-based dyspraxia. She has poor body awareness because she is not obtaining adequate input from her tactile and proprioceptive systems. Thus, her "body maps" are lacking and her spontaneous ability to use her body to play, learn, socialize, and engage in daily life activities is delayed. In addition, Sophie demonstrates poor vestibular processing, which impacts on her postural and ocular control and balance. As a result, Sophie does not have adequate awareness and orientation of herself in space, and does not have the mature postural and balance reactions needed to support the movement needed to act and interact with her environment.

Goals for Intervention

Following the assessment, a parent meeting was held to relate the results of the assessment to her presenting problems. Given the extent of her somatosensory concerns and her poor praxis on all subtests of the SIPT, it was felt that her difficulty in eating dinner was directly related to her difficulty with both postural abilities and praxis, contributed to by poor underlying somatosensory discrimination problems. In addition, her difficulty with pencil and scissor use was also related to this poor somatosensory awareness of her hands and her poor ability to plan her movements with these tools.

Her difficulty with dressing in the morning was also related to her poor somatosensory processing and poor praxis. Her social participation difficulties also seemed related to her poor overall praxis as she appeared to have to use cognition to do many motor tasks that other children in her age could do easily and automatically. In addition, she did not yet have some of the basic coordination skills that her peers had such as pumping a swing, skipping, or galloping, resulting from her somatosensory and vestibular problems. Therefore she did not have the same repertoire of skills many others had on the playground or within the classroom or physical education class.

Thus, Sophie's goals focused on (1) improving sensory processing (tactile, vestibular, and proprioceptive) and body awareness and (2) facilitation of praxis as a basis for improved participation in activities of daily living (such as eating and dressing), school (such as handwriting and other learning activities), and play/socialization with her peers.

The Intervention Plan

Within each session, the activity warm-up phase was rich with somatosensory and vestibular sensations. The goal was to increase arousal and improve sensory registration and processing of input to enhance Sophie's body awareness. Sophie would often enter the session seeming to be tired or in a state of lower arousal. However, with opportunities for strong sensory input such as lying on top of an air pillow and trying to maintain her position while being bounced by her therapist as she sang "Pop Goes The Weasel" and then eventually crashing onto nearby large pillows, Sophie's affect would increase as would her state of arousal and she would show more initiation in the subsequent activities.

The next phase of the intervention focused on sensory motor play that would promote praxis. The therapist focused on improving postural control using vestibular activities that included a "just right" postural challenge. Often, the next activity would typically involve working on whole body flexion while seated on the Flexion Disc swing to provide an "achievable challenge" for total body flexion as Sophie used flexion to hold on and stay on the swing (Figure 6.25). The therapist chose to keep the swing positioned close to the ground and provide slight bounces provided by a bungee cord to further increase arousal and vestibular input. The deep touch pressure and proprioception from this activity helped to activate the flexor muscles to help her develop the postural skills needed to stay on the swing. Getting on and off the swing was the initial praxis challenge. Over time, Sophie developed successful motor plans and ideas for getting her body on and off the swing, even when the therapist adjusted the challenge by moving the swing higher. Eventually, the therapist also jostled and swung the swing more fully to challenge Sophie's posture and praxis, and Sophie could eventually reach out with one

FIGURE 6.25 For children with low arousal, movement in various planes can help facilitate posture, muscle tone, body awareness, and increase arousal level.

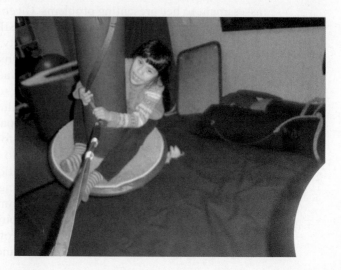

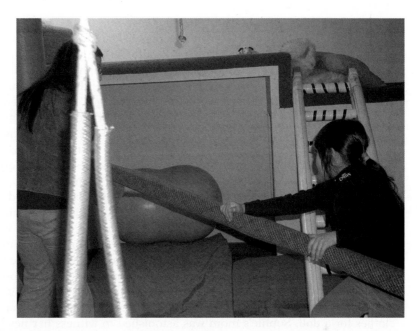

FIGURE 6.26 Increasing the load on muscles facilitates the proprioceptors and provides additional input from muscles, tendons, and joints.

hand and try to hit punching bags or "space aliens" hanging nearby. This allowed her to work on more and more sophisticated praxis skills with large objects (Figure 6.26). After further improvement occurred, Sophie was able to reach onto the mat below her for bean bags and throw them to a large teddy bear inside of an inner tube "feeding the bear" while swinging. The therapist continued to increase the challenge as Sophie's skills improved. Sophie eventually chose different swings that required greater postural control, including trunk rotation, and increased ocular skills to track where the bean bags were placed on the floor.

At the end of the session, Sophie and her therapist would have a snack to work on the sequencing of simple food preparation, the use of utensils, and socialization with a peer when available. Because Sophie was involved in many sensory-rich activities during the therapy session, she was able to have more success with the fork and spoon at the end of the session than she did at school or at home. Over time, however, as her body awareness, body scheme, postural and praxis improved, she began to spontaneously use utensils competently in other environments.

Progress

Over time, Sophie began to engage with peers as she no longer had to think about all of her motor actions, but could move more automatically to plan and sequence activities. This skill was addressed in therapy first by having Sophie set up and sequence several pieces of equipment in the clinic to create an obstacle course. As her praxis abilities improved, the therapist adjusted the challenge and invited peers to participate in the obstacle course with Sophie. This helped Sophie learn to "watch and do" simultaneously. In addition, snack time provided an opportunity for the peers to model social interactions with Sophie within the context of an activity. Thus, Sophie was again using her improved body awareness, body scheme, and praxis to "watch and do" simultaneously. Eventually, Sophie was able to laugh and socialize while engaged in structured activity, and over time this began to generalize to more unstructured activities on the playground and during play dates at home with classmates. Sophie's parents learned to "scaffold the environment" or set up activities that were sensory rich and at the "just right" level for Sophie. For example, they might set up a large mattress on the floor of the playroom for a jumping activity, or use a spray bottle filled with color water to spray on large pieces of paper hanging on their fence outside. They were so pleased that other children were actively asking Sophie for play dates. Eventually, the parents did not need to set up the play activities, as Sophie began to participate in reciprocal play with her peers.

Sophie's fine motor skills also improved through therapy. The clinic therapist worked in collaboration with the school-based therapist to address both the underlying sensory motor issues that impacted on Sophie's fine motor skills, as well as providing "just right" opportunities to use her emerging fine motor skills to play, learn, and participate in craft activities. One weekend, Sophie surprised her mom when she used scrap fabric to cut out clothes for a doll. Sophie's mom was astonished to witness her newly emerged scissor skills, as well as her improved ability to create, initiate, and carry out a constructional plan (praxis) that was quite accurate—the clothing was a near correct fit for her doll. This was a huge step forward for Sophie and the ultimate goal for her therapy—using her newly developed skills to participate in age-appropriate, meaningful activities.

 Summary

These case studies help elucidate the relation between sensory integrative dysfunction and participation in daily life occupations. Michael and Sophie presented with different types of sensory processing problems that impact on their daily occupations in unique ways, yet both benefited from occupational therapy using a sensory integrative approach. Their treatment was individualized based on age, the nature of the dysfunction, the role and participation of their families, and the availability of environmental supports. Michael and Sophie's cases provide anecdotal evidence that support the impact of sensory integration on the acquisition of developmentally appropriate skills and abilities. Empirical evidence is also emerging in the literature that provides further support of the effectiveness of the sensory integration frame of reference on shaping the lives and development of children with sensory integrative dysfunctions (Miller, Coll, & Schoen, 2007; Schaaf & Nightlinger, 2007).

REFERENCES

Anzalone, M. E., & Williamson, G. G. (2000). Sensory processing and motor performance in autism spectrum disorders. In A. M. Wetherby, & B. M. Prizant (Eds). *Autism Spectrum Disorders: A Transactional Developmental Approach* (pp. 143–166). Baltimore, MD: Brooks Publishing.

Ayres, A. J. (1965). Patterns of perceptual-motor dysfunction in children: A factor analytic study. *Perceptual and Motor Skills, 20*, 335–368.

Ayres, A. J. (1966). Interrelationships among perceptual-motor functions in children. *American Journal of Occupational Therapy, 20*(2), 68–71.

Ayres, A. J. (1969). Relation between gesell developmental quotients and later perceptual-motor performance. *American Journal of Occupational Therapy, 23*(1), 11–17.

Ayres, A. J. (1971). Characteristics of types of sensory integrative dysfunction. *The American Journal of Occupational Therapy, 25*(7), 329–334.

Ayres, A. J. (1972a). *Sensory Integration and Learning disorders*. Los Angeles, CA: Western Psychological Services.

Ayres, A. J. (1972b). Types of sensory integrative dysfunction among disabled learners. *The American Journal of Occupational Therapy, 26*(1), 13–18.

Ayres, A. J. (1972c). *Southern California Sensory Integration Test Manual*, Los Angeles: Psychological Services.

Ayres, A. J. (1976). *The Effect of Sensory Integrative Therapy on Learning Disabled Children: The Final Report of a Research Project*, Los Angeles, CA: University of South California.

Ayres, A. J. (1977). Cluster analyses of measures of sensory integration. *The American Journal of Occupational Therapy, 31*(6), 362–366.

Ayres, A. J. (1979). *Sensory Integration and the Child*. Los Angeles, CA: Western Psychological Services.

Ayres, A. J. (1985). *Developmental Dyspraxia and Adult Onset Apraxia*. Torrance, CA: Sensory Integration International.

Ayres, A. J. (1986). *Sensory Integration Dysfunction: Test Score Constellations. Part II of a Final Report*. Torrance, CA: Sensory Integration International.

Ayres, A. J. (1989). *The Sensory Integration and Praxis Tests*. Los Angeles, CA: Western Psychological Services.

Ayres, A. J. (2003). *Sensory Integration and Praxis Test Manual, Revised*. Los Angeles, CA: Western Psychological Services.

Ayres, A. J. (2005). *Sensory Integration and the Child, 25th Anniversary Edition*. Los Angeles, CA: Western Psychological Services.

Ayres, A. J., Mailloux, Z., & Wendler, C. L. (1987). Developmental dyspraxia: Is it a unitary function? *Occupational Therapy Journal of Research, 7*, 93–110.

Ayres, A. J., & Tickle, L. S. (1980). Hyper-responsivity to touch and vestibular stimuli as a predictor of positive response to sensory integration procedures by autistic children. *American Journal of Occupational Therapy, 34*(6), 375–381.

Bar-Shalita, T., Goldstand, S., Hahn-Markowitz, J., & Parush, S. (2005). Typical children's responsivity patterns of the tactile and vestibular systems. *American Journal of Occupational Therapy, 59*(2), 148–156.

Blanche, E. I. (2002). *Observations Based on Sensory Integration Theory*. Torrance, CA: Pediatric Therapy Network.

Blanche, E. I. (2006). Clinical reasoning in action: designing intervention. In R. C. Schaaf, & S. Smith Roley (Eds). *Sensory Integration: Applying Clinical Reasoning to Practice with Diverse Populations* (pp. 91–106). Austin, TX: Pysch Corp.

Blanche, E. I. Botticelli, T. M., & Hallway, M. K. (1995). *Combining Neuro-Developmental Treatment and Sensory Integration Principles: An Approach to Pediatric Therapy*. San Antonio, TX: Therapy Skill Builders.

Blanche, E. I., & Schaaf, R. C. (2001). Proprioception: a cornerstone of sensory integrative intervention. In S. Smith Roley, E. I. Blanche, & R. C. Schaaf (Eds). *Understanding the Nature of Sensory Integration with Diverse Populations* (pp. 109–124). San Antonio, TX: Therapy Skill Builders.

Brown, J. P., Cooper-Kuhn, C. M., Kempermann, G., & Van Praag, H. (2003). Enriched environment and physical activity stimulate hippocampal but not olfactory bulb neurogenesis. *European Journal of Neuroscience, 17*, 2042–2046.

Bundy, A. C., & Koomar, J. A. (2002). Orchestrating intervention: the art of practice. In A. C. Bundy, S. L. Lane, & E. A. Murray (Eds). *Sensory Integration Theory and Practice* (2nd ed., pp. 261–309). Philadelphia, PA: FA Davis Co.

Bundy, A. C., Lane, S. L., & Murray, E. A. (2002). *Sensory Integration: Theory and Practice* (2nd ed.). Philadelphia, PA: FA Davis Co.

Cermack, S. A. (2001). The effects of deprivation on processing, play, and praxis. In S. Smith Roley, E. Blanche, & R. Schaaf (Eds). *Understanding the Nature of Sensory Integration with Diverse Populations*. San Antonio, TX: Therapy Skill Builders.

Cohn, E., & Miller, L. J. (2000). Parental hopes for therapy outcomes: Children with sensory modulation disorders. *American Journal of Occupational Therapy, 54*(1), 36–43.

Conrad, K. E., Cermak, S. A., & Drake, C. (1983). Differentiation of praxis among children. *American Journal of Occupational Therapy, 37*(7), 466–473.

Cummins, R. A. (1991). Sensory integration and learning disabilities: Ayres' factor analyses reappraised. *Journal of learning disabilities, 24*(3), 160–168.

DeGangi, G. (2000). *Pediatric Disorders of Regulation in Affect and Behavior*. San Diego, CA: Academic Press.

Dewey, D. (2002). Subtypes of DCD. In S. Cermack, & D. Larkin (Eds). *Developmental Coordination Disorder* (pp. 40–53). Albany, NY: Delmar.

Dunn, W. (1999a). *The Sensory Profile*. San Antonio, TX: Psychological Cooperation.

Dunn, W. (1999b). *The Sensory Profile: Examiner's Manual*. San Antonio, TX: Psychological Cooperation.

Floeter, M. K., & Greenough, W. T. (1979). Cerebellar plasticity: Modification of Purkinje cell structure by differential rearing in monkeys. *Science, 206*(4415), 227–229.

Gibson, J. J. (1979). *The Ecological Approach to Visual Perception*. Boston, MA: Houghton-Mifflin Company.

Grandin, T. (1995). *Thinking in Pictures*. New York: Doubleday.

Greenough, W. T., Black, J. E., & Wallace, C. S. (1987). Experience and brain development. *Child Development, 58*, 539–559.

Hoehn, T. P., & Baumeister, A. A. (1994). A critique of the application of sensory integration therapy to children with learning disabilities. *Journal of Learning Disabilities, 27*(6), 338–350.

Huebner, R. A. (2001). *Autism: A Sensorimotor Approach to Management*. Gaithersburg, MD: Aspen.

Interdisciplinary Council on Developmental and Learning Disorders (ICDL). (2005). *Diagnostic Manual for Infancy and Early Childhood: Mental Heath, Developmental, Regulatory-Sensory Processing, and Language Disorders and Learning Challenges (ICDL-DMIC)*. Bethesda, MD: ICDL.

Jacobs, S. E., & Schneider, M. L. (2001). Neuroplasticity and the environment: implications for sensory integration. In S. Smith Roley, E. I. Blanche, & R. C. Schaaf (Eds). *Understanding the Nature of Sensory Integration with Diverse Populations* (pp. 29–42). San Antonio, TX: Therapy Skill Builders.

Kandel, E. R., Schwartz, J. H., & Jessell, T. M. (1995). In E. R. Kandel, J. H. Schwartz, T.M. Jessell (Eds). *Essentials of Neural Science and Behavior*. Norwalk, CT: Appleton & Lange.

Kempermann, G., & Gage, F. H. (1999). New nerve cells for the adult brain. *Scientific American, 280*, 48–53.

Kientz, M. A., & Dunn, W. (1997). A comparison of the performance of children with and without autism on the sensory profile. *American Journal of Occupational Therapy, 51*(7), 530–537.

Knickerbocker, B. M. (1980). *A Holistic Approach to the Treatment of Learning Disabilities*. Thorofare, NJ: Slack Inc.

Kraemer, G. W. (2001). Developmental neuroplasticity: a foundation for sensory integration. In S. Smith Roley, E. Imperatore Blanche, & R. C. Schaaf (Eds). *Understanding the Nature of Sensory Integration with Diverse Populations* (pp. 43–56). San Antonio, TX: The Psychological Corporation.

Lai, J., Fisher, A. G., Magalhaes, L. C., & Bundy, A. C. (1996). Construct validity of the sensory integration and praxis tests. *Occupational Therapy Journal of Research, 16*(2), 75–97.

Lane, S. J. (2002). Sensory modulation. In A. C. Bundy, S. J. Lane, & E. A. Murrary (Eds). *Sensory Integration: Theory and Practice* (2nd ed., pp. 101–123). Philadelphia, PA: FA Davis Co.

Mailloux, Z. (2001). Sensory integrative principles in intervention with children with autistic disorder. In S. Smith Roley, E. Imperatore Blanche, & R. C. Schaaf (Eds). *Understanding the Nature of Sensory Integration with Diverse Populations* (pp. 365–382). San Antonio, TX: The Psychological Corporation.

Mailloux, Z. (2006). Setting goals and objectives around sensory integration concerns. In R. C. Schaaf, & S. Smith Roley (Eds). *Sensory Integration: Applying Clinical Reasoning to Practice with Diverse Populations* (pp. 63–70). Austin, TX: PyschCorp.

Mailloux, Z., & Smith Roley, S. (2001). Sensory integration. In H. Miller-Kuhaneck (Ed). *Autism: A Comprehensive Occupational Therapy Approach*. Bethesda, MD: American Occupational Therapy Association.

May-Benson, T. (2005). Examining ideational abilities in children with dyspraxia, Unpublished doctoral dissertation. Boston University, Boston, MA.

May-Benson, T. A., & Cermak, S. A. (2007). Development of an assessment for ideational praxis. *American Journal of Occupational Therapy, 61*(2), 148–153.

May-Benson, T. A., & Koomar, J. A. (2007). Identifying gravitational insecurity in children: A pilot study. *American Journal of Occupational Therapy, 61*(2), 148–153.

McIntosh, D. N., Miller, L. J., & Hagerman, R. J. (1999). Sensory modulation disruption, electrodermal responses and functional behaviors. *Developmental medicine and child neurology, 41*, 608–615.

Merzenich, M. M., Nelson, R. J., Stryker, M. P., & Cynader, M. S. (1984). Somatosensory cortical map changes following digit amputation in adult monkeys. *Journal of Comparative Neurology, 224*(4), 591–605.

Miller, L. J., Anzalone, M. E., Lane, S. J., & Cermak, S. A. (2007). Concept evolution in sensory integration: A proposed nosology for diagnosis. *American Journal of Occupational Therapy, 61*(2), 135–140.

Miller, L. J., Coll, J. R., & Schoen, S. A. (2007). A randomized controlled pilot study of the effectiveness of occupational therapy for children with sensory processing disorder. *American Journal of Occupational Therapy, 61*(2), 228–238.

Miller, L. J., James, K., & Schaaf, R. C. (2007). Phenotypes with sensory modulation dysfunction, Manuscript in preparation.

Miller-Kuhaneck, H., Henry, D. A., Glennon, T. J., & Mu, K. (2007). Development of the sensory processing measure—school: Initial studies of reliability and validity. *American Journal of Occupational Therapy, 61*(2), 170–175.

Miller, L. J., Reisman, J. E. McIntosh, D. N., & Simon, J. (2001). An ecological model of sensory integration: performance of children with fragile X syndrome, autistic disorder, attention-deficit/hyperactivity disorder, and sensory modulation dysfunction. In S. Smith Roley, E. I Blanche, & R. C. Schaaf (Eds). *Understanding the Nature of Sensory Integration with Diverse Populations* (pp. 57–88). San Antonio, TX: Therapy Skill Builders.

Miller, L. J., Wilbarger, J. L., Stackhouse, T. M., & Trunnell, S. L. (2002). Use of clinical reasoning in occupational therapy: the STEP-SI model of treatment of sensory modulation dysfunction. In A. C. Bundy, S. J. Lane, & E. A. Murray (Eds). *Sensory Integration: Theory and Practice* (2nd ed., pp. 435–451). Philadelphia, PA: FA Davis Co.

Mulligan, S. (1996). An analysis of score patterns of children with attention disorders on the sensory integration and praxis tests. *American Journal of Occupational Therapy, 50*(8), 647–654.

Mulligan, S. (1998). Patterns of sensory integration dysfunction: A confirmatory factor analysis. *American Journal of Occupational Therapy, 52*(10), 819–828.

Mulligan, S. (2000). Cluster analysis of scores of children on the sensory integration and praxis tests. *Occupational Therapy Journal of Research, 20*(4), 256–270.

Mulligan, S. (2002). Advances in sensory integration research. In A. C. Bundy, S. L. Lane, & E. A. Murray (Eds). *Sensory Integration: Theory and Practice* (2nd ed., pp. 397–411). Philadelphia, PA: FA Davis Co.

Neumann, E. A. (1971). *The Elements of Play*. New York: MSS Information.

Ognibene, T. C. (2002). Distinguishing sensory modulation dysfunction from attention-deficit/hyperactivity disorder: Sensory habituation and response inhibition processes, Unpublished manuscript, University of Denver, Denver, CO.

O'Neill, M., & Jones, R. S. P. (1997). Sensory-perceptual abnormalities in autism: A case for more research? *Journal of Autism and Developmental Disorders, 27*(3), 283–294.

Parham, L. D. Ecker, C. Kuhaneck, H. M., & Henry, D. A. (2007). *Sensory Processing Measure Manual*. Los Angeles, CA: Western Psychological Services.

Parham, D., & Mailloux, Z. (1995). Sensory integrative principles in intervention with children with autistic disorder. In J. Case-Smith, A. S. Allen, & P. N. Pratt (Eds). *Occupational Therapy for Children* (3rd ed., pp. 329–382). St. Louis, MO: Mosby.

Parham, L. D., & Mailloux, Z. (2001). Sensory integration. In J. Case-Smith (Ed). *Occupational Therapy for Children* (4th ed., pp. 329–381). St. Louis, MO: Mosby.

Parham, L. D., & Mailloux, Z. (2005). Sensory integration. In J. Case-Smith, A. S. Allen, & P. N. Pratt (Eds). *Occupational Therapy for Children* (5th ed., pp. 356–411). St, Louis, MO: Elsevier Science.

Reeves, G. D., & Cermak, S. A. (2002). Disorders of praxis. In A. C. Bundy, S. L. Lane & E. A. Murray (Eds). *Sensory Integration: Theory and Practice* (2nd ed., pp. 71–100). Philadelphia, PA: FA Davis Co.

Rogers, S. J., & Ozonoff, S. (2005). Annotation: What do we know about sensory dysfunction in autism? A critical review of empirical evidence. *Journal of Child Psychology and Psychiatry, 46*(12), 1255–1268.

Roley, S. (2006). Sensory integration theory revisited. In R. C. Schaaf, & S. Smith Roley (Eds). *SI: Applying Clinical Reasoning to Practice with Diverse Populations* (pp. 15–36). San Antonio, TX: PsychCorp.

Rosblad, B. (2002). Visual perception in children with *developmental coordination disorder*. In S. Cermak, & D. Larkin (Eds). *Developmental Coordination Disorder*. Albany, NY: Delmar.

Royeen, C. B., & Lane, S. J. (1991). Tactile processing and sensory defensiveness. In A. Fisher, E. A. Murray, & A. C. Bundy (Eds). *Sensory Integration Theory and Practice*. Philadelphia, PA: FA Davis Co.

Schaaf, R. C., & Miller, L. J. (2005). Novel Therapies for Developmental Disabilities: Occupational Therapy using a Sensory Integrative Approach. *Journal of Mental Retardation and Developmental Disabilities, 11*, 143–148.

Schaaf, R. C., & Nightlinger, K. M. (2007). Occupational therapy using a sensory integrative approach: A case study of effectiveness. *American Journal of Occupational Therapy, 61*(2), 239–246.

Schaaf, R. C., & Smith Roley, S. (2006). *SI: Applying Clinical Reasoning to Practice with Diverse Populations*. San Antonio, TX: PsychCorp.

Schneider, M. (2005). What is sensory integration? In A. J. Ayres, (Eds). *Sensory Integration and the Child 25th Anniversary Edition* (pp. 169–170). Los Angeles, CA: Western Psychological Services.

Schneider, M. (2006). Environmental toxicants, stress, and genes: Effects on sensory processing in a primate model. R2 R: Research Symposium, Long Beach, CA.

Smith Roley, S. (2006). Evaluating sensory integration function and dysfunction. In R. C. Schaaf, & S. Smith Roley (Eds). *SI: Applying Clinical Reasoning to Practice with Diverse Populations* (pp. 15–36). San Antonio, TX: PsychCorp.

Smith Roley, S., Blanche, E., & Schaaf, R. C. (2001). *Understanding the Nature of Sensory Integration with Diverse Populations*. San Antonio, TX: Therapy Skill Builders.

Spitzer, S. L., & Smith Roley, S. (2001). Sensory integration revisited: a philosophy of practice. In S. Smith Roley, E. Blanche, & R. Schaaf (Eds). *Understanding the Nature of Sensory Integration with Diverse Populations*. San Antonio, TX: Therapy Skill Builders.

Stein, B. (2007). Multi-sensory integration. November, Paper presented at the Sensory Processing Disorder Foundation Research and Intervention Conference, New York.

Tomchek, S. D., & Dunn, W. (2007). Sensory processing in children with and without autism: a comparative study using the short sensory profile. *American Journal of Occupational Therapy, 61*(2), 190–200.

Volkmar, F. R., & Greenough, W. T. (1972). Rearing complexity affects branching of dendrites in the visual cortex of the rat. *Science, 176*, 1445–1447.

West, R. W., & Greenough, W. T. (1972). Effect of environmental complexity on cortical synapses of rats: preliminary results. *Behavioral Biology, 7*(2), 279–284.

Williams, D. (1992). *Nobody Nowhere: The Extraordinary Autobiography of an Autistic*. New York: Times Books.

Windsor, M. M., Smith Roley, S., & Szklut, S. (2001). Assessment of sensory integration and praxis. In S. Smith Roley, E. I. Blanche, & R. C. Schaaf (Eds). *Understanding the Nature of Sensory Integration with Diverse Populations* (pp. 215–246). San Antonio, TX: Therapy Skill Builders.

Yochman, A., Parush, S., & Ornoy, A. (2004). Responses of preschool children with and without ADHD to sensory events in daily life. *American Journal of Occupational Therapy, 58*(3), 294–302.

Zero to Three. (2005). *Diagnostic Classification of Mental Health and Developmental Disorders of Infancy and Early Childhood, Revised (DC:0-3 R)*. Arlington, VA: Zero to three: National Center for Clinical Infant Programs.

CHAPTER 7

A Frame of Reference for Neuro-Developmental Treatment

KIMBERLY A. BARTHEL

The Neuro-Developmental Treatment (NDT) frame of reference is a dynamic hands-on treatment approach guiding occupational therapists globally in their assessment and intervention of pediatric clients who experience posture and movement impairments. This client-centered perspective provides an individualized, problem-solving framework for managing the motor skill challenges that limit the child's participation in life roles. Sensorimotor techniques are the fundamental applications of this frame of reference, focusing on prevention, remediation, and reeducation of movement within a functional context.

HISTORY

Berta Bobath, physiotherapist and her husband, Dr. Karel Bobath first developed the "Bobath approach" in the 1940s. This approach was later identified in the scientific literature as the NDT approach for children with cerebral palsy (Howle, 2002). Mrs. Bobath proposed that with guided movement experiences, children with cerebral palsy could change their muscle strength and length leading to changes in functional performance (Bobath, 1948). Through NDT intervention, Mrs. Bobath detected observable and palpable changes in the neuromotor systems of her patients with cerebral palsy.

In developing a theoretical framework for their treatment approach, the Bobaths looked to dominant neurophysiological theories of the 1940s. Early motor control theories emphasized a hierarchical, reflex model of motor control, offering an elementary explanation for the movement challenges experienced by children with cerebral palsy. Over the last 60 years, the understanding of typical and atypical motor control has advanced through prolific neurophysiological and motor control research. Subsequently, these original motor control theories have expanded, resulting in revised evidence supporting the rationale for NDT.

As the early NDT theory evolved, core concepts of "typical movement analysis" were incorporated into the theoretical foundations. These concepts have remained consistent over time, maintaining the belief that *typical* movement patterns can be learned, altering the existing *atypical* motor control patterns of children with neuromotor challenges

Domains

Dimension	Functional Domain	Disability Domain
A. Body structure and functions	Structual and functional integrity	Impairments A. Primary B. Secondary
B. Motor functions	Effective posture and movement	Ineffective posture and movement
C. Individual functions	Functional activities	Functional activity limitations
D. Social functions	Participation	Participation restriction

Dimensions

FIGURE 7.1 The NDT enablement classification of health and disability. NDT, Neuro-Developmental Treatment.

(Howle, 2002). Through the provision of artful handling of NDT techniques, facilitation of typical motor patterns is combined together with simultaneous inhibition of atypical movements. Mrs. Bobath emphasized the need for treatment techniques to be based upon moment-to-moment observations of client reactions during treatment interaction. The approach insists upon flexible and adaptable treatment intervention that is based upon a consistent knowledge base (Howle, 2002).

In the late 1990s the Neuro-Developmental Treatment Association (NDTA) adopted a model of practice entitled the "NDTA Enablement Model of Health and Disability" guided by the World Health Organization's International Classification of Functioning, Disability and Health Model. The Enablement/Disablement model of NDT considers the "whole" person, recognizing both competencies and limitations in a wide variety of domains (Figure 7.1). The model encompasses body systems integrity and impairments, individual functional activities and activity limitations, and participation in life roles and participation restrictions. Unique to the NDT Enablement/Disablement model is the focus upon the domain of *motor function* as the key contribution of the NDT frame of reference to the occupational performance of the client (Howle, 2002).

THEORETICAL BASE

An intimate understanding of typical motor development directs the occupational therapist in the assessment and treatment of children with neuromotor challenges. Through careful analysis and knowledge of typically developing infants, therapists internalize kinesiological and biomechanical principles of typical movement execution. These principles are embedded within handling and positioning techniques provided throughout NDT sessions teaching the client typical adaptive motor patterns for function.

Motor development theories have been refined and expanded over the last 60 years, reflecting the findings of current motor control research. Previous hierarchical, developmental theories of typical motor development have been modified to emphasize an interactive, spiraling continuum of motor skill acquisition that occurs in context. Motor patterns are observed to endure continuous modification and alteration in response to continuously changing environmental conditions. Movement patterns are no longer considered to arise as an outcome of maturation.

An important characteristic of motor development is the simultaneous emergence of competing movement patterns in typically developing infants. Typically, competing patterns of movement coexist without the domination of one particular pattern of movement over the other. Typical movement repertoires are fluid, flexible, and interactive. Babies rehearse these competing patterns of movement continuously dependent upon their positional relationship to gravity. For example, when placed in supine, the 4- to 5-month-old infant reaches against gravity developing his or her antigravity flexor muscles. When the same baby is placed prone, the infant will practice antigravity extension, moving his or her neck, shoulders, and trunk up off of the support surface. These two competing motor patterns develop simultaneously, creating core trunk stability and postural control. NDT compares and contrasts these typical findings with the observed atypical patterns of movement demonstrated by children with neuropathology where competing patterns of movement develop in an asynchronous fashion.

Secondly, typically developing patterns of movement require the experience of a previously acquired pattern, building upon skills through practice and interaction with the environment. As these new patterns of movement emerge, they can temporarily dominate the baby's repertoire, destabilizing the organization of motor skill performance. In time, and with practice, the baby reorganizes movements into a broader spectrum of function. NDT recognizes that children with neuropathology experience challenges with this natural process of continuous reorganization of motor skills and require direct assistance in the learning of new functional repertoires.

NDT applies these concepts of typical motor skill acquisition into the teaching of movements to the atypical neuromotor system. As children with atypical movement patterns learn *typical* movements, old patterns are superseded, destabilized, and modified. Through handling and movement experiences in a functional context, the therapist attempts to integrate and assimilate competing patterns of movement into a balanced interaction for movement and postural control development.

Despite the emphasis upon typical development, the Bobaths stated "Treatment should not attempt to follow the typical developmental sequence, regardless of the age and physical condition of the individual child. Whatever function a child requires most urgently at any one stage is the priority of the established treatment goals" (Howle, 2002, p. 40).

Development of Reach and Grasp

Historically, the occupational therapist has specialized in treatment pertaining to upper extremity function within the NDT frame of reference. As a result, explicit examination of typically developing reach and grasp is emphasized.

Consistent with the development of all motor skills, reaching skills progressively evolve through experience and interaction with task and environment. Newborns exhibit a distinct reaching pattern similar to the more advanced reaching behaviors observed in a 5-month-old infant. This suggests that reach is a "centrally programmed" function imprinted in human behavior (von Hofsten & Rönnqvist, 1993). Similar to the development of other motor skills infants begin with a preferred reaching pattern, which becomes progressively restructured with experience, eventually maturing to a smooth and efficient trajectory of reaching movements (Thelen et al., 1993). Understanding that reach develops in relationship to the objects inviting reach, the occupational therapist carefully selects a wide variety of toys and stimuli to entice movements of the arm and hand in varying orientations in space.

Muscles on the ventral side of the body "come on line" to counteract the force of the muscles on the dorsal side of the body as the body is displaced away from the center of gravity during reaching movements (van der Heide, 2004). This basic activation enables the upright posture to "hold on and stay put" against the perturbations of the center of body mass during reach. Postural control is then finely tuned and modified, refining the postural mechanisms generated. Processes of postural control and refined motor control work collaboratively to produce accurate and appropriate adjustments to the postural control system during reaching tasks (Barthel, 2004). The link between postural control and efficient upper extremity function demands the occupational therapist to treat the body as a "linked" system for alterations in functional upper extremity control.

Grasp depends on appropriate hand orientation and the ability to switch between various forms of grip. The hand's ability to be functional during manipulation depends upon the balance between the long finger flexors and extensors, the capability for alignment between the wrist and hand, mobility of the carpal and metacarpal bones, and the activity of the intrinsic muscles of the hand (Howle, 2002). The weight-bearing and weight-shifting activities observed in typically developing infants elongate and prepare upper extremity musculature, setting the stage for biomechanical activation of arm and hand muscle synergies.

The production of precision hand movements relies upon a distinct neuromotor pathway of the central nervous system (CNS). The corticospinal tract is a direct pathway from the cortex to the motor units of the hand affording this precision and movement specificity. This discrete channel of communication proves challenging for the occupational therapist rehabilitating hand movements due to the neurological constraints upon the production of selective fractionated movements. Through careful selection of tasks demanding the development of isolated finger movements, combined with appropriate handling supports, opportunities are provided to train precision control within context.

Kinesiological and Biomechanical Concepts

NDT draws upon kinesiological and biomechanical concepts as a theoretical foundation for analysis and treatment of posture and movement impairments. Important concepts are planes of movement, alignment, range of motion (ROM), base of support, muscle strength, postural control, weight shifts, and mobility.

Planes of movement refer to motor action in the anatomical planes of the body. NDT recognizes that movement of the body occurs in three planes of space. Kinesiological studies demonstrate that motor control begins in sagittal plane with babies rehearsing flexion and extension movements of their bodies against gravity. Movements in the frontal plane begin to integrate with sagittal plane movements as the baby's torso muscles become active and biomechanically competent in producing forces against gravity. Transverse plane movements are the most sophisticated motor patterns of typical development requiring interplay of the musculature developed in the sagittal and frontal plane. Movement in the transverse plane enables rotation around the body axis necessary for developing balance and posture in space.

Alignment of the body refers to the arrangement of these bodily segments relative to each other with reference to the force of gravity, the base of support, and the nature of the task (Howle, 2002). The human body is a "linked system," with each segment biomechanically relating to all other bodily segments within the system. Alignment of body segments over the base of support determines the amount of effort required to support the body against gravity. Synergistic activation of muscle systems relies upon these biomechanical relationships to produce accurate and efficient functional movement.

Range of motion is the joint flexibility allowed at a joint. Normal voluntary, active joint ROM is also required for movement production. In the musculoskeletal system, muscles generate and transmit force via tendons to bones. When muscles generate sufficient force, bones will move (Lieber, 2002). Joints that are limited in ROM due to intrinsic properties such as muscle stiffness, soft tissue contracture, or fascial restrictions prevent muscles from generating sufficient force to move the bones for competent functional engagement with the environment. The amount of length, speed, and force produced by a muscle for a given task requires that a joint be moveable into the "just right angle" for the task desired (Lieber, 2002). Contractile properties of muscles are most efficient when joint segments are biomechanically aligned with available degrees of freedom, or several motor elements (Sabari, 2002).

The base of support is the area of the body that is in contact with the support surface. Biomechanical principles indicate that the reaction forces applied to the body, as well as the center of pressure, depend upon the characteristics of the base of support. Muscles work in relationship to the base of support using ground reaction forces, inertia, and surface frictional characteristics to assist in their activation (Bouisset & Le Bozec, 2002). In sitting position, the base of support includes the pelvis, hips, and femurs. In standing, the feet are the base of support. The base of support functions as a "point of initiation and stability" for movement. Stability is the ability to maintain a posture against opposing forces (Schoen & Anderson, 1999). Postural activity is initiated at the base of support (Hartbourne, Giuhani, & MacNeela, 1993). Postural responses in standing are initiated at the ankles followed by motor activity progressively more proximally working off the base of support (Nashner & McCollum, 1985). Typical postural development is characterized by the ability to gradually narrow the base of support in conjunction with refinement of movement against gravity. Changes in the base of support impact the alignment of all body segments demanding changing interaction of muscle synergies. Examination of the base of support and the alignment of the body segments in relationship to the base of support is integral to NDT intervention.

Muscle strength requires an understanding of the intimate interaction between muscle and joint properties. Strength is not simply "force generated" within a muscle, but force applied within the musculoskeletal system that acts upon a rotating joint axis (torque) (Lieber, 2002). All properties of the musculoskeletal system (muscle fibers, tendons, joint ROM, connective tissue mobility) must be intact for "muscle strength" to be an available property of movement (Lieber, 2002). This statement has profound implications for children with neuropathology who may experience disruption in function of any or all elements within their motor system. Typical developing babies accrue strength through movement of the body system against gravity. Muscle lengthening and elongation set the stage for the physiological contractile properties for muscles to fire appropriately. Basic biophysical properties of muscle (increased force during active lengthening) demonstrate the necessity of elongation for the promotion of muscle fiber activation (Lieber, 2002). Eccentric contractions (lengthening of an activated muscle) result in higher muscle force production potentially increasing muscle strength. NDT recognizes the importance of muscle elongation combined with strengthening muscle synergies for the production of functional motor performance.

Postural control involves controlling the body's position in space for the dual purposes of stability and orientation (Shumway-Cook & Woollacott, 2007). Postural orientation is defined as the ability to maintain an appropriate relationship between the body segments, and between the body and the environment for a task (Horak, 1991). The term "posture" is often used to describe both the biomechanical alignment of the body and the orientation of the body to the environment (Shumway-Cook & Woollacott, 2007). Essentially, the production of postural control requires ROM, alignment, muscle recruitment, strength, and the ability to move off the base of support. Handling and treatment intervention encourage postural control through experiences of facilitation, weight bearing, weight shifts, and movement in space.

Weight shifts and mobility off the center of mass is required for a person to be able to meet varying demands of task performance. Movement of the body in space requires a shift of weight off the center of mass in one of the various planes of movement. Some tasks place importance on maintaining an appropriate orientation at the expense of stability. For example, the successful blocking of a goal in soccer or catching a fly ball in baseball requires that the player always remains oriented with respect to the ball, sometimes falling to the ground in an effort to block the goal or catch the ball. Stability and mobility demands change within each task (Shumway-Cook & Woollacott, 2007). The potential for shifting weight and movement off the center of mass allows the body system to meet the varying demands of task performance.

Movement Dysfunction

Evaluation of competing typical and atypical patterns of movement demonstrated by children with neuromotor impairment is fundamental to NDT. NDT recognizes that atypical movements in individuals with CNS pathology result from (1) damage to specific (discrete or diffuse) neural tissue, (2) the attempt of the developing nervous system to compensate for the initial lesion, (3) the interaction between the impaired nervous system with other body systems and the environment resulting in inefficient functional performance, and (4) the inability of the impaired CNS to readily adapt to the opportunities afforded by the environment (Howle, 2002).

Infants with brain injury begin their motor development process with an already compromised repertoire of movements resulting in cascading outcomes of compensatory motor activation to accomplish movement problems. As the infant with neuromotor challenges reinforces these limited repertoires, over time patterns of movement become tightly linked and constrain possible expansion of additional motor skills. Stereotypical patterns of posture and movement become hardwired within the nervous system and persist as a dominant motor expression in varying movement conditions and contexts.

In attempts to move the body against gravity, infants with challenged neuromotor systems may reduce their "degrees of freedom" at selective joints, using inappropriate muscle synergies to accomplish their motor goal. Predominance of "fixing" patterns prevents dissociation and uncoupling of interlimb–intralimb relationships diminish flexibility of movement responses.

Identification of atypical patterns of movement helps the therapist select appropriate intervention techniques. Without intervention, it is assumed that atypical compensatory movements will become the dominant habitual motor strategy for function. For example, infants who begin with an extensor muscle tone bias and excessive neck hyperextension with concomitant weakness of counteracting antigravity neck flexor control may select a shoulder girdle elevation compensation strategy to minimize the effort of holding the head in midline. After prolonged recruitment of this neck hyperextension and shoulder girdle elevation strategy, the motor synergy will become hardwired within the nervous system as a preferred method for the achievement of head control, limiting the potential for upper extremity performance (Bly, 1980). Although infants and children who have abnormal patterns of movement certainly may attain some degree of independence in functional activities, their skill levels are compromised due to excessive reliance upon compensatory patterns of movement (Schoen & Anderson, 1999).

Within the NDT frame of reference, atypical movements are classified as *primary* or *secondary* impairments that limit participation in life roles. Primary impairments are identified as the components representing the major constraints upon movement and posture. Impairments of the neuromuscular and musculoskeletal systems can occur as either "positive" or "negative" signs of pathology (Howle, 2002). Primary positive signs are directly produced by upper motor neuron lesions and present as "atypical" behaviors. Primary negative signs represent the *loss* of typical behaviors and capacities. Primary positive and negative signs of impairment include the following: atypical muscle tone (spasticity), impaired muscle activation, excessive coactivation, ineffective, stereotyped muscle synergies, impaired motor execution, atypical scaling of muscle forces, excessive overflow of intralimb and interlimb contractions, and timing and sequencing impairments (Howle, 2002). Interlimb coordination is the ability to coordinate movements between individual limbs necessary for efficient movement. Interlimb coordination is impaired by challenges with muscle inactivation, inefficient muscle synergy patterns, limitations in timing and sequencing of movements between limb segments. Intralimb coordination is the behavior of two or more joints within a single limb in relationship to each other necessary to produce skilled movements. Coordination of these joint segments is also impaired by poor muscle activation, muscle stiffness, inefficient muscle synergy patterns, and limitations in timing and sequencing of individual muscles acting upon a joint.

A secondary impairment is a challenge in function that arises "secondarily" from the atypical interaction between the neuromuscular system and structural–functional changes in the musculoskeletal system. Secondary impairments affect a client's level of disability by adding extra physical, cognitive, or emotional difficulties that further affect the person's ability to cope with the primary impairments.

Atypical Muscle Tone

Although children with cerebral palsy and other neuropathologies demonstrate atypical movement patterns for various reasons, one aspect of the motor system that is important to a therapist is the feature of muscle tone (Barthel, 2004). Clinically, therapists have been taught to observe and feel the "tone" of their clients and have regarded this phenomenon as a significant problem interfering with motor control.

But what is muscle tone and how exactly do we measure it? Normal muscle tone is regarded as the muscle's resistance to being lengthened; its general overall stiffness. Normal muscle stiffness is the result of both neural and non-neural components. The mechanical elastic characteristics of the muscle and connective tissue participate in this so-called resistance to movement. The neural basis for stiffness reflects the degree of motor unit activity and most importantly the stretch reflex generated muscle activity that resists muscle lengthening. Bleck describes tone as "the state of partial contraction in which muscles maintain their posture without fully relaxing" (Bleck, 1987, p. 100). Muscle tone changes readily with position, posture, activity (resting or during movement), excitement, illness, and other factors that affect overall state (Barthel, 2004).

Spasticity is defined as a "motor disorder characterized by a velocity dependent increase in the tonic stretch reflexes (muscle tone) with exaggerated tendon jerks, resulting from the hyper excitability of the stretch reflex, as one component of the upper motor neuron syndrome" (Shumway-Cook & Woollacott, 2007). Resistance to externally imposed movement increases with increasing speed of stretch and varies with the direction of joint movement (Sanger et al., 2007). The Bobath definition of spasticity traditionally included hypertonus caused by tonic reflexes, muscle cocontraction and combined with abnormal movement patterns of movement (Giuliani, 2003). The Bobaths used the term "spasticity" to describe all of the encompassing atypical movement patterns noted in the cerebral palsy population (Howle, 2002).

In addition to spasticity, NDT considers other muscle tone disturbances such as dystonia, ataxia, rigidity, and hypotonia. Dystonia is defined as a movement disorder in which involuntary sustained or intermittent muscle contractions cause twisting and repetitive movements, abnormal postures, or both (Sanger et al., 2007). Ataxia is a lack of muscle coordination during voluntary movements. Rigidity is hypertonia demonstrated as resistance to externally imposed joint movements that occur at very low speeds. Rigidity presents as simultaneous cocontraction of agonist and antagonist muscles, which is reflected as an immediate resistance to a reversal of the direction of movement around a joint. Alternately, hypotonia is characterized by diminished resting muscle tension and decreased ability to generate voluntary muscle force. Excessive flexibility and postural instability are also aspects of hypotonia. Researchers have not currently identified a particular neural lesion responsible for the production of hypotonia (Howle, 2002).

NDT views atypical muscle tone as a primary impairment of the neural system contributing to the impairments of posture and motor performance observed in children with neuromotor challenges.

Impaired Muscle Activation

Excessive cocontraction of muscles occurs when the child with neuromotor impairment activates too many muscles, so that both the correct muscles and additional inappropriate muscles simultaneously contract to produce a single action (Barthel, 2004). Biomechanically, coactivation can purposefully increase joint stiffness, occurring under normal conditions that require both eccentric and concentric contractions for increased joint stability and precision movement. Cocontraction reduces degrees of freedom at a joint, increasing stability and motor control at that joint. Although coactivation is a common typical motor control strategy from a mechanical standpoint, coactivation can be an inefficient use of muscle forces when used as a strategy on a long-term basis. Excessive coactivation does not typically occur during skilled posture and movement control. Normal neuromuscular systems have the capacity to scale the amount of agonist and antagonist muscle activation into a harmonious relationship, adjusted by sensory information grading motor responses to task demands (Howle, 2002). Prolonged overuse of coactivation as a muscle recruitment strategy has the cost of decreased energy, which further affects functional performance of the neurologically impaired child (Damiano, 1993).

Impaired Muscle Synergies

In addition to excessive coactivation, children with neuropathology also recruit ineffective muscle synergies as their stereotyped patterns of movement. These limited movement repertoires are resistant to change and difficult to adapt to changing movement requirements. As previously stated, synergies function to simplify the demands upon the CNS creating possibility for more efficient motor production. Normal muscle synergies that are hardwired through practice and experience represent the best possible solution for functional motor problems. Children with cerebral palsy are able to generate their functional movements with *inefficient* synergies leaving them unable to adapt to varying conditions requiring alteration in velocity, force, timing, and sequencing of muscle execution as demanded by varying tasks (Howle, 2002).

For example, atypical muscle synergies are often recruited by the child with cerebral palsy when attempting to reach. When reaching away from the body, the child's center of mass is disturbed often creating the need for recruitment of "extra" muscles to sustain balanced postural control during the arm movements. Alterations in muscle tone, postural tone, postural control, and poor alignment of the body segments in relationship to the base of support may be impairments contributing to the emergence of these atypical synergies. Biomechanically, maladaptive alignment predisposes certain muscle groups to be at an advantage for ease of recruitment helping to provide a stable yet immobile postural strategy in the trunk and extremities. When attempting to reach, the child may produce a counterproductive muscle synergy to reaching by prioritizing "holding on and staying put" against the forces of gravity (Figure 7.2). This counterproductive muscle synergy is frequently seen as the combined activation of shoulder girdle elevation, humeral extension and internal rotation, elbow flexion, forearm pronation, and tightened grasp. This pattern may be observed bilaterally or unilaterally. Repeated use of this muscle synergy pattern will reinforce the frequency of its use as a strategy for movement.

Impaired Timing, Sequencing, and Scaling of Forces in Motor Execution

Children with cerebral palsy often demonstrate limited ability to modulate and adapt the muscular forces necessary for specific tasks. This challenge with force modulation reduces accuracy and interjoint coordination. Children with neuropathology can produce too much or too little muscle activation in anticipation of movement, selecting too many muscle groups during a movement, or use inappropriate types of muscle contraction, demonstrating excessive muscle force rather than selective and precise motor control within task (Howle, 2002).

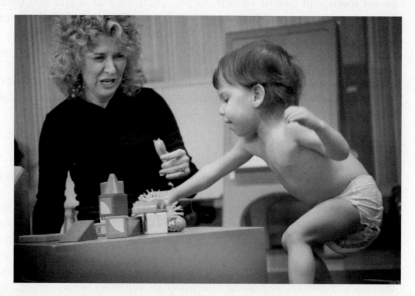

FIGURE 7.2 Atypical muscle synergy pattern observed in the left upper extremity as the child attempts to reach forward in space. Shoulder girdle elevation, humeral extension, elbow flexion, and subtle hand closure are noted, employed as a compensatory synergy to sustain body posture with forward displacement in the sagittal plane.

Many children with cerebral palsy not only experience difficulty with generating force within a muscle but also with the ability to *time* the application of forces of these muscles in concert. Latency in initiation, slowness in performance, and problems terminating muscle contractions are common challenges resulting in difficulty turning on and turning off patterns of muscle execution, impairing the adaptation of movement for function (Howle, 2002).

Children with cerebral palsy may also activate their muscles within the wrong sequence for a motor task further impairing the quality of movement production. Challenges with timing, sequencing, and scaling coincide with varying atypical muscle tone patterns and distribution. This phenomenon is especially observable in children experiencing dystonia.

Excessive Overflow of Intralimb and Interlimb Contractions

Overflow of contractile activity in multiple muscles is often evident in children with neuropathology. This motor control challenge produces a widespread motor response in muscles of the same body segment and/or in muscles far removed from the prime movers involved in the action. Overflow is observed during normal movement production, typically as a movement is first learned or performed with effort. Michael Jordan, one of the most famous basketball players of our time, uses overflow movements in his tongue to help him produce his best shots on basket. In typical movement systems this contractile overflow can be overridden and dampened as needed, permitting the right amount of movement in relationship to the movement goal (Howle, 2002). The inability to override the tendency to use more muscles than necessary to accomplish a task is an indicator of atypical movement. Overflow is noted in children with cerebral palsy when they "self-initiate" a movement or use excessive effort to move their body. Overflow is most obviously observed in children who experience stiffness that is predominantly distributed on one side of the body (hemiplegia). Attempts to use the stiffened hand will often produce simultaneous overflow in the opposite hand.

Insufficient Force Generation

Weakness is the inability to generate sufficient levels of force in a muscle for the purpose of posture and movement (Howle, 2002). Strength results from both properties of the muscles themselves and the appropriate recruitment of motor units and the timing of their activation. Neural aspects of force production reflect (1) the number of motor units recruited, (2) the type of units recruited, and (3) the discharge frequency (Shumway-Cook & Woollacott, 2007). An insufficient input from descending motor pathways can result in loss of strength of voluntary muscle action (Howle, 2002).

Insufficient force generation is generally considered a primary impairment of cerebral palsy; however, it can also result from secondary changes in the musculoskeletal system. Prolonged upper motor neuron weakness produces changes in the morphology and mechanical properties of the muscles demonstrating atrophy and hypertrophy of muscle fibers. Changes in connective tissue properties have also been noted (Lieber, 2002).

Changes in muscle and tissue length can also contribute to weakness. Muscles that are maintained in a constant lengthened position can be more difficult to contract than they would be if movements were initiated in the midrange or the shortened position (Howle, 2002). Addressing biomechanical constraints to the production of muscle contractions is a definite consideration of NDT.

Muscle weakness and imbalance between agonists and antagonists lead to an inability in the performance of movement sequences, encouraging reliance upon the compensatory movement patterns typically observed in the child with cerebral palsy. Weakness is associated with all varieties and distributions of atypical muscle tone. Muscle weakness is one of the most significant motor control impairments limiting participation in functional activity (Barthel, 2004).

Impaired Anticipatory Postural Control

Both clinical observation and motor control research suggest that children with cerebral palsy lack relevant functional activity in the primary cortical and subcortical neuronal networks, resulting in problems with initiating and timing anticipatory muscle activity for postural control (Hirschfield, 1992). Anticipatory postural adjustments create inertial forces within the neuromuscular system, which, when the time comes, will counterbalance the disturbance due to the forthcoming intentional movement. Considerable motor control research has indicated that children with cerebral palsy experience difficulty with proactive recruitment of their postural muscles, relying instead on reactive recruitment of their muscles (Woollacott & Sveistrup, 2002).

Poverty of Movement

Children with cerebral palsy demonstrate hypokinesia, where spontaneous movements have a monotonous quality, lacking fluidity, adaptability, variety, and complexity. The ranges of movements are small and often limited to repertoires of movement in the sagittal plane. Hypokinesia further contributes to the stereotypical patterns of movement observed in the neurologically impaired child (Howle, 2002).

Loss of Fractionated or Dissociated Movements

Loss of fractionated movement is observed as difficulty making precise, independent joint movements, particularly of the fingers, thumb and hand, resulting in poor dexterity when attempting fine manipulation. Dissociation is the ability to differentiate movements between different parts of the body. Movement patterns that are inappropriately coupled together are indicators of dysfunction. Muscle synergies enlisted to reduce degrees of freedom at joints create fixed stability often minimizing the ability to dissociate the segments of those joints. These tightly coupled cocontraction synergies prevent flexibility and adaptability in movement; limiting abilities to perform independent functions, such as necessary weight shifts in and out of positions. Bunny hopping is a movement pattern used for mobility in place of reciprocal crawling and is an example of a poorly dissociated movement pattern occurring between the spinal segments, pelvis, and femurs. In the upper extremities, hand movements are often coupled with arm movements demonstrating limited dissociation between the intralimb segments of the upper extremity.

Sensory Processing Impairments

Children with neuromotor challenges often experience the inability to appropriately detect and identify incoming sensory information. These sensory processing impairments can have a vast effect upon motor control production. Inability to interpret single-sensory or multisensory information in anticipation of movement, or during motor production, can result in incorrect postural orientation and movement. Many children experience the inability to modulate sensory input and to match necessary state changes required for varying tasks. Sensory integration processes can potentially interfere with motor control, by altering perception, arousal state, and alertness (Barthel, 2004).

Secondary Impairments in the Neuromuscular and Musculoskeletal Systems

Secondary impairments *indirectly* result from CNS pathology and develop as a consequence of primary impairments and environmental influences (World Health Organization, 1999). Secondary impairments contribute to the client's functional limitations as significantly as primary impairments by adding physical constraint to the motor control system. Two secondary impairments are flexibility and skeletal.

Problems with flexibility occur in joints, soft tissues, ligaments, tendons, and muscles secondary to the primary impairments of motor control. Mobility issues seen at the joints are present as either hypermobile or hypomobile. Hypermobile joints are described as lax with excessive ROM. Hypermobility often correlates with hypotonia and muscle weakness observed as insufficient musculoskeletal support at a joint. Alternately, hypomobility is typically demonstrated as joint stiffness and decreased ROM. Hypomobility frequently contributes to maladaptive changes in joint alignment, deformities, and pain (Howle, 2002). Flexibility problems occur in soft tissues and muscles as well as joints. Soft tissues lose length and flexibility as a secondary complication to changes in muscle tone and muscle strength; this further contributes to challenges with joint alignment. Creating flexibility in soft tissue length and increasing muscle length is important for the prevention of orthopedic impairments later in life (Howle, 2002).

Mechanical and neuromuscular forces of imbalanced muscle and spasticity can affect growth and change in the skeletal system. Skeletal changes are typically observed in the spine, lower extremities, wrists, and hands. Deformation of bone further contributes to ongoing challenges related to alignment of bony segments within the body. Asymmetric muscle forces affect the shaping of the bones by stimulating growth in noncompressed areas, while inhibiting bone development in areas of bone compression (Gajdosik & Gajdoski, 2000).

Assumptions

NDT has listed the following ten assumptions posed by the Bobaths that are core to its theoretical base.

1. Impaired patterns of postural control and movement coordination are the primary problems in clients with cerebral palsy.

2. Identifiable system impairments are changeable, and overall function improves when the problems of motor coordination are treated directly addressing neuromotor and postural control abnormalities in a task-specific context.
3. Sensorimotor impairments affect the whole individual—the person's function, place in the family and community, independence, and overall quality of life.
4. A working knowledge of typical adaptive motor development and how it changes across the lifespan provides the framework for assessing functions and planning intervention.
5. NDT focuses on changing movement strategies as a means to achieve the best energy-efficient performance for the individual within the context of age-appropriate tasks and in anticipation of future functional tasks.
6. Movement is linked to sensory processing in two distinct ways (feedback and feedforward/anticipatory control).
7. Intervention strategies involve the individual's active initiation and participation, often combined with the therapist's manual guidance and direct handling.
8. NDT utilizes movement analysis to identify missing or atypical elements that link functional limitations to system impairments.
9. Ongoing evaluation occurs throughout every treatment session.
10. The aim of NDT is to optimize function.

As the frame of reference has evolved, additional assumptions have been accepted. Howle (2002, pp. 3–8) in the text *Neuro-Developmental Treatment Approach: Theoretical Foundations and Principles of Clinical Practice* outlines additional assumptions. The assumptions are reproduced with permission.

- NDT accepts that human motor behavior and function emerge from ongoing interaction amongst the individual, the task characteristics, and the specific environmental context.
- Movement is organized around behavioral goals.
- All individuals have competencies and strengths in various systems.
- A hallmark of efficient motor function is the ability of the individual to select and match various global neuronal maps with the potentially infinite number of movement combinations that are attuned to the forces of gravity, forces generated by contracting muscles, and constraints posed by various environmental conditions.
- NDT uses a model of enablement/disablement based on the International Classification of Functioning, Disability and Health (World Health Organization, 2001) developed by the World Health Organization to categorize the individual's health and disability.
- Clinicians can best design intervention by establishing functional outcomes in partnership with clients and caregivers.
- Intervention programs are designed to serve clients throughout their lifetime.
- Learning or relearning motor skills and improving performance requires both practice and experience.
- Treatment is most effective during recovery or phase transition.
- NDT clinicians assume the responsibility to provide clients with the available evidence related to all intervention methods, outcomes, and service delivery systems.

Current Theoretical Foundations

As a "living concept," NDT draws upon the knowledge of evolving contemporary science. Movement analysis, problem solving, and handling intervention prevail as primary constructs aimed at the influence of posture and movement skills in pediatric clients. Primary concepts of therapeutic exercise, biomechanics, and kinesiology contribute to core NDT theoretical foundations.

The specific and unique focus of the NDT frame of reference is the production of change in functional posture and movement skills. Lesions in the CNS are assumed to produce these postural and movement problem encountered by children with neuropathology. Together with features of atypical qualities of muscle tone and muscle activation, clients experience resulting impairments in occupational performance. To effect change in functional posture and movement skills, current theoretical foundations of NDT include aspects of the Dynamic Systems Theory of Motor Control, the Neuronal Group Selection Theory, Sensory Contributions, and Motor Learning.

Dynamic Systems Theory of Motor Control

NDT has embraced the *Dynamic Systems approach* as a theoretical foundation emphasizing the notion that movement is an interactive process between multiple systems (Darrah & Bartlett, 1995). Collectively, diverse systems shape the production of functional movement skills. Typical control of posture and movement relies upon interplay between elements of the various neural and body systems, the task, the individual, and the context of the task.

The Dynamic Systems perspective rejects the hierarchical "top-down" perception of the nervous system operating as a control center over the production of motor skills (Figure 7.3). Advanced technology has clarified that all physical parameters (muscles, ligaments, joints, brain, etc.) contribute to the production of movement in an interconnected manner, demanding consideration of all variables. The nervous system codes and learns movements related to task and environmental conditions. Movements having functional relevance to a person are stored as a "dynamic system" of information processing. When one element in the movement system is altered, change is observed in the entire movement system.

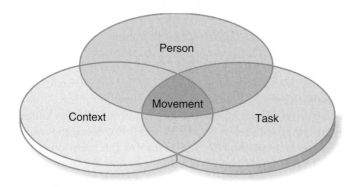

FIGURE 7.3 Dynamic systems model of motor control.

The Dynamic Systems approach ensures examination of all systems involved in movement production (Kamm, Thelan, & Jensen, 1990; Smith & Thelen, 1993). Identification of movement "constraints" or "limiting factors," terms used within Dynamic Systems approach, assists the therapist in problem solving the selection of optimum treatment strategies. Constraint factors limiting movement production might include bony restrictions, limited flexibility in soft tissues and fascia, varying level of arousal, poor sensory processing, and movement impairments created by faulty timing and lack of coordinative firing of muscles attempting to work cooperatively together (Howle, 2002).

Dynamic Systems Theory recognizes that each individual movement subsystem develops at its own rate, but is constrained (or supported) by physical and environmental elements. Any component that prevents the success of a functional task can be considered a "rate-limiting" factor. For example, the mass of an infant's head relative to the body size limits the rate of the developmental head lifting. Consequentially, *NDT no longer considers rate of development as an outcome measure of an NDT program*. Currently, importance is placed upon reducing or influencing the various rate-limiting factors with the goal of improving function. Therapists analyze and problem solve, choosing the optimal variables within the movement system for manipulation enhancing opportunity for motor skill development (Howle, 2002).

The Dynamic Systems approach proposes that motor development is a self-organizing phenomenon that appears to occur naturally as children experience their environment. Through practice and repetition, different elements of the movement system "come together," integrating information to form a distinct movement synergy. Movement synergies are depicted as pieces "assembled" together within the nervous system, resulting in a distinct movement outcome facilitating quick and efficient interaction with the environment (Thelen et al., 1993). When learning new movements, children actively "solve movement problems" through their engagement with the environment, practicing a wide variety of movement strategies prior to selecting the single "best" solution to their movement problem. The development of compensatory motor synergies observed in children with neuropathology are often established as a "problem-solving" strategies to their movement problems.

Trial and error provides feedback to the motor learning system, allowing for adjustment and refinement of motor skills within a context. NDT captures this element of the Dynamic Systems Theory during treatment sessions by inviting the child to actively problem solve new movement opportunities which are repeated and reinforced in various contexts and tasks.

NDT and the Dynamic Systems Theory share the value of creating "chaos" in the movement systems as mechanism for promoting the evolution of new motor behaviors. Transitions from a stable state of being to an unstable state are natural occurrences of learning and necessary for the development of skilled movement. During typical development, motor behaviors naturally shift and change in "phase," moving toward increased stability or toward destabilization. During these episodes of change and chaos, new forms of movement emerge (Thelen, 1992). When influencing the motor strategies employed by children with neuropathology, sensorimotor interventions potentially create episodes of destabilization and "chaos" making way for the growth of new motor patterns and behaviors.

The Neuronal Group Selection Theory

NDT also incorporates the theoretical foundations of the Neuronal Group Selection Theory (Hadders-Algra, 2000). This theory provides the occupational therapist with an understanding of the neuronal interactions inside the CNS contributing to movement production. According to Neuronal Group Selection Theory, the brain is dynamically organized into neural networks or neuronal groups that share connections related to their function. Engagement with the environment and tasks shape these neuronal groups, creating networks of hardwired neurons engrammed through repeated experience. These functional neuronal units "come on line" jointly as a coded synergy of information producing efficient and integrated interaction with the environment.

The nervous system possesses an inherent mechanism recognizing the distinct value that a particular movement or behavior has to each person. This built-in mechanism fuels the hardwiring process with neurochemistry reinforcing the connection of these neural synergies within the CNS (Edelman, 1987). Factors such as cognition, motivation, and temperament prime the nervous system for this selective organizational process. The architecture of each individual's nervous system is shaped by the distinct and unique experiences of that individual, accomplished by a selective neurobiological process known as "pruning." Similar to pruning a hedge, the nervous system selectively cuts back on neural connections that are unnecessary while trimming and organizing the connections of value.

NDT subscribes to the principles of the Neuronal Group Selection Theory by repeating valuable adaptive movement experiences in therapy with the aspiration of creating new neuronal maps easing future access to these "motor files" within the CNS. NDT uses handling as its "key" treatment strategy correlating enhanced somatosensory input with movement, loading the nervous system with additional neurochemical information to reinforce the neural mapping process.

Sensory Contributions

NDT recognizes two distinct types of complementary sensory systems contributing to the production of well-coordinated movement (Howle, 2002). The feedforward sensory system is a proactive sensory system that anticipates and initiates movements intrinsic to the person, while the complementary feedback sensory system reacts to the environment, regulating and adapting motor execution. Together these sensory systems interact within the CNS fueling the motor system with information about the movement, the task, and the environment.

Sensory processing is the ability to receive, register, and organize sensory input for use, facilitating creative and adaptive responses to the surrounding environment (Howle, 2002). The acquisition of complex, intentional, and accurate coordinated movements requires precise registration and interpretation of sensory feedback received from the movement and the environment. Registration of this sensory information within the nervous system serves as an internal mechanism for detection of movement errors, the learning of new movements, motor planning, and skilled motor execution. Movements created by an individual's motor system in the absence of sensory feedback from the body or the environment are derived from the feedforward sensory system, preparing the motor system with appropriate sensory information in advance of muscle recruitment. NDT provides the child with enriched motor experience and opportunity to practice movements emphasizing sensorimotor feedback and providing possibilities for problem-solving movement strategies using anticipatory motor control.

Motor Learning

NDT also assimilates principles of motor learning theory into its primary theoretical foundations. Motor learning theory is a set of processes that directly relate to practice or experience leading to relatively permanent changes in the capability for movement (Larin, 2000; Schmidt & Lee, 1999). NDT intervention structures motor learning experiences eliciting active movement participation from the client. Physical and cognitive, verbal and nonverbal *guidance* as well as verbal and nonverbal *feedback* in relationship to performance are shared elements of motor learning theory and NDT intervention. Transfer of newly learned skills into daily life settings is an inherent feature of the NDT approach (Howle, 2002).

FUNCTION–DYSFUNCTION CONTINUA

Function–dysfunction continua provide therapists with descriptions of observable behaviors that are clinically relevant and identify the presence of function and dysfunction in children (Schoen & Anderson, 1999). There are five key function–dysfunction continua, essential for the clinical assessment process that provides therapists with descriptions of observable behaviors. The continua are ROM and dissociation of movement, postural alignment and patterns of weight bearing, muscle tone/postural tone, balance and postural control, and coordination.

Indicators of Function and Dysfunction: Range of Movement and Dissociation of Movement

Typically developing infants do not yet demonstrate full ROM at all of their joints. Infants gradually increase the ROM at each of their joints by practicing varieties of movements in all three planes of movement—sagittal, frontal, and transverse (Bly, 1999) (Table 7.1). As the constraints on joint range and muscle strength become more flexible with maturation and experience, the movements and muscle activity involved in motor control also become more adaptive (Howle, 2002).

Infants with CNS pathology do not practice movements on all three planes. They maintain a few positions and rarely alternate between positions. This poor variation of movement manifests as a limited repertoire of general movement. Infants with CNS pathology typically move in a sagittal plane and subsequently develop stereotyped, limited repertoires of motor behavior. These limited motor repertoires restrict opportunity to elongate and activate muscles, preventing the experience of full ROM of the joints. If these motor limitations continue throughout time, the child becomes vulnerable to the development of muscular contractures and skeletal deformities (Bly, 1999).

TABLE 7.1 Indicators of Function and Dysfunction for Range of Motion and Dissociation of Movement	
Full Passive Range of Motion	***Contractures or Deformities***
FUNCTION: Ability for the child to be moved through passive range of motion	*DYSFUNCTION:* Contractures, deformities, limiting passive range of motion
Indicators of Function	**Indicators of Dysfunction**
Full passive range of motion	Contractures
	Deformities
Dissociation of Movement	***Associated Movement Patterns***
Indicators of Function	**Indicators of Dysfunction**
Rolls with rotation between shoulders and pelvis	Log rolling
Use of reciprocal leg movements in creeping and crawling	Bunny hopping
Orients head in all planes in space	Pull to stand with lower extremities in extension, adduction, and internal rotation
Holds toy in one hand and manipulates with another	Hand closing associated with flexion of the arm and extension of the arm

Indicators of Function and Dysfunction: Alignment and Patterns of Weight Bearing

Normal alignment is defined as alignment of the body segments necessary for anticipation and organization of movements for a task. As previously stated, the alignment of the body segments over the base of support determines the amount of effort required to support the body against gravity (Howle, 2002).

Atypical postural alignment in any or all of the three planes of movement is an indicator of dysfunction (Schoen & Anderson, 1999). Abnormal alignment can occur due to changes in muscle tone, strength imbalances, or skeletal problems related to growth. The limited capacity of children with neuromotor challenges to "line up" the spinal segments places muscular activation at a biomechanical disadvantage resulting in subsequent postural control difficulties. Limited postural control necessary to sustain the alignment of spinal segments automatically alters the center of mass over the base of support, changing the forces of gravitational pull upon both intrasegmental and intersegmental joint relationships (Table 7.2). Limited segmental alignment can be observed in a sagittal plane (posterior pelvic tilt/flexor bias or anterior pelvic tilt/extensor bias), the frontal plane (asymmetry), and/or in a transverse plane (rotation of segments upon each other).

Atypical patterns of weight bearing are a particular alignment dysfunction arising from the abnormal distribution of the body weight at rest in relation to the support surface and in anticipation of movement (Figure 7.4). Efficient contact with the support surface through weight bearing is necessary for the typical initiation of muscle contraction and effective movement (Howle, 2002). Children with neuromotor challenges are often unable to conform to the support surface. Limitation in pressure distribution between the body part and the support surface hinders the child's ability to generate the

TABLE 7.2 Indicators of Function and Dysfunction for Alignment and Patterns of Weight Bearing

Postural Alignment	Lack of Postural Alignment

FUNCTION: Postural alignment and appropriate distribution of weight in relationship to the base of support during weight bearing
Indicators of Function
  Alignment of body parts in relation to each other and to position in space
	DYSFUNCTION: Lack of postural alignment and abnormal patterns of weight bearing
	Indicators of Dysfunction
	  Malalignment of spinal segments in frontal, sagittal, or transverse planes
	  Posterior pelvic tilt, spinal flexion
	  Anterior pelvic tilt, spinal hyperextension
	  Asymmetrical posture
	  Skeletal deformities (scoliosis, kyphosis)
	  Narrow or widened base of support resulting in maladaptive weight bearing patterns

necessary force to push off against the base of support to get up off the floor or initiate transitional movements in and out of positions (Howle, 2002).

Indicators of Function and Dysfunction: Muscle Tone

"Muscle tone" is a term describing the stiffness or tension with which a muscle resists being lengthened. "Stiffness," a term often used interchangeably with spasticity, describes

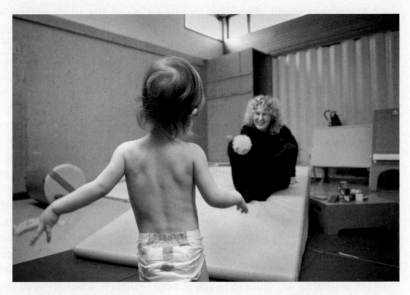

FIGURE 7.4 Atypical alignment of the joint segments in the frontal plane.

the elastic characteristics of muscles. Like spasticity, stiffness is a measure of the resistance to motion. Stiffness is the amount of force required to produce a change in length. If a great amount of force is needed to produce a change in length, then the muscle is said to have increased stiffness (Holt, Butcher, & Fonesca, 2000).

Hypotonia is evident when there is a disruption in recruitment patterns causing inefficient muscle activation or abnormal timing in recruitment of the agonists and antagonists, producing ineffective muscle contractions (Carr & Shepherd, 2000). Muscles that are hypotonic create a problem in effective motor execution because they are either unable to reach the threshold for muscle fiber firing or are unable to recruit enough motor units to initiate movement (Howle, 2002).

Children with neuromotor challenges demonstrate an uneven distribution of muscle tone throughout their body. For example, children identified with cerebral palsy affecting all four extremities (child with spastic quadriplegia) often exhibit increased stiffness in a distal distribution of their bodies. Children with cerebral palsy affecting only the lower extremities (child with spastic diplegia) typically exhibit increased stiffness in the lower extremities relative to the upper extremities. Differences in muscle tone can also be observed between the right and left sides of the body (asymmetry). The distribution of muscle tone is also generally influenced by state of arousal, health, and by position of the body in relationship to gravity (Table 7.3).

Indicators of Function and Dysfunction: Postural Tone

Postural tone is the actual distribution of muscle tone among specific muscle groups that are "constrained" together to maintain posture against the force of gravity and must simultaneously adapt their internal stiffness to allow for the flexibility necessary

TABLE 7.3 Indicators of Function and Dysfunction for Muscle Tone

Normal Muscle Tone	Atypical Muscle Tone

FUNCTION: Active state of muscle readiness to move
Indicators of Function
  Developmentally appropriate use of limbs for support and finer adjustments during skilled activity
	DYSFUNCTION: Trunk or extremities stiff or floppy interfering with antigravity movements
	Indicators of Dysfunction
	  Hypermobility and hyperextendability of joints
	  Decreased degree of tension in muscles
	  Limbs feel heavy on passive range of motion
	  Limbs and body sink into any support surface
	  Presence of varying degrees of stiffness in various joints interfering with antigravity movement
	  Presence of involuntary movements, or fluctuations in muscle activation
	  Increased degree of tension in muscles
	  Resistance to passive range of motion
	  Areas of the body with increased stiffness withdraw from contact with the support surface

for movement (Shumway-Cook & Woollacott, 2007). Postural tone is observed in the muscles of the trunk and the supporting extremities. The amount of tone and the muscle groups constrained at any one time change with the individual's position, counteracting the force of gravity for orientation and stability.

The term "postural tone" has been traditionally used in NDT literature to describe the background tone for movement. The term "fixing" used in the context of examining postural tone specifically addresses the muscle activity around a joint that is used to degrees of freedom for stability, supporting postural control. In other words, "fixing" is a means of gaining postural control for movement.

Children with neuromotor challenges experience impairments of postural tone. These abnormalities in muscle tone, while sustaining a posture, are observed in various systems affecting motor control. As previously noted, mechanical properties of muscle tone may be altered prohibiting active muscle contraction for sustained postural control (Stockmeyer, 2000). An example of abnormal postural tone is observed when a child exhibits the inability to organize and integrate somatosensory input from the muscles of the neck, resulting in changes in muscle tone patterns in relationship to head movements (Shea, Guadagnoli, & Dean, 1995). Varying systems within the motor system interact collectively to produce postural control and disturbance in any one system affects motor execution. A challenge in processing of sensory information from the vestibular and visual systems diminishes the organization of postural tone for active movement against gravity (Figure 7.5).

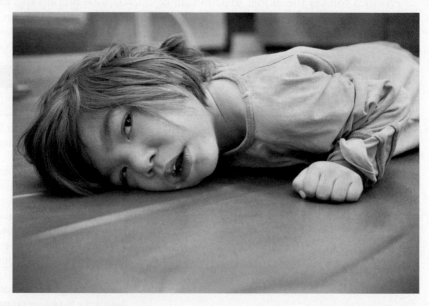

FIGURE 7.5 Limitations in postural tone prevent antigravity movements away from the support surface. This child is unable to push her body up off the support surface against the forces of gravity due to decreased postural tone.

TABLE 7.4 Indicators of Function and Dysfunction for Postural Tone	
Normal Postural Tone	*Atypical Postural Tone*
FUNCTION: Ability to sustain muscle activation for postural support against gravity	*DYSFUNCTION*: Inability to sustain muscle activation for postural support against gravity
Indicators of Function	**Indicators of Dysfunction**
Adapt muscle stiffness providing flexible movement synergies	Excessive stiffness in trunk and/or extremities when attempting to sustain posture against gravity
Sufficient muscle force production to counter-act forces of gravity	Excessive floppiness in trunk and/or limbs when attempting to sustain posture against gravity
	Presence of "fixing" or compensatory muscle synergies when attempting to sustain posture against gravity
	Increased postural tone or stiffness to "hold on and stay put" at the expense of movement against gravity
	Postural control predominantly static
	Stereotypical movement patterns

Postural tone can change in nature along a continuum ranging from either low to normal, normal to high or all the way from low to high depending upon the position of the body, the nature of the task and environmental factors (Schoen & Anderson, 1999) (Table 7.4).

Indicators of Function and Dysfunction: Balance and Postural Control

Postural control is the ability to assume and maintain body positions during static and dynamic movement. As is observed in all movement acquisition, the development of typical postural control involves multisystems within the body and arises through experience and interaction between the individual, the task, and the environment (Table 7.5).

To achieve postural control, the body must have the capacity to maintain a stable position or "steady-state of balance" maintaining the center of mass within the limits of the base of support. The body must also have the capacity to react and adjust to perturbation, exhibiting equilibrium reactions that are flexible and varied in response to the environment (Howle, 2002).

Difficulties with scaling or the ability to match the size of muscle response to the size of perturbation are additional features often observed in children with neuropathology, contributing to postural control difficulties. Postural responses are often too large for the displacement, thereby creating struggle in equilibrium reactions (Howle, 2002).

Indicators of Function and Dysfunction: Coordination

Coordination is the temporal–spatial quality of task execution. Being "well-coordinated" means having movements that are accurate, reliable, efficient, quick, and adaptable

TABLE 7.5 Indicators of Function and Dysfunction for Balance and Postural Control

Active Balance and Postural Reactions Both Anticipatory and Reactive	*Atypical Postural and Balance Reactions*
FUNCTION: Dynamic postural control	*DYSFUNCTION*: Compensatory postural control
Indicators of Function	**Indicators of Dysfunction**
Maintains and moves in and out of developmental positions	Lack of accommodation of body segments to base of support
Anticipates postural orientation and prepares body for task interaction	Wide or excessively narrow base of support
Ability to assume and maintain positions during static and dynamic movement	Attempts to gain postural control by moving away from the base of support
	Use of upper extremities for stability beyond developmentally appropriate age
	Use of compensatory patterns such as persistence of the upper extremities in high guard position for maintaining or regaining balance during a weight shift; excessive reliance on protective reactions during weight shifting; persistence of asymmetrical patterns; various fixation patterns present (i.e., hand fisting, toe clawing)
	Exclusive use of "w" sitting position for postural control in sitting

(Table 7.6). Coordination also requires an efficient musculoskeletal system, including the properties of the muscles and tendons. Impaired coordination refers to movements that appear awkward, uneven, clumsy, or inaccurate and results from the disruption of the activation, sequencing, timing, and scaling of muscle activity (Howle, 2002).

One of the major sources of interference with interlimb coordination involves the temporal structures of the actions that the child is trying to coordinate. Discrete tasks

TABLE 7.6 Indicators of Function and Dysfunction for Coordination

Stereotypical Movement Patterns	*Various Movement Patterns*
FUNCTION: Various movement patterns	*DYSFUNCTION*: Stereotypical movement patterns that are consistent compensations in various positions and tasks
Indicators of Function	**Indicators of Dysfunction**
Use of varied repertoire of movement patterns based on the demands of the activity	Stereotypically, one or both lower extremities persist with extension, adduction, and internal rotation in all positions
	Stereotypically, one or both upper extremities persist with shoulder elevation and retraction in all positions

have definite start and end points with considerable planning necessary for preparing the body to move (Howle, 2002). Coordination is an additional characteristic of movement that helps therapists identify function and dysfunction in children.

GUIDE TO EVALUATION

The NDT problem-solving model guides occupational therapists through evaluation and goal setting to intervention implementation (Howle, 2002). The core premise of NDT evaluation is centered upon the analysis of posture and movement as it relates to functional skill performance. The NDT examination process is an individualized method, evaluating each child as a unique person with multiple competencies and limitations. Assessment is provided within the context of the child, the family and the environment in which the child engages in occupational behaviors. The NDT evaluation initiates the problem-solving process based upon evidence from clinical research, therapeutic experience, and clinical reasoning skills. This examination incorporates principles from the study of motor control, motor learning, and motor development, providing structure to the therapist's clinical reasoning process.

During the handling process, the therapist gathers further data for their assessment based upon the reactions of the child's body and movements provided to sensorimotor input and to positioning that optimizes the child's maximum functional performance. Therapists evaluate and hypothesize potential effects of posture and motor control limitations upon occupational performance. Identification of consistent posture and movement problems in various positions and functions helps the occupational therapist establish priorities for intervention.

Clinicians observe spontaneous posture and movements produced by the child during functional activities, noting the frequency with which specific postural and movement strategies are repeated. The child's variability of movement strategies is noted, reflecting the stability and adaptability within the child's motor system. Components of movement that are either atypical or missing entirely are identified. Particular attention to the *repeated* use of particular compensatory strategies within varying positions and tasks guides the therapist's clinical reasoning for intervention. Focus upon the elements of alignment, weight bearing, balance, coordination, muscle and postural tone, and movement components utilized by the child. Handling further provides assessment information with respect to the child's capacity to use sensorimotor information in alteration of current movement strategies.

A complete occupational therapy evaluation might include evaluation of oral-motor and feeding skills, gross and fine motor skills, sensory deficits, social–emotional factors, and cognitive skills. Not all of these areas, however, are addressed in this chapter. Other frames of reference in this book may be applicable to these areas (Schoen & Anderson, 1999).

NDT emphasizes the need for informal, ongoing examination as part of treatment to identify the success of treatment strategies. NDT does not have a standardized assessment format. Lack of standardization and minimal relative evidence has encouraged some critics of the NDT approach to label it as an ineffective treatment approach. Therapists agree it is difficult to quantify this type of child's condition and improvements. Indeed, it is widely recognized that there are challenges with standardization that arise due to the heterogeneity of the population of children with CNS pathology.

NDT evaluation is predominantly concerned with the "quality" of how movements are performed within a functional context. Currently, most evaluations of motor skill performance are focused upon acquisition of skills in a quantitative manner, so they do not necessarily reflect the whole picture of the child's abilities or their changes in abilities following therapeutic intervention.

The entry-level therapist develops skills in this type of assessment by following a more structured evaluation approach under the supervision of an experienced therapist (Schoen & Anderson, 1999). The outline presented provides some structured guidelines for NDT assessment (Figure 7.6).

Overall Assessment of Functional Skills

In addition to the evaluation of posture and movement, contributing elements to functional skills are also assessed. Factors such as motivation, arousal, perception, and cognition are examined in relationship to movement production.

The occupational therapist is also concerned with assessing upper extremity occupational behavior. These skills relate to the child's ability to use the arms for weight bearing, provide support during transitions, as well as facilitate reach, grasp, manipulation, and release of objects in various positions.

Gross motor and upper extremity functional performance skills contribute to the ability to perform activities of daily living (ADL). Within NDT, ADL is a distinct area of functional skills, often an end result of the combination of gross motor and upper extremity function. ADL includes participation in feeding, dressing, and self-care, as well as the ability to explore, play, and then learn from the environment (Schoen & Anderson, 1999). Of particular importance to the occupational therapist is the impact of abnormal movement and posture on the child's use of his or her upper extremities as they relate to independent tool use and self-care.

Evaluation of Posture and Movement

Specific to NDT is the evaluation of posture and movement. Qualities of the function–dysfunction continuum are assessed within this analysis process. Attention is paid to the quality of muscle tone at rest and postural tone changes that occur during stable and mobile task demands. To assist with evaluating posture and movement, the therapist notes postural alignment in all three planes of movement. Joint ROM and postural control in relationship to the base of support are also evaluated. Interlimb and intralimb coupling are both assessed to determine the dissociation of one body part from another. For example, many children with cerebral palsy experience restrictions in their hamstrings and hip flexors, demonstrating a "tightly linked" intralimb coupling relationship between the pelvis and the femur. Additionally, children may demonstrate an intralimb relationship between wrist flexion and radial deviation that is tightly constrained,

I. Examination of functional task/potential for change
  1. Gross motor abilities/movements through space
  2. Fine motor/task-directed functions
  3. Activities of daily living
  4. Communication
  5. Oral-motor functions
  6. Social skills/behavior
II. Examination of posture and movement
  1. Alignment
  2. Relationship of base of support and center of mass
  3. Postural control and balance
    a. Anticipatory (proactive)/weight shift
    b. Steady-state balance
    c. Equilibrium (reactive)
  4. Movement strategies and compensations
  5. Muscle and postural tone/distribution of hypertonia and hypotonia
  6. Symmetry/asymmetry
  7. Kinesiological and biomechanical components of mpvement
  8. Coordination
  9. Description analysis of specific motor functions (gait, handwriting, chewing)
III. Examination of system integrity and impairments
  1. Neuromuscular
    a. Muscle activation and execution
      i) Timing initiating, sustaining, terminating muscle activity
      ii) Generation of force/tension
      iii) Coactivation/reciprocal relationships
      iv) Intralimb and interlimb dynamics
      v) Modulation and scaling of forces
    b. Coordination of postural stability with movement
    c. Synergies
    d. Spasticity
    e. Extraneous movements
    f. Fractionated or dissociated movements
    g. Hypokinesia
	2. Musculoskeletal
	    a. Range of motion; joint and soft tissue
	    b. Muscle extensibility, functional range
	    c. Muscle strength and endurance
	    d. Skeletal abnormalities
	  3. Sensory
	    a. Vision
	    b. Auditory
	    c. Gustatory
	    d. Vestibular
	    e. Somatosensory (tactile and proprioceptive)
	    f. Sensory processing and modulation
	  4. Regulatory
	    a. Arousal
	    b. State regulation
	    c. Emotional regulation and control
	  5. Perceptual/cognitive
	    a. Intelligence
	    b. Attention
	    c. Memory
	    d. Adaptability
	    e. Motor planning (gestalt of task, perception of position in space, and spatial relationships)
	    f. Executive functions (goal setting, inhibit impulsiveness, understanding consequences of actions)
	  6. Other systems
	    a. Integumentary
	    b. Respiratory
	    c. Cardiovascular
	    d. Gastrointestinal
	  7. Changes in performance and capacity, basedon response to facilitation, modification of task, or environment

Reproduced with permission from Howle, J. M. (2002). *Neuro-Developmental treatment approach: Theoretical foundations and principles of clinical practice.* Laguna Beach, CA. NDTA.

FIGURE 7.6 Guideline for neurodevelopmental assessment.

thereby preventing "dissociation" of these joint segments. The relationship between body segments needs to be analyzed to assist in the planning of treatment implementation.

The therapist also observes the postural control patterns and synergies of muscle activation used by the child to maintain positions in space or to move the body from place to place. For example, a child with hypotonia and decreased strength in the trunk musculature may use the upper extremities as a support for the body to maintain an erect posture, limiting the availability of upper extremity freedom for function. Reduced opportunities for play, hand exploration, ADL, and tool use may result from this dominating postural strategy.

POSTULATES REGARDING CHANGE

Postulates for creating change in functional performance guide the therapist in developing strategies and methods of intervention to facilitate that change. When the results of evaluation indicate dysfunction, intervention focuses on the qualitative aspects of movement that interfere with the child's ability to develop skills or functional abilities. Varying movement and postural problems may require different handling approaches. As previously emphasized, the primary technique of intervention during NDT is therapeutic handling provided by the therapist. The following postulates assist the therapist in treatment facilitation.

General Postulates Relating Change

The development of a wide variety of movements is influenced by the child's human and nonhuman environment. The occupational therapist's use of objects and activities maximizes the child's motivation to engage in therapy and, ultimately, improve motor abilities.

1. If movement achieved through handling is used in functional interaction within the environment, then the child has the greatest opportunity to develop functional skills.
2. If the therapist adapts the environment to take into account the child's developmental level, needs, and interests, then the maximum amount of stimulation will be provided to encourage motor skills.
3. If the therapist uses handling techniques when a child's attention is focused on a play activity, then it is often easier for the child to respond with an automatic movement pattern.
4. If the occupational therapist is responsive to the child's needs (i.e., sensitivity to movement, familiarity with situation or environment) and encourages the child to initiate movement during treatment, then therapeutic handling will be an interactive and meaningful process and the child will be more likely to initiate active movement to engage in purposeful activities.
5. If preventative measures such as adaptive equipment and orthotic devices are provided, then the child will receive consistent input to prevent or reduce the occurrence of secondary deformities and limitations (Schoen & Anderson, 1999).

Postulates Relating to Range of Motion and Dissociation of Movement

There are two general postulates regarding change in this frame of reference:

1. If the therapist prepares the client's muscle length and joint ROM with various forms of handling, potential to increase muscle activation is facilitated. Traction combined with joint alignment into end ranges of joint mobility may potentially prepare the muscle length and soft tissue mobility for muscle recruitment. Speed, position of the child's body, and direction of handling cues vary depending on the child's conditions of stiffness, hypotonia, and soft tissue/bony restrictions.
2. If the therapist provides handling to promote weight shifts and transitional movements, alignment and dissociation of joint segments are supported as the child moves in and out of positions with proper alignment.

Postulates Relating to Postural Alignment and Patterns of Weight Bearing

There are six postulates regarding change related to postural alignment and patterns of weight bearing:

1. If the therapist facilitates postural alignment in preparation for initiation of movement, then the child will have the potential to use appropriate muscle activation to maintain postural control during activities.
2. If the therapist maintains alignment throughout an active movement sequence within a functional task, the child will have the potential to sustain muscle activation for posture and movement with greater independence and energy efficiency.
3. If the therapist facilitates cocontraction of musculature around a joint through aligned weight-bearing experiences, potential to develop proximal muscle strength, timing, and sequencing of muscle contractions will be afforded. The therapist may add sensory input to the weight-bearing experience with deep pressure, joint compression, or weight shifts enhancing motor control in an aligned position.
4. If the therapist provides sensory input such as deep pressure down toward the child's base of support when the body segments are aligned, this pattern of weight bearing will facilitate the initiation of movement from the base of support using the benefit of ground force reactions to aiding in muscle activation.
5. If the therapist provides weight bearing through an aligned body segment, sensory feedback from the weight-bearing experience potentially relaxes muscle activation and prepares the body segment for active engagement in task.
6. If the therapist provides handling to promote weight shifts and transitional movements to support alignment and dissociation of coupled joint segments, then the child will likely learn to move in and out of positions with proper alignment.

Postulates Relating to Muscle Tone/Postural Tone

There are four postulates regarding change related to muscle tone/postural tone:

1. If the therapist is able to feel the child's muscle activation/relaxation and the therapist can grade his or her touch and directional cues accordingly, then the child

will receive enhanced sensory input preparing the body for active participation in movement activity.

2. If the therapist is able to monitor the child's reactions to handling, then handling techniques may be modified in accordance to the child's changing needs for sensory information.

3. If the child has atypical muscle tone/postural tone, the therapist uses graded sensory input. This sensory input includes combinations of tactile, vestibular, and proprioceptive stimulation provided at different rates, rhythms, speeds, positions, and directions. Distal and proximal key points of control are used with varying ranges to modulate tonal properties. The goal of this handling is to reduce the use of compensatory muscle synergies and "fixation" of muscle patterns for stability and reduced degrees of freedom.

4. If the therapist is able to alter the impact of gravity through handling, positioning, or equipment, then the child will experience potential muscle activation under conditions of either reduced or increased resistive forces within a movement task.

Postulates Relating to Balance and Postural Control

There are six postulates regarding change related to balance and postural control:

1. If the therapist facilitates smooth interplay between agonist and antagonist muscles, then the child will potentially be able to achieve postural control in relationship to gravity.

2. If the therapist selects the appropriate position, equipment, and therapeutic handling techniques, facilitating opportunities for isometric, sustained holding of the trunk against gravity the potential to improve postural control is afforded.

3. If the therapist facilitates postural control during functional movement activities, and provides the child with repeated opportunity to experience these movement patterns in context, potentially the child will integrate these movement patterns into neuronal groups within the CNS.

4. If the therapist uses graded handling techniques combined with analysis of the child's response to sensory input over time, the child will potentially develop greater strength, stability, and control during increasingly complex movement sequences.

5. If the therapist includes facilitation in all three planes of movement with specific facilitation of weight shifts into the transverse plane, then the child will experience the potential for axial rotation, elongation of multiple muscular systems simultaneously, dissociation of intralimb/interlimb couples, and activation of postural control synergies.

6. If the therapist provides concentric and eccentric muscle work throughout aligned joint range, motor strength and control are potentially increased and graded during functional movement tasks.

Postulates Regarding Coordination

There are two postulates regarding change related to coordination:

1. If the therapist provides support to the performance of isolated movements requiring precision potentially increased dissociation and fractionated movements will be available to the child.
2. If the therapist facilitates bimanual coordination through the choice of appropriate tasks demanding coordination, the child will potentially develop patterns of integrated interlimb movements.

APPLICATION TO PRACTICE

The NDT theoretical base constitutes essential knowledge for entry-level occupational therapists who work with children experiencing neurological impairment. The application of these concepts requires skill and practice. Translating these concepts into treatment may also be learned effectively through supervision from an experienced therapist. Specialized training, through continuing education workshops—ranging from 2-day introductory courses to 8-week basic courses—is available through the NDTA, providing a comprehensive understanding and application of this frame of reference (www.ndta.org; Schoen & Anderson, 1999).

The ideal application of NDT incorporates a team approach including occupational therapy, physical therapy, speech therapy, special education, and the family. In each setting, such as school, home, clinic, or private practice, the occupational therapist must establish treatment priorities. The role and responsibilities of the occupational therapist may vary, depending on the setting and the other disciplines involved and the therapist's individual skills (Schoen & Anderson, 1999).

Following an in-depth evaluation of the child's consistent competencies and challenges, a treatment plan is established anticipating outcomes that can be observable within a specific time frame under specific environmental conditions. The emphasis of NDT is to establish a purposeful relationship between sensory input and motor output. This is accomplished through the inclusion of precise therapeutic handling, which includes facilitation of posture and movement combined with inhibition of the child's limiting movement repertoires. NDT involves the following components of handling which are often interactive: preparation, facilitation, and inhibition.

Handling

Therapeutic handling is the primary intervention technique of NDT. When handling, the therapist places his or her hands purposefully and precisely upon the child's body to specifically influence posture and movement (Howle, 2002). Graded application of manual external forces is provided to the child's body through the therapist's hands.

Combined with directional cues the child can potentially feel and learn new movement patterns. As determined in the moment by clinical reasoning, grading of handling is achieved by changing hand placements, directions or forces, and the amount of sensory information provided (Howle, 2002). Handling directs, regulates and organizes tactile, vestibular, and proprioceptive contributions of movement production. Handling changes the alignment of the body in relationship to the base of support and with respect to the forces of gravity before and during movement sequences. Through handling, the child is guided to decrease the amount of excessive muscle force used to stabilize the body segments. As the child develops independent motor control, the therapist diminishes handling support as the child assumes greater internal control of his or her movement strategies (Howle, 2002).

Handling is based upon principles of biomechanics, laws of physics, and knowledge of anatomy and kinesiology. Correction of alignment and muscle length tension relationships allows the client to bring muscles "on line" with greater ease. Handling progresses from passive elongation and alignment to active assisted movement and resistive activities, which ensures desired muscle synergy during task performance (Bly & Whiteside, 1997).

The placement of the therapist's hands needs to be preplanned and monitored ensuring against unnecessary and potentially confusing sensory information. Light pressure touch may leave the child feeling insecure or confused about the movement expectations. If the pressure is too heavy, however, movement may be "blocked" or minimized by the therapist's excessive sensory information (Bly & Whiteside, 1997).

Therapists new to the handling process may be tempted to grip onto body parts, imposing pushing, pulling, or lifting forces upon the child. The therapist's hands serve to guide rather than control movements. The therapist's hands can be placed across joints to ensure alignment, facilitate movement, or initiate weight shifts from that body segment. The therapist's hands are also placed directly on muscles to recruit muscle activity. The child feels the therapist initiate or block certain movements, learning from these sensations. Initially, hands-on placement may be necessary for the execution of all of the child's movements. In time as the child develops greater internal motor control, the therapist reduces the pressure and handling intensity promoting increasingly independent problem solving and motor execution.

Mrs. Bobath called the hand placement used during facilitation "key points of control." Key points may be proximal (such as the shoulder girdle, trunk, and pelvis) or distal (such as the head, hands, and feet) (Figure 7.7). Proximal hand placements can provide stability with some techniques, or mobility if the technique demands active movement of distal segments.

The therapist can also facilitate movements from joints or muscles that are distal to the trunk. Distal key points of control are only effective when the child possesses sufficient proximal control to organize a whole body movement from such a distal point of facilitation (Figure 7.8). Therapists must be very conscientious not to pull on an extremity that is subluxed, flaccid, or out of alignment when facilitating movement with a distal hand placement (Howle, 2002) (Figure 7.9).

During handling, each hand may possess a distinct role offering different forms of sensory input to the child's body while facilitating movement experiences. One hand

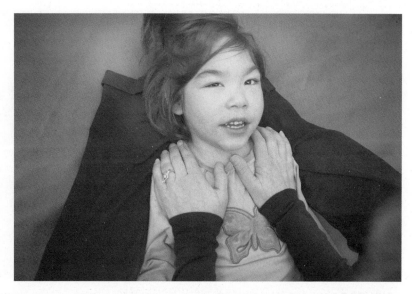

FIGURE 7.7 Therapist places her hands on a proximal key point of control providing downward compression from the superior surface of the shoulder girdle in an inferior direction toward the pelvis. This proximal key point of control elongates the neck/shoulder girdle musculature creating possibility for the development of active head control.

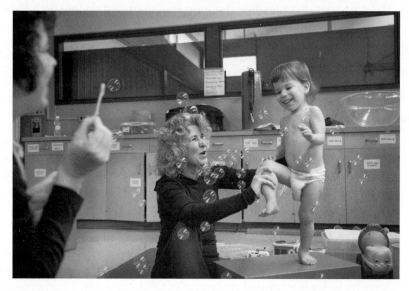

FIGURE 7.8 Therapist provides handling at a distal key point of control by placing her guiding hand on the child's leg, creating weight shift of the center of mass combined with increased proximal muscle strength and motor control at the trunk, pelvis, and hips.

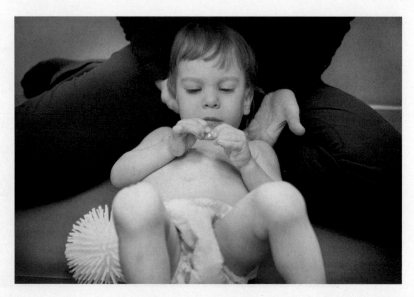

FIGURE 7.9 Using the head as a distal key point, the therapist creates a sense of midline orientation for the child facilitating eye–hand coordination and bilateral fine motor skills.

may be required to guide movement, while the other hand assists. The guiding hand has the primary task of leading the movement sequence while both hands work together to attain and maintain alignment of the body and individual joint segments. The guiding hand initiates weight shifts and provides stability to the body throughout a movement sequence (Bly & Whiteside, 1997). The role of each hand may shift numerous times throughout a handling session, depending upon the varying conditions (Howle, 2002).

Qualities of Touch

The levels of touch provided during handling are direct and contoured, shaped to the child's body. Depth of touch varies depending upon the type of sensory input required to elicit an active movement. Light touch is best used when the child demonstrates greater degrees of independent motor control and deep touch provides increased support and direction.

Compression and traction provide sensory data through both the touch and proprioceptive systems modifying tonal properties, alignment, and muscle activation. This touch cue adds a directional component to the cueing system signaling the direction of potential weight shifts. Compression is often employed to create cocontraction of muscles to anchor created alignment of joint segments. Compression can either relax or activate muscles depending upon their state of origination (Figures 7.10 and 7.11). Traction is often introduced to elongate stiff muscles, align joint segments, or facilitate the initiation of movement (Figure 7.12). Together, these changing forces applied to joints and muscles create changes in alignment and activation of muscle synergies for function.

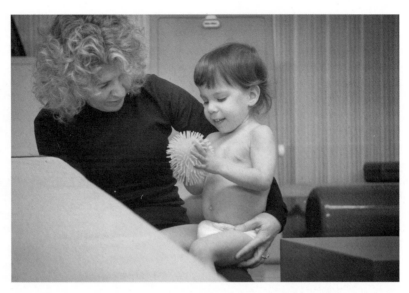

FIGURE 7.10 Compression forces in a downward direction provide deep sensory input to the muscles of the hips increasing contact with the base of support to enable muscular activation initiating erect trunk posture. With stable and active postural control in the trunk the upper extremities are free for bilateral play.

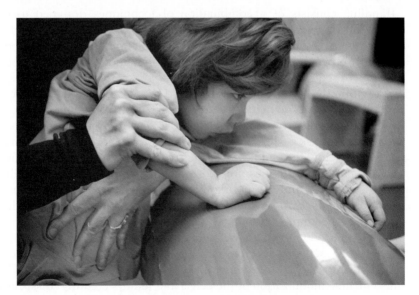

FIGURE 7.11 Compression forces directed from the elbow joint toward the hand with an aligned wrist provide deep sensory input to the hand against the support surface. This technique potentially relaxes the musculature of the hand in preparation for active weight bearing through an open hand.

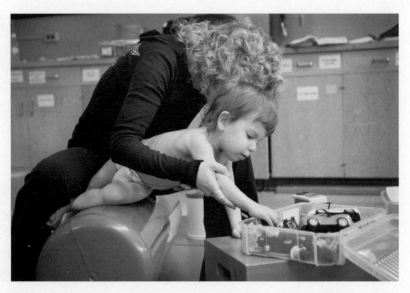

FIGURE 7.12 Traction along the length of the humerus creates an elongating force to the musculature between the scapula and the humerus extending the excursion of reach.

Preparation, Facilitation, and Inhibition

Handling consists of a combination of techniques designed to prepare the child's body, facilitate active movement, and inhibit unwanted movement patterns. At times, preparation techniques are provided in isolation, readying the body for movement, while at other times, preparation, facilitation, and inhibition meld and merge within a treatment sequence.

Within the context of NDT, the child is not expected to improve function simply by practicing a skilled activity. Children with neuromotor challenges do not have the capacity to independently select or activate the new appropriate motor patterns required for independent task performance. Often the components of a movement sequence must be prepared before the child can put them together in a functional sequence (Howle, 2002).

Preparatory activities are those techniques that involve mobilizing or elongating tight structures and promoting alignment of body segments to each another and in relationship to gravity. Whenever possible, treatment strategies mesh preparation within a task. For example, a therapist may have greater success elongating the child's trunk muscles and mobilizing the scapula on the thoracic wall, if the child is simultaneously engaged in active reach (Howle, 2002). The end result of preparation is a state of readiness for active initiation of posture and movement (Figure 7.13). Preparation may also include mobilization of the pelvis and femurs creating "dissociation" between joint segments to relax cocontracted muscles around those joints.

Facilitation is a handling strategy designed to ease the production of appropriate and efficient posture and movement patterns. Following preparatory activities, active or automatic movement patterns are facilitated, or invited into action, using therapeutic

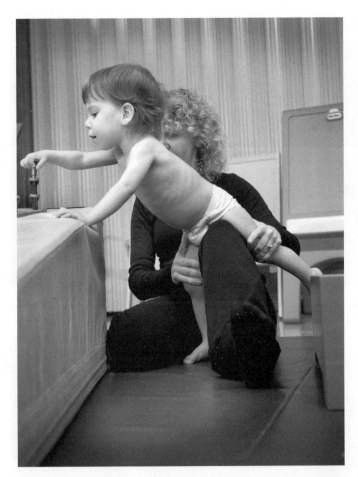

FIGURE 7.13 Creating dissociation between the lower extremities prepares the legs for reciprocal gait. Preparation is provided by combining a traction force to the left leg, relaxing left hip musculature, with downward compression to the right leg activating hip musculature.

sensorimotor input at various key points of control. Most often, preparation and facilitation techniques merge together as a single treatment sequence. For example, compression can be applied to the trunk, rib cage, or scapula inviting "stable" muscle activation of the proximal musculature. At the same time, "facilitation" is evident when the occupational therapist provides gentle traction on the humerus to invite active reach (Figure 7.14). This is an example of a dual intention achieved concurrently through handling; the promotion of both stability and mobility.

The child with high tone often benefits from facilitation that uses full ranges of movement and varieties of movement patterns. Generally, handling of the child with stiffness involves an interaction of techniques reducing tightness while facilitating active movement. Alternately but not exclusively, the child with low tone often benefits from slow, controlled movements in limited ranges, demanding increased muscle stiffness and activation. The hypotonic child often benefits from treatment provided in higher level antigravity positions, such as sitting and standing, requiring increased activation of proximal musculature (Figure 7.15).

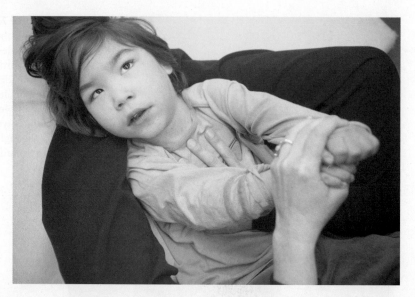

FIGURE 7.14 Handling techniques combine preparation to the trunk for stability with facilitation to the upper extremities for reach.

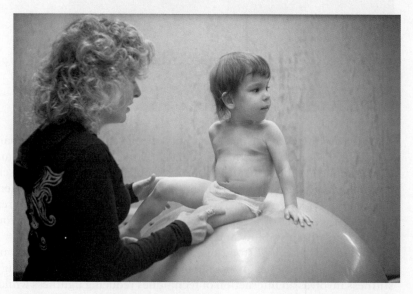

FIGURE 7.15 Handling and positioning with higher level antigravity forces facilitating active postural control in the hypotonic trunk.

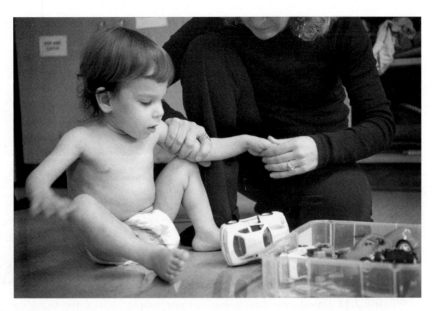

FIGURE 7.16 Handling techniques to facilitate reach and grasp for functional play.

Occupational therapists are often specifically concerned with the facilitation of upper extremity movements such as reaching, grasping, releasing of objects, and in-hand manipulation skills (Figure 7.16). Handling is also incorporated by the occupational therapist during self-care activities such as feeding, dressing, toileting, and personal hygiene.

Facilitation also includes the principles of weight bearing and weight shifting to activate motor control (Figure 7.17). All postural movements, whether gross or subtle, occur with a shift of weight. Shifts in weight, therefore, may occur in degrees of amplitude and in various planes (e.g., anterior–posterior, laterally, and diagonally). Children who experience problems in postural tone often have difficulty initiating, controlling, or grading weight shifts. The hypertonic child often has difficulty initiating a weight shift, whereas the hypotonic child tends to have greater difficulty grading weight shifts (Schoen & Anderson, 1999).

Weight bearing occurs when a child's body part or extremity maintains contact with and exerts pressure against a support surface such as the ground, therapy equipment, or even the therapist's body. Weight bearing assists in the developing cocontraction of stabilizing muscles around a joint with the intention of enhancing proximal stability. This phenomenon is observed in typical development when children bear weight in quadruped and weight shift over extended arms as they move in and out of sitting or four-point positions.

Deep compression to the large muscles of the trunk toward the weight-bearing surface is a specific facilitation technique enlisted to increase stability and postural control using ground force reactions to assist the initiation of muscle activation from the base of support (Figure 7.18). Applying pressure downward to the child's torso

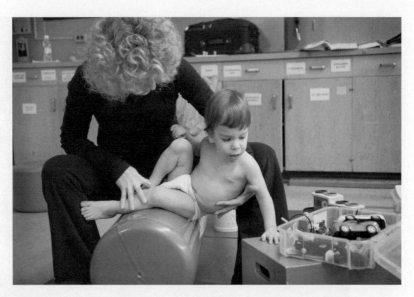

FIGURE 7.17 Therapeutic handling to initiate weight shift of the trunk combined with weight bearing through upper extremity for support.

inward and downward potentially assists the child in holding his or her trunk more independently or in moving his or her limbs actively.

Weight bearing and weight shifting are important in the development of both proximal and distal control. Therefore, weight bearing may be alternated in a treatment sequence with graded reaching or hand activities. If movement is not initiated by the child, the therapist can either alter the environment to encourage motivation, or change the therapeutic input. For example, a more visually stimulating toy can be used to motivate the child to reach. In addition, graded therapeutic stimulation can be provided at different rates and speeds to stimulate more active participation (Schoen & Anderson, 1999).

Rotational movements are often emphasized in facilitation sequences as they combine the movements of both sagittal and frontal planes. Movements in and out of the transverse plane offer elongation and activation of many muscle groups simultaneously (Figure 7.19).

The child benefits from the introduction of facilitation techniques to both sides of the body regardless of the client's diagnosis. Transitional movements from one side to the other move the body through the midline which is a starting point for all movement patterns (Bly & Whiteside, 1997). Many children with neurological disorders experience a diminished sense of midline and maintain asymmetrical postures. Treatment of both sides of the body irrespective of diagnosis can enhance structural alignment, body image, and sensory awareness.

Facilitation can be slow, moderate, or fast in speed. Slow movement is optimum when a child is fearful of movement in space or when sustained muscle contractions are required. For some, slow movements can be boring and inappropriate, however,

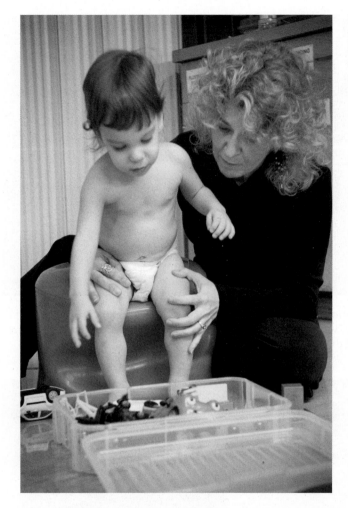

FIGURE 7.18 Deep pressure touch combined with weight bearing and weight shifting enlists active initiation from the muscles connected to the base of support.

causing certain children to be unmotivated or not aroused. Fast movement can be used to alert a nervous system that is not aroused or to create enjoyment when the child seeks speed of movement. Fast movements are contraindicated for children who are posturally insecure or who experience latency in their response to sensory information. In time, all clients need to experience varying speeds of movement to develop responses to multiple variables within their environment.

Inhibition is provided coincidentally with facilitation, altering abnormal stiffness and ineffective motor strategies that interfere with task completion. The term "inhibition" refers to the reduction of specific underlying impairments that interfere with function. Inhibition is targeted toward the prevention or redirection of components of movement that are unnecessary and/or interfering with intentional coordinated actions. Inhibitory positions and feedback through handling constrain degrees of freedom, decreasing the amount of force the child uses to stabilize the posture (Figure 7.20).

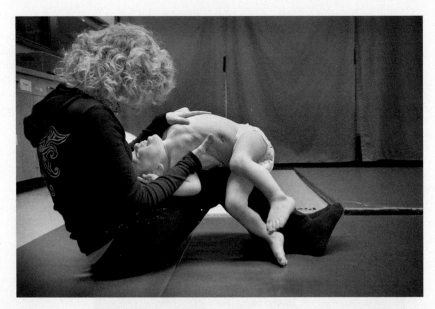

FIGURE 7.19 Facilitation of movement into the transverse plane elongates muscles of the lengthened side of the trunk while simultaneously enlisting muscle recruitment of the shortened trunk muscles in a diagonal direction.

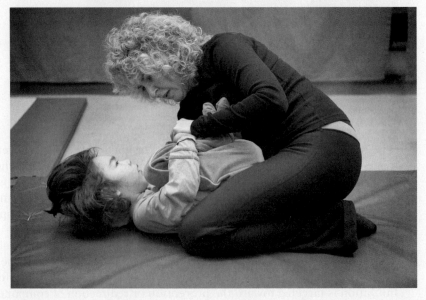

FIGURE 7.20 Positioning the body into total flexion promotes inhibition of the extensor tone bias in the trunk combining facilitation of the trunk antigravity flexor muscles.

Learning the Process of Therapeutic Handling

The therapist must be able to conceptualize a movement sequence before the actual execution of the handling facilitation. This is an example of feedforward anticipation on the part of the therapist. The therapist's ability to motor plan and predict the child's movements in advance is also important for the child's safety. The therapists must be able to put their hands on the child's body at one location and visualize the whole body's response in their mind's eye (Bly & Whiteside, 1997). When first learning, therapists may find their eyes overly focused upon the placement of their hands. Later as their skills develop, the therapist learns to "see" the whole movement of the child's body with a soft gaze, and the process becomes intuitive and natural (Bly & Whiteside, 1997).

We know that the goal of handling is ultimately to provide the child with the experience of independent, smooth, and efficient movement within a functional outcome. However, to observers of NDT that is performed in an artful and connected manner, the process looks smooth and effortless.

Integration of Neuro-Developmental Treatment into Activity

Activities that facilitate function constitute the essence of occupational therapy. As play is the primary occupation of the child, play activities for therapists are key because children who have motor impairments frequently have limited or altered play experiences (Figure 7.21). Because play drives movement for children it is therefore an essential component of NDT. In addition to being a motivator, play supports cognition, perception, creativity, and self-esteem. Play activities are chosen sensitively by the therapist to

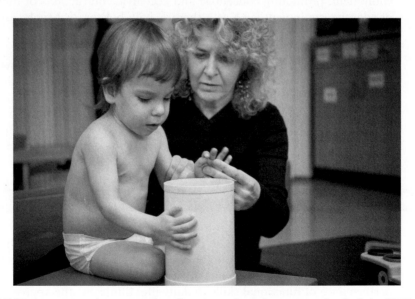

FIGURE 7.21 Integrating therapeutic handling into play schema is an "art" of the NDT process. NDT, Neuro-Developmental Treatment.

facilitate the child's feelings of success and fun. Movement goals are embedded into a play schema, allowing the child to maintain focus upon the play activity while simultaneously experiencing competency in occupation. The therapist carefully selects the play activity to avoid the influence of excessive effort by the child, which may result in associated reactions or inappropriate muscle cocontraction. The therapist modifies handling input in the background of an activity to support the "whole" movement within the play sequence.

Movements used during play schemes are often the same movement patterns required for other tasks in daily life. The use of play activities during treatment may in fact *simulate* movements required for ADL activities. For example, facilitating bilateral hand movement patterns during play activities such as drawing in shaving cream on the mirror simulate the same movement synergies required for ADL tasks such as personal hygiene, feeding, and dressing.

To create generalization of skills, the therapist must continuously alter the demands of the environment to assist the child in learning to perform new movements in various contexts. Activities refined in therapy must be practiced at home and/or in school environment to support the carryover of newly learned skills.

Positioning and Adaptive Equipment

Adaptive equipment is used as an adjunct to handling, altering gravitational forces, challenging posture and movement strategies, supporting the child's weight and/or accommodating structural deformities. As the therapist works for dynamic stability in postural control, small displacements of movement can be created with moving equipment, promoting concentric and eccentric contractions of musculature. The use of adaptive equipment such as a therapy ball, bolster, or bench can be of tremendous support in achieving incremental components of motor control.

Positioning on equipment can also facilitate postural alignment and stability without hands-on contact by the therapist. The external stabilization provided by the equipment potentially facilitates greater independence of movement in distal body segments. Equipment is also designed to reduce the likelihood of deformities and contractures that develop with habitual abnormal posturing and movement. Through the use of positioning, adaptive equipment, and orthotic devices designed specifically for the child's needs, the goals of therapy can be reinforced by parents and other professionals (Whiteside, 1997).

 Summary

The NDT frame of reference is based upon the work of Berta and Karel Bobath developed in the 1940s. Other professionals in the field of pediatric rehabilitation have contributed extensively to this body of knowledge over the last 60 years. This approach uses a "hands-on" method to facilitate the movement patterns required for performance of functional skills in daily life. Clinically, the approach is individualized, providing concepts and treatment principles that are applicable for children with varying diagnoses and developmental skills.

The theoretical basis of NDT has evolved with the emergence of contemporary motor control and neural sciences. Functional movement is known to require intimate interaction between an individual, the environment, and a task. Practice and experience are essential to the learning and adaptation of motor skills. An in-depth analysis of individuals' motor impairments and competencies guides the therapist in developing appropriate intervention strategies. Therapeutic handling is integral to the NDT approach as the primary method of intervention.

There are five key function–dysfunction continua, essential for the clinical assessment process that provides therapists with descriptions of observable behaviors. Postulates regarding the creation of functional change delineate the requirements for environmental modifications and the necessary therapeutic techniques used to facilitate the change. NDT postulates for change emphasize the following: the importance of consistent handling, the active participation of the child, the responsivity of the therapist to the child's needs, the creation of a motivating environment, the use of ongoing assessment, the incorporation of movement into functional activities, the maximization of sensory feedback to reinforce motor learning, and the use of preventative strategies such as adaptive equipment and orthotic devices (Schoen & Anderson, 1999).

NDT is often embedded in play, thereby setting the stage for engagement, motivation, cognition, and perceptual demand. As a result, the child potentially acquires the movement components needed to achieve their greatest independence in developmentally appropriate areas of play, self-care, and school performance.

Application of the NDT frame of reference is most effectively learned through practice under the supervision of an experienced mentor. NDT continuing education courses can also support the therapist's learning and growth, when combined with these opportunities for mentorship and supervision.

The purpose of NDT is to facilitate a child's maximum participation in his or her life's roles. Contributions of the NDT approach are most empowering when therapeutic intervention is integrated into the child's everyday life.

ACKNOWLEDGMENTS

Photos by Helene Cyr, photographer. Victoria, British Columbia, 2007.

REFERENCES

Barthel, K. (2004). *Evidence and Art: Merging Forces in Pediatric Therapy*. Victoria, BC: Labyrinth Journeys.

Bleck, E. E. (1987). Orthopaedic management in cerebral palsy. *Clinics in Developmental Medicine*, Vol. 99-100 (pp. 1–16). Oxford: MacKeith Press.

Bly, L. (1980). Abnormal motor development. In D. Slaton (Ed). *Development of Movement in Infancy*. University of North Carolina at Chapel Hill, Division of Physical Therapy, May 19-22, 1980.

Bly, L. (1999). *Baby Treatment Based on NDT Principles*. San Antonio, TX: Therapy Skill Builders.

Bly, L., & Whiteside, A. (1997). *Facilitation Techniques*. San Antonio, TX: Therapy Skill Builders.

Bobath, B. (1948). The importance of the reduction of muscle tone and the control of mass reflex action in the treatment of spasticity. *Occupational Therapy and Rehabilitation*, 27(5), 371–383.

Bouisset, S., & Le Bozec, S. (2002). Posturo-kinetic capacity and postural function in voluntary movements. In M. Latash (Ed). *Progress in Motor Control*. Champaign, IL: Human Kinetics.

Carr, J., & Shepherd, R. (2000). A motor learning model for rehabilitation. In J. Carr, & R. Shepherd (Eds). *Movement Science: Foundations for Physical Therapy in Rehabilitation* (2nd ed., pp. 33–110). Gaithersburg, MD: Aspen Publishers.

Damiano, D. L. (1993). Reviewing muscle co-contraction: Is it developmental, pathological or motor control issues? *Physical and Occupational Therapy in Pediatrics, 12*(4), 3–20.

Darrah, J., & Bartlett, D. (1995). Dynamic systems theory and management of children with CP: Unresolved issues. *Infants and Children, 8*(1), 52–59.

Edelman, G. M. (1987). *Neural Darwinism: The Theory of Neuronal Group Selection*. New York: Basic Books.

Gajdosik, C. G., & Gajdosik, R. L. (2000). Musculoskeletal development and adaptation. In S. K. Campbell (Ed). *Physical Therapy for Children* (2nd ed., pp. 117–197). Philadelphia, PA: WB Saunders.

Giuliani, C. A. (2003). Spasticity and motor control. In B. Connolly, & P Montgomery (Eds). *Clinical Applications for Motor Control* (pp. 309–334). Memphis, TN: Slack Inc.

Hadders-Algra, M. (2000). The neuronal group selection theory: Promising principles for understanding and treating developmental motor disorders. *Developmental Medicine and Child Neurology, 24*(10), 707–715.

Hartbourne, R., Giuhani, C. A., & NacNeela, J. (1993). Kinematic and electromyographic analysis of the development of sitting posture in infants. *Developmental Psychobiology, 26*, 51–64.

van der Heide, J. (2004). Postural control during reaching in preterm children with cerebral palsy. *Developmental Medicine and Child Neurology, 46*, 253–266.

von Hofsten, C., & Rönnqvist, L. (1993). The structuring of neonatal arm movements. *Child Development, 64*, 1047–1057.

Holt, K., Butcher, R., & Fonesca, S. T. (2000). Limb stiffness in active leg swinging of children with spastic hemiplegic cerebral palsy. *Pediatric Physical Therapy, 12*, 50–61.

Horak, F. (1991). Assumptions underlying motor control for neurological rehabilitation. In M. J. Lister (Ed). *Contemporary Management of Motor Control Problems: Proceeding of the II Step Conference* (pp. 11–27). Alexandria, VA: American Physical Therapy Association.

Howle, J. M. (2002). *Neuro-Developmental Treatment Approach: Theoretical Foundations and Principles of Clinical Practice*. Laguna Beach, CA: NDTA.

Kamm, K., Thelan, E., & Jensen, J. (1990). A dynamical systems approach to motor development. *Physical Therapy, 70*, 763–775.

Larin, H. (2000). Motor learning: theories and strategies for the practitioner. In S. K. Campbell, D. W. Vander Linden, & R. J. Palisano (Eds). *Physical Therapy for Children* (2nd ed., pp. 170–197). Philadelphia, PA: WB Saunders.

Lieber, R. (2002). *Skeletal Muscle Structure, Function and Plasticity*. Baltimore, MD: Lippincott Williams & Wilkins.

Nashner, L. M., & McCollum, G. (1985). The organization of human postural movements: A formal basis and experimental system. *Behavioral Brain Science, 8*, 135–172.

Sabari, J. S. (2002). Optimizing motor skill using task related training. In M. V. Radomski, & C. A. T. Latham (Eds). *Occupational Therapy for Physical Dysfunction* (5th ed., pp. 618–639). Philadelphia, PA: Lippincott Williams & Wilkins.

Schmidt, R. A., & Lee, T. D. (1999). *Motor Control and Learning: A Behavioral Emphasis* (3rd ed.). Champaign, IL: Human Kinetics.

Schoen, S., & Anderson, J. (1999). NeuroDevelopmental Treatment frame of reference. In P. Kramer, & J. Hinojosa (Eds). *Frames of Reference for Pediatric Occupational Therapy* (2nd ed., pp. 83–118). Philadelphia, PA: Lippincott Williams & Wilkins.

Smith, L., & Thelen, E. (1993). *A Dynamic Systems Approach to Development*. Cambridge, MA: The MIT Press.

Shea, C. H., Guadagnoli, M. A., & Dean, M. (1995). Response biases: Tonic neck response and aftercontraction phenomenon. *Journal of Motor Behavior, 27*(1), 41–51.

Shumway-Cook, A., & Woollacott, M. H. (2007). *Motor Control: Translating Research into Clinical Practice* (3rd ed.). Philadelphia, PA: Lippincott Williams & Wilkins.

Stockmeyer, S. (2000). What about tone? Paper presented at the meeting of the Neuro-Developmental Treatment Association Conference, Cincinnati, OH.

Thelen, E. (1992). Development of locomotion from a dynamical systems approach. In H. Forssberg, & H. Hirschfeld (Eds). *Movement disorders in children*, Vol. 36 (pp. 169–173). Basel, Switzerland: Medicine and Sport Science, Karger.

Thelen, E., Corbella, D., Kamm, K., & Spencer, J. P. (1993). The transition to reaching: Mapping intentional and intrinsic dynamics. *Child Development, 64,* 1058–1097.

Whiteside, A. C. (1997). *Clinical Goals and Application of NDT Facilitation* (pp. 1–14). NDT Network.

Woollacott, M., & Sveistrup, H. (1992). Changes in the sequencing and timing of muscle response coordination associated with developmental transitions in balance abilities. *Human Movement Science, 11,* 23–36.

World Health Organization. (2001). *ICF: International Classification of Functioning, Disability and Health.* Geneva, Switzerland: WHO.

CHAPTER 8

A Frame of Reference to Enhance Teaching-Learning: The Four-Quadrant Model of Facilitated Learning

CRAIG GREBER • JENNY ZIVIANI

A part from being a profession in its own right, teaching is a strategy. Coaches, trainers, consultants, and therapists all utilize elements of teaching to facilitate skill acquisition. In doing so, they do not reproduce the wide and varied roles of professional teachers. Rather, they use effective teaching–learning strategies in ways that enhance their own competencies in attaining outcomes for those with whom they work. This chapter explores the ways occupational therapists can use teaching and learning to enable their clients to attain autonomy in skills that lead to enhanced occupational performance. In this chapter, the learner is the child and the facilitator refers to the therapist.

Facilitating learning is a complex behavior that includes what we do, as well as how we do it. The four-quadrant model of facilitated learning (4QM) (Greber, Ziviani, & Rodger, 2007a, b) has been advanced as one way of informing the selection of effective learning strategies based on the changing needs of the learner when acquiring a new skill. Grouped into four broad clusters, these strategies provide a scaffold for identifying and attending to a child's various learning needs throughout the skill acquisition process. In this chapter, the theoretical base of the 4QM will be outlined, the concepts contained in the model will be defined, function and dysfunction will be identified, and evaluation procedures will be linked to the indicators of function and dysfunction. To establish the relationship between theory and practice, a case example will illustrate how the 4QM can be used as a frame of reference to guide teaching–learning interventions in occupational therapy.

THEORETICAL BASE

This section presents the underlying theoretical base of the 4QM. First, the assumptions that validate teaching and learning as a useful intervention in occupational therapy will be reviewed. Then, the theoretical postulates that illustrate the relationship between essential concepts embedded in the 4QM will be described.

Occupational therapists use teaching and learning as an intervention when the acquisition of skills is viewed as an important step in occupational goal attainment. To begin to understand how teaching and learning can be used, it is first necessary to understand how such an intervention embodies the core principles of occupational therapy. When a therapist identifies the learning of key skills as central to enhancing a child's occupational performance, there are several interventions available. When a specific task is difficult to perform, the use of adaptive equipment might make it easier. For example, when fitting a shoe is problematic, the use of a shoehorn can simplify the process. Alternatively, when the entire activity is too difficult for the child, a compensatory approach can be used to find an easier alternative (e.g., a child who is unable to tie shoelaces might perform more autonomously when using Velcro straps instead). In both these cases, repeated practice can be used to enhance the acquisition and performance of the key skills. The acquisition of new skills is pivotal in both cases; however, the skills come together in a way that changes the performance of the original occupation. Although a degree of teaching and learning is necessary to acquire these skills, these interventions are slightly different to those wherein the skills are central to occupational performance.

Occupational therapists routinely utilize teaching and learning as a prominent method of intervention in pediatric practice to enhance self-care, productivity, and leisure occupations (Rodger, Brown, & Brown, 2005). The efficacy of teaching and learning depends on understanding the theoretical base. This requires becoming familiar with the range of strategies used to facilitate learning and embracing the factors that determine the selection of strategies for an individual on a given task at various stages of the learning process.

In his seminal work, developmental psychologist Lev Vygotsky proposed a process by which children with superficial competencies could develop advanced abilities through guidance from a facilitator. Vygotsky identified a principle of learning called the "zone of proximal development" (Vygotsky, 1978). The zone of proximal development represented a stage of learning where a learner required support to perform a task successfully. In Vygotsky's theory, progress toward autonomy was made possible through systematic facilitator supports called "scaffolds." As the learner became increasingly competent, Vygotsky observed the initiation of scaffolding to move from the facilitator to the child. Similarly, the use of prompts transitioned from being overt to covert. Vygotsky's person-centered approach to learning provides an appropriate theoretical framework on which to draw for occupational therapists.

Direct instruction teaching methods have been contrasted with more indirect inductive approaches in conceptualizations of the teaching–learning process (e.g., Joyce, Calhoun, & Hopkins, 2002; Woolfolk, 2004). Mosston and Ashworth (2002) positioned a range of teaching styles on a continuum from "command style" at one extreme to "self-teaching" at the other, based on the cognitive focus of the style. More direct styles informed the learner of key elements of the task or the response required, while those styles that encouraged the learner to consider barriers to performance facilitated the learner to arrive at solutions. These latter strategies were seen to engage the learner to a greater extent in the decision-making process.

The Four-Quadrant Model of Facilitated Learning

When therapists choose teaching and learning as an intervention strategy, they take on the role of facilitator, with the child as learner. The 4QM provides a means of understanding, planning, and coordinating the use of learning strategies in occupational therapy but also lends itself to multidisciplinary use by others involved with the child, such as teachers, teaching assistants, and parents.

The 4QM groups the various cognitive and physical learning strategies useful in leading children to perform occupational tasks more autonomously. As Mosston and Ashworth (2002) theorized, some learning strategies are more direct and overt than others. For instance, learning can be based on telling the child what to do, or how to do it. These direct strategies serve the need for knowledge, they provide information about the characteristics of the task, or the response required. Less direct strategies (such as provision of feedback) engage the learner to a greater extent in the decision-making process. These strategies encourage the learner to be more active in planning, executing, and evaluating performance. Direct strategies can be viewed as being at one extreme of a continuum of teaching–learning styles, with indirect strategies at the other end.

Approaches to teaching and learning vary not only in their directness, but also on the basis of the person initiating the strategy. Some learning strategies are initiated by the person facilitating the learning (in this case, the therapist), while others utilize the learner as a source of initiation through discovery methodologies. The source of initiation of learning strategies can be viewed as a progression in the relationship between facilitator-initiated strategies and learner-initiated strategies.

When the approaches to teaching and learning and the person initiating the strategy are integrated, four distinct clusters of learning strategies become apparent, each serving a different learner need. Those strategies that are direct and initiated by a facilitator (quadrant 1) specify the characteristics of the task and/or the performance required. Other strategies that are indirect in nature, yet still facilitator initiated, fall into quadrant 2. These are useful in encouraging decision making by the learner. Quadrant 3 groups those overt self-prompting strategies initiated by the learner that help him or her to recall key points essential to task performance. A range of self-regulatory strategies that are not obvious to observers underpins autonomy and these strategies are grouped in quadrant 4. The 4QM helps a therapist to coordinate the learning strategies used to promote autonomy by alerting him or her to learner needs and providing a structure that allows the therapist to respond to these needs as skill acquisition proceeds. Within each quadrant, specific learning strategies that demonstrate the characteristics relevant to that quadrant can be positioned. When these are added, the complete 4QM (Figure 8.1) becomes a useful frame of reference to guide therapists in implementing teaching and learning as a method of invention.

Assumptions

Many professions use teaching and learning as an approach to their professional duties. Occupational therapists use teaching and learning in ways that are at once both similar and different to how they are used in other professions. The relationship between

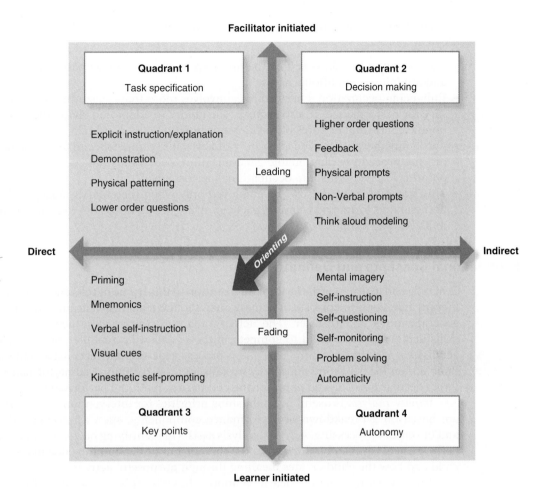

FIGURE 8.1 The four-quadrant model of facilitated learning.

teaching and learning and the overarching theoretical principles of occupational therapy is central to the 4QM. This relationship is based on the assumption that enhancing a child's repertoire of skills can enable him or her to perform target occupations more autonomously. By enabling a child to enhance his or her occupation-relevant skills, the triangular interaction between person, occupation, and environment becomes more congruent, improving occupational performance. The learning of key skills fundamental to the target occupation can be facilitated by either structuring practice routines to optimize skill mastery, altering the activity to simplify its performance, or by invoking specific teaching and learning strategies to facilitate learning of the skills essential to occupational performance. Although these three options are sometimes combined, it is this third aspect with which the 4QM is specifically concerned, using specific teaching and learning strategies to facilitate learning.

The following assumptions about the development of autonomy are important to the 4QM.

- Acquisition of key skills is only the first step in improving occupational performance and attaining occupational goals.
- Enhancing occupational performance involves more than mastering the skills necessary for performance. It also requires the ability to adapt and shape the skills to the unique contextual features of the target occupation.
- Autonomy therefore includes mastery of key skills, competence in using the decision-making procedures that enable generalization, and contextual competence in incorporating learned skills into occupational performance.
- This frame of reference can be employed only when the child is judged to have the necessary performance components (e.g., strength and dexterity) to complete the task in its current form.

Foundational Concepts and Definitions

Teaching and learning is the basis of intervention in this frame of reference. Occupational therapy intervention consists of activity analysis, the teaching–learning encounter, and generalizations and transfer. The activity analysis supports the acquisition of core skills and enables the child to compete in those skills in a real-life context. While the acquisition of skills is a central part of this process, teaching and learning as a therapeutic intervention looks beyond autonomy in skills and toward improved performance in the target occupation. The end point for the child is occupational performance.

Activity analysis is useful in establishing priorities for intervention when constraints are based on a breakdown of performance components, such as strength, dexterity, and/or sensory processing. Activity analysis assists in identifying barriers to occupational performance. Ultimately, this allows the therapist to understand the occupations of the child and how the child creates meaning through purposeful activity.

When selecting teaching–learning approaches, therapists typically address barriers to occupational performance created by lack of proficiency in specific tasks. By enabling the child to learn the necessary tasks, occupational performance components are not enhanced through other therapeutic means. Rather, through teaching and learning the essential activities for attaining occupational goals are mastered. For example, when reviewing a child's mealtime occupations, the use of knife and fork might be a central activity. Activity analysis helps the therapist to identify the child's ability to perform specific tasks (such as holding the fork steady, or making the sawing action with the knife) that are potential barriers to performing the activity, and hence limit performance of the child's mealtime occupations. The teaching–learning approach has the appeal of directness. It requires a thorough understanding of the occupation, the activities that comprise it, and the tasks that are necessary to facilitate performance. In this approach, emphasis is not placed on performance components such as strength, dexterity, or bilateral coordination that might be targeted when using other frames of reference.

To assist a child to acquire a skill, it is first necessary to identify the components of the skill that require tutelage. Activity analysis is a means through which this can occur and is a core skill in occupational therapy. Activity analysis should provide the therapist with a thorough understanding of the activity, and the knowledge base for facilitating the child to learn to perform it. Activity analysis, therefore, forms an important basis for clinical reasoning when using teaching–learning approaches.

The teaching–learning encounter involves the interaction between the therapist and the child. The therapist can set about designing interventions that will support learning, after key tasks that are barriers to performance have been identified. The teaching–learning encounter is a complex procedure that requires the therapist to be responsive to the changing needs of the learner and adapt the strategies employed to respond to these needs. Within this context a range of child and therapist characteristics, such as preferred learning style, communication mode, and interpersonal factors should be considered.

For the acquisition of skills to occur, the learner needs to understand the task and the performance requirements, engage effective decision making to modify performance in response to errors, recall the key elements of successful performance, and monitor performance through both concurrent and reflective analyses. Once a skill is acquired, these processes might become automatic, but during the learning phase, strategies that establish competence in these processes need to be developed.

The strategies employed by a therapist during intervention must therefore match not only the characteristics of the learner, task, and environment but also the learning needs of the child at any point in time. Each child has unique learning requirements that change as skill acquisition proceeds, and so their needs cannot always be predicted. Therein lies a challenge for therapists. They are faced with the task of developing an intervention that depends on high levels of teaching skill and degrees of knowledge about the teaching–learning process of which they may not have in-depth knowledge. In this sense, knowledge of effective teaching–learning strategies, and the ability to match them with a learner's needs, is paramount to the outcomes for the child. The 4QM supports the therapist's reasoning in this process.

Generalization and transfer of learned skills to the target occupation is a key role of the therapist. Teaching the essential skills within a real-life context minimizes the adaptation a child needs to make to the contextual features of his or her occupational performance. For example, teaching a child to use a knife and fork during mealtime enables the child to generalize those skills to other mealtime environments more easily. This is preferable to teaching knife and fork use when cutting play dough in a play-based setting. Autonomy in occupational performance is attained when a child has the necessary knowledge of the task, decides on an appropriate course of action, and is able to independently enact, monitor, and mediate performance in such varied contexts as the occupation might entail.

To illustrate the point, consider a child who has a goal to brush his or her teeth before going to bed. The therapist might facilitate learning of the fundamental skills for toothbrushing—putting toothpaste on the brush, grasping and manipulating the brush, rinsing, and so on (Figure 8.2). The child then develops performance autonomy—competence in the skills required to brush his or her teeth. To engage in toothbrushing, however, the child must orient to the features of performance, such as locating the toothbrush, judging the amount of paste and the temperature of rinsing

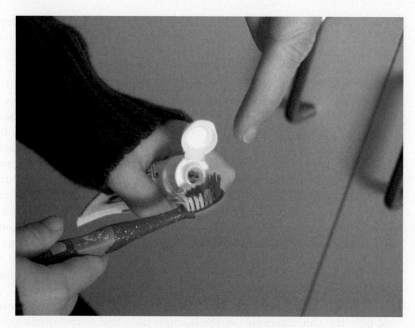

FIGURE 8.2 A child putting toothpaste on a toothbrush with cueing.

water, and completing the task in an appropriate amount of time. Making decisions about these variables engages the child in procedural autonomy—autonomy in transfer of learned skills to the real-life context. The closer the learning context is to that of the goal occupation, the fewer adaptations needed. Intervention that takes place in the child's own bathroom, for example, minimizes the degree of transfer of skills needed.

Becoming "able" is an important stage in developing occupational autonomy; however, if the child expects to be reminded to brush his or her teeth (as often develops when a child has become reliant on help from others), complete autonomy has not yet been attained. Implementing strategies that encourage the child to recognize the appropriate time to brush teeth, and engage in the occupation without prompting can help develop initiative in using learned skills. Only when the child initiates the use of skills in ways that respond to changing contexts can he or she become truly autonomous in the goal occupation.

Key Concepts and Definitions

The 4QM builds upon the integration of the directness and source of initiation continua by detailing the various learning strategies that can be used to address learner needs in each of the four quadrants. The complete 4QM is illustrated in Figure 8.1. For a child to acquire a skill, he or she must understand the task, decide on a plan of action, recall the important features of performance, and monitor the outcomes of each effort. When a child finds particular parts of this process troublesome, the 4QM can assist the therapist to identify strategies relevant to the child's needs. Each of these strategies conceptualizes a mode of scaffolding that can be used to attain successful performance of the target skill. In the various theories that have been used to inform the development of the 4QM, these concepts have sometimes been given different names in the many bodies of knowledge that refer to the same phenomena. The labels used in the 4QM represent a consolidation of these many names into terms that are best understood by occupational therapists.

To establish each of the learning strategies in the 4QM as separate and discrete entities, it is necessary to define and exemplify each. This enables distinctions to be made between the strategies available to the therapist and enables him or her to select the most meritorious approach for a learner at a given time and on a given task, and to effectively link or combine those strategies used throughout the learning process.

Quadrant 1 — Direct, Facilitator-Initiated Strategies

Quadrant 1 strategies use direct instruction methods to communicate information from the facilitator to the learner to inform the learner of the goal of the task, the task requirements, and/or the nature of performance. Therapists can use explicit instruction and explanation, demonstration, physical patterning and/or lower order questions to provide this information. Each of these strategies involves the facilitator providing the learner with direct prompts, which provide task-specific information in a way that encourages the learner to reproduce previously learned responses. They inform or remind the learner what to do to complete the task.

Explicit instruction and explanation provide the learner with descriptions of various characteristics of the task itself, and/or the expected response. Such strategies can be used to inform the learner of the requirements of the task ("Do this") or key features of performance ("Do it this way"). Verbal, print, and technology-based forms of instruction may all provide the same type of information if their purpose is specifically to impart information. A therapist is using explicit instruction and explanation when he or she says:

- "You need to hold the food still with your fork while you cut to stop it sliding around."
- "Push your arm through the sleeve."
- "Turn the paper with your left hand and open and close the scissors with your right hand."

Explicit instruction and explanation is frequently used in conjunction with demonstration to provide the learner with a clear understanding of what is required.

Demonstration occurs when a therapist provides an example of the expected response or performance (Figure 8.3). It can be used to highlight specific points of technique, clarify ambiguity in verbal instructions, and/or provide a reference of correctness for the learner's efforts. Demonstration usually uses visual modalities, but can also be used to model appropriate verbal responses (e.g., in social interaction). Demonstration can occur when:

- The therapist shows the learner how to perform the task.
- The learner views a videotape of the task being performed.

FIGURE 8.3 The therapist demonstrating for a child how to put on a sweater in quadrant 1.

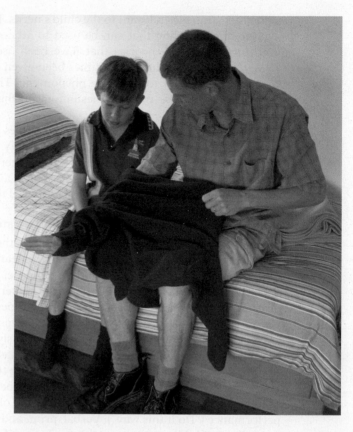

- A simulated task is shown using audiovisual technology (e.g., cartoon) as an example of the expected response.
- The facilitator models a verbal response such as a response to a question.

Physical patterning (Greber, Ziviani, & Rodger, 2007a, b) has been used to identify a specific element of physical manipulation of the learner's body. The terms "physical assistance," "physical guidance," and "manual guidance" have variously been used in the literature to describe a range of physical facilitations, from partial prompts to complete patterning (Carr & Shepherd, 1998; Chen et al., 2001; Schmidt & Wrisberg, 2000). In understanding how these strategies might be employed in skill acquisition, it is useful to draw a distinction between those strategies that manipulate the child through the entire movement (*physical patterning*) (Figure 8.4), those that direct but do not control the movement (*physical guidance*), and intermittent strategies that use tactile and kinesthetic prompts to ensure motor accuracy (*physical prompts*) (Figure 8.5). Each of these strategies involves the learner to a different degree in planning and executing the movement, and consequently supports different outcomes. These three labels have been used in the 4QM to identify particular learning strategies based on physical input by the facilitator.

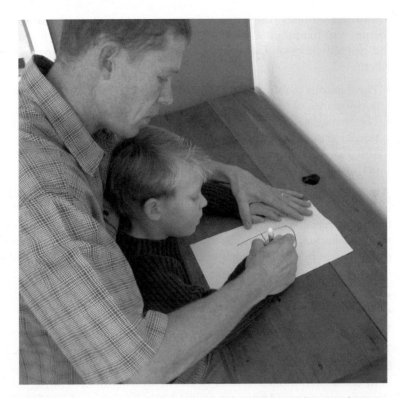

FIGURE 8.4 The therapist using physical patterning for a writing task in quadrant 1.

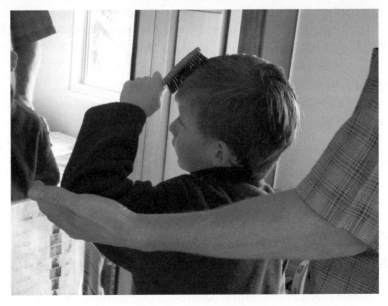

FIGURE 8.5 The therapist demonstrating physical prompts for a grooming task in quadrant 1.

In this strategy, the learner does not contribute to the movement, but allows the therapist to manipulate the body part. Physical patterning might be used to establish the general form or the spatial characteristics of the movement. This might occur when:

- The therapist manipulates the learner's limbs to provide an example of the appropriate performance of the task
- The therapist works hand over hand with the learner to perform a task, while the learner remains passive
- The therapist moves the learner's limb through the range of motion required to perform the task to provide a general feel for the movement

"Lower order questions" is a term that describes questions used to assess the learner's understanding of the task and/or performance by focusing recall and recognition of factual material. This type of questioning ensures that the learner's interpretation of the task is accurate. It can also be used to focus the learner's attention on key aspects of performance by challenging him or her to recall previously learned material. Examples of lower order questions include the following:

- "What do you do next?"
- "Where should you look?"
- "How should you be standing?"

The use of questions has received considerable attention in many bodies of literature. One way of distinguishing the various types of questions a therapist might ask a child is to use a hierarchical system of distinguishing the cognitive skills involved, such as Bloom's taxonomy (Anderson et al., 2001; Bloom et al., 1956). Several authors have used this taxonomy to discriminate questions that evoke lower level processes, such as recalling and understanding, from those that stimulate higher order productive cognitions (e.g., Bissell & Lemons, 2006; Johnson, 2000; Marzano, Pickering, & Pollock, 2001). The use of this taxonomy in the 4QM has resulted in the use of the labels *lower order questions* (quadrant 1) and *higher order questions* (quadrant 2).

Quadrant 2 — Indirect, Facilitator-Initiated Strategies

When the learner understands the task requirements, but is unable to generate an effective plan for performing the task, different learning tools are necessary. Strategies that engage the learner in decision making have different features to those that specify the task. Although they remain facilitator initiated, they are less direct in nature. These strategies are represented in quadrant 2. They involve a hint of suggestion, rather than a specific instruction. Strategies such as higher order questions, feedback, physical prompts, nonverbal prompts, and think-aloud modeling all serve this purpose. Each of these approaches encourages the learner to make appropriate decisions about his or her own performance.

Higher order questions are used to provoke thought and draw the learner's attention to elements of the skill that need to be considered. This type of question requires the application of knowledge to engage the learner in analysis, problem solving, judgment, reasoning, and/or evaluation. Questions that facilitate the use of higher order cognitive skills, such as "Why did that happen?" stimulate the production of new cognitions rather than the recall of old ones. For example:

- "What might be the problem here?"
- "How could you do it differently?"
- "Why did that happen?"
- "How does that look?"

Statements such as "I wonder why that happened," though not phrased as a question, still imply one. They function to engage the learner in analysis, problem solving, and critical evaluation; therefore, statements such as these can be considered higher order questions.

Feedback (Schmidt & Lee, 2005) can be intrinsic; it can also be provided by others observing performance to support the learner by orienting him or her to the use of self-regulatory procedures. Feedback therefore reports the therapist's observations to the learner, but does not instruct the learner what to do, or what to change (this would be akin to explicit instruction). For example, a therapist might comment:

- "You really moved smoothly that time."
- "Uh-oh, I think there's a problem."
- "You're leaning a little to the left."

Symbolic representations that record or evaluate performance, such as checklists, can also provide useful feedback to learners in a visual form.

Physical prompts (Thompson et al., 2004) are touch that promotes the initiation of movement, or provides direction at various points during the response (Figure 8.6). Such strategies support the learner to make successful efforts, without detracting from his or her ability to plan and execute a response. Physical prompts can include tapping or pushing a limb in response to delayed movement initiation. With complex activities, it may be necessary to provide physical prompts on various subtasks, rather than just at the commencement of movement. For example, prompts may be used sequentially to initiate grasping the spoon, loading it, transporting food to the mouth, and then replacing the spoon in the bowl. Physical prompts challenge the learner to plan, monitor, and execute movements in ways that physical facilitation does not do.

Nonverbal prompts are facial expression, eye gaze, and gestures used by the therapist. Learner performance can be initiated, modified, and terminated by an array of nonverbal inputs by the facilitator. For example, a therapist might:

- Give a quizzical look to indicate a need to reassess performance
- Point at a potential hazard
- Direct eye gaze at key objects involved in task

Think-aloud modeling (Polatajko & Mandich, 2004) is the verbalization of physical skills and guidance on the use of cognitive strategies. In this strategy, the therapist audibly describes the decision-making processes that are occurring as he or she performs the task. While demonstration (from quadrant 1) of physical skills provides the learner with task specific information, think-aloud modeling shows the learner how to engage in higher cognitive processes. The dialogue can model the recognition of errors (e.g., "Uh-oh,

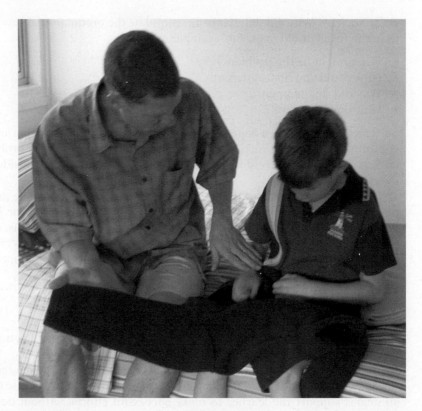

FIGURE 8.6 The therapist demonstrating physical prompts for a dressing task in quadrant 2.

something's gone wrong"), describe the problem-solving process, and/or exemplify self-monitoring procedures. A therapist might comment:

• "That doesn't seem right. What went wrong there? Maybe if I concentrate on keeping my hand a bit steadier."
• "What happens if I put it on there? Oh no, it fell off. Where else could I put it? Maybe over here."

Performance of the task while describing the associated cognitions aloud combines the use of two strategies: demonstration (from quadrant 1) and think-aloud modeling (from quadrant 2). The visual representation of the response is considered demonstration, while the verbalization is think-aloud modeling.

Quadrant 3 — Direct, Learner-Initiated Strategies

Strategies that involve the learner reminding or prompting himself or herself using strategies that are observable to others are grouped in quadrant 3. Learners might use any of the several strategies to recall key points about the task to perform successfully. Priming strategies, mnemonics, verbal self-instruction, visual cues, and kinesthetic self-prompting all serve this purpose. It is noteworthy that the terms "verbal self-guidance" and "rote script" (Polatajko & Mandich, 2004) have been used to distinguish two types of self-talk strategies encouraged by occupational therapists working with children. Because both procedures serve the same purpose of talking oneself through a difficult task, they are described collectively in the 4QM as *verbal self-instruction*.

Priming (Greber, Ziviani, & Rodger, 2007a, b) are learner-initiated strategies that involve verbal rehearsal. Priming differs from strategies that involve repeating procedures that were already learned. Priming strategies bring together the various skills involved in a performance as a type of rehearsal of previously learned procedures to ensure that the intended response is the correct one. An example of priming is when the child verbally rehearses what he or she will say to a cashier while waiting in line, or do a "dry run" of a task before performing it. The goal of priming, then, is to prepare for performance rather than improve it. Priming strategies can use various modalities to organize general response schemas to meet the temporal and contextual demands of the imminent performance. The key element here is the *intention* of priming. If the goal is to prepare and optimize the response, rather than to provide an avenue for improving mastery, the strategy can be considered to be a priming one. Practice is an opportunity to implement previously acquired strategies to refine and improve specific skills.

Mnemonics (Joyce, Calhoun, & Hopkins, 2002) are a type of associative learning that enables learners to increase their capacity to store and retrieve information. Mnemonics aid the recall of key features, processes, facts, and procedural steps. They include the use of link words, acronyms, nonsense phrases, and rhymes. Although a facilitator might aid in the development of a mnemonic, its use becomes the responsibility of the learner, making it a learner-initiated strategy. For instance, a learner might use the nonsense phrase "Every Good Boy Deserves Fun" to prompt the recall of the notes E, G, B, D, and F in musical notation. Alternatively, a child might say, "Nose over toes and up she goes" to focus on body position during transition to standing. Mnemonics use simple and/or symbolic language to focus on key elements of the task.

Verbal self-instruction (Greber, Ziviani, & Rodger, 2007a, b); Martini & Polatajko, 1998) is when a child uses verbal strategies to engage in the problem-solving process or to recall the steps involved in performance. Complex tasks are not easily reduced to a few key points represented in a mnemonic. Sometimes, a child might find it more valuable to think out loud, describing the task and the decisions necessary to perform it. On occasion, a formal rote script might be recited to guide the child through the task. The use of verbal self-instruction and tools such as a formal script support both cognitive (e.g., memory) and metacognitive (e.g., self-monitoring) processes. Some examples of verbal self-instruction include a child saying to himself or herself:

- "I hold it like this and tip it in like that."
- "What happens if put it on there. Oh dear, it fell off. Where else could I put it?"
- "Put my feet on here. Put my hands on here. Ready to push. Go. Whoops, I have to try to stay balanced."

Visual cues (Greber, Ziviani, & Rodger, 2007a, b; Hudson, Lignugaris-Kraft, & Miller, 1993) prompt the learner to recall steps in a task or prompt action. It can include picture cues, computer-generated visual prompts, real-object cues, mind maps, graphic organizers, visual displays, and computer-assisted instruction. Mirrors and video recordings can also be useful visual prompts to enhance performance. Simple examples of visual cues include picture charts that remind the learner to engage in particular behaviors and a sequence of pictures that guide the learner through the steps of a task.

Kinesthetic self-prompting (Greber, Ziviani, & Rodger, 2007a, b) strategies enhance or direct the child's attention to a particular action or body part during learning. When a child touches or rubs his or her hemiplegic arm as a reminder to use it to stabilize an object, he or she is using a kinesthetic prompting strategy.

Quadrant 4 — Indirect, Learner-Initiated Strategies

Internalized strategies for monitoring and evaluating performance are not observable to onlookers, but are necessary for autonomous performance. Because they are not overtly observable, these strategies can be deemed indirect in nature. Such strategies and processes are assessable only by learner self-reports, making the content of strategies in quadrant 4 somewhat speculative. Sinha and Sharma (2001) described a series of covert cognitive processes that underpin autonomous performance as *self-instruction, self-questioning, and self-monitoring*. Additionally, *mental imagery* and *problem solving* aid in preparation for performance, as well as in overcoming barriers (Schmidt & Wrisberg, 2000; Sinha & Sharma, 2001). Schmidt and Lee (2005) used the term "automaticity" to describe a final stage of learning that is independent of the cognitive processes that mark earlier stages. This label has been adopted in the 4QM.

Mental imagery (Schmidt & Wrisberg, 2000) can support decision making, planning, and other cognitive strategies. Although mental imagery may exhibit subtle signs of engagement (e.g., closing eyes, failing to respond to stimuli), it is a process that occurs entirely within the learner's mind, making it unobservable to onlookers. Mental imagery is a higher order process, and is often a useful strategy to recall the visual cues used in quadrant 3.

Self-instruction (Montague, 1992), the use of inner speech to direct the learner's actions, is symbolic of the internalization of verbal self-instruction strategies. Wherein verbal self-instruction is an observable learning strategy, self-instruction provides no signs of engagement. Self-instruction helps to identify and direct the use of problem-solving strategies. It is particularly useful in recalling procedural steps involved in a performance.

Self-questioning (Montague, 1992) utilizes internal dialogue to analyze information and regulate the use of cognitive strategies through reflective thinking. The distinction between self-instruction and self-questioning is an academic one because neither process is obvious to the observer. Reports from the learner can be used to identify the characteristics of internal dialogue if this is likely to be helpful to the learning process, and if the learner has sufficient insight to distinguish the strategies used. As with self-instruction, inner speech can be used to engage in silent reviews of performance, development and critique of plans of action, and clarification of goals.

Self-monitoring (Vaidya, 1999) supports the appropriate use of specific strategies, analyzes their effectiveness, critiques performance, and assesses the need for modification. Self-monitoring enables the child to assess the extent to which his or her performance matches the anticipated response. Once again, this is an internal process that is not observable.

Problem solving (Sinha & Sharma, 2001) includes various cognitive processes that are employed to plan, judge, and reason. Individually, each of these processes can be used in either observable or unobservable ways to overcome difficulties in performance. Collectively, the synthesis of these processes in deciding on a course of action is a covert process termed "problem solving." To the therapist, it becomes obvious that problem solving is occurring when a child overcomes barriers to performance independently.

Automaticity (Schmidt & Lee, 2005) is the spontaneous ability to perform a task autonomously (Figure 8.7). It is the ultimate outcome when performance is not attention demanding, and is unregulated by cognitive or metacognitive activity. As automaticity develops, processing occurs without the forms of internalized self-prompting that mediated earlier autonomous stages. Responses become routine, consistent and predictable, and occur in the absence of conscious planning.

Intermediate Strategies through Quadrants

Those strategies exhibiting characteristics of adjoining quadrants can be considered *intermediate strategies*. They might perform dual functions, or link the content of one quadrant to that of another. Three forms of intermediate strategies are discernable: *leading strategies* (bridging quadrant 1 and quadrant 2), *orienting strategies* (linking quadrant 2 and quadrant 3), and *fading strategies* (used to move from quadrant 3 to quadrant 4) (Figure 8.1).

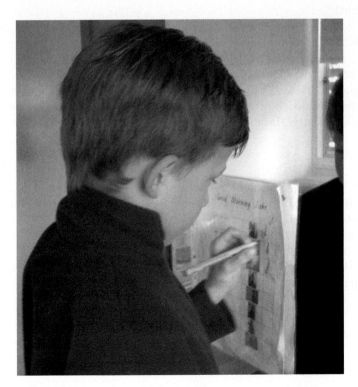

FIGURE 8.7 A child demonstrating automaticity in quadrant 4.

Leading strategies are forms of questions, incomplete statements, and physical guidance reflect characteristics of both task specification (quadrant 1) and facilitation of problem-solving processes (quadrant 2). These strategies might provide effective links between information giving strategies of quadrant 1 and the cognitive processes of quadrant 2. Examples of leading strategies include the following:

- "Cloze," a test of reading comprehension that involves having the person supply a word that has been systematically deleted from the text (Merriam Webster on-line retrieved 6/1/07) (incomplete statements), such as "Next, you need to ... (pause)"
- Guiding a child's reach and positioning the wrist to enable grasp of an object by working hand over hand (physical guidance)
- Questions that stimulate both higher and lower order cognitive processes (e.g., "What part of your body should you use to overcome that problem?")
- Partial demonstration of the expected response

Orienting strategies include verbal and nonverbal strategies that provide no information to the child apart from a reminder to use self-prompting procedures. These strategies share the characteristics of quadrant 2 (engaging the learner in decision-making processes) and quadrant 3 (remembering the key features of performance), which help orient learners to the need for self-regulated instruction. For instance, a therapist might orient a child to the use of verbal self-instruction strategies by asking, "What could you say to remind yourself what to do next?" or direct to a visual cue by pointing to the child's picture prompt card.

Fading is a gradual process involving internalization of the overt self-regulatory strategies of quadrant 3. Some forms of self-prompting can become less obvious to observers, yet are not representative of the covert self-instruction of quadrant 4. Strategies such as subvocalization (whispering) are on the margin of both quadrants. Similarly, when a child begins to orient to only a few of the steps in a picture sequence, it is clear the child is internalizing some of the procedures, but is not yet able to do without the visual prompt. In these cases, fading of overt self-prompting strategies is occurring.

Theoretical Postulates

The 4QM embeds Vygotsky's notion of the zone of proximal development as a period in skill acquisition wherein learning and performance can be scaffolded by self and others. The relationship between quadrants enables scaffolds to be systematically reduced as the learner proceeds toward skill acquisition. As Vygotsky (1978) theorized, learning and performance can be enabled by provision of appropriate learning supports.

In the 4QM, these supports are specific learning strategies that are appropriate to the learner's needs at a given point in time.

- In earlier stages, the learner's efforts are shaped by information from the facilitator (quadrant 1).
- Stimuli are used to prompt appropriate decisions about performance (quadrant 2).
- Later stages of mastery are characterized by the gradual internalization of self-mediated prompts (quadrants 3 and 4).

- Intermediate strategies are used to move the child from one quadrant to another and from facilitator initiated to learner initiated.
- A facilitator of learning needs to respond to the child's needs in a way that is fluid and adaptable.

Within the 4QM, specific learning strategies are grouped together based on the learner needs they support. At the same time, strategies in one quadrant are closely related to those in other quadrants. For example, physical patterning in quadrant 1 is aligned with physical prompts in quadrant 2 and kinesthetic self-prompting in quadrant 3. Similarly, explicit instruction and explanation (quadrant 1) has similarities to think-aloud modeling in quadrant 2 and verbal self-instruction in quadrant 3. In this way, learning strategies used in different parts of the learning process can be coordinated.

FUNCTION–DYSFUNCTION CONTINUUM

As a child develops competency in the key skills that underpin occupational performance, the type of scaffolding requires to enable performance changes. Four broad types of scaffolding have been described earlier: task specification, decision making, key points, and autonomy. Each of these corresponds to a different quadrant in the 4QM, and illustrates varied levels of function and dysfunction on the target skill. These indicators are discussed below. It is important to note that the learner can enter the learning encounter exhibiting need for any or all of these scaffolds. Although he or she might generally be expected to move through the quadrants sequentially, in practice, this might not be the case. The learner might move quickly toward autonomous performance after the task and corresponding performance have been explained. Alternatively, some learners might require varied levels of scaffolding within a single learning encounter, or even on a single trial. For some children, performance will always be marked by a need for facilitator support or overt self-mediation. Such children may never develop autonomy on the task.

The 4QM has one function–dysfunction continuum, autonomous task performance (Table 8.1). The functional end of the continuum is able to perform successfully and autonomously, while the dysfunctional end of the continuum would be unable to perform a task without facilitator-initiated strategies. It should be noted that while the identified points of function and dysfunction mark two ends of the continuum, there are really two groups of behaviors in between these two end points. They are respectively (as you move from function to dysfunction) the ability to use externally obvious self-mediating strategies for successful performance and the need for external facilitation to stimulate successful performance. In the 4QM, the continuum is not truly linear, as one moves from dysfunction to function, the path is more like a Z, as illustrated in Figure 8.8.

Within the one continuum, four groups of behaviors indicate the characteristics of function and dysfunction, based on the discussion above. These characteristics can be used as the basis for evaluation of autonomy in the target skill.

A child may not demonstrate all behaviors in a quadrant.

TABLE 8.1 Indicators of Function and Dysfunction for Autonomous Task Performance	
Autonomous Performance	**Performance Requires Direct Facilitation**
FUNCTION: Able to perform a task successfully and autonomously through the use of self-initiated strategies	*DYSFUNCTION*: Unable to perform a task without facilitator-initiated strategies
Indicators of Function	**Indicators of Dysfunction**
Successfully uses mental imagery to complete a task	Requires explicit instruction or explanation to complete a task
Successfully uses self-instruction to complete a task	Requires demonstration to complete a task
Successfully uses self-monitoring to complete a task	Requires physical patterning to complete a task
Successfully uses self-instruction to complete a task	Require lower order questions to complete a task
Successfully problem solves to complete a task	
Successfully uses automaticity to complete a task	

GUIDE FOR EVALUATION

Activity analysis can be useful both in identifying the core tasks that need to be mastered to enhance occupational performance, and also in establishing the characteristics of the person's current performance. Notably, a person's performance can change not only from one occasion to the next, but even during sustained performance of the same task (such as when maintaining balance while transferring from the toilet). Through the process of activity analysis, the therapist needs to ascertain that the child had the necessary performance components, such as strength and dexterity, to successfully complete the task.

In establishing the learning strategies that are likely to be most appropriate for a child, the therapist must maintain a fluid view of the child's learning needs, systematically guiding him or her through various stages of the learning process. Understanding the characteristics of performance that indicate the learner's needs leads the therapist to select learning strategies most likely to enable successful performance. This dynamic approach to the use of activity analysis leads to the coordinated use of learning strategies, which is essential in developing autonomy. A therapist might pose specific questions when evaluating a child's learning needs as delineated in Figure 8.9. The answer to each question helps establish the child's learning status, and consequently the quadrant from which appropriate learning strategies might be drawn. Repeated use of these questions throughout the learning encounter ensures that the child's learning needs are met and skill acquisition is optimized.

While characteristics of the child's performance can be indicative of the quadrant most likely to serve his or her needs, activity analysis provides other important

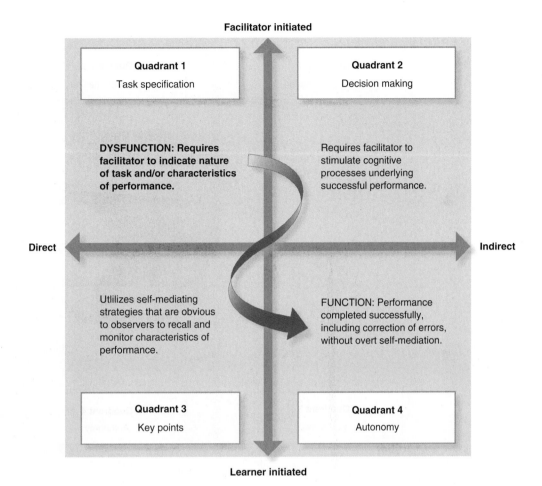

FIGURE 8.8 The features of function and dysfunction on the 4QM.

information. Characteristics of the task itself can determine the approach a learning strategy should take. Motor, cognitive, and social activities each have unique characteristics that require the selection of optimal learning strategies. For example, while physical tasks lend themselves to demonstration and physical facilitation, cognitive and verbal tasks may be better served by higher order questioning and think-aloud modeling.

In various cases, the physical environment may or may not support the use of particular learning strategies. For example, it might not be socially appropriate to use verbal self-instruction strategies if the environment is an inherently quiet one. Similarly, visual prompts such as picture sequences might not be able to be used in environments that do not have a location for affixing them. Consideration of the environment in which the occupation takes place enables the therapist to select strategies that are socially valid.

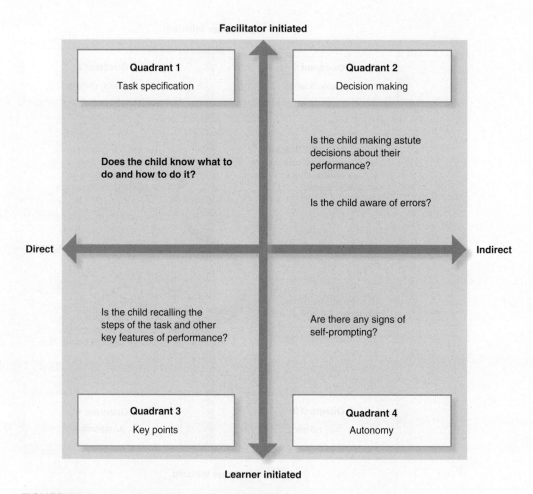

FIGURE 8.9 Guideline for evaluating learning needs.

A synthesis of these factors provides the therapist with the basis for selecting and using learning strategies that are appropriate to the needs of the learner, the characteristics of the environment, and the target occupation.

POSTULATES REGARDING CHANGE

At the center of the 4QM frame of reference are three general postulates regarding change:

1. Learning can be enhanced by appropriately scaffolding performance so that the learner achieves a successful outcome. In this way, the social environment can be manipulated to enhance performance and learning as proposed by Vygotsky (1978).

2. When a therapist dually seeks to facilitate skill acquisition and maximize self-mediation he or she will be most effective by moving from those strategies that are facilitator initiated and involve the child in reproductive cognitions (quadrant 1) toward those that are covert and learner initiated (quadrant 4).
3. To enable a child to progress through the stages of skill acquisition, and hence advance through the quadrants, it is useful to employ intermediate strategies that straddle two quadrants.

Specific Postulates Regarding Change

The various learning strategies in the 4QM have been described and defined earlier. In order to put the general postulates above into action, they must be linked to provide a pathway toward autonomy, while at the same time maintaining the flexibility to respond to individual learning needs on a temporal and contextual basis. This can be effectively achieved by using the concepts in the 4QM in a well-directed and coordinated fashion. Accepting the general postulates regarding change to be true, several specific postulates regarding change enable the 4QM to be implemented.

1. If the therapist employs facilitator-initiated methods such as explicit instruction explanation, physical patterning, and lower order questions, then the child will be able to understand the characteristics of the task and/or the performance required.
2. If the therapist employs additional facilitator-initiated methods such as higher order questions, feedback, physical prompts, no verbal prompts, and thinking aloud modeling, then the child will be encouraged to make decisions about the task.
3. If the therapist encourages the child to engage in learner-initiated strategies such as priming, mnemonics, verbal self-instruction visual cues, and kinesthetic self-prompting, then the child will be able to recall key points essential to task performance.
4. If the therapist encourages the child to use learner-initiated strategies such as mental imagery, self-instruction, self-questioning, self-monitoring, problem solving, and automaticity, then the child will be able to perform the task autonomously.
5. If the therapist uses intermediate strategies to move the child from facilitator initiated to learner initiated and from direct strategies to indirect strategies, then the child will be able to move form one quadrant to the next quadrant.

APPLICATION TO PRACTICE

This frame of reference can be employed only when the child is judged to have the necessary performance components (e.g., strength, dexterity) to complete the task in its current form. Each strategy in the 4QM reflects a body of knowledge about the way that learning occurs, and has been validated as an effective method of facilitating learning. These are grouped into various quadrants based on shared characteristics.

To provide only as much scaffolding as necessary, it may be necessary for the therapist to work backwards to determine where to begin the intervention. A therapist should first provide sufficient time for a child to perform the task autonomously, and if that is not possible, use orienting strategies to remind the child of the self-prompting strategies in quadrant 3. If the child still fails to embrace quadrant 3 strategies, the therapist should utilize indirect prompts, employing more direct prompts only as necessary. This process eliminates the likelihood of dependent behaviors that can develop when therapists anticipate failure, assume the need for guidance, and provide scaffolds that are not required.

When the 4QM frame of reference is used, the therapist integrates knowledge of the task, child, environment, and his or her own skills to develop specific learning strategies that will result in enhanced occupational performance for the child. One way of approaching the task of developing specific strategies for a child is to begin by identifying the features of autonomous performance. Using knowledge of the child's characteristics, and those of the environment and task itself, the therapist can then work backwards through the model to identify effective strategies in earlier quadrants that will be useful in establishing autonomy.

It is helpful to use a "What if?" scenario to frame strategy development for intervention. The strategy works backwards from quadrant 4 to quadrant 1 to identify where the child is having a problem with the task. For example, with a child learning to tie shoelaces (quadrant 4) the therapist might ask, "What could she do to remind herself if she forgets the sequence of movements?" (quadrant 3). Next, the therapist might ask, "What would she do if she was internalizing her self-prompting strategies?" (Fading strategy). After that, he or she could ask, "What could I say if she forgets her prompts?" (Orienting strategy). Subsequently, he or she might ask, "What will I do to help her decide what to do if she doesn't use self-prompting?" (quadrant 2), and then, "What will I do if she forgets what she should do and can't figure it out?" (quadrant 1). Finally, the therapist might ask, "What could I do if she is reluctant to attempt the task without direct prompting?" (Leading strategies). Armed with these questions, the therapist can construct an individualized set of strategies that relate directly to a barrier to occupational performance in a coordinated and sequential way.

To understand how the 4QM might be implemented in practice, it is useful to consider its application in the following case example:

Implementing the 4QM: A Case Study

Imogen is a young girl who lives with her mother in an inner city apartment block. She is in her first year of schooling and enjoys school immensely. Because Imogen's mother works full time, mornings are a very busy time. Although she is left to get ready for school by herself, Imogen has difficulty dressing and usually her mother does this activity for her. Imogen's developmental delay has resulted in difficulties mastering some of the basic skills required in dressing. Her occupational therapist responds to Imogen and her mother's request to target her dressing skills as a way of enhancing self-care occupations in getting ready for school.

The occupational therapist begins by analyzing the occupation. Getting ready for school engages Imogen in a range of self-care occupations. She finds meaning in being able to perform these occupations independently. Dressing, however, has resulted in ongoing difficulty and repeated failure, and she has become less enthusiastic about completing the task unless her mother helps her. Although Imogen has indicated a desire to learn to dress herself, she has also indicated some doubts that she will be able to develop the necessary skills.

An activity analysis identifies that in fact Imogen can perform most of the tasks required to dress. She can orientate the garments and put them on, and she is able to don her slip-on shoes without problems. In fact, only two barriers limit her being able to get ready for school independently: difficulty with buttons and problems aligning the two sides of the garment. Because she prefers to wear open front blouses this has become a constant source of frustration for Imogen, and this frustration has led to the belief that she cannot dress herself. At this stage, she refuses to try and waits for her mother to do the buttons for her.

The therapist considers several directions for intervention. She could encourage Imogen to wear only pullover clothing; however, this would likely limit Imogen's performance of other dressing occupations when buttons were essential. The therapist could encourage Imogen's mother to button the blouses as she puts them away, allowing Imogen to simply slip the garment on over her head. However, Imogen has identified that she would like to learn to dress independently because all her friends are able to do so. With these factors in mind, the therapist observes Imogen's attempts at doing up buttons and believes Imogen's fine motor strength and dexterity are adequate to learn the skill of buttoning. The therapist decides to facilitate Imogen's acquisition of the skill so that she can learn to button her blouse independently when she dresses for school.

To intervene in this case, the therapist identifies the following three key theoretical postulates:

1. That Imogen lacks the necessary skills to dress herself
2. That her strength, endurance, fine and gross motor skills are sufficient to perform dressing tasks
3. That with appropriate use of teaching–learning strategies, Imogen will be able to master the skills required for dressing and generalize those skills to the home environment when getting ready for school

The therapist focuses specifically on two tasks she perceives as barriers to occupational performance: aligning the two sides of the blouse and fastening buttons. This leads her to select the 4QM as a frame of reference to guide teaching–learning strategies. The therapist uses a series of questions to determine Imogen's learning needs.

- Does she know what needs to be done and how to begin buttoning?
- Is she aware when she has inserted the button into the wrong buttonhole?
- Is she choosing appropriate tactics for grasping and manipulating the buttons?
- Can she recall the steps of buttoning, or does she omit/repeat some steps?
- Is she using any obvious strategies to remember how to use buttons effectively?
- Are there any signs that she requires self-prompting to perform?

Additionally, the therapist uses other questions to guide the selection of appropriate strategies in each quadrant of the 4QM.

- What type of activity is this? Physical? Verbal? Cognitive? Sensory?
- What are the characteristics of the learner (physical, cognitive, verbal)?
- Are there environmental features that make it difficult to use particular strategies (e.g., space, noise, distractibility)?
- What psychological factors need to be considered (e.g., learned helplessness, attribution of success/failure, risk-taking behaviors, response to praise)?

The occupational therapy service available to Imogen allows therapy to take place in the home environment. Although it is not possible to time the sessions to correspond with getting ready for school, home-based therapy sessions will help minimize the transfer of skills necessary to the target occupation. Features of the environment in which therapy takes place will be consistent with those inherent in performance of the occupation; however, Imogen will still have to manage time restrictions on school mornings.

With these factors in mind, the therapist develops several coordinated learning strategies and records them in each quadrant of the 4QM. She does so by working backward through the model beginning in quadrant 4, linking each of the learning strategies directly with the target skill.

Quadrant 4 represents autonomous performance. The therapist begins by identifying what the features of autonomous performance will be. As a physical activity, it will be easy to observe when performance using only covert self-prompting is occurring. Working in the home will allow the therapist to identify any potential sources of distraction. The therapist collaborates with Imogen to identify several central features of performance. Imogen will correctly locate and align each button with the buttonhole, then grasp the button using index finger and thumb on her right hand and open the hole by pushing her left thumb partially through. Imogen will then push the button through the hole, grasp it between her left index finger and thumb, and pull it through. To engage in autonomous performance, Imogen will need to have a clear image of the task, and covertly instruct and monitor her own performance. The therapist will also observe Imogen's responses to difficulties encountered, and review the use of reinforcers if necessary. By identifying what autonomous performance will look like, the therapist is then able to identify the key features of the performance that need to be mastered (Figure 8.10, quadrant 4).

Quadrant 3 strategies are useful in helping the learner to remind himself or herself of the key features of performance. In developing appropriate strategies for quadrant 3, the therapist takes into account Imogen's strength in verbal recall, particularly of simple rhymes and songs. She enjoys dance and action songs that link verbal and physical activities. This suggests she will be able to use verbal self-prompting strategies. Firstly, the therapist identifies a verbal self-instruction strategy that will enable Imogen to remember to line up the two sides of the blouse before proceeding with buttoning. Imogen will say aloud, "Are the two sides lined up?" In collaboration with Imogen, the therapist will develop a simple mnemonic

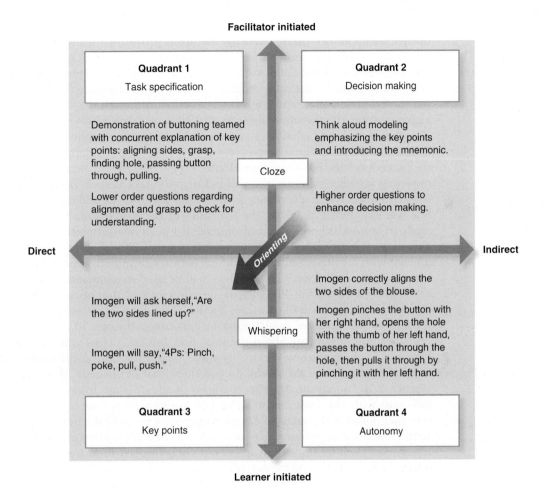

Facilitator initiated

Quadrant 1

Task specification

Demonstration of buttoning teamed with concurrent explanation of key points: aligning sides, grasp, finding hole, passing button through, pulling.

Lower order questions regarding alignment and grasp to check for understanding.

Cloze

Quadrant 2

Decision making

Think aloud modeling emphasizing the key points and introducing the mnemonic.

Higher order questions to enhance decision making.

Direct ← → **Indirect**

Orienting

Imogen will ask herself,"Are the two sides lined up?"

Imogen will say,"4Ps: Pinch, poke, pull, push."

Whispering

Imogen correctly aligns the two sides of the blouse.

Imogen pinches the button with her right hand, opens the hole with the thumb of her left hand, passes the button through the hole, then pulls it through by pinching it with her left hand.

Quadrant 3

Key points

Quadrant 4

Autonomy

Learner initiated

FIGURE 8.10 Imogen's 4QM for buttoning her blouse.

that Imogen can say to herself as she buttons her blouse: "4 Ps: pinch, poke, push, pull." This jingle encapsulates all of the key points of the task identified in quadrant 4: grasp of the button, opening the buttonhole, passing the button through, and then pulling it out the other side. Although the use of verbalization could prove intrusive (and even embarrassing) in some environments, the target occupation occurs in the home, making these more appropriate strategies in this instance. If Imogen does not spontaneously use her mnemonic, the therapist might use an orienting prompt such as "What could you say to yourself to help you remember?" As Imogen moves from the overt self-prompting strategies of quadrant 3, to the covert ones of quadrant 4, she may naturally choose to whisper the jingle rather than say it aloud (Fading). Quadrant 3, Orienting and Fading strategies are all detailed in Figure 8.10.

Whereas quadrant 3 strategies are initiated by the child, quadrant 2 strategies involve the facilitator (in this case the therapist) providing the impetus for learning. Strategies in this quadrant should be congruent with those in quadrant 3, so that they naturally lead the child to become more self-directed. Quadrant 3 strategies engage the child in decision making, fostering the cognitive skills necessary to select, organize, and monitor a course of action. Although the skill of buttoning is a physical one, the therapist observes that Imogen's difficulties are often the result of not understanding what to do, rather than not having the physical competencies to perform the task. The therapist chooses two strategies to enable Imogen to learn the procedures for buttoning her blouse. Firstly, the therapist plans a think-aloud modeling strategy, wherein she will perform the task herself, describing aloud to Imogen the decisions she makes as she aligns the buttons and does up the blouse. She will say things like, "Are the two sides of the blouse even? Oh yes. Now I'm ready to button. Where's that buttonhole? If I push my thumb through a bit I'll be able to see it better. That's it. Now, push it through. Woops! that's a bit clumsy, I'll pinch it with my finger and thumb. Much better. Now pinch, open, push, and pull it through. There, all done." This strategy will be used to emphasize key points, such as the grip on the button, and also the decision making that occurs following error. The other strategy used in quadrant 2 will be higher order questions. The therapist recognizes the value of questioning to encourage Imogen to make appropriate decisions and judgments about the task. She will ask, "How will you know if the button is in the right hole?" and, "Is your grip on the button the same with both hands?" She will also ask, "Why do you think that happened?" if an error occurs (Figure 8.10, quadrant 2). The therapist is aware that Imogen's longstanding difficulty with the task might make her hesitant to answer such questions, so she also develops a series of simpler questions to scaffold Imogen's answers if such reluctance eventuates. The development of a supportive and nonjudgmental relationship will be important in encouraging Imogen to answer questions, even when she is uncertain of the correct answer.

Strategies in quadrant 1 provide information about either the task itself or the anticipated response. Although Imogen has attempted buttoning on previous occasions, her understanding of the critical features of performance could be poor. The therapist establishes a series of strategies to clarify the characteristics of the task. The home environment, as a safe and secure one, is optimal for the use of more direct learning strategies. Although it is a physical task, the therapist's experience in teaching fine motor skills leads her to believe that little will be gained in this instance from hand over hand physical facilitation. In addition, from her observations, she believes Imogen has a general understanding of the task parameters. However, demonstration teamed with direct instruction will provide Imogen with a clear picture of the critical features of buttoning on which success depends. The therapist decides it might be necessary to demonstrate buttoning a blouse, clearly showing how to align the two sides, hold the buttons, open the buttonhole, and pull it through. She develops a concise description of each step to accompany the demonstration. Lower order questions such as, "How should you hold the button?" or "How do you know when the holes are lined up?" can be used following demonstration to check for understanding. With quadrant 1 strategies established, the therapist develops some leading strategies that bridge quadrant 1 and quadrant 2, such as cloze sentences like "I pinch the button with my finger and ... (pause)" and "Push the button through and then ... (pause)." Imogen will consider the process and identify the next step when the therapist pauses. These strategies are identified in Figure 8.10, quadrant 1.

The therapist has now developed a complete 4QM that will guide her through the intervention process.

Intervention takes place in the home environment. The therapist begins by establishing Imogen's knowledge of the task. She observes Imogen attempting to button her blouse and asks her questions about the procedure ("What should you do first?"), technique ("What do you think is the best way to hold the button?"), and outcome ("Why do you need to do the right buttons in the right holes?"). This gives an indication of Imogen's orientation to the task. The answers to these questions indicate that although Imogen understands the task at a general level, she has not acquired an appreciation of the key features of the task that determine success, such as the importance of aligning the two sides first, and the various grasp patterns required.

The therapist uses demonstration and concurrent explanation to draw Imogen's attention to the need to keep the two sides of the blouse equal (Figure 8.11), and to use pincer grasp to hold and manipulate the buttons (Figure 8.12). Answers to lower order questions indicate that Imogen is able to recall the key features when

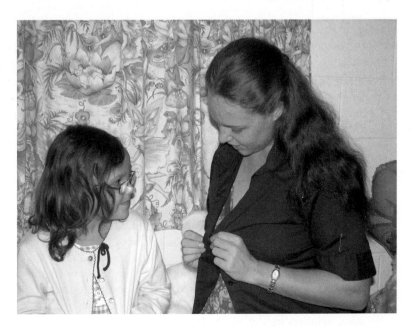

FIGURE 8.11 The therapist demonstrates aligning both side of the blouse and buttoning the buttons.

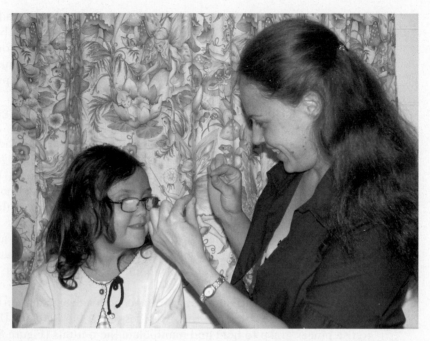

FIGURE 8.12 The therapist demonstrates the pincer grasp needed for buttoning.

prompted. The therapist then begins to use incomplete instructions (cloze) during her demonstrations, and Imogen is able to complete them.

The therapist then changes her demonstration to illustrate the decision-making process, rather than the critical physical skills, by using think-aloud modeling. Imogen is able to see not only how the task is performed but also the essential cognitive skills that underpin performance. Imogen then takes a turn at buttoning her blouse. The therapist poses higher order questions to stimulate Imogen's decision making. After some practice, Imogen is able to perform the task with ongoing support from the therapist, but continues to have difficulty recalling how to perform the specific stages of the task. Over the course of a few sessions, Imogen becomes able to use self-initiated (quadrant 3) strategies to instruct herself to align the garment, and a mnemonic to remember the key aspects of the buttoning task (Figure 8.13). Occasionally, she forgets to use these strategies, and the therapist uses an orienting strategy to remind her to say it to herself. Over time, Imogen begins to whisper these instructions to herself, eventually becoming able to button her blouse independently.

At this point, Imogen demonstrates autonomy in the performance of some key tasks (Figure 8.14). When rushed to complete the activity however, as occurs when getting ready for school, this performance breaks down. Using the strategies detailed in the 4QM, Imogen's mother, and others involved with Imogen, can easily take on the role of facilitator, using consistent learning strategies to

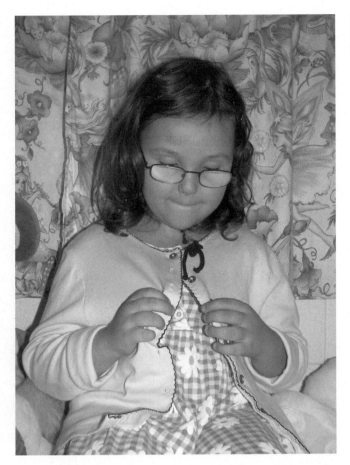

FIGURE 8.13 Imogen practices aligning both sides of her blouse.

promote the acquisition of skills. The use of quadrant 3 (self-prompting) strategies, and exposure to higher order questions (quadrant 2), enable Imogen to make astute decisions about the contextual demands of the occupation. When the task becomes difficult due to time restrictions, or wearing a different garment with slightly smaller buttons, Imogen could retreat into her previously learned dependent patterns, waiting for her mother to dress her or help her through the problem. Instead, her mother uses orienting strategies to encourage Imogen to use the self-mediating strategies of quadrant 3 to think and talk her way through difficult situations, demonstrating an ability to initiate processes that will enable occupational performance.

As the result of a carefully thought through intervention process, Imogen has been able to learn the skills necessary to dress herself without assistance when getting ready for school. Through attention to the many factors that influence the mastery and generalization of skills, her therapist has used the 4QM as a frame of reference in enabling Imogen to develop occupational autonomy.

FIGURE 8.14 Imogen practices buttoning the buttons of her blouse.

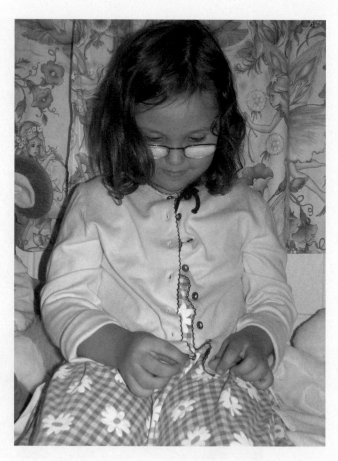

REFERENCES

Anderson, L. W., Krathwohl, D. R., & Bloom, B. S. (2001). *A Taxonomy for Learning, Teaching, and Assessing: A revision of Bloom's Taxonomy of Educational Objectives*. New York: Longman.

Bissell, A. N., & Lemons, P. P. (2006). A new method for assessing critical thinking in the classroom. *Bioscience, 56*(1), 66–72.

Bloom, B., Englehart, M. B., Furst, E. J., & Hill, W. H. (1956). *Taxonomy of Educational Objectives: The Classification of Educational Goals. Handbook 1: The Cognitive Domain*. New York: Longman.

Carr, J. H., & Shepherd, R. B. (1998). *Neurological Rehabilitation: Optimising Motor Performance*. Oxford: Butterworth Heinemann.

Chen, S., Zhang, J., Lange, E., & Miko, P. (2001). Progressive time delay procedure for teaching motor skills to adults with severe mental retardation. *Adapted Physical Activity Quarterly, 18*(1), 35–48.

Greber, C., Ziviani, J., & Rodger, S. (2007a). The four-quadrant model of facilitated learning (Part 1): Using teaching–learning approaches in occupational therapy. *Australian Occupational Therapy Journal, 54*(s1), S31–S39.

Greber, C., Ziviani, J., & Rodger, S. (2007b). The four-quadrant model of facilitated learning (Part 2): Strategies and applications. *Australian Occupational Therapy Journal, 54*(s1), S40–S48.

Hudson, P., Lignugaris-Kraft, B., & Miller, T. (1993). Using content enhancements to improve the performance of adolescents with learning disabilities in content classes. *Learning Disabilities Research and Practice, 8*(2), 106–126.

Johnson, S. (2000). How would you code your questions? *Gifted Child Today, 23*(2), 5.

Joyce, B. R., Calhoun, E., & Hopkins, D. (2002). *Models of Learning: Tools for Teaching* (2nd ed.). Buckingham, Philadelphia, PA: Open University.

Martini, R., & Polatajko, H. J. (1998). Verbal self-guidance as a treatment approach for children with developmental coordination disorder: A systematic replication study. *Occupational Therapy Journal of Research*, *18*(4), 157–181.

Marzano, R. J., Pickering, D. J., & Pollock, J. E. (2001). *Classroom Instruction that Works: Research-Based Strategies for Increasing Student Achievement*. Alexandria, VA: Association for Supervision and Curriculum Development.

Montague, M. (1992). The effects of cognitive and metacognitive strategy instruction on the mathematical problem solving of middle school students with learning disabilities. *Journal of Learning Disabilities*, *25*(4), 230–248.

Mosston, M., and Ashworth, S. (2002). *Teaching Physical Education* (5th ed.). San Francisco, CA: Benjamin/Cummings Publishers.

Polatajko, H. J., & Mandich, A. (2004). *Enabling Occupation in Children: The Cognitive Orientation to Daily Occupational Performance (CO-OP) Approach*. Ottawa, ON: Canadian Association of Occupational Therapists.

Rodger, S., Brown, G. T., & Brown, A. (2005). Profile of paediatric occupational therapy practice in Australia. *Australian Occupational Therapy Journal*, *52*(4), 311–325.

Schmidt, R. A., & Lee, T. D. (2005). *Motor Learning and Control: A Behavioral Emphasis* (4th ed.). Campaign, IL: Human Kinetics.

Schmidt, R. A., & Wrisberg, C. A. (2000). *Motor Learning and Performance: A Problem-Based Learning Approach* (2nd ed.). Champaign, IL: Human Kinetics.

Sinha, S. P., & Sharma, A. (2001). Cognitive strategy instruction approach of problem solving for learning disabled children. *Journal of Indian Psychology*, *19*(1-2), 33–38.

Thompson, R. H., McKerchar, P. M., Paige, M., & Dancho, K. A. (2004). The effects of delayed physical prompts and reinforcement on infant sign language acquisition. *Journal of Applied Behavior Analysis*, *37*(3), 379–383.

Vaidya, S. R. (1999). Metacognitive learning strategies for students with learning disabilities. *Education*, *120*(1), 186–191.

Vygotsky, L. S. (1978). Mind in society: the development of higher psychological processes. In R. W. Reiber, & D. K. Robinson (Eds.) (Translated by M. Cole, S. Scribner, V John-Steiner, & E. Souberman), *The essential Vygotsky* (pp. 345–400). New York: Kluwer Academic Publishers.

Woolfolk, A. E. (2004). *Educational Psychology* (9th ed.). Boston, MA: Allyn & Bacon.

CHAPTER 9

A Frame of Reference to Enhance Childhood Occupations: SCOPE-IT

KRISTINE HAERTL

Children construct their individual and collective identities through occupational engagement. Preparing for school, playing baseball with friends, reading a book, and cooking with a parent all represent activities and occupations used to create the self through daily experiences. Consideration of how children create and interpret their worlds is crucial to the understanding of development and childhood occupations (Lawlor, 2003).

The understanding and therapeutic application of occupation has been central to the core of occupational therapy since its inception. In 1917, the National Society for the Promotion of Occupational Therapy, the preceding professional association to the American Occupational Therapy Association (AOTA), emphasized the importance of "curative occupations" in the therapeutic application of occupational therapy (AOTA, 2007). Although the importance of occupation is emphasized throughout our profession, each theoretical model and frame of reference has its own emphasis, yet the concept of occupation is not always the primary focus in the application of every frame of reference. As emphasis on the therapeutic value of occupation has reemerged in recent years (AOTA, 2002; Cottrell, 2005) occupation-based theoretical models and frameworks have been developed for occupational therapy intervention throughout the life span (e.g., Christiansen & Baum, 1997; Dunn, Brown, & McGuigan, 1994; Kielhofner, 1983a). Within the frame of reference to enhance childhood occupations, the primary focus is on the unique relationship between the person, environment, and occupation. The focus is on occupation as the primary means and ends to therapy. This chapter outlines the application of one particular occupation-based theoretical model, the SCOPE-IT model (Poulsen & Zivani, 2004a,b) to pediatric practice. Underlying assumptions of this frame of reference are discussed, along with the theoretical base, and a framework for applying SCOPE-IT to occupational therapy evaluation and intervention.

THEORETICAL BASE

The work of pioneers such as Reilly (1962), Yerxa (1967), and Kielhofner (1983a, 1995) emphasize the importance of occupation as the foundation of our profession. Personal interests, values, goals, skills, habits, and roles were viewed as integral to the occupations chosen and the resulting *occupational behavior* (Kielhofner, 1995). Adaptive *occupational behavior* is the outcome of an individual's ability to organize behavior in time with personally and culturally meaningful activities in areas such as work, rest, play, and self-care (Kielhofner, 1983b; Reilly, 1966). The frame of reference to enhance childhood occupations considers the child's growth and maturity in occupational engagement through the natural course of development (Figure 9.1). Children are viewed as developing dynamically through participation in daily activities. Person, environment, social, and cultural variables influence development and occupational behavior. *Occupation* is "culturally valued, coherent patterns of actions that emerge through transactions between the child and environment and as activities the child either wants to do or is expected to perform" (Humphry, 2002, p. 172). Occupational behavior changes over time and is influenced by genetic and environmental factors that naturally occur in the child's developmental process.

Occupational development is the progressive change that occurs in occupational behavior as a result of an individual's interaction with the environment over time (Wiseman, Davis, & Polatajko, 2005). Inherent within this definition are the influences of personal motivation, will, and social engagement. Characteristics of the person, environment, and occupational opportunities shape the course of occupational development through growth and maturation (Davis & Polatajko, 2004). Factors that influence change and occupational development include (1) community and caregiving practices

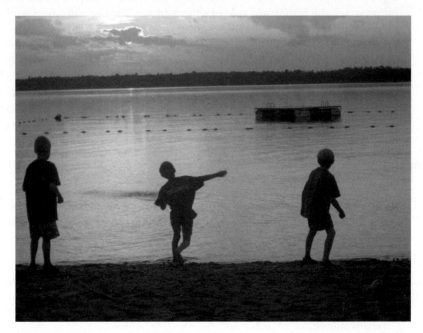

FIGURE 9.1 "I like to skip rocks because each time they can go farther" (Alex, age 9). These children demonstrate the quest for mastery during occupational engagement.

that create occupational opportunities, (2) the social and interpersonal transactions that surround activities, and (3) the self-organizing process that underlies occupational engagement (Humphry & Wakeford, 2006).

Within this frame of reference to enhance childhood occupations, the therapist takes on the role of facilitator of occupational engagement through use of *occupation as a means* to achieve the desired therapy outcomes, and *occupation as an ends* to maximize occupational performance of the child. *Occupation as a means* involves the use of occupation as a therapeutic agent to promote transformation of the person (Trombly, 1995), whereas *occupation as an ends* refers to the product of therapy and may include goals related to improving occupational performance. For instance, when treating Andy, a 13-year-old male with a recent L4 spinal cord injury, the therapist may capitalize on Andy's love of sports and use games involving the throwing and catching of balls to improve mobility and upper extremity strength (*occupation as a means*) in order to work toward Andy's expressed goal of playing wheelchair basketball (*occupation as an ends*). The therapist capitalizes on Andy's strengths and interests in using activities that are meaningful to him, to work toward the end goal of participating in adaptive sports. Additional methods used to achieve the occupational end goal may also include fitting Andy with a specialized lightweight wheelchair, and collaborating with Andy and his family to secure community resources that would help him achieve his goals.

Consistent with Deci and Ryan's self-determination theory (Deci & Ryan, 2000; Ryan & Deci 2000a,b) children are intrinsically driven to seek challenge, master and integrate experience, and work toward personal objectives. Self-determination theory emphasizes the important role of others in facilitating autonomy and reaching personal goals (Williams et al., 2006). Therefore, *motivation* is a key concept in the frame of reference to enhance childhood occupations. Work toward establishing autonomy through the child's engagement in activities involves collaboration with families, educators, and communities (Figure 9.2). Teachers and parents have been shown as effective mediators in facilitating engagement, autonomy, and motivation through use of behavioral feedback and personal support as well as through educating the child on the relevance of a particular task (Assor, Kaplan, & Roth, 2002; Assor, Roth, & Deci, 2004).

Assumptions

The frame of reference to enhance childhood occupations has six assumptions. Assumptions are consistent with the understanding of the study of occupation, as we have come to know it through the contributions of researchers in occupational therapy and occupational science.

- Children are occupational and social beings.
- The use of occupation is the underlying foundation of occupational therapy and is equally important both as a means and as an ends.
- Personal, environmental, social, cultural, and temporal factors influence occupational performance.
- Occupational development occurs through a dynamic process involving innate drives and guided participation.

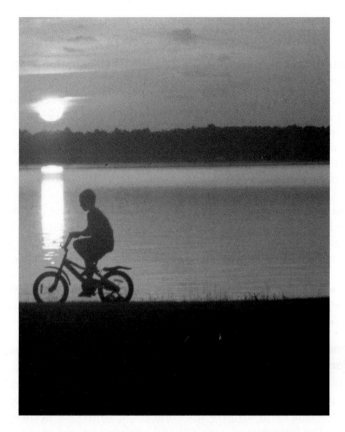

FIGURE 9.2 "I like riding my bike because it takes me wherever I want to go!" (Cole, age 7, demonstrating the importance of autonomy in the development of a child).

- Engagement in occupation brings about change.
- Occupational engagement influences health and well-being.

Children are Occupational and Social Beings

The familiar sight of children running toward a playground illustrates the innate drive toward action that is perceived as meaningful and motivating for the child. Kielhofner (2002a) wrote, "whatever else characterizes being human-our spiritual yearnings, our capacity for love-we also share an innate occupational nature" (p. 1). Through interaction with the world, we maintain balance in our daily lives by active engagement and active use through time (Meyer, 1922). This frame of reference, which enhances childhood occupations, views the child as intrinsically motivated toward meaningful occupational engagement in a social world. Children are viewed as "socially occupied beings" (Lawlor, 2003, p. 424). Such engagement occurs in a context influenced by the sociocultural environment. Lawlor (2003) stressed that conceptualizations of the study of childhood occupations need to be framed in the understanding of children as socially occupied beings. Engagement with caregivers, peers, and therapists provide an emotional and social context by which children participate in occupation. The understanding of significant relationships (e.g., parents, peers, teachers, and therapists) and their effect on the child is crucial to the foundations of occupation-based pediatric practice.

The Use of Occupation is the Underlying Foundation of Occupational Therapy and is Equally Important both as a Means and as an End

Occupation is relevant to the therapeutic process both as a *means* to serve as a change agent and achieve goals, and as an *end* goal of therapy (Trombly, 1995). Occupation as a means is viewed as a remedial approach to using purposeful activity to address goals. The use of occupation as a therapeutic agent should advance an individual toward an "occupational outcome," one that provides meaning in the therapeutic environment (Gray, 1998). Such use of meaningful occupation serves as a catalyst to the healing and change process.

Occupation as an ends focuses on a therapeutic approach to achieve an occupational goal. The therapist who focuses on *occupation as an ends* may use a direct skill training approach to achieving an end occupational goal (e.g., dressing following a traumatic brain injury) or may use additional techniques (e.g., lifting weights to enhance function) in order to address underlying deficits to achieve the end goal. When focusing on occupation as the end goal, the means to achieve that goal should remain relevant, occupational, and meaningful; therefore, the focus on occupation is held throughout the therapeutic process from evaluation to intervention (Gray, 1998).

Personal, Environmental, Social, Cultural, and Temporal Factors Influence Occupational Performance

O*ccupational form is* "the composition of objective physical and sociocultural circumstances external to the person that influences his or her *occupational performance*" (Nelson, 1988, p. 776). This form involves the contexts in which the occupation takes place. The focus is on the influence of personal and environmental factors on occupational performance. Environments provide occupational opportunities or barriers, in conjunction with social and cultural influences to structure the context of occupational engagement through time. An emphasis is on the interaction between the person and the environment and its influence on occupational performance. Each environment offers unique resources, opportunities, and constraints that interact with the individual's values, interests, roles, habits, and performance capacities (Kielhofner, 1985, 1995, 2002b). It is critical to consider the unique influence of the environment on performance (Christiansen & Baum, 1991, 1997, 2004; Dunn, Brown, & McGuigan, 1994). Viewing individual abilities and life roles from a contextual perspective, the emphasis is on the inter-relationship between the person and environment and its impact on an identified potential "performance range" (Dunn, Brown, & McGuigan, 1994). Thus, context is a key variable in assessment and intervention in order to determine contextual opportunities and barriers and to identify personal goals within the performance range. For instance, a child may have the intellectual and musical capacity to be a great musician, yet if environmental barriers such as lack of adequate opportunities for instruction or lack of resources exist, then the child's potential may not be met. Considerations are intrinsic factors such as psychological, cognitive, physiological, and neurobehavioral characteristics of an individual and the extrinsic environmental factors such as physical, cultural, social, and societal influences (Law, Baum, & Dunn, 2005). The interaction between the person and the environment influences choice of time use and is affected by the developmental stage, chronological age, and period of time in which the occupational engagement occurs.

Occupational Development Occurs through a Dynamic Process Involving Innate Drives and Guided Participation

The study of occupation assumes that character and competence are formed through childhood occupations (Clark et al., 1991; Primeau, Clark, & Pierce, 1989). Historically, developmental theorists emphasized the innate drive toward active engagement and learning in children. Piaget stressed the importance of the child's inborn curiosity and drive toward active acquisition of knowledge, whereas Vygotsky emphasized the importance of an adult or mentor's role in facilitating learning through guided participation (Berger, 2004). This developmental process of learning and growth occurs through social and occupational engagement. A child's innate drives are occupationally driven and influenced upon by the environment (Clark et al., 1991; Humphry, 2002). Humphry stressed the reciprocal process of innate child factors, the drive toward occupational engagement, and the transactional time-specific process (Humphry, 2002; Humphry & Wakeford, 2006). Social influences of adult mentors affect occupational development as "experiences in occupation and influence of others' modeling, performance expectations, and assistance with difficult elements given equal importance as intrinsic changes" (Humphry & Wakeford, 2006, p. 259). The dynamic interaction between the child's curiosity and inner drive along with the cultural expectations and guided participation plays an integral role in occupational development.

The Engagement in Occupation Brings About Change

Consideration of the therapeutic process and product of occupation is integral to evaluation and intervention. The process of occupational engagement creates growth and change. The therapeutic value of occupation is a "change agent to remediate impaired abilities or capacities" (Trombly, 1995, p. 963). Yet the participation in occupation goes beyond remediation and facilitates a dynamic process that fosters change both in the individual and the environment. On the basis of the underlying assumption that occupational engagement creates change, use of a frame of reference to enhance childhood occupations identifies specific therapeutic aspects of occupation (e.g., through an activity analysis), in conjunction with client and environmental factors, and plans intervention in a systematic way to work toward identified therapeutic goals.

Adaptive Occupational Engagement Influences Health and Well-Being

The foundations of occupational therapy rest on the therapeutic influence of meaningful doing. Reilly (1962) asserted that "man, through the use of his hands as energized by his mind and will can influence the state of his own health" (p. 2). Thus, the personal occupational choices we make influence our present state of health and well-being. Occupational engagement is linked to health and survival (Wilcock, 1998). Given that survival is an innate drive, humans are intrinsically driven toward participation in activities to meet physical, mental, and social needs. On the basis of the premise that occupational engagement brings about change, the frame of reference to enhance childhood occupations seeks to apply occupation in a therapeutic way in order to promote health and well-being. Further, there is a reciprocal relationship in that occupation influences health, and personal and societal health influences occupational participation and performance.

Synthesis of Child, Occupational, Performance, and Environment-In Time (*SCOPE-IT* Model)

The Synthesis of Child, Occupational, Performance, and Environment-In Time (SCOPE-IT model, Poulsen & Ziviani, 2004a,b) is based on Primeau and Fergusen's description of the occupational frame of reference (1999), as well as theoretical models that focus on the person, environment, and occupational performance; that is, Person–Environment–Occupation–Performance Model (Christiansen & Baum, 1997), Human Ecology Model (Dunn, Brown, & McGuigan, 1994), Model of Human Occupation (Kielhofner, 1997) (Figure 9.3). The occupational frame of reference according to Primeau and Ferguson focuses on enabling occupation through the use of client-centered practice. The emphasis of this frame of reference is improvement of occupational performance through maximization of the child–environment fit within

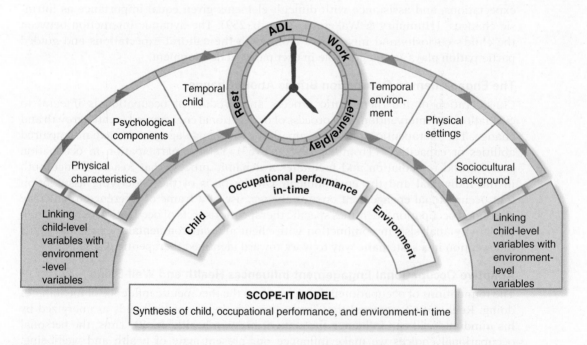

FIGURE 9.3 SCOPE-IT model. (Reprinted with permission from: Poulsen, A. A., & Ziviani, J. M. (2004). Health enhancing physical activity: factors influencing engagement patterns in children. *Australian Occupational Therapy Journal, 51,* 72.)

the scope of time. Within the frame of reference to enhance childhood occupations, the SCOPE-IT model emphasizes personal effort and choice as it is synthesized with child, environment, and temporal factors in order to influence occupational performance.

The SCOPE-IT model is pictorially symbolized as a watch band with a focal point of the face of the watch emphasizing balance of work, rest, activities of daily living (ADL), and leisure or play. In the center of the face, importance is placed on the individual's personal choice and effort in the temporal context of time.

The central concepts of the SCOPE-IT model, time, and occupation are based on Adolf Meyer's work emphasizing balance in the daily rhythms of life (Poulsen & Ziviani, 2004b). Occupational engagement, as measured quantifiably and qualitatively, considers how children structure time in daily life. The temporal context includes features of the individual (i.e., age, developmental stage, life cycle, and health status) as well as temporal features of the task (sequential structure, duration, when the task takes place, rate of recurrence, and structure) (Dunn, Brown, & Youngstrom, 2003). At the environmental level, physical, geographical, social, cultural, economic, occupational, and political factors influence the child's occupational performance (Kielhofner, 2002b; Pierce, 2003; Primeau & Ferguson, 1999). Consideration of the temporal and environmental contexts along with the child's physical and psychological characteristics helps the therapist design evaluation and intervention strategies aimed at overall improvement of occupational performance.

Health and Wellness Continuum

Health, wellness, and personal well-being are distinct but related concepts that underlie the occupational therapy process. The application of the frame of reference to enhance childhood occupations occurs along the health–wellness function/dysfunction continuum. Historically, the term *health* was rooted in the old English word "heolth" which typically referred to a sound state physically and denoted the condition of the body (Dolfman, 1973). Yet conceptualizations of health in recent years have become more holistic as health increasingly is equated with a state of well-being. Over a half century ago health was defined by the World Health Organization (WHO) as "a complete state of physical, mental, and social well-being, and not merely the absence of disease or infirmity" (WHO, 1946). This definition continues as the official definition of the WHO and affirms the connection between the state of the mind–body–spirit and personal well-being.

Concepts of health, wellness, and personal well-being are integral throughout the life span. Within the SCOPE-IT model, the facilitation of adaptive responses in the child and promotion of health satisfaction, well-being, efficacy, and quality of life are the desired outcomes of therapy. Subjective *well-being* includes an individual's perception of life, the presence of positive emotional states, and absence of negative ones (Diener, 1994). Diener et al. (1999) expanded this definition to include life satisfaction and personal satisfaction on specific life domains. Conceptualizations of well-being include various components including measures of satisfaction, balance, happiness, stress, and personal evaluation of the state of one's life (Kim-Prieto et al., 2005). When children are younger, although they are not of the developmental level to conceptualize ideas of personal well-being, their interactions with the environment, caregivers, and their occupations

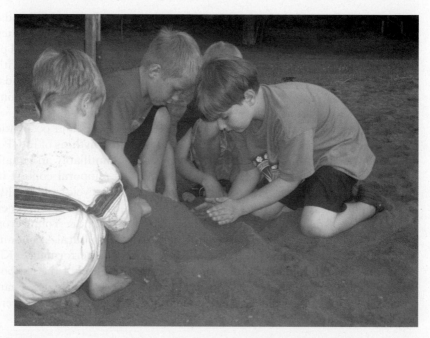

FIGURE 9.4 "Playing in the sand is fun because you get to build things!!" (Andrew, age 7). These children spontaneously adapt the environment (sand volleyball court) to engage in building a sand castle.

influence personal identity, their sense of efficacy and mastery, satisfaction, and overall health (Figure 9.4).

A distinct but related term "wellness" is a state of being evolving through a process that occurs throughout the life journey (Jonas, 2005). This process involves personal choices that influence our state of health and life satisfaction. According to the National Wellness Institute (2007), wellness involves six dimensions including the following:

1. A person's contribution to the environment, community, and how to build improved living spaces and social networks
2. Life enrichment through work and its connection to living and playing
3. The development of belief systems, values, and the creation of a worldview
4. The benefits of healthy choices including physical activity, healthy eating, health, strength and vitality, personal responsibility, self-care, and seeking medical attention when needed.
5. Self-esteem, self-control, and determination influencing life direction
6. Creative stimulating mental activities and sharing of personal gifts and talents with others

The engagement of healthy choices leads to improved personal wellness and may enhance quality of life. Starting from a very young age, parental influences, the sociocultural environment, and personal experiences influence a child's personal choices related

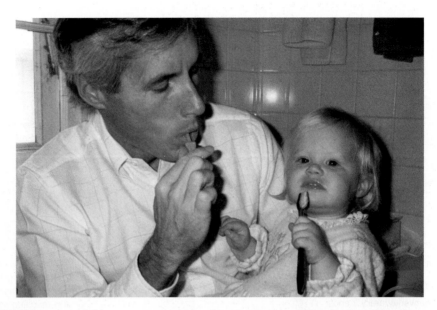

FIGURE 9.5 Parent–child interaction is integral to developing skills, values, and habits.

to health, wellness, and occupational engagement (Figure 9.5). Within the frame of reference to enhance childhood occupations, the therapist chooses occupational interventions aimed at engaging the child in meaningful activity to improve overall personal function, occupational performance, wellness, and life satisfaction.

Persons with chronic and severe illness can still have personal well-being and life satisfaction (i.e., Matthews et al., 2002; Mulkana & Hailey, 2001). For instance, an adolescent may have personal wellness in one of the dimensions (i.e., making healthy eating choices and maintaining good physical health) but may be lacking in other areas (i.e., strong social connections). The SCOPE-IT model views wellness more holistically to include concepts of effort, choice, and time as they create a unique rhythm within the child's occupational engagement in areas of rest, ADL, work, and leisure or play (Figure 9.6). Integrating concepts from the SCOPE-IT model along with the National Wellness Institute's (2007) dimension of wellness and Diener's (1994) emphasis on individual self-perception, a more holistic conceptualization of individual wellness and well-being should be dynamic, multidimensional, and applicable throughout the life span.

In a dynamic representation of well-being, all dimensions influence one another and contribute to an individual's overall health, wellness, and perceived well-being. Within the frame of reference to enhance childhood occupations, therapists work with children in all dimensions utilizing a client-centered focus and creating occupational opportunities for personal success and growth. Through use of meaningful occupations, the identified outcomes of the SCOPE-IT model aim to increase adaptive responses leading to health, satisfaction, sense of well-being, flow, efficacy experiences, quality of life, and a sense of identity (Poulsen & Ziviani, 2004b).

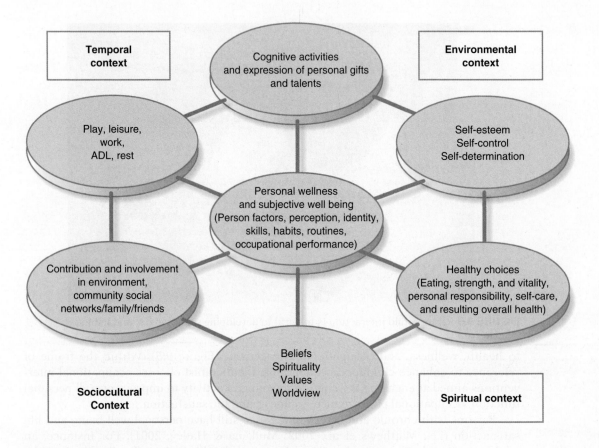

FIGURE 9.6 Dynamic representation of personal wellness and well-being.

FUNCTION–DYSFUNCTION CONTINUA

Within the spectrum of health and wellness, individuals move throughout life along a continuum of function–dysfunction in areas of occupational performance. Applying the SCOPE-IT model within the frame of reference to enhance childhood occupations, functional indicators are considered within the occupational performance areas of (1) work and productivity, (2) play and leisure, (3) ADL and self-care, and (4) rest and sleep. These are in no particular order and all are of equal importance. Human performance is not static; its complexity is dynamic and performance along each continuum ranges is based on the interaction of personal, environmental, and temporal factors. Occupational behavior may be functional in one set of circumstances, but not in another. Therefore, although the following charts indicate guidelines for function–dysfunction, it is important to remember the variability that occurs based on personal motivation, choice, effort, time, and environmental context.

Indicators of Function and Dysfunction for Work and Productivity

Although play is often referred to as the work of the child, there are several contexts in which children engage in productive work behaviors. Household chores, schoolwork, and beginning vocations as an adolescent all fall under the category of work. The function of children's work serves to "foster development and occupational competence, assist in household labor, and foster social relationships" (Larson, 2004, p. 373). Children's conceptualization of work develops early and is heavily influenced by observation and participation of adults, especially within their families (Brown, 2002; Galinsky, 1999). The development of work ethics, performance skills, and personal value of productivity all influence the child's choice, effort, and time spent in work-related behaviors. Productive activities and the development of work habits through weekly routines serve to develop skills and educate the child in the sociocultural expectations of work within the environmental contexts of the family, school, community, and society. The development of work skills within the child is largely influenced within the school and family contexts. Expectations for on-task behaviors and completion of homework influence the child at school, whereas family participation in household responsibilities and routines facilitates work skills at home (Table 9.1). Occupational scaffolding is a means by which parents foster their children's competence as adults through techniques that use play in order to foster work-related task behaviors (Primeau, 1998). Within the family, work and play are frequently embedded and therefore are often blended experiences without clear distinct lines of whether an activity constitutes work or play (Primeau, 1998).

Work-related occupations (i.e., for school) involve various physical, cognitive, and psychological skills. If a child has difficulty with a particular skill such as attending to a task, challenges result in successfully performing the desired task. Within the frame of reference to enhance childhood occupations, therapists identify enablers and barriers to

TABLE 9.1 Indicators of Function and Dysfunction for Work/Productivity Initiating Behaviors	
Engages in Productive Work Tasks	*Does Not Engage in Productive Work Tasks*

FUNCTION: Ability to engage in productive work tasks in the home, school, and community
Indicators of Function
  Sustains attention for task completion
  Demonstrates adequate physical and psychological skills to meet task demands
  Manipulates and uses materials in a productive manner to engage in work behaviors
  Performs to age-level expectations in work-related activities in the home, school, and community
	DYSFUNCTION: Inability to engage in productive work tasks in the home, school, and community
	Indicators of Dysfunction
	  Inability to sustain attention for task completion
	  Impaired skills in one or more areas cause difficulty with task demands
	  Difficulty with manipulating and using materials in a productive manner
	  Does not perform to age-level expectations in work-related activities in the home, school, and community

productive work performance and develop intervention plans with the child and family to maximize strengths, minimize barriers, build on resources, and improve occupational performance.

Indicators of Function and Dysfunction for Play and Leisure

Play is a major means by which children develop competence and mastery (Rodger & Ziviani, 1999). Through exploration of the environment and spontaneous engagement in meaningful activity, children develop social, emotional, cognitive and physical skills that provide the foundation for later role expectations. *Play* is a spontaneous or organized activity that produces enjoyment, entertainment, amusement, or diversion and involves an attitude or mode of experience driven by intrinsic motivation (Parham & Fazio, 1997). The emphasis is on the process rather than the product and is driven by internal rather than external control. Stagnitti, (2004, p. 5) synthesized dispositional concepts of play into the following characteristics:

1. Is more internally than externally motivated
2. Transcends reality as well as reflects reality
3. Is controlled by the player
4. Involves more attention to the process than product
5. Is safe
6. Is usually fun, unpredictable, and pleasurable
7. Is spontaneous and involves nonobligatory active engagement

Within the play context or setting, children are intrinsically driven and take on the role of *player*, which infers active occupational participation in play (Table 9.2). Forms of play may be individual, parallel (next to another individual), didactic (with another individual), or group play. Expectations of the player often include participation based on rules, skills, and habits that lay the foundation for additional roles later in life (Burke, 1993; Parham & Primeau, 1997). Occupational therapists work to foster adaptive play

TABLE 9.2 Indicators of Function and Dysfunction for Play and Leisure

Engages in Play and Leisure	Does Not Engage in Play and Leisure
FUNCTION: Ability to engage in play and leisure to developmental expectations	DYSFUNCTION: Inability to engage in play and leisure to developmental expectations
Indicators of Function	**Indicators of Dysfunction**
Initiates play behaviors	Failure to initiate play
Demonstrates adequate physical and psychological skills to meet task demands	Impaired skills in one or more areas cause difficulty with task demands
Manipulates and uses materials in a creative manner to engage in play behaviors	Difficulty with manipulating and using materials necessary for play
Maintains safety within play behaviors	Plays in an unsafe manner
Performs to age-level expectations in individual, dyadic, and group play and leisure	Does not perform to age-level expectations in individual, dyadic, and group play and leisure

skills through analysis of the child's skills, the environmental context, and the nature of the play occupation.

A similar but distinct term to play, "leisure," typically denotes individual choice in time use for the purposes of personal pleasure or psychological need that may or may not be structured (i.e., a hobby or specific craft). Within pediatric practice, developing leisure skills becomes increasingly important as the child ages and enters the adolescent years. Stebbins (1997) identified two types of leisure: casual and serious leisure, the latter of which often requires more structure and often a specific skill set, such as in a hobby. Stebbins (2005) challenged the concept of freedom to choose one's leisure given the fact that there are various sociocultural and leisure constraints that inhibit an individual's choice of leisure (i.e., an individual from a lower socioeconomic background may be limited in the ability to participate in downhill skiing because of limited funds). Given inherent barriers to complete choice of leisure pursuits, Stebbins identified leisure as "uncoerced activity undertaken during free time where such activity is something people want to do, and, at a personally satisfying level using their abilities and resources they succeed in doing" (p. 350). As children develop, peer and family interactions along with contextual opportunities (i.e., a nearby baseball field) influence leisure pursuits.

Indicators of Function and Dysfunction for Activities of Daily Living and Self-Care

An integral part of occupational development is the learning of self-care skills necessary for daily living (Table 9.3). Child factors interact with environmental and temporal contexts affecting occupational performance. Values, interest level, and motivation to engage in personal self-care facilitate skill development and are heavily influenced by caregivers. ADLs include bathing, bowel and bladder management, toilet hygiene, dressing, eating, feeding, functional mobility, personal device care, personal hygiene,

TABLE 9.3 Indicators of Function and Dysfunction for Activities of Daily Living (ADL) and Instrumental Activities of Daily Living (IADL)

Participates in ADL and IADL	Does Not Participate in ADL and IADL
FUNCTION: Ability to complete self-care activities to developmental expectations	*DYSFUNCTION*: Inability to complete self-care activities to developmental expectations
Indicators of Function	**Indicators of Dysfunction**
Meets personal, familial, and societal expectations for completion of self care	Difficulty meeting expectations for completion of self-care
Demonstrates physical and psychological skills to meet task demands	Impaired skills in one or more areas cause difficulty with task demands
Manipulates and uses materials to successfully complete self-cares	Inability to manipulate and use materials for successful completion of self-cares
Demonstrates awareness and follow through regarding the purpose of self-cares	Lack of understanding regarding the purpose of self-care activities
Participation in necessary daily routines related to personal health and hygiene	Difficulty following through with expected self-care routines

sexual activity, and sleep or rest. Instrumental activities of daily living (IADL) include care of others, care of pets, child rearing, communication device use, community mobility, financial management, health management and maintenance, home establishment and management, meal preparation and clean up, safety procedures, and shopping (AOTA, 2002). Given the broad scope of ADL and IADL, therapists must work with the child and family to holistically assess self-care occupational function in the home, school, and community and set priorities related to intervention planning.

Indicators of Function and Dysfunction for Rest and Sleep

The consideration of sleep as an occupation is controversial because it is not equated with action (Christiansen & Townsend, 2004), yet sleep and rest are integral to health and well-being. Sleep–rest patterns and habits are heavily influenced biologically and contextually through the impact of cultural practices and familial daily routines. Inability to obtain proper rest and sleep may result in impaired mood, cognition, immune function, and overall health (Owens, 2004).

The participation in rest and sleep ventures beyond the act and requires the development of routines and habits surrounding sleep preparation, daily rhythms and naps, regulation of arousal, and an awareness of the need for sleep and rest (Table 9.4). Daily occupations related to sleep and rest include preparation (i.e., evening self-care routine, putting on pajamas, and reading a book) followed by the calming of one's physical and emotional state to engage in the rest behaviors. Integral to the development of sleep–rest behaviors is the responsiveness and attitude of the parents; research has indicated that the attitude and under- or over-responsiveness of parents may influence sleep behaviors (Thunstrom, 1999). Within the family there is a dynamic relationship whereby the parental expectations and practices influence child behaviors related to sleep and rest; yet conversely, a child who does not sleep well may cause stress within the family, thereby developing a vicious cycle and impairing a healthy sleep and rest routine. Applying the SCOPE-IT model within this frame of reference to enhance childhood occupations, therapists emphasize sleep and rest as an integral routine in daily life.

TABLE 9.4 Indicators of Function and Dysfunction for Sleep and Rest	
Adequate Sleep and Rest	*Inadequate Sleep and Rest*
FUNCTION: Ability to engage in daily sleep and rest necessary for optimal health	*DYSFUNCTION*: Inability to engage in daily sleep and rest necessary for optimal health
Indicators of Function	**Indicators of Dysfunction**
Follow through with daily routines surrounding sleep and rest	Difficulty following through with daily sleep and rest routines
Ability to regulate emotional and arousal states necessary for sleep and rest	Emotional dysregulation and inability to regulate arousal states necessary for sleep and rest
Engagement in restful occupations that promote health and balance in daily life as age appropriate (e.g., reading a book before bed)	Difficulty with restful occupations

GUIDE FOR EVALUATION

Applying Poulsen & Ziviani's (2004a,b) SCOPE-IT model within the frame of reference to enhance childhood occupations, therapists emphasize top-down approaches to assess overall performance, yet effort is made to look dynamically from both top-down and bottom-up perspectives by considering the synthesis of (1) the child's occupational performance components, (2) the child's occupational engagement, and (3) the environmental context within the scope of time. "The focus is not on the underpinning components of performance but on the balance and quality of time spent engaging in daily occupations" (Poulsen & Ziviani, 2004a, p. 73). As the therapist considers the dynamic exchange of the child, environment, and occupational performance, attempts are made to identify strengths, barriers, and motivational factors in order to develop the intervention plan and to work toward adaptive occupational development, engagement, and performance.

Evaluation methods within this frame of reference to enhance childhood occupations are holistic and include history taking; caregiver and client interviews (depending on the age and function of the child); observation; and use of standardized and nonstandardized tools and techniques to identify the child's occupational performance in work, leisure or play, ADL, and rest. The use of a client-centered approach within the evaluation process attempts to identify the motivations and goals of both the child and the caregivers. In addition, a client-centered occupation-based assessment with the child ideally takes place in the natural setting utilizing meaningful activities and occupations that are motivating to the child (Poulsen, Rodger, & Ziviani, 2006; Primeau, 1999). General questions that the therapist may explore prior to and during the evaluation process include the following:

- What is the reason for the evaluation?
- What are the desired outcomes of this evaluation?
- Which tools and methods will provide a holistic picture of the child's occupational performance and environment within the scope of time?
- How do I make the evaluation process meaningful to the child?
- Is it possible to evaluate this child in his or her natural home, school, or community environment?
- What are the child's wishes and motivations for the evaluation process?
- What are the parents', caregivers', and educators' wishes and motivations for the evaluation process?
- What are the individual and contextual strengths and barriers to performance?
- How can we work from a client-centered focus to maximize occupational performance and elicit adaptive outcomes such as health, satisfaction, sense of well-being, flow, efficacy experiences, quality of life, and positive identity? (Poulsen & Ziviani, 2004b)

Evaluating the Child

Within the evaluation process, the therapist considers a child's habits, routines, roles, skills, and underlying personal characteristics that affect occupational performance in areas of work, productivity, play, leisure, ADL, and rest. A top-down approach considers

TABLE 9.5	Three Levels of Doing
Levels of Doing	**Examples**
Occupational participation	Self-grooming
	Playing on playground
	Completing homework
Occupational performance	Washing face
	Combing hair
	Swinging on a swing
	Jumping rope
	Writing a paper
	Mathematical equations
Occupational skill	Sequencing
	Reaching
	Manipulating coordinating limbs
	Socializing
	Jumping
	Thinking
	Problem solving
	Sequencing

(Adapted from Kielhofner, G. [Ed]. [2002b]. Dimensions of doing. *Model of Human Occupation* [3rd ed., pp. 1–19]. Baltimore, MD: Lippincott Williams & Wilkins.)

overall function first, yet does not lose sight of underlying child factors that affect performance or the *doing* of an activity.

The concept of *doing* has three levels, (1) occupational participation, (2) occupational performance, and (3) occupational skill (Kielhofner, 2002b) (Table 9.5). Occupational participation is viewed in the broadest sense (i.e., self-grooming), whereas occupational performance involves the specific tasks within the participation (i.e., taking a bath, brushing teeth, and getting dressed). Occupational skill relates to the component requirements of the activity (i.e., reaching, manipulating, and problem solving). As the therapist evaluates the child's occupational participation, performance, and skill, observations are made regarding personal motivation, occupational and social engagement, and contextual influences.

Kielhofner (2002b) asserted that occupational participation is influenced by (1) performance capacities, (2) habituation, (3) volition, and (4) environmental conditions. As a result, standardized evaluations should be paired with additional means of evaluation including interviews and observation.

Specific child factors as influenced by the temporal, physical, and sociocultural contexts affect occupational participation, performance, and skill. A child's performance components include (1) *temporal factors* (the child's chronological age, developmental maturity, life history, and internal clocks), (2) *physical characteristics* (gender, neuromuscular, sensorimotor, perceptual, health, appearance, and biological), and

(3) *psychological characteristics* (cognitive, affective, self-concept, motivation, beliefs, interests, goals, intentions, and spirituality) (Poulsen & Ziviani, 2004b). The therapist approaches evaluation holistically, considering the child as an open dynamic system. Underlying foundations of evaluation acknowledge the complex synthesis of child factors as interrelated with the environment to influence occupational engagement and performance. Ideally, the child is evaluated using occupation-based assessment tools within natural performance environments. Client strengths and barriers are identified along with temporal characteristics that take into consideration the child's chronological and developmental performance expectations. Examples of common assessment tools used to identify child factors in everyday occupational performance include the *Pediatric Evaluation of Disability Inventory* (PEDI) (Haley et al., 1992), the *Functional Independence Measure* (*FIM*) (Guide for the Uniform Data Set for Medical Rehabilitation, 1999), *Functional Independence Measure for Children* (*Wee FIM II*) (Hamilton & Granger, 2000), the *Vineland Adaptive Behavioral Scales II* (Sparrow, Cichetti, & Balla, 2005), the *School Function Assessment* (Coster et al., 1998), the *Assessment of Motor and Process Skills* (*AMPS*) (Fisher, 2003), and the *School Assessment of Motor and Process Skills* (Fisher & Bryze, 2005) (Figure 9.7).

Key questions considered in the evaluative process as related to child factors include:

- What is the life history of this child?
- What are the age and developmental expectations of this child?
- What strengths and needs does the child have in occupational performance areas?
- What temporal, physical, and psychological occupational performance components influence this child's engagement and performance in work and productivity, play and leisure, ADL, or self-care and rest?

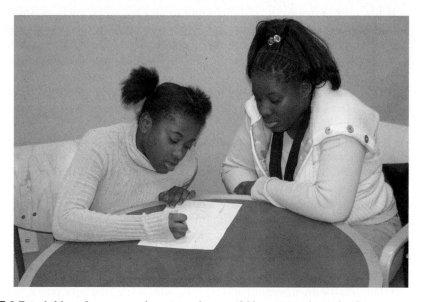

FIGURE 9.7 A child performs a work activity that would be expected in school.

- What individual characteristics influence this child's performance and how are they related to social, temporal, and physical contexts?

Evaluating Occupational Performance In-Time

A unique feature of the SCOPE-IT model is the emphasis of temporal factors (individual and environmental) as they influence quality and quantity of time spent in daily activity. Choice, time, and effort are focal points within the model (Poulsen & Ziviani, 2004a,b) and are integral to overall balance and quality of performance. Inner drive and perceived opportunities along with past occupational experiences affect the child's choice, participation, and engagement. Occupational choice is influenced by individual and societal forces including personal causation, values, interests, degree of control, perceived efficacy, resources, motivations, opportunities, and social encouragement (Kielhofner, 2002c; Poulsen & Ziviani, 2004b; Wiseman, Davis, & Polatajko, 2005). As the therapist evaluates the child, daily patterns of activity are assessed along with level of participation, engagement, and motivation. Underlying factors related to the child's environmental and social surroundings (i.e. parents, teachers, peers, siblings) are considered along with strengths and barriers to establishing balance and rhythm to foster adaptive responses and promote overall health and development.

Evaluation techniques used to assess personal motivation, choice, and daily patterns of activity may include the use of observation, interviews, time-use charts, interest checklists, and occupation-based tools. An example of an assessment used to identify volitional influences on choice and engagement is the *Pediatric Volitional Questionnaire* (PVQ) (Geist et al., 2002), an observational tool that identifies specific behaviors that influence choice, engagement, and performance. The client is rated on a scale (P-passive; H-hesitant; I-involved; and S-spontaneous) in areas such as initiation, engagement, mastery, pleasure expression, problem solving, and activity completion. The use of observational tools such as the PVQ enables the therapist to evaluate client motivation, choice, and quantity and quality of time spent in occupational activities. Additional assessments such as the *Knox Preschool Play Scale* (Knox, 1997), *Test of Playfulness* (Bundy, 1997), *The Adolescent Role Assessment* (Black, 1976), the *Volitional Questionnaire* (De las Heras et al., 2002), the *Child Occupational Self-Assessment* (Federico & Kielhofner, 2002), the *Canadian Occupational Performance Measure* (either with the parents or child depending on the age and function) (Law et al., 1998), the *Pediatric Interest Profiles* (Henry, 2000), and the *Occupational Therapy Psychosocial Assessment of Learning* (Townsend et al., 2001) are examples of instruments that may be used to evaluate choice, time, effort, and patterns of engagement.

Key questions considered in the evaluative process as related to occupational performance in-time include the following:

- What is the child's discretionary and nondiscretionary use of time and how is it affected by perceived efficacy, control, and performance?
- What influences this child's motivation, choice, effort, and will?
- How do the environment and social contexts (i.e., parents, peers, teachers, and siblings) influence the child's motivation, choice, engagement, and performance?

- What are the environmental and temporal enablers and barriers that influence the child's occupational performance in the scope of time?
- Do the daily rhythm and patterns of engagement contribute to developmental expectations, adaptive occupational performance, and overall health and well-being?
- What are the strengths and the needs in the child's daily pattern of engagement and time use?

Evaluating the Environment

A child's socialization with peers on the playground, performance in household chores, and completion of required school activities are affected by the context in which they are performed. The interaction between the child and the environment influences one another in the scope of time. Environmental contexts offer opportunities and pose barriers to occupational development and performance (Dunn, Brown, & McGuigan, 1994; Primeau, 1999). If a child has several friends, has numerous opportunities for community sports leagues, and is reinforced by success experiences participating in a sporting activity, motivation increases, time spent in the activity may increase, and performance is enhanced. Conversely, if the child is teased by peers, gets poor grades in homework because of familial stressors, and lacks supports necessary for success, performance may suffer as a direct result of environmental constraints.

Evaluation of performance in current contexts must be considered along with future environmental demands to adequately predict present function and future needs (Batavia, 1992). *Context* (cultural, physical, social, personal, spiritual, temporal, and virtual) is a "variety of interrelated conditions within and surrounding the client that influence performance" (AOTA, 2002, p. 623). Occupational performance contexts as identified in the SCOPE-IT model (Poulsen & Ziviani, 2004a,b) include the *temporal environment* (days, weeks, months, year, past, present, future, weekends, and other external time structures), the *physical settings* (location, climate, physical structures, facilities, materials and resources, barriers and supports), and *sociocultural background* (peers, family members, community influences, social norms, roles and cultural expectations, institutions, policies, and mass media).

Evaluation techniques used to assess the environmental performance contexts include the use of history taking, interviews, observations, occupation-based activity analysis, visits to the school and home settings, classroom checklists, and the use of formal tools. Given the underlying premise of the transactional nature between the individual and environment in the SCOPE-IT model, emphasis is placed on the use of natural environments for the evaluation process (Figure 9.8). The use of natural environments may add meaning and motivation to the client (Battari et al., 2006) and provide an opportunity to assess not only client performance but also environmental opportunities and constraints.

Examples of tools used to assess context include the *School Function Assessment* (Coster et al., 1998), the *Classroom Environment Scale* (Moos & Trickett, 2002), the *Social Skills Rating System* (Gresham & Elliot, 1990), the *Home Observation for Measurement of the Environment* (*HOME*) (Caldwell & Bradley, 1984), and the *Infant-Toddler Environment Rating Scale-Revised* (Harms, Cryer, & Clifford, 2003). In addition, an evaluation of

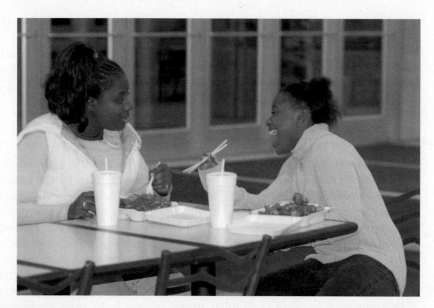

FIGURE 9.8 Eating Chinese food in the school cafeteria provides an opportunity to master specific motor and social skills.

the client–environment–occupation fit must consider the occupational demands within the context. Occupation-based activity analysis differs from a standard activity analysis in that it is highly individualized and embedded in the perspective of the client, the occupational performance strengths and needs, and the performance context (Crepeau, 2003).

The evaluative process takes into account environmental accessibility, enablers, and barriers to adaptive occupational performance. It is important to move beyond the physical context and integrate temporal and sociocultural considerations and their influence upon the child's occupational performance. Key questions for consideration include the following:

- Who are the important individuals in the child's life (i.e., parents, peers, siblings, and teachers) and how does social engagement foster or hinder adaptive occupational performance?
- What are the strengths and barriers in the child's home, school, and community environments and how do they influence occupational development and performance?
- Do the physical environments meet the needs of the child? What strengths, resources, and barriers are there to facilitating performance?
- What is the quality of the child's relationship with the caregiver, teacher, and other important persons in the child's life?
- Are there barriers and influences in the child's environment that contribute to maladaptive occupational behavior? If so, how may they be addressed?
- What are the societal, temporal, and physical influences on the child?

- How do the parental and teacher expectations and goals relate to the child's expectations and goals?
- How can the intervention plan support the expectations of the child, family, teachers, and other important individuals?

Evaluation Synthesis

The synthesis of the evaluation involves a summary of information from both informal and formal evaluation techniques. Given the dynamic nature of the SCOPE-IT model, the therapist considers the complex influences and reciprocal interactions between the child and environment as related to developmental patterns of engagement and performance (Poulsen & Ziviani, 2006). Intervention is planned from evaluation results acknowledging the child–environment–occupation interactions as an open system, ever changing and continuously influenced by the child's internal and external factors. The therapist works with the child and caregivers to identify goals and develop meaningful occupation-based strategies for intervention.

POSTULATES REGARDING CHANGE

Intervention within this frame of reference, using the SCOPE-IT model (Poulsen & Ziviani, 2004a,b), is built upon the underlying premises that enhancing childhood occupations requires that the therapist maximize the child–environment–occupation fit (Primeau & Ferguson, 1999). Focus is placed on areas of occupational performance within the context, particularly in work, sleep or rest, ADL, and leisure or play. Efforts are made to establish a rhythm and balance that lead to the desired outcomes: (1) health, (2) satisfaction, (3) sense of well-being, (4) flow, (5) efficacy experiences, (6) quality of life, and (7) sense of identity (Poulsen & Ziviani, 2004b).

The following are the postulates regarding change:

1. There is a dynamic interaction between the child–environment–occupation that elicits constant change.
2. A client-centered occupation-based approach considers the child and important individuals in his or her life (i.e., parents, teachers, and siblings) as the primary change agents in the therapeutic process.
3. The use of occupation as a means within therapy enhances occupation as an ends, resulting in improved occupational performance.
4. Therapeutic doing that involves true occupational engagement facilitates greater adaptive change than contrived activities.
5. The facilitation of intrinsically motivated goal-directed activities within a therapeutic environment enhances engagement and leads to adaptation and growth.
6. Activities that are within the scope of the child's capacities, and that have personal meaning, will lead to greater motivation, practice, skill development, adaptation, and improved occupational performance.

7. The creation of occupational opportunities for success enhances engagement, effort, motivation, and mastery.
8. Intervention within real-life environments promotes contextual specific skill development and improved occupational performance.
9. The adaptation, creation, and facilitation of optimal environments and occupational opportunities within occupational therapy intervention results in improved client–environment–occupation fit and enhanced occupational performance.
10. The establishment of healthy life patterns of habits, routines, and time use facilitates improved well-being and quality of life.
11. If the therapist works with the child and significant persons (i.e., parents and teachers) to establish an optimal child–environment–occupation fit, then occupational performance will improve and desired outcomes (health, satisfaction, sense of well-being, flow, efficacy, quality of life, and identity formation) will be met.

APPLICATION TO PRACTICE

Improved occupational performance and quality of life are accomplished through a multidimensional approach that acknowledges the ever-changing relationship between child factors, occupational engagement, and the context in which they occur (Poulsen & Ziviani, 2004b). Within this frame of reference, the use of occupation as a means is essential to therapeutic outcomes and therefore attempts are made to identify areas of meaning and motivation to the client. Intrinsic and extrinsic motivators are viewed as integral to the child's engagement (Poulsen, Rodger, & Ziviani, 2006; Poulsen & Ziviani, 2006), and efforts are made to collaborate with the child and family to maximize the child–environmental fit, which in turn maximizes occupational development and performance (Letts et al., 1994; Primeau, 1999). When applying an occupational approach to intervention, (Poulsen, Rodger, & Ziviani 2006) emphasized three basic needs (1) autonomy, (2) competence, and (3) relatedness to facilitate intrinsic motivation with the child. "Intrinsic motivation means engaging in authentic, self-authored and personally endorsed activities. When individuals are intrinsically motivated they have high levels of spontaneous interest, excitement, confidence, persistence, and creativity" (p. 287). Such motivation increases engagement, enjoyment, and well-being.

Within the frame of reference to enhance childhood occupations, the therapist works with the child to foster autonomy and mastery through (1) the use of affirming environments; (2) education of the child, caregivers, and teachers; (3) the use of occupation-based interventions in natural environments; (4) the selection, creation, and modification of the task to fit the child; and (5) the use of interventions designed to adapt and create empowering environments. Competence is developed through (1) maximizing the child–environment fit, (2) providing opportunities for occupational engagement, and (3) through the facilitation of adaptive changes within the therapeutic process (Figure 9.9). Self-perception of competence leads to increased willingness to engage in an activity over time (Poulsen, Rodger, & Ziviani, 2006).

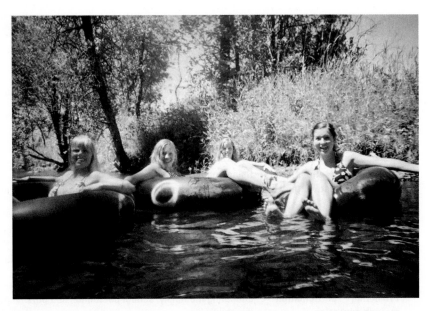

FIGURE 9.9 Activities in the natural environment foster autonomy and mastery.

The Child–Environment–Occupation Fit

The relationship between person and environmental factors influence the quality and quantity of time spent within daily occupations (Poulsen & Ziviani, 2004b). Interventions aimed at maximizing the child–environment–occupation fit focus on a top-down occupational perspective, yet acknowledge that the component processes affect overall performance (Table 9.6). Strategies to achieve goals include (1) improving occupational performance, (2) adapting occupations or providing assistive technology, (3) modifying the environment, and (4) promoting occupational participation through the use of education (Case-Smith, Richardson, & Schultz-Krohn, 2005). Guiding questions for intervention include the following:

- What was the reason for referral and what are the family's, child's, and significant persons' (i.e., teachers, caregivers, etc.) priorities for intervention?
- How will information from the evaluation be used to achieve goals?
- Given the time and resources available, who, what, where, and how will intervention occur?
- What is the child's developmental stage, current developmental performance, and expected developmental trajectory?
- What are the strengths and barriers of the child, environment, and occupational requirements for successful performance?
- What education is needed for the family, child, and significant persons?
- How can empowering environments be adapted and created to maximize the child–environmental fit?

TABLE 9.6 Intervention Purposes and Strategies	
Improving performance	Using occupation as a means Selecting motivating developmentally relevant occupations to provide the "just right challenge" Utilizing occupation to address the underlying component processes that affect performance Use of cueing, facilitation, and feedback Promoting positive social supports Therapeutic use of self
Adapting occupations and providing assistive technology	Using compensatory strategies Identification of assistive devices to maximize performance Adaptation of the occupation/activity
Creation and modification of environments	Consideration of strengths and barriers in the home, school, and community Analysis of the resource, safety, and accessibility of the environment Consideration of the sociocultural and familial values, influences, and beliefs that influence occupational performance
Promoting participation through education	Educating the family, school personnel, and other important individuals in the child's life The use of micro (person) level education and macro (systems/community) level education

(Adapted from Case-Smith, J., Richardson, P., & Schultz-Krohn, W. [2005]. An overview of occupational therapy for children. In J. Case-Smith (Ed). *Occupational Therapy for Children* [5th ed., pp. 2–31]. St. Louis, MO: Elsevier Science.)

- How can a rhythm and balance be optimized in the child's daily occupational patterns to enhance overall health and well-being?

When selecting occupations for interventions, an occupation-based analysis places the client's interests first and considers interest, goals, abilities, task demands, and contexts (Crepeau, 2003).

Work and Productivity

Although work is a key area of childhood occupational performance, little is written on occupational therapy interventions related to the work skills of children. At a very young age, children learn concepts of work by observing family members and receiving caregiver feedback on the importance of helping out with household tasks. Preschool children may attend environments that require school tasks, and within the home environment they may be expected to take on simple chores such as helping to clean up the play area, or put silverware in a dish tray. Work and play are imbedded in some contexts (Primeau, 1998), yet in other areas such as household chores and schoolwork, the delineation may be more apparent. Larson's (2004) review of various definitions of childhood work reveals work as a mandatory or strongly guided activity, whereas play is often in the context of free time.

Improving Performance

Occupational performance in the area of work for a child differs from that of adult in that the focus is on (1) work skills, (2) homework, and (3) chores, rather than a paid activity designed to create social capital. Children learn of the importance of work through occupational engagement within the familial and sociocultural expectations. Within the frame of reference to enhance childhood occupations, the therapist acknowledges that children learn to perform household work through observation and participation and therefore daily routines and habits are established encouraging work-related occupations. Primeau (1998) demonstrated that work concepts and skills are often introduced by parents through scaffolding techniques through the use of (1) cues, (2) feedback, (3) anticipation of needs and problems, and (4) providing graded assistance. Therapists consider the nature of the work, child factors, and the context in which the work behaviors take place. Occupational therapy intervention in childhood work supports the importance of (1) keeping the task consistent with the child's concept of work, (2) considering the nature of the disability and readiness for work tasks, and (3) providing adequate time for children to practice, master skills, and develop expectations and routines for the completion of work tasks (Larson, 2004). Additional suggestions include social participation in work tasks with the family, use of guided participation, and gradual transfer of the work responsibilities from the parent to the child (Dunn, 2004). Similar to household chores, intervention surrounding homework attempts to provide the supports necessary and grade the activity for success. Developing homework routines, creating a value in academic success and learning, and identifying areas of strengths are all strategies to maximize the child–occupation–environment fit.

Adapting Occupations, Environments, and Providing Assistive Technology

The use of environmental and task modifications is common in school settings, yet strategies used at schools should be reinforced at home. Augmentative communication devices, communication boards, computers, and adapted learning materials (i.e., books on tape and enlarged print) are common strategies to enhance work performance. Additional modifications within the school environment include (1) consideration of placement, (2) minimization of distractions, (3) the use of adaptive seating devices, (4) the use of assistive writing devices, (5) the implementation of breaks in the daily routine, (6) the use of learning activities to accommodate multiple learning styles, (7) adapted assignments, (8) tutor/peer help, and (9) modified writing utensils. Home adaptations include (1) environmental modifications, (2) task gradation, and (3) the use of structured routines.

Education

Collaboration with the home and school is integral in the therapy process. Reinforcement of work expectations, the development of consistent routines, and the promotion of work values are important (Figure 9.10). The treatment setting may choose to use additional frames of reference when addressing work, including sensory integrative, biomechanical, and behavioral approaches. The use of a behavioral approach paired with the frame of reference to enhance childhood occupations should always keep in mind the underlying

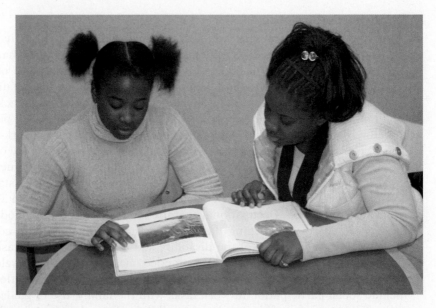

FIGURE 9.10 Sharing a reading assignment at home fosters a value for education.

premise of child-directed activity and should maintain consistency of expectations between the home, school, and community.

Play and Leisure

Play and leisure interventions are aimed at exploration and participation. Exploration relates to identifying appropriate play and leisure activities to maximize the person–occupation fit, whereas participation focuses on the engagement in the play and leisure activities with an emphasis on maintaining a balance with other areas of occupation (AOTA, 2002). While both play and leisure are important, the emphasis in this section will be on play.

Play is a primary means by which children develop competence and learn roles of player and friend (Burke, 1993; Rodger & Ziviani, 1999). Interventions are aimed at occupation as a means (the use of play within therapy) and occupation as an ends (developing underlying social skills necessary for play and interaction) (Figure 9.11). Therapists work with the child as well as the parents to facilitate the "just right challenge" in order to match the child's skill with the environment and play activity.

Improving Performance

There are various types of play including (1) object play, (2) pretend/imitative play, (3) active play (or sporting activities), (4) construction/manipulative play, and (5) creative play. Children participate in play activities alone, through parallel (side-by-side) play, or through dyadic or group play. The use of play as a therapeutic means differs from free play in that goals and objectives are established by the therapist and parents, and when

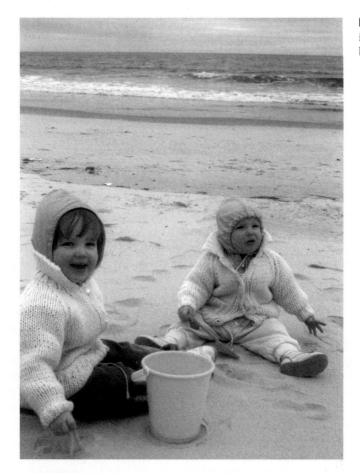

FIGURE 9.11 Children enjoying a natural activity on the beach.

possible the child as well (Knox, 2005). The established goals guide the type of play used in therapy, and emphasize child-directed activities.

Therapists use play in four ways during therapy: (1) as a reward for performance that creates therapeutic change; (2) to facilitate acquisition of the developmental components necessary for play; (3) to facilitate the ability to negotiate temporal, spatial, and social dimensions in the environment; and (4) to facilitate an alteration of occupational patterns (Pierce, 1997). Motivation is a key element in play and efforts are made to facilitate playfulness within the child. Suggestions by Knox (2005) to facilitate play in a child include the following:

1. The application of play theories
2. The use of activity/play analysis
3. Let the child lead
4. Empathize
5. Demonstrate spontaneity
6. Display creativity

Within the frame of reference to enhance childhood occupations, the therapist may use play as a therapeutic tool and as an end goal. The focus is top-down, yet the therapist may use additional frame of references such as the sensory integration frame of reference and the biomechanical frame of reference to remediate underlying component deficits. When possible, play is facilitated in natural play environments (i.e., home, school, and community) and contexts are adapted to (1) provide the just right challenge, (2) to facilitate intrinsic motivation and success, and (3) to create adaptive responses. The facilitation of playfulness and occupational patterns that promote play create mastery and dynamically interact with the child to increase motivation for additional play experiences.

Adapting Occupations, Environments, and Providing Assistive Technology

Through the use of activity analysis matched with the child's strengths and needs, play and leisure activities and play environments are adapted to maximize the child–environment–occupation fit. The use of low-technology solutions such as modification of seating positions, adaptation of rules, use of Dycem and lap tables to hold toys, and enlarged toy and game pieces may be paired with high-technology assistive technology solutions such as computers, augmentative communication systems, mobility devices, adaptive sports equipment, and structural modifications (i.e., adapted play environments). The use of novel arrangements, adaptable play areas (i.e., moveable chairs and tables), and the introduction of new toys are often helpful to facilitate intrinsic motivation and encourage playfulness (Rodger & Ziviani, 1999). Consideration of the child's needs, resources available, and play contexts determine the focus of adaptation. Information on the American Diabetes Association (ADA) guidelines for play areas may be located at: http://www.access-board.gov/play/guide/intro.htm.

Education

The play interactions between parent and infants are integral to promoting play behaviors (Okimoto, Bundy, & Hanzlik, 2000). Play is dynamically intertwined with a child's learning process (Samuelsson & Johansson, 2006). Yet parents and teachers are not always familiar with the means to facilitate adaptive play. The use of family-directed education and intervention may include observation, in-home evaluation and intervention, incorporation of the caregivers into therapy, and consideration of means to maximize the home environment to promote play behaviors. Additional education of teachers, family members, and systemic work (i.e., schools and group homes) are incorporated to reinforce the importance of the child–environment–occupation fit.

Activities of Daily Living

Children are expected in society to master self-care skills. Familial and sociocultural expectations influence performance expectations along with developmental and child factors. Children typically develop self-care skills in relation to complexity of task and environmental supports. For instance, a child with a mother who is an avid cook may learn higher level cooking skills earlier than most of her peers, but may lag behind in

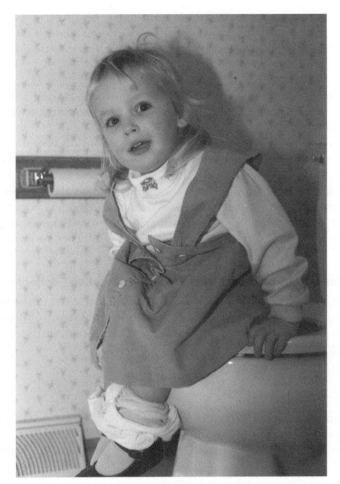

FIGURE 9.12 Child practicing potty training.

learning simple budgeting because it is not reinforced within the familial context. In the infant-toddler years, children learn to self-feed, dress, toilet, and perform simple grooming skills (Figure 9.12). As the child reaches school age, increased expectations are placed on basic ADLs, socialization, grooming, and functional communication (Shepherd, 2005). Beginning skills for higher level cooking, money management, and safety skills are also developed. During adolescence, the child typically becomes more independent in all ADLs and IADLs including areas related to emancipation and freedom such as driving, managing personal finances, and taking responsibility for living areas.

Improving Performance

Interventions related to improvement of ADL performance considers the child's development, physical and psychological structures and functions, and the nature of the task demands and contextual barriers and supports. Efforts are made to identify client and family priorities in order to promote skill development, yet foster balance and quality of life. For instance, Sue, a 13-year-old, with a recent injury resulting in quadriplegia, takes 3 hours to get dressed with assistance. She may determine along with the family and therapist that it would be advantageous for her to have a personal care attendant so that her time could be better spent completing other occupations that take on more meaning for her.

Interventions aimed at improving performance often focus on the use of training techniques along with the use of adaptive equipment and modified environments. Occupation-based ADL teaching strategies may include the use of (1) prompts and feedback, (2) instructional cues, (3) grading of the activity, and (4) repeated opportunities for practice within the daily or weekly routine. When possible the training is completed in the natural environment and reinforced in multiple environments where appropriate (i.e., making change at the store). Additional remedial strategies may be paired with the occupation frame of reference to address underlying factors that affect performance. Strategies to influence motivation include the development of personal value in self-care completion and the use of behavioral approaches to reinforce task completion.

Adapting Occupations, Environments, and Providing Assistive Technology

Assistive devices for ADL include low-technology items such as a tub seat, swivel spoon, or pill box, and high-technology devices such as computers, communication, and mobility devices. Some of the key considerations in selecting assistive technology include the following:

- What are the priorities of the family and child?
- What resources are available?
- What are the child's strengths and needs?
- What will be accomplished with the use of technology? How will developmental and disability/health changes influence technology selection?
- How much training is required for the technology and what are the maintenance requirements?
- How portable is the product and what is its overall utility?
- Are there major safety and maintenance considerations?
- How well does the product fit with the child, the environmental context, and the occupations to be performed?

Additional adaptations may be made to the ADL task and the environment (i.e., accessible areas within the home, school, and community).

Education

Personal self-care expectations may vary from setting to setting. For instance, for a teenager struggling with major depression and attention deficit disorder, the motivation to complete self-grooming may be a challenge. Expectations regarding appearance at home may be very different than at a work setting. Collaboration, communication, and education between the therapist, client, family, and other significant persons are important in setting up clear expectations, providing the necessary environmental supports, and in establishing self-care routines.

Rest and Sleep

The focus of balance and rhythm within the SCOPE-IT model acknowledges the importance of sleep and rest as a vital part of daily occupational patterns. In addition to personal biological rhythms, sleep–rest patterns and habits are heavily influenced by the familial and sociocultural contexts. Sleep disturbances are widespread in children resulting in impact on mood, cognition, and significant performance impairments (Owens, 2004). Physical and emotional distress often negatively affects sleep and rest and therefore attempts are made to design occupational patterns and provide environmental contexts conducive to sleep and rest.

Improving Performance

Strategies used to improve sleep and rest include the establishment of routines around bedtime (i.e., brushing teeth, washing face, and reading a book), the use of calming techniques paired with sleep and rest (massage and warm blankets), and the inclusion of calming quiet occupations into the daily schedule. Therapists may pair additional frames of references such as Neuro-Developmental Treatment, Cognitive Behavioral Strategies, and Sensory Integration in order to affect alert/arousal levels; yet within the frame of reference to enhance childhood occupations, focus is on the daily patterns and rhythms. An analysis of temporal factors related to time use may be completed and suggestions may be made regarding the types of activities performed throughout the day. The therapist, client, and family may have limited control over external factors such as school start times, work requirements, and school/sport-related functions, yet the timing of daily activities is important, particularly as related to the bedtime. For instance, Andy, a 9-year-old child with autism was having considerable difficulty getting to bed by 9 p.m. and was unable to get up at 7 a.m. to prepare for school. A review of his daily occupational pattern revealed that every night at around 7:30 p.m. he liked to go downstairs to listen to his older brother practice on the electric guitar. Typically, Andy would run around, dance, and ask to try out the guitar. A slight revision to his daily schedule, and work with the family and Andy's brother to alter practice times, significantly helped him reduce his arousal level and get to bed closer to the 9 p.m. goal.

Adapting Occupations, Environments, and Providing Assistive Technology

In addition to the establishment of habits and rituals around rest and sleep, environments can be designed to promote restfulness. The environmental surrounding, bedding, and sleeping arrangement may all affect rest and sleep patterns (Owens, 2004). According to the National Sleep Foundation (2007), children who watch more TV traditionally have less rest, and recommendations for sleep environments include removing the television and computer from the child's room. Additional environmental modifications to promote rest times during the day may include the addition of a quiet area at school or home, equipped with lower lighting, comfortable chairs, and quiet activities.

Education

Perhaps one of the most important roles the therapist plays in the area of sleep and rest is that of an educator. Parents and families should be educated about the importance of routine and establishment of balanced occupational patterns; teachers and educational systems should be educated regarding the importance of rhythm within the daily schedule. Children often need breaks after several hours of sitting, and the daily academic and home schedule should include both high-arousal and low-arousal activities.

Occupational Patterns

A synthesis of the intervention approach within the occupation-based frame of reference is the maximization of the child–environment–occupation fit to promote healthy habits, routines, and patterns. Collaboration occurs with the family, educators, and those within the child's daily environment. A focal point within the SCOPE-IT model relates to the amount of time and daily rhythm the child spends in work, play, rest, and ADL. Personal choice and motivation affect the amount and quality of time spent in each area of occupational performance and therefore efforts are made to provide empowering environments, create motivating occupational opportunities, and work with the child to develop occupational patterns that create health and well-being. The use of meaningful occupation and the promotion of mastery enhance occupational development and provide a client-centered occupation-based approach in working toward the desired therapeutic outcomes.

Case Example of Shonda

Shonda is a 14-year-old female with a history of fetal alcohol syndrome (FAS), depression, and cognitive deficits secondary to the FAS and head trauma suffered under abuse from her biological father. Shonda was referred to an outpatient clinic that specializes in working with individuals and families affected by FAS. Shonda was placed in foster care at the age of 3 and was adopted at 9 years. She has had marginal success with her adoptive family and frequently gets into physical and verbal altercations with her 11-year-old stepsister and 7-year-old stepbrother. She is fairly athletic and active in a local Special Olympic program and has shown some promise as a swimmer and runner. Recently Shonda has had ongoing difficulties at school because of repeated suspensions for aggressive behaviors. In addition, her teachers report concern that she is not "applying" herself in the classroom. She is mainstreamed in the classroom but does have tutorial support and attends a special afternoon program for high-risk kids. Difficulties at home include an increase in altercations with her siblings, unwillingness to partake in household chores, and spending excessive time watching TV and playing video games. Shonda was referred to the occupational therapy for an evaluation and consideration for 1:1 intervention as well as a possible referral to the adolescent group (Figure 9.13). The group is designed to provide an interactive, fun atmosphere to teach social skills, assertiveness, and healthy ways of coping.

Using the SCOPE-IT model within this frame of reference to enhance childhood occupations, the therapist conducts an evaluation. This includes a home visit, a family interview, a chart review, and an observation of Shonda engaging in a

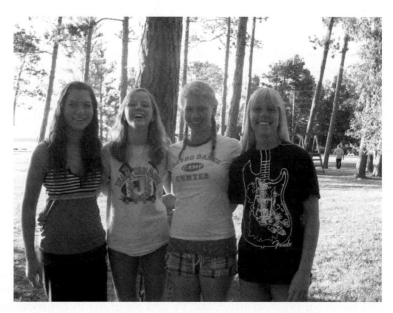

FIGURE 9.13 Children are occupational and social beings. Peer interaction is a key element of development during the adolescent years.

board game with her siblings. It would also include administration of the *Canadian Occupational Performance Measure* (Law et al., 1998), the *Piers Harris Self Concept Scale 2* (Piers & Herzberg, 2002), the *Adolescent Leisure Interest Profile* (Henry, 2000), the *Vineland Adaptive Behavior Scales II* (Sparrow, Cichetti, & Balla, 2005).

Information from the family and individual interviews revealed that Shonda is fairly active at home, school, and in Special Olympics. She likes activity but, with the exception of her participation in sports, she seems to have difficulty focusing on occupations for more than a few minutes at a time. She performs basic ADLs with minimal assistance but requires moderate assistance with IADLs including money management, cooking, and community mobility. Her father has indicated concern regarding her safety and judgment as well as concerns that at times she is "running with the wrong crowd." Sleep and rest patterns are erratic given Shonda's preference for late night television. In addition, she has developed a fixation with Internet games and spends hours at a time playing online games.

Results of the Vineland suggested that Shonda's communication, daily living skills, and socialization were low as compared with her peers, with motor skills scoring as adequate. Paired with the other assessment tools and observations, the results of the Vineland revealed that Shonda appears to have low self-esteem and places high expectations upon herself as related to her peers and siblings. Sensory issues (based on former occupational therapy reports) as well as Shonda's continued attempts to be accepted by her peers and family exacerbate aggressive behaviors. In addition, although her adoptive parents have positive intentions, they often appear to put pressure on Shonda related to school and home performance and do not seem to fully understand the implications of cognitive, sensory, and developmental challenges secondary to her FAS and history of head trauma. The home observation further revealed that although Shonda appears to genuinely like her siblings, power struggles relate to the vying for attention from her parents, and the desire to outperform her siblings in games and competitive activities.

On the basis of the evaluation, Shonda has cognitive, sensory, and psychological challenges that interfere with her daily occupational performance. Her developmental age of adolescence is marked by high personal expectations and desires to be accepted by peers. Given her developmental disability, her self-esteem suffers when comparing herself with classmates. Strengths include her willingness to partake in several daily activities, her high level of attendance to the after school program and Special Olympics, and her performance in motor activities. Difficulties in occupational performance include poor sleep and wake habits, refusal to complete assigned homework, and performance and safety issues with IADLs.

Shonda has a supportive family but feels personal and familial pressure to perform at a level higher than her current capabilities. The home environment, a three-bedroom ranch with a large back yard and a basketball hoop, seems to fit her needs for physical space, but TV and computer in her room cause distraction and encourage overuse. In addition, she currently shares a room with her 11-year-old sister and conflicts arise regarding use of the TV and computer, and disagreement regarding bedtime. At school, Shonda feels continued peer pressure and therefore the plans include a school environment assessment as well as an interview with her teachers.

Shonda's choice of activities includes both social (after school program and Special Olympics) and solo occupations (television and computer). While she does participate in work, rest, play, and ADL, she favors activities that she feels competent in (i.e., motor activities and computer games) often spending excess time on the computer and watching TV at the expense of participation in expected work behaviors (chores and schoolwork). Her level of engagement and persistence with homework and higher level ADLs is low, and when frustrated her behaviors escalate often resulting in verbal or physical aggression.

On the basis of the evaluation results, Shonda, the therapist, and the family developed goals related to (1) improved socialization marked by an increase in positive social participation and decrease in aggressive behaviors, (2) development of positive coping skills, (3) increasing independence in higher level IADLs including safety and basic money management, and (4) the development of a healthy daily schedule promoting balance in ADL, rest, work, and play. Additional school-based goals would be developed along with the teacher following further evaluation. To build on her interests and strengths, continued involvement with Special Olympics was recommended, and Shonda agreed to participate in the adolescent social skills group. Strategies used to maximize the child–environment–occupation fit included suggestions for environmental modifications including a separate living space within the home for Shonda, and the removal of the television and computer from her room. Additional frames of references including the use of behavioral reinforcements for decrease in negative behaviors paired with a sensory integrative frame of reference to deal with underlying sensory problems were also implemented. Efforts were made to adapt familial expectations regarding performance, and a strategy involving a daily schedule proved helpful. Predictable daily routines were implemented and Shonda was encouraged to participate in writing out her daily schedule. With time, an educational approach was used to teach Shonda concepts of healthy daily choices in time use and balance of work, play, leisure, ADL, and rest. A behavioral reinforcement system paired with the educational approach worked well to teach her the concepts stressed in the SCOPE-IT model.

Shonda also met individually with the therapist to work on personal safety and simple budgeting. Building on Shonda's interests, she was encouraged to help plan and implement the Special Olympics bake sale and under supervision took care of the cash drawer. Although some social strains continued at both home and school, with time the predictable schedule, involvement in the adolescent group, personal skill training, and environmental adaptations proved helpful. Shonda developed basic coping strategies, decreased her negative behaviors, and was able to spend more time in rest and work occupations providing a healthier overall balance to her daily life. As she felt more confident, she made plans to join a prework group in order to explore future areas of work interest.

CONCLUSION

The use of a model such as SCOPE-IT (Poulsen & Ziviani, 2004a,b; Poulsen & Ziviani, 2006) within this frame of reference to enhance childhood occupations provides a holistic view of promoting adaptive occupational performance through the maximization of the child–environment–occupation fit. Therapists utilize occupation as both a means and ends to achieve desired outcomes. Child-level variables interact with environmental contexts to influence effort, choice, and the quality of time spent in work, play, ADL, and rest. Evaluation and intervention within the frame of reference to enhance childhood occupations involves synthesis of multiple factors influencing the child's occupational engagement.

Function–dysfunction continua are considered along with an understanding of the dynamic influence of child–environment–occupation variables within the scope of time. Through the use of strategies to enhance performance, adapt environments and occupations, and educate at the micro (family, teachers, and caregivers) and macro (systems) levels, therapists work with the child toward the desired outcomes of maximizing adaptive responses, promoting health, well-being, and improving quality of life.

ACKNOWLEDGMENTS

Special thanks to Anne Poulsen, PhD, BOccThy (HONS), for her research in pediatric practice leading to the development of SCOPE-IT model. Ms. Poulsen has been generous in the sharing of her research publications that have contributed greatly to the development of this chapter. Heartfelt thanks to my colleague and friend Linda Buxell, MAOT, OTR/L, for providing her insight, expertise, and feedback regarding the development of the chapter. I am deeply grateful.

REFERENCES

American Occupational Therapy Association. (2002). Occupational therapy practice framework: Domain and process. *American Journal of Occupational Therapy, 56*, 609–639.

American Occupational Therapy Association. (2007). *History of AOTA accreditation*. Retrieved April 27, 2007 from the world wide web: http://www.aota.org/nonmembers/area13/links/LINK15.asp.

Assor, A., Kaplan, H., & Roth, G. (2002). Autonomy-enhancing and suppressing teacher behaviours predicting students' engagement in schoolwork. *British Journal of Educational Psychology, 72*, 261–278.

Assor, A., Roth, G., & Deci, E. L. (2004). The emotional costs of parent's conditional regard: A self-determination theory analysis. *Journal of Personality, 72*, 47–88.

Batavia, A. I. (1992). Assessing the function of functional assessments: a consumer perspective. *Disability and Rehabilitation, 14*, 156–160.

Battari, C., Dutil, E., Dassa, C., & Rainville, C. (2006). Choosing the most appropriate environment to evaluate independence in everyday activities: Home or clinic? *Australian Occupational Therapy Journal, 53*, 98–106.

Berger, K. (2004). *The Developing Person Through the Life Span* (6th ed.). New York: Worth Publishers.

Black, M. M. (1976). Adolescent role assessment. *American Journal of Occupational Therapy, 30*, 73–79.

Brown, D. (2002). The role of work and cultural values in occupational choice, satisfaction, and success. *The Journal of Counseling and Development, 80*, 48–56.

Bundy, A. (1997). Play and playfulness: what to look for. In L. D. Parham, & L. S. Fazio (Eds). *Play in Occupational Therapy for Children* (pp. 52–66). St. Louis, MO: Mosby.

Burke, J. P. (1993). Play: the life role of the infant and young child. In J. Case-Smith (Ed). *Pediatric occupational therapy and early intervention* (pp. 198–224). Boston, MA: Andover Medical Publications.

Caldwell, B., & Bradley, R. H. (1984). *Home Observation for Measure of the Environment*, revised ed. Little Rock, AR: University of Arkansas.

Case-Smith, J., Richardson, P., & Schultz-Krohn, W. (2005). An overview of occupational therapy for children. In J. Case-Smith (Ed). *Occupational Therapy for Children* (5th ed., pp. 2–31). St. Louis, MO: Elsevier Science.

Christiansen, C., & Baum, C. (1991). Occupational therapy: intervention for life performance. In C. Christiansen, & C. Baum (Eds). *Occupational Therapy: Overcoming Human Performance Deficits* (pp. 4–43). Thorofare, NJ: Slack Inc.

Christiansen, C., & Baum, C. (1997). Person-environment occupational performance: a conceptual model for practice. In C. Christiansen, & C. Baum (Eds). *Occupational Therapy: Enabling Function and Well Being* (2nd ed., pp. 47–70). Thorofare, NJ: Slack Inc.

Christiansen, C., & Townsend, E. (2004). An introduction to occupation. In C. Christiansen, & E. Townsend (Eds). *Introduction to Occupation: The Art and Science of Living*. Upper Saddle River, NJ: Prentice-Hall.

Clark, F., Parham, D., Carlson, M. E., Frank, G., Jackson, J., Pierce, D., Wolre, R. J., & Zemke, R. (1991). Occupational science: academic innovation in the service of occupational therapy's future. *American Journal of Occupational Therapy, 45*, 300–310.

Coster, W. J., Deeney, T. A., Haltiwanger, J. T., & Haley, S. M. (1998). *School Function Assessment (SFA). Standardized version*. Boston, MA: Boston University.

Cottrell, R. P. (2005). Occupational therapy's heritage: historical and philosophical foundations for best practice. In R. Fleming Cottrell (Ed). *Perspectives for Occupation-Based Practice: Foundation and Future of Occupational Therapy* (pp. 1–4). Bethesda, MD: AOTA Press.

Crepeau, E. B. (2003). Analyzing occupation and activity: a way of thinking about occupational Performance. In E. B. Crepeau, E. S., Cohn, & B. A. Schell (Eds). *Willard & Spackman's Occupational Therapy* (10th ed., pp. 189–198). Philadelphia, PA: Lippincott Williams & Wilkins.

Davis, J. A., & Polatajko, H. J. (2004). Occupational development. In C. Christiansen, & E. Townsend (Eds). *Introduction to Occupation: The Art and Science of Living* (pp. 91–119). Upper Saddle River, NJ: Pearson Education.

Deci, E. L., & Ryan, R. M. (2000). The 'what' and 'why' of goal pursuits: Human needs and the self determination of behavior. *Psychological Inquiry, 11*, 226–228.

De las Heras, C. G., Geist, R., Kielhofner, G., & Li, Y. (2002). *The Volitional Questionnaire (VQ) (Version 4.0)*. Chicago, IL: Model of Human Occupation Clearinghouse, Department of Occupational Therapy, College of Applied Health Sciences, University of Illinois at Chicago.

Diener, E. (1994). Assessing subjective well-being: Progress and opportunities. *Social Indicators Research, 31*, 103–157.

Diener, E., Suh, E. M., Lucas, R. E., & Smith, H. L. (1999). Subjective well-being: Three decades of progress. *Psychological Bulletin, 125*, 276–302.

Dolfman, M. (1973). The concept of health: An historic and analytic examination. *Journal of School Health, 43*, 491–497.

Dunn, L. (2004). Validation of the CHORES: A measure of school-aged children's participation in household tasks. *Scandinavian Journal of Occupational Therapy, 11*, 179–190.

Dunn, W., Brown, C., & McGuigan, A. (1994). The ecology of human performance: a framework for considering the effect of context. *American Journal of Occupational Therapy, 48*, 595–607.

Dunn, W., Brown, C., & Youngstrom, M. J. (2003). Ecological model of occupation. In P. Kramer, J. Hinojosa, & C. Royeen (Eds). *Perspectives in Human Occupation* (pp. 222–263). Philadelphia, PA: Lippincott Williams & Wilkins.

Federico, J., & Kielhofner, G. (2002). *The Child Occupational Self Assessment (COSA) (Version 1.0)*. Chicago, IL: Model of Human Occupation Clearinghouse, Department of Occupational Therapy, College of Applied Health Science, University of Illinois at Chicago.

Fisher, A. G. (2003). *Assessment of Motor and Process Skills. Development, Standardization and Administration Manual* (5th ed.). Fort Collins, Colorado: Three Star Press.

Fisher, A. G., & Bryze, K. (2005). *School AMPS: School Version of the Assessment of Motor and Process Skills*. Fort Collins, CO: Three Star Press.

Galinsky, E. (1999). Today's kids, tomorrow's employees: What children are learning about work. *HR Magazine, 44*, 75–84.

Geist, R., Kielhofner, G., Basu, S., & Kafkes, A. (2002). *The Pediatric Volitional Questionnaire (PVQ) (Version 2.0)*. Chicago, IL: Model of Human Occupation Clearinghouse, Department of Occupational Therapy, College of Applied Health Sciences, University of Illinois at Chicago.

Gray, J. M. (1998). Putting occupation into practice: Occupation as ends, occupation as means. *American Journal of Occupational Therapy, 52*, 354–364.

Gresham, F. M., & Elliot, S. N. (1990). *Social Skills Rating System*. Circle Pines, MN: American Guidance Services.

(1999). *Guide for the Uniform Data Set for Medical Rehabilitation (FIM™ instrument), Version 5*. Buffalo, NY: University at Buffalo.

Haley, S. M., Coster, W. J., Ludlow, L. H., Haltiwanger, J. T., & Andrellos, P. J. (1992). Pediatric Evaluation of Disability Inventory (PEDI). *Development Standardization and Administration Manual*. Boston, MA: Boston University.

Harms, T., Cryer, D., & Clifford, R. M. (2003). *Infant/Toddler Environment Rating Scale-Revised*. New York: Teachers College Press.

Hamilton, B. B., & Granger, C. V. (2000). *Functional Independence Measure for Children (WeeFIM II)*. Buffalo, NY: Research Foundation of the State University of New York.

Henry, A. D. (2000). *The Pediatric Interest Profiles: Surveys of Play for Children and Adolescents*. San Antonio, TX: Therapy Skill Builders.

Humphry, R. (2002). Young children's occupations: Explicating the dynamics of developmental processes. *American Journal of Occupational Therapy, 56*, 171–179.

Humphry, R., & Wakeford, L. (2006). An occupation-centered discussion of development and implications for practice. *American Journal of Occupational Therapy, 60*, 258–267.

Jonas, S. (2005). The wellness process for healthy living: A mental tool for facilitating progress through the stages of change. *American Medical Athletic Association Journal, 18*, 5–7.

Kielhofner, G. (1983a). *Health Through Occupation*. Philadelphia, PA: FA Davis Co.

Kielhofner, G. (1983b). Components and determinants of human occupation. In G. Kielhofner (Ed). *Health Through Occupation* (pp. 93–124). Philadelphia, PA: FA Davis Co.

Kielhofner, G. (Ed). (1985). *A Model of Human Occupation: Theory and Application*. Baltimore, MD: Williams & Wilkins.

Kielhofner G. (Ed). (1995). *A Model of Human Occupation: Theory and Application* (2nd ed.). Baltimore, MD: Williams & Wilkins.

Kielhofner, G. (1997). *Conceptual Foundations of Occupational Therapy* (2nd ed.). Philadelphia, PA: FA Davis Co.

Kielhofner, G. (Ed). (2002a). Introduction to the model of human occupation. *Model of Human Occupation* (3rd ed., 1–9). Baltimore, MD: Lippincott Williams & Wilkins.

Kielhofner, G. (Ed). (2002b). Dimensions of doing. *Model of Human Occupation* (3rd ed., 114–123). Baltimore, MD: Lippincott Williams & Wilkins.

Kielhofner, G. (Ed). (2002c). Volition. *Model of Human Occupation* (3rd ed., 44–62). Baltimore, MD: Lippincott Williams & Wilkins.

Kim-Prieto, C., Diener, E., Tamir, M., Scollon, C., & Diener, M. (2005). Integrating the diverse definitions of happiness: A time-sequential framework of subjective well-being. *Journal of Happiness Studies, 6*, 261–300.

Knox, S. (1997). Development and current use of the Knox Preschool Play Scale. In L. D. Parham, & L. S. Fazio (Eds). *Play in Occupational Therapy for Children* (pp. 35–51). St. Louis, MO: Mosby.

Knox, S. (2005). Play. In J. Case-Smith (Ed). *Occupational Therapy for Children* (5th ed., pp. 571–586). St. Louis, MO: Elsevier.

Larson, L. A. (2004). Children's work: the less-considered childhood occupation. *American Journal of Occupational Therapy, 58*, 369–379.

Law, M., Baptiste, S., Carswell, A., McColl, M. A., Polotajiko, H., & Pollack, N. (1998). *Canadian Occupational Performance Measure* (3rd ed.). Toronto, ON: Canadian Association of Occupational Therapists.

Law, M., Baum, C., & Dunn, W. (2005). *Measuring Occupational Performance: Supporting Best Practice in Occupational Therapy* (2nd ed.). Thorofare, NJ: Slack Inc.

Lawlor, M. C. (2003). The significance of being occupied: The social construction of childhood occupations. *American Journal of Occupational Therapy, 57*, 424–434.

Letts, L., Law, M., Rigby, P., Cooper, B., Steward, D., & Strong, S. (1994). Person-Environment assessments in occupational therapy. *American Journal of Occupational Therapy, 48*, 608–618.

Matthews, B. A., Baker, F., Hanne, D. M., Denniston, M., & Smith, T. G. (2002). Health status and life satisfaction among breast cancer survivor peer support volunteers. *Psycho-Oncology, 11*, 199–211.

Meyer, A. (1922-1977). The philosophy of occupation therapy. *American Journal of Occupational Therapy, 31*, 639–642, Original work published 1922.

Moos, R., & Trickett, E. J. (2002). *Classroom Environment Scale* (3rd ed.). Menlo Park, CA: Mindgarden.

Mulkana, S., & Hailey, B. J. (2001). The role of optimism in health-enhancing behavior. *American Journal of Health Behavior, 25*, 388–395.

National Sleep Foundation (2007). *Waking America to the importance of sleep.* Retrieved June 9, 2007 from the world wide web: http://www.sleepfoundation.org/site/c.huIXKjM0IxF/b.2419303/k.27B0/The_Sleep_Of_Americas_Children.htm.

National Wellness Institute. (2007). *Defining wellness.* Retrieved May 25, 2007 from the world wide web: http://www.nationalwellness.org/index.php?id=390&id_tier=81.

Nelson, D. (1988). Occupation: form and performance. *American Journal of Occupational Therapy, 42*, 633–641.

Okimoto, A. M., Bundy, A., & Hanzlik, J. (2000). Playfulness in children with and without disability: Measurement and intervention. *American Journal of Occupational Therapy, 54*, 73–82.

Owens, J. A. (2004). Sleep in children: Cross cultural perspectives. *Sleep and Biological Rhythms, 2*, 165–173.

Parham, L. D., & Fazio, L. S. (1997). *Play in Occupational Therapy with Children.* St Louis, MO: Mosby.

Parham, L. D., & Primeau, L. (1997). Play and occupational therapy. In L. D. Parham, & L. Fazio (Eds). *Play in Occupational Therapy with Children* (pp. 2–21). St. Louis, MO: Mosby.

Pierce, D. (1997). The power of object play for infants and toddlers at risk for developmental delays. In L. D. Parham, & L. S. Fazio (Eds). *Play in Occupational Therapy for Children* (pp. 86–111). St. Louis, MO: Mosby.

Pierce, D. (2003). *Occupation by Design: Building Therapeutic Power.* Philadelphia, PA: FA Davis Co.

Piers, E. V., & Herzberg, D. S. (2002). *Piers-Harris 2: Piers-Harris children's Self-Concept Scale* (2nd ed.). Los Angeles, CA: Western Psychological Services.

Poulsen, A. A., Rodger, S., & Ziviani, J. M. (2006). Understanding children's motivation from a self-determination theoretical perspective: Implications for practice. *Australian Occupational Therapy Journal, 53*, 78–86.

Poulsen, A. A., & Ziviani, J. M. (2004a). Health enhancing physical activity: Factors influencing engagement patterns in children. *Australian Occupational Therapy Journal, 51*, 69–79.

Poulsen, A. A., & Ziviani, J. M. (2004b). Can I play too? Physical activity engagement of children with developmental coordination disorders. *Canadian Journal of Occupational Therapy, 71*, 100–107.

Poulsen, A. A., & Ziviani, J. M. (2006). Participation beyond the school grounds. In S. Rodger, & J. Ziviani (Eds). *Occupational Therapy with Children: Understanding Children's Occupations and Enabling Participation* (pp. 280–298). Oxford: Blackwell Science.

Primeau, L. A. (1998). Orchestration of work and play within families. *American Journal of Occupational Therapy, 52*, 188–195.

Primeau, L. A., Clark, F., & Pierce, D. (1989). Occupational science alone has looked upon occupation: Future applications of occupational science to the health care needs of parents and children. *Occupational therapy in health care, 6*, 10–32.

Primeau, L. A., & Ferguson, J. M. (1999). Occupational frame of reference. In P. Kramer, & J. Hinjosa (Eds). *Frames of Reference for Pediatric Occupational Therapy*, (pp. 496–516). Philadelphia, PA: Lippincott Williams & Wilkins.

Reilly, M. (1962). Occupational therapy can be one of the great ideas of 20th century medicine. *American Journal of Occupational Therapy, 16*, 1–9.

Reilly, M. A. (1966). A psychiatric occupational therapy program as a teaching model. *American Journal of Occupational Therapy, 20*, 61–67.

Rodger, S., & Ziviani, J. (1999). Play-based occupational therapy. *International Journal of Disability, Development and Education, 46*, 337–365.

Ryan, R. M., & Deci, E. L. (2000a). Self-determination theory and the facilitation of intrinsic motivation, social development, and well being. *American Psychologist, 55*, 68–78.

Ryan, R. M., & Deci, E. L. (2000b). Intrinsic and extrinsic motivations: Classic definitions and new directions. *Contemporary Educational Psychology, 25*, 54–67.

Samuelsson, I. P., & Johansson, E. (2006). Play and learning: inseparable dimensions in preschool practice. *Early Child Development and Care, 176*, 47–65.

Shepherd, J. (2005). Activities of daily living and adaptations for independent living. In J. Case-Smith (Ed). *Occupational Therapy for Children* (5th ed., pp. 521–570). St. Louis, MO: Elsevier Science.

Sparrow, S., Cichetti, D., & Balla, D. (2005). *Vineland Adaptive Behavior Scales*. Circle Pines, MN: American Guidance Services.

Stagnitti, K. (2004). Understanding play: the implications for play assessment. *Australian Journal of Occupational Therapy, 51*, 3–12.

Stebbins, R. A. (1997). Casual leisure: a conceptual statement. *Leisure Studies, 16*, 17–25.

Stebbins, R. A. (2005). Research reflections: choice and experiential definitions of leisure. *Leisure Studies, 27*, 349–352.

Thunstrom, M. (1999). Severe sleep problems among infants in a normal population in Sweden: Prevalence, severity, and correlates. *Acta Paedatrica, 88*, 1356–1363.

Townsend, S. C., Carey, P. D., Hollins, N. L., Helfrich, C., Blondis, M., Hoffman, A., Collins, L., Knudson, J., & Blackwell, A. (2001). *The Occupational Therapy Psychosocial Assessment of Learning (OT PAL), (Version 1.0)*. Chicago, IL: Model of Human Occupation Clearinghouse, Department of Occupational Therapy. University of Illinois, Chicago.

Trombly, C. A. (1995). 1995 Eleanor Clarke Slagle lecture: Occupation: Purposefulness and meaningfulness as therapeutic mechanisms. *American Journal of Occupational Therapy, 49*, 960–972.

Wilcock, A. A. (1998). *An Occupational Perspective of Health*. Thorofare, NJ: Slack Inc.

Williams, G. C., Lynch, M., McGregor, H. A., Ryan, R. M., Sharp, D., & Deci, E. L. (2006). Validation of the "important other" climate questionnaire: Assessing autonomy support for health related change. *Families, Systems and Health: The Journal of Collaborative Family Health Care, 24*, 179–194.

Wiseman, J. O., Davis, J. A., & Polatajko, H. J. (2005). *Journal of Occupational Science, 12*, 26–44.

World Health Organization. (1946). Preamble to the constitution of the World Health Organization. Adopted by the International Health Conference (19–22), New York.

Yerxa, E. J. (1967). Authentic occupational therapy. *American Journal of Occupational Therapy, 21*, 1–9.

CHAPTER 10

A Frame of Reference to Enhance Social Participation

LAURETTE JOAN OLSON

This frame of reference is designed to be useful to occupational therapists working in a variety of school-based and community settings to support the social participation of children who have a range of physical or psychiatric disabilities and have typical to mildly deficient cognitive functioning. Social participation is "organized patterns of behavior that are characteristic and expected of an individual in a given position with a social system" (AOTA, 2002, p. 621). Children's social participation within Western society requires them to have organized patterns of behavior to participate in their families, in academic settings, and communities. Studies show that children with social and emotional deficits are at high risk for problematic family relationships, academic failure, as well as difficulties in their occupational functioning as adolescents and adults (Dishion & Stormshak, 2007; Maag, 2006).

Public policy related to education has historically focused on children's mastery of academic skills and content. Researchers and educators now consider social and emotional development as important as academic development in children's education (Coolahan et al., 2000; Fantuzzo & McWayne, 2002; Raver, 2002; Zins, Weissberg, & Wang, 2004).

Occupational therapists can play a key role in supporting children's social participation. The expertise of occupational therapists is sought to help children with a range of disabilities increase participation and improve their performance in family, academic, and community-based occupations. It is important that occupational therapists assess and intervene with the social aspects of children's occupational participation as fully as they address the sensory and motor aspects of occupational performance. Children engage with others in all types of settings. If a particular child cannot relate to other children or adults, the therapist considers whether it is the social context, the demands of the activity or occupation, or whether the child has skill deficits that inhibit social participation in the activity or occupation.

This frame of reference is based on acquisitional and behavioral theories that conceptualize how children learn to participate effectively in social situations and how to promote development of the skills necessary for social participation. The primary concern of the frame of reference is with children who are not effectively participating in the social contexts of their daily lives. This frame of reference also describes how the tasks or the contexts for social participation may need to be adjusted in the interest of increasing children's opportunities for social participation.

THEORETICAL BASE

The theoretical base begins with the importance of children's social development and how early relationships influence their skill and habit formation for social participation. Children's skills, habits, and routines are then discussed relative to how they affect peer interaction and friendship in early and middle childhood.

Interaction between Caregivers and Children

Occupational therapists, like other professionals, have an optimal impact on children when they work with the people who have the most influential relationships with children. Generally, parents and caregivers have these relationships with the children. Caregivers determine the objects and people that children can access. This is done by promoting or limiting activity participation. They also shape children's social ecology by promoting habits and routines. The presence of habits and routines in the family's daily living promotes competence in caregivers and children alike.

Children's relationships with primary caregivers in infancy and early childhood provide the foundation for their social development. Through these relationships, children learn how to attract other people for physical survival as well as for comfort and companionship. Typically, mothers and infants are in tune to one another's emotional signals. They respond to each other in ways that reflect the emotional message of the other, amplify, or modify the emotion and behavior exhibited by the other. When an infant coos at his or her mother, a mother typically responds back in kind. When a mother focuses on feeding an infant, but the infant cries, a mother typically shifts to working to lessen the infant's discomfort before continuing the feeding activity. The emotional exchange and regulation between caregiver and child maintain interaction and optimally, a harmonious, mutually growth-promoting relationship (Cole, Martin, & Dennis, 2004).

Children give meaning to their own emotional experiences and learn strategies for regulating their emotional states on the basis of responses from people and environmental conditions and resources. If a mother introduces calming input to reorganize a child overwhelmed by physiological needs or states, a child first learns that distress can be relieved by his or her mother's behavior. Over time, the children learn to decrease their own distress with a mother's absence by seeking out the blanket, stuffed animal, or a glass of hot milk that the mother may have previously provided.

Children also regulate their caregiver's behaviors by how receptive they are to their attempts to engage them in interactions. They approach or withdraw from the stimuli provided by their caregivers. Through this reciprocal interaction of emotional regulation, children gradually learn how to regulate their own emotions and how to regulate the emotions of others in social interaction (Cole, Martin, & Dennis, 2004; Denham, 1993,

Feldman, Greenbaum, & Yirmiya, 1999). Greenspan & Wieder (2006) have articulated stages of emotional development that are helpful in analyzing children's first interactions and relationship with their parents or other first caregivers. The stages are attention, mutual engagement, intentional and purposeful communication, elaborating on ideas, and emotional thinking.

Temperament is a constitutionally based individual style of emotional, motor and attentional reactivity, and self-regulation (Rothbart et al. 2001). Specific behavior patterns of temperament that are evident even in the first days of life are activity level, regularity of biological functions, approach/withdrawal tendencies for new situations, adaptability to change, sensory thresholds, quality of moods, intensity of mood expression, distractibility, and persistence and attention span (Chess & Thomas, 1984). Some infants are easy to please and adapt readily to their environments. They have regular eating and sleeping patterns and are generally attentive and cheerful with their care providers. Other infants may be similar in their reaction when their environments are consistent, but may withdraw and become anxious when faced with change; their adaptation is slow. Still other infants are labeled difficult; they are difficult to please, have frequent and strong displays of negative moods, have irregular eating and sleeping patterns, and are less likely to respond to care providers in a warm, cuddly fashion. Some infants may demonstrate hyperactivity, hypersensitivity, distractibility, emotional lability, or insatiability. These temperamentally difficult infants may experience their physical and social world as very stressful; similarly, their caregivers may view interactions with them as equally stressful.

Recently, theorists (Rothbart & Bates, 1998) have further conceptualized temperament by subdividing its components into reactive and self-regulatory categories. The reactive category of temperament develops in the first year of life. This includes the factors of activity level, sociability, impulsivity, intensity of mood, as well as the negative effect factors of fear, anger/frustration, discomfort, and sadness. Rothbart et al. (2001) have labeled an additional category of temperament, effortful control. Effortful control is the capacity to inhibit an impulse in favor of exhibiting another response that may support social acceptance or may allow an individual to plan a response that will be able to meet individual and environmental needs and demands (Rothbart & Bates, 1998).

In typically developing children, effortful control allows children to voluntarily focus attention, take in different sources of information, and more actively learn and use coping strategies to control their own behavior and emotions (Figure 10.1). Effortful control, which typically develops during toddler and preschool years, includes inhibitory control, the ability to focus and shift attention, and sensitivity to and pleasure in low-intensity stimuli. When young children are playing and are asked to clean up by a caregiver, they must inhibit the impulse to keep on playing in favor of responding to the caregiver's request to clean up and to transition to another activity. The expectation of social approval and harmony is sufficiently rewarding to override the impulse to continue playing.

Skill at regulating emotions in challenging situations makes social problem solving possible. If children can manage their emotional reactions, they can access and evaluate several potential responses before acting. Good regulators may be more likely to consider

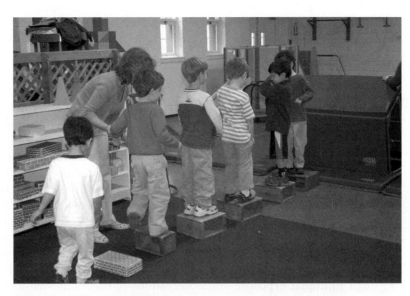

FIGURE 10.1 Group leader using blocks to support children in lining up in an organized way as they wait their turn to participate in an activity.

a situation from multiple cognitive and affective perspectives, thus facilitating their selection of a competent response.

Interaction between Caregivers and Children with Disabilities

Children with disabilities are more likely to exhibit difficulty with the reactive categories of temperament from birth as a result of their impaired ability to modulate their physiological state, cognitive, and/or physical deficits. They are more likely to have biological rhythms that are asynchronous with the natural rhythms of their caregivers, may be more active, less attentive, and may not persevere in tasks. They may also experience emotions more intensely. As a result, these children may be more physically disorganized and less able to focus on the directions provided by adults, resulting in interchanges that are more negative with adults.

Children with disabilities are likely to develop effortful control (self-regulation) more slowly than those without disabilities. In a social occupation such as participating in an academic group lesson, these children may be unable to maintain their focus on a group lesson. When they experience the impulse to move and are not able to regulate their physiological and emotional state, they are not likely to consider their options for managing their impulses or to weigh out the consequences of getting up and disrupting their teacher and classmates.

Effortful control has been related to children's development of social competence (Lemerise & Arsenio, 2000). Low levels of effortful control have been associated with higher levels of disruptive behavior (Rothbart et al., 2001). A combination of regulatory abilities and low emotionality predicted social competence concurrently and longitudinally. High emotionality with poor regulation predicts poorer social functioning while children with high emotionality and good regulatory were not at risk for behavior problems (Eisenberg et al., 2003).

Developing Habits and Routines

Children must develop habits and routines to facilitate their acceptance by others to successfully participate in society. Habits of social interaction include behaviors such as making eye contact to engage others before speaking and scanning the faces of others to gather nonverbal cues about openness and emotional states of others. Most children imitate the behaviors of caregivers and the behaviors quickly become habitual ways that children use to engage or maintain engagement with others. Social routines are complex sequences of behavior such as the series of behavior that people consistently use to engage others and maintain their everyday social exchanges. Adults and children develop typical ways of approaching and organizing familiar games or activities to allow for the harmonious participation of multiple participants. Children learn social routines through continual exposure and observations of others as well as through caregivers' direct teaching and reinforcement of their appropriate behaviors as children participate in routine family, school, or community activities.

Children who are successful in social interaction have developed culturally appropriate habits and routines to engage and maintain positive interaction with others. Routines define and direct behavior, as well as provide comfort and confidence in the stability of one's daily life. The organization that they provide supports children's abilities to process the cognitive and social information needed for developing skills for other social situations. They allow tasks to be completed with minimal stress and without excessive thinking or planning.

Socially competent children recognize the different social routines that are accepted in different environments that they encounter over the course of daily living. They are accepted by social partners in these varied environments without excess effort. Basic rhythms for social interaction are intuitively understood and coordinated so that cognitive energies can be focused on the individual or group tasks at hand. These children are more likely to be accepted by peers and caregivers in their families, schools, and communities.

Routines for toddlers allow families to provide children's care in the most efficient and least stressful manner. Routines present a context for social engagement between parents and children thereby providing critical opportunities for the building of a strong parent–child relationship (Kubicek, 2002). Children of mothers who provided structure to family life through their daily routines more likely have a stronger sense of temporal adaptation and may fare better academically than children who are in less structured family situations (Norton, 1993). Children from families who participate in Head Start and have predictable family routines have demonstrated greater preschool social competence including more interest and participation in school and more cooperative and compliant behavior than children whose families did not have consistent routines (Keltner, 1990).

Children can also develop inattention and avoidant or aversive responses through regular maladaptive interactions in family routines over the course of time (Dishion & Stormshak, 2007). Caregivers may respond angrily to children's attempts to participate in family routines or be impatient with children slowing down the speed of a routine. Routines may be too fast paced or not be adapted to children's level of skill development.

Some of the routines of a family develop into rituals that strengthen the family identity and its interest in activities. Rituals extend beyond routines; they convey meaning about the family's identity and the special connections among its members (Figure 10.2). Families with young children typically have bedtime rituals in addition to bedtime routines. There may be predictable requests for stories or a snack that are special events for caregivers and children. Leisure occupations are often integral parts of family rituals and often help its members develop, sustain, and strengthen relationships (Olson & O'Herron, 2004). Families may have particular holiday or seasonal rituals to which members look forward to year after year. They may be as simple as summer barbeques in a local park or playing board games outside on hot summer nights or as complex as planning family vacations to exotic locations. Rituals arouse strong positive emotions. They have a powerful influence on family members long after their occurrence; memories of one's family participation in them provide comfort and reassurance throughout life.

Developing Habits and Routines for Children with Disabilities

The development of habits and routines are particularly important for children with disabilities. Children with disabilities may not learn and adapt to the routines of caregivers as typically developing children do, purely by the nature of their atypical

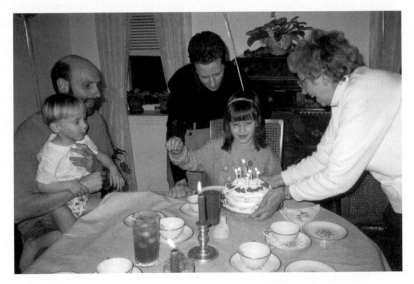

FIGURE 10.2 Families typically develop rituals around children's birthdays.

cognitive and/or physical development. Children with difficult temperaments may also experience the same problem. They may resist participation in family routines, which may discourage parents from setting limits and providing structure for children's productive participation in daily occupations resulting in inconsistent family routines.

When meaningful family rituals are disrupted or lose their affective connections for family members, young children may experience difficulty engaging in their everyday occupations or may exhibit decreased skills in the routine activities that the rituals supported (Fiese, 2002). Children may have difficulty preparing for bed and sleeping soundly when bedtime rituals are disrupted because of family or parental stressors. Additionally, the stress of a child's disabilities may interfere with a family's development of rituals or a family's regular participation in valued activities. A family's daily living routines may be disrupted by children's frequent illnesses or habits of avoidance including withdrawal or disruptive behavior.

Social Participation with Peers

The developmental significance of social acceptance in the preschool and school-age years is well documented (Guralnick, 2006; Odom et al., 2006; Raver, 2002). Children who experience social acceptance from peers are more likely to succeed as preschool and elementary school students and to have positive transitions through childhood and adolescence. Being socially accepted and having the opportunities to interact with peers are precursors to the development of friendships. Having friends has been associated with children's positive self-esteem, and reported experience of emotional security and social support. Friendship can support adaptive social processing skills including perspective taking and the development of social skills important for interacting in many social environments. Friendships can lessen the tendency for negative, uncomfortable, or distressing emotions that accompany stressful peer experiences and as a result support emotional regulation. Emotional regulation refers to the ability to take action by changing behavior to modify feeling states for the purpose of accomplishing interpersonal goals (Eisenberg & Spinrad, 2004; Guralnick, 2006). It involves effortful control and responding. Children may feel frustrated and feel the impulse to grab blocks from another child to build a fort, but they may ask the other child to build a fort with them and hence support sharing and cooperative play. Emotional regulation facilitates focusing attention and problem solving. Flexibility in emotional situations is critical; it requires both control over one's expressivity and sensitivity to the situation from multiple perspectives. Intensity with which children experience emotions influences their capacity to regulate emotion and subsequently the types of goals that they pursue in social encounters. If children can control the intensity of emotions triggered by their desires and impulses, they will more likely consider that their peers may also have similar desires and interests. Poor regulatory abilities may interfere with assessing a situation from different cognitive and affective perspectives and prevent a flexible approach to goal selection.

Friendships place new demands on young children's social skills as friendship is different in content, construction, and symmetry from adult–child relationships. They require children to suspend a self-centered viewpoint and embrace the importance of the viewpoints of their friends as equal to their own. Though friends help and support one another, children's friendships are typically based on mutual sharing of activities and interests. Friendships are different in content, construction, and symmetry from adult–child relationships. They require children to suspend a self-centered viewpoint and embrace the importance of the viewpoints of their friends as equal to their own. Children are concerned with participation in activities of mutual interest. Although friends help and support one another, children's friendships are typically based on mutual sharing of activities and interests. Conflicts may be resolved through negotiation or through one child asserting power over the other. To have a positive and enjoyable interaction with a friend, socioemotional coregulation is important (Figure 10.3). This requires that both parties are aware and responsive to the mood state and behavior of the other and then have a mutually shared meaning of the activity. Both children adjust and coordinate their mutual participation in activity. To do this, children need to be socially oriented and not physically, cognitively, or emotionally withdrawn. If both parties are successful at orienting to one another and adjusting their own rhythm and degree of participation in the activities to support the participation of the other, the dyad is likely to experience enjoyment in the activity.

Children with Disabilities: Social Participation with Peers

In a qualitative study of three children with disabilities, Richardson (2002) found that the children's interactions with typically developing peers centered on their needs

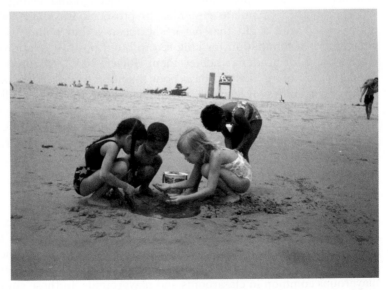

FIGURE 10.3 To develop friends, children coordinate their activity participation in the interest of group harmony.

and that these children had few opportunities to reciprocate help. As a precursor to helping these children develop friendships, Richardson suggested that it is important to adjust the balance of helping and being helped for children with disabilities in inclusive classrooms. Similarly, Meyers and Vipond (2005) reported that children with disabilities typically do not experience reciprocal play with their siblings as they take on subordinate roles in play with siblings. They recommended that occupational therapists work to increase role symmetry and social reciprocity in the sibling play of children with disabilities.

It is important to understand the concept of social competence to help children with disabilities to first gain acceptance from peers and then to develop friendships. One definition is that a socially competent child exhibits the social-cognitive and emotion regulation skills necessary to select and engage in social behaviors sensitively and appropriately in different situations (Fraser et al., 2005). Social-cognitive skills are the abilities to process social information; to understand the thought, feelings, and intentions of others; to consider alternative plans of action; to anticipate social consequences; and to evaluate outcomes (Rubin, Daniels-Beirness, & Bream, 1984).

Reading the emotional cues of others and sending emotional cues to others are important social-cognitive skills and precursors to emotional regulation. If children have difficulty reading and sending emotional cues, they are more likely to resort to rigid approaches to manage the situation. Children need to recognize and label the different emotions that they experience as well as observe in others. This provides a powerful socioemotional tool as children can talk through rather than act out feelings of anger, sadness, or frustration. Some children have difficulty identifying their own emotional states as well as the emotional states of others. They may misinterpret social situations and then respond inappropriately leading to rejection and feeling disliked.

The ability to regulate emotions in prosocial ways (i.e., when a child is very disappointed with a gift that he or she receives, but politely says thank you to the gift giver) is a foundation for children to build positive relationships with peers and teachers and for academic achievement (Raver, 2002). Children with poor emotional regulation are more likely to have poor attention to task. They also may not use peer group opportunities for learning within their classroom successfully. Such children may be challenging in a classroom situation. Consequently, they are likely to receive less positive feedback than their peers receive, influencing their interest in participation. Besides the immediate negative implications of their behavior, children with poor emotional regulation lose the benefits that positive, supportive relationships can provide to the development of their emotional and social skills.

Friendships grow out of opportunities to interact and play with peers. An important factor in the development of friendships in some children with disabilities is the opportunities to participate in various classroom activities with their typically developing peers (Buysse, Goldman, & Skinner, 2002). Contrary to what is typically the practice in classroom settings, children with disabilities may need time to exclusively play with one child to develop a friendship as opposed to more open-ended and shifting playgroups common in classrooms and playgrounds. In these situations, children must negotiate with other children moving in and out of interaction with them (Buysse, Goldman, & Skinner, 2003). It may be too difficult for some children with disabilities to focus attention on their preferred social partner while simultaneously attempting to coordinate their social behavior with other children joining their play.

Key behaviors influencing whether children with disabilities are successful in social relationships are their cognitive, social problem solving, and emotional regulation capacities (Odom et al., 2006). The friendship difficulties that exist for some children with disabilities were related to the absence of appropriate social strategies and poor conflict resolution (Guralnick, 2006). Other children with disabilities engage in less social interaction and exhibit less adaptive and more negative interaction styles with peers. These children tended to have disabilities that impacted their communication skills (Guralnick et al., 2006). Although an inclusive environment may provide the optimal role models for children with disabilities to learn communication and social skills for social participation, they are also likely to be rejected if they do not have skills for social activity participation (Odom et al., 2006).

Dynamic Theories that Support Social Participation

This frame of reference recognizes the power of emotion to motivate and engage persons with each other. That power drives activity choice in intervention. Therapists plan interventions consistent with behavioral, social learning, and cognitive theories to facilitate change in children's social participation. Behavioral (Skinner, 1974), social learning (Bandura, 1977, 1997; Dishion & Stormshak 2007; Guralnick et al., 2006; Prochaska, 1995), and cognitive theories (Vygotsky, 1978) are used in this frame of reference to promote change in children's social participation. Understanding and promoting emotional engagement is critical to motivate caregivers and children in the change process. Therapists need to be cognizant of how meaningful assessment and intervention activities are for children and caregivers. It is crucial that parents and/or caregivers and children generally enjoy their interactions with one another so that they continuously seek interactions with one another, and then seek out social interaction outside of the family (Figure 10.4).

People seek reinforcement and their behaviors are learned or changed as a result of that reinforcement (Skinner, 1974). Behavioral theory explains how a person's environment, including the social environment, results in learning. To increase the frequency with which children exhibit positive social behaviors that they have already learned, a therapist considers how behaviors are reinforced in their environments. When children need to learn new social behaviors, successive approximations of the correct behavior are positively reinforced until the child can exhibit the new behavior.

Social learning theory highlights the importance of observing the behavior of others and then modeling one's behavior upon what is observed to be successful or unsuccessful about the behaviors of others (Bandura, 1977). To promote positive change in children's capacities for social participation, the importance of positive social role models is emphasized in this frame of reference.

Prochaska (1995) identified useful stages that people seem to go through to change. In the first stage, precontemplation, persons may be aware of a problem, but see it as primarily a problem that is caused by others and does not recognize their own role

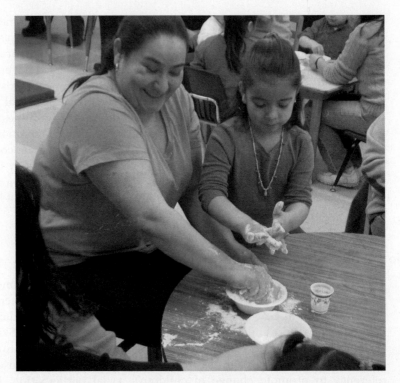

FIGURE 10.4 Mother and child making Play-Doh together in a preschool-based family activity program.

in causing or maintaining a problematic situation. In this case, caregivers may see a problem as solely children's behavior and as change needing to occur by changing the children only. Caregivers in the second stage, contemplation, may recognize that they may need to change to reduce a problematic situation or improve the quality of their lives, but have not committed to changing. They are ready to weigh out the positives and negatives of change strategies, but are not ready for action; the costs of change may still seem too high. In the preparation stage, caregivers may be open to discuss changing family or classroom routines or the structure of the environment, but may not be ready to implement those changes. As the benefits of committing to change outweigh the personal sacrifices of working toward change, people begin to prepare for change by exploring and implementing change strategies in a tentative way. In the action stage, persons are committed to a plan for change and work hard to carry out change strategies that seem most effective for them. Once change has been achieved, persons work to maintain the change. This often requires managing environmental situations or persons who may interfere with maintenance of change.

Dishion & Stormshak (2007) identify the steps for motivating change. The steps are to provide an engaging rationale for change, break content into teachable units, and shape success by tailoring steps leading to change to skill level, resources, culture, and ecology of family or institution.

Guralnick et al. (2006) recommended that to promote the friendships for children with disabilities in inclusive classrooms, professionals should pair children with compatible peers, select toys and activities of high interest, create circumstances to minimize conflict and to provide support and guidance in children's activities. A study by Odom et al. (2006) suggested that intervention strategies that systematically teach socially competent peers to engage children with disabilities in positive playful activities might have substantial effects on the social skills of children with disabilities. Brown, Odom, & Conroy (2001) recommended that to create classroom environments that support social interaction and friendship development among children with and without disabilities, opportunities for mutual play interaction and social problem solving must be created. They also stress the importance of children participating in an inclusive classroom learn about disabilities, discuss misconceptions and stereotypes about people with disabilities, and have the opportunity to explore adaptive equipment.

Vygotsky's theory of cognitive development (1978) is also critical to the change process advocated in this chapter. Vygotsky addressed the central role of caregivers and more competent peers in children's learning process for all skill development. Children learn through supported problem-solving experiences with others. A more skilled person mediates the learning experience for a particular child. He stated that understanding what a particular child can do with help or support is crucial to support a child's learning. Vygotsky also highlighted the importance of understanding how a caregiver teaches children to recognize problems and how to solve those problems. Children learn through problem-solving experiences with others. A more skilled person mediates the learning experience for the child. This frame of reference emphasizes the importance of therapists supporting and teaching caregivers optimal ways of helping children understand, organize, and use social information in their environments in the process of developing effective habits and routines for social participation. Therapists also provide direct input to children relative to social understanding and problem solving in their individual and group interventions.

FUNCTION–DYSFUNCTION CONTINUUMS

There are seven function–dysfunction continua found in this frame of reference.

Temperament

Temperament is a person's innate style of emotional, motor and attention reactivity to environments, events, and people. As a child experiences and acclimates to the daily environments, he or she learns what to expect. His or her everyday life becomes routinized to some degree, and reactive facets of his or her temperament become modulated. When the child is able to focus attention on social tasks as needed and manage impulses for productive social participation, he or she can effectively adapt to family, school, and community social demands.

A child may have difficulty regulating his or her activity level and attention span to participate in the required activities when a child's temperament is difficult. Such a

TABLE 10.1 Indicators of Function and Dysfunction for Temperament Adaptation

Expected Self-Regulatory Capacities	*Poor Self-Regulatory Capacities*
FUNCTION: Exhibits developmentally expected ability to regulate emotional, motor, and attentional reactivity as well as age-expected self-regulatory capacities	*DYSFUNCTION*: Does not exhibit developmentally expected abilities to regulate emotional, motor, and attentional reactivity as well as developmentally expected self-regulatory capacities
Indicators of Function	**Indicators of Dysfunction**
Focuses attention	Cannot focus attention
Manages activity level and impulses with caregiver support given age and situation	Cannot manage activity level and impulses with caregiver support given age and situation
Orients to relevant sensory input	Does not orient to relevant sensory input
Able to ignore environmental distractions	Cannot ignore environmental distractions
Adjusts to the daily routines of home, school, and community environments	Does not adjust to daily routines of home, school, and community environments
Appropriately shifts attention in activity and conversation	Cannot shift attention in activity and conversation
Is sensitive and responsive to the demands of the environment and can put aside favored activities to respond appropriately to environmental demands	Is not sensitive or responsive to environmental demands and cannot put aside favored activities to respond appropriately
Persists in tasks as expected developmentally	Is not persistent in tasks as expected developmentally

child may struggle with new situations or adapting to changes in routines (Table 10.1). This will likely interfere with the child's ability to fit in and be accepted by other persons within his or her environment. A child who has not learned to modulate the reactive facets of his or her temperament and who has not developed effortful control may not be open to learning in his or her environment (Table 10.2). Such a child may not respond appropriately to nurturing and guidance, or may have difficulty participating in peer play groups.

TABLE 10.2 Indicators of Function and Dysfunction for Emotional Regulation

Modifies Feelings	*Unable to Modify Feelings*
FUNCTION: Given age and development, can take action to modify feeling states to accomplish interpersonal goals	*DYSFUNCTION*: Given age and development, cannot take action to modify feeling states to accomplish interpersonal goals
Indicators of Function	**Indicators of Dysfunction**
Can identify emotional states in self and others	Cannot identify emotional states in self and others
Is aware of own emotional signals	Is not aware of own emotional signals
Recognizes the emotional signals of others	Does not recognize the emotional signals of others
Exhibits capacity to control emotional expression to support prosocial goals	Does not exhibit capacity to control emotional expression to support prosocial goals

Habits and Routines

A family has functional habits and routines when they are able to complete daily living activities while maintaining harmonious relationships among members. Children participate in these daily living routines according to their functional and/or developmental levels. Caregivers provide instruction, support, and assistance to children as needed and they positively respond to caregivers' instructions. Children demonstrate the basic habits for social interaction within these daily family routines including making eye contact, and verbally and nonverbally responding to questions and directions (Table 10.3). Families who exhibit function in this area also report regular participation in mutual activities that are pleasurable to family members (Figure 10.5). These activities recur at regular intervals (daily, weekly, or seasonally).

Families that exhibit dysfunction in this area do not have daily family living routines or routines for daily activities are excessively stressful, causing disharmony among family members. Children do not participate in daily living routines. Children do not respond to caregiver's instruction, support, or assistance. Children do not demonstrate the basic habits for social interaction within family activities. Families do not report regular participation in mutual activities that are pleasurable to family members.

Environment

At the functional end of the continuum, a home environment provides safety, security, support, and developmental stimulation to the child (Table 10.4). The physical living space of the home is safe from intruders, has no safety hazards, and is relatively clean. It includes materials for participating in developmentally appropriate activities.

TABLE 10.3 Indicators of Function and Dysfunction for Family Habits and Routines

Effective Family Routines	Inadequate Family Routines
FUNCTION: Family routines allow members to complete daily living activities while maintaining harmonious relationships among members	*DYSFUNCTION*: Family routines do not exist or do not support family members completing daily living activities while maintaining harmonious relationships
Indicators of Function	**Indicators of Dysfunction**
Participates in family routines according to functional or developmental level	Does not participate in family routines according to functional or developmental levels
Caregivers provide instruction, support, and assistance to children as needed	Caregivers do not provide instruction, support, and assistance to children as needed
Positively responds to caregivers' instructions in family routines	Negative or nonresponsive to caregiver instructions in family routines
Demonstrates the basic habits for social interaction within family routines	Does not demonstrate the basic habits for social interaction with family routines
Caregivers report that the family regularly participates in mutual activities that are pleasurable to family members	Caregivers report that family does not regularly participate in mutual activities that are pleasurable to family members

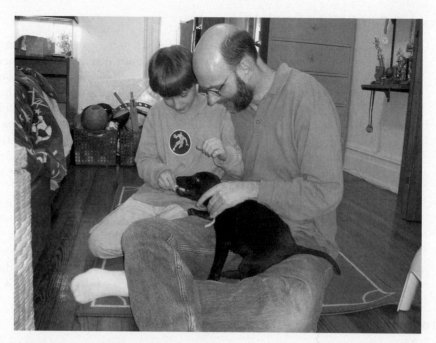

FIGURE 10.5 Father teaching son to care for his puppy's teeth.

The caregivers are interested and focused on keeping a child safe and meeting his or her developmental needs. Problems in this area are evident when there is an unsafe physical environment, or the caregivers are not meeting the developmental needs of the child.

Functional school environments include teachers who support the child's development of academic, social, and living skills. A functional school environment is safe

TABLE 10.4 Indicators of Function and Dysfunction for Environmental Supports

Supportive Home	Nonsupportive Home
FUNCTION: Child's home provides safety, security, support, and developmental stimulation to the child	DYSFUNCTION: Child's home does not provide safety, security, support, and developmental stimulation
Indicators of Function	**Indicators of Dysfunction**
Physical home environment is physically safe and has sufficient materials to engage child in developmentally appropriate activities	Physical home is not physically safe and does not have sufficient materials to engage child in developmentally appropriate activities
Responds to caregivers nurturing and responsiveness	Does not respond to caregivers nurturing and responsiveness
Demonstrates appropriate behaviors as role modeled by caregivers	Does not demonstrate appropriate behaviors as role modeled by caregivers

TABLE 10.5 Indicators of Function and Dysfunction for Social Participation in School	
Supportive School	**Nonsupportive School**
FUNCTION: School environment is safe, provides the nonhuman and human support for successful academic achievement	*DYSFUNCTION*: School environment is not safe, does not provide the nonhuman and human support for successful academic achievement
Indicators of Function	**Indicators of Dysfunction**
Physical environment is safe and has adequate space and materials for learning	Physical environment is not safe and does not have adequate space and materials for learning
Positive interactions with other children facilitated by teachers and staff	Unable to positive interact with other children even when facilitated by teachers and staff
Benefits from individualized teaching and interactional styles of teachers and staff	Difficulty with individualized teaching and interactional styles of teacher and staff

and has adequate space and materials for learning. Teachers facilitate and support positive interactions among children and adjust their teaching styles sensitive to the learning needs of various children (Table 10.5). Problems in the school environment arise when space and materials are inadequate for learning or when a teacher is unable to facilitate positive interactions among children and has an inflexible teaching style.

Within a functional environment for peer interaction, a child has opportunities to participate in various activities with peers and the opportunity to help his or her peers as well as to receive help from them in their mutual activity (Table 10.6). The child also has time and space to develop friendships with preferred peers. Caregivers support the child as he or she learns to manage conflict and the ability to negotiate with peers (Figure 10.6). In a dysfunctional environment for peer interaction, a child does not have opportunities to participate in various activities with peers and does not have the

TABLE 10.6 Indicators of Function and Dysfunction for Environments for Peer Interaction	
Supportive Environments for Peer Interaction	**Nonsupportive Environment for Peer Interaction**
FUNCTION: Access to environments where the child can interact with peers in positive, prosocial ways regularly	*DYSFUNCTION*: Does not have access to environments where the child can interact with peers in positive, prosocial ways on a regular basis
Indicators of Function	**Indicators of Dysfunction**
Participates in opportunities to participate in various activities with peers	Does not have opportunities to participate in various activities with peers
Has time and space to develop friendships with preferred peers	Does not have time and space to develop friendships with preferred peers
Has caregivers to support learning of conflict and negotiation with peers	Does not have caregivers to support learning of conflict and negotiation with peers

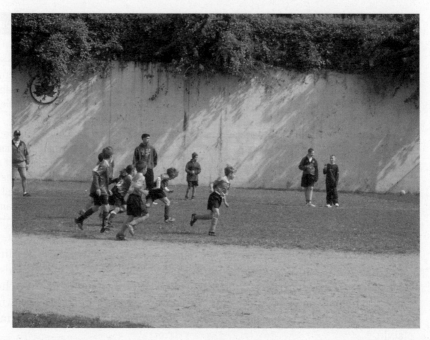

FIGURE 10.6 Through organized programs such as sports leagues, children have the opportunity to share common interests, develop skills, and friendships.

opportunity to reciprocally help and be helped by peers in activities. Children are not afforded the time or space to develop friendships with preferred peers.

Peer Interaction

Functional peer interaction is exhibited when a child is accepted by other children in age-appropriate and/or developmentally appropriate groups (Table 10.7). The child approaches peers in a positive way to initiate activity interaction and responds positively to most friendly overtures. The child exhibits social orientation through his physical posture, cognitive attention, and emotion state. In the interest of becoming involved in group play, the child takes turns and increasingly develops the skills of compromise, cooperation, and negotiation. The child is responsive to the verbal and nonverbal cues that peers give to indicate their emotional states and their reactions to the child. The child can change his or her approach to succeed in a social situation if the cues the child receives from others suggest a need for change. Willingness to help peers in play and to accept help are also skills that the child exhibits. These behaviors facilitate closer bonds with peers and lead to the child's development of friendships. Through friendships, a child receives emotional support and companionship that facilitates the child's emotional well-being and competence in daily activities.

The inability to respond to peers appropriately leads to being ignored or rejected. The child may be socially isolated as a result of poor peer interaction skills. He or she

TABLE 10.7 Indicators of Function and Dysfunction for Peer Interaction	
Constructive Peer Interactions	*Unconstructive Peer Interactions*
FUNCTION: Child is accepted in an age-appropriate and/or developmentally appropriate peer group	*DYSFUNCTION*: Child is not accepted in an age-appropriate and/or developmentally appropriate peer group
Indicators of Function	**Indicators of Dysfunction**
Can approach peers in a positive way to initiate activity interaction	Does not approach peers in a positive way to initiate activity interaction
Responds positively to most friendly overtures	Does not respond positively to most friendly overtures
Exhibits social orientation through physical posture, cognitive attention, and emotional state	Does not exhibit social orientation through physical posture, cognitive attention, and emotional state
Responsive to the verbal and nonverbal cues of peers	Not responsive to the verbal and nonverbal cues of peers
Can shift approach in response to cues from others	Cannot shift approach in response to cues from others
Accepts and follows implicit and explicit rules for group-play activities	Does not accept and follow the implicit and explicit rules for group-play activities
Takes turns with peers in group activities	Does not take turns with peers in group activities
As developmentally appropriate, child exhibits skills of compromise, cooperation, and negotiation	Does not exhibit skills of cooperative, compromise, and negotiation as developmentally expected

may not initiate activity interaction in a positive way. A child may attempt to bully peers or may be intrusive to get his or her needs met. Another reaction may be that a child is overly dependent and passive, and therefore is rejected by peers because he or she is considered immature. The child ignores or is insensitive to social cues from others and, therefore, does not alter unsuccessful methods of peer engagement. Help from peers may not be accepted or the child may excessively seek help from peers. The child may not offer to help peers or may be overly intrusive or domineering when trying to help. The end result is a lack of friendships.

GUIDE TO EVALUATION

Assessing Caregivers' Needs for Support in Increasing Children's Social Participation

An occupational therapist must actively engage children's caregivers in any assessment and intervention to effectively design an approach to increase children's social participation. Caregivers create children's social ecology. Their own values, beliefs, habits, and routines relative to social participation as well as their desire for change are critical for helping children increase the quality and/or quantity of their social participation.

Once children reach school age, in addition to considering children's primary caregivers, teachers become important secondary caregivers.

An occupational therapist must identify what social demands caregivers place on children and their vision for children's social occupational performance. It is important to identify what caregivers believe is important for children's social participation in everyday environments. A therapist will be better positioned to help caregivers support a child's social participation if he or she understands the current structure that caregivers provide for children's activities, as well as the skills and methods that they use to teach and reinforce children's skill development within those activities.

Assessment of Children's Social Participation

An occupational therapist interested in facilitating a particular child's social participation creates an occupational profile related to the child's activities so that the therapist can then develop an effective plan for intervention that may include foci on promoting change in the child, tasks for social participation, and/or the child's human or nonhuman environment for social participation. When creating a profile, the *Pediatric Interest Profiles* (Henry, 2000) assist a therapist in assessing children's leisure participation from their own point of view relative to their preferences, actual participation, and their perceptions about that participation. The *Children's Assessment of Participation and Enjoyment and Preferences for Activities of Children* (CAPE/PAC, King et al., 2004) similarly structures a practitioner in systematically gathering and organizing information from children about their activity preferences, the diversity and intensity of their participation, with whom and where they participate, as well as their degree of enjoyment of each activity. The *Occupational Therapy Psychosocial Assessment of Learning* (Townsend et al., 1999) helps a practitioner collect and organize a great deal of information related to children's school environment, activities, and social behavior.

A therapist may also decide to use the *Social Skills Rating System* (*SSRS*, Gresham & Elliott, 1989) to gather information from teachers and parents who have had opportunity to observe children's social participation over time. The SSRS is a teacher and parent questionnaire designed to gather specific information about caregivers' perception about children's social competence. Caregivers identify their perceptions of the frequencies that a particular child exhibits specific social skills and the importance of each social skill in the child's social environments. From this assessment, a therapist can identify the specific social skills that children need to develop or skills that children need to exhibit more frequently to be socially competent in their environments.

There are several occupational therapy assessments that address children's social participation as well as other areas of occupational performance. Using one of these tools may be most efficacious as occupational therapists often are initially consulted because of concerns about children's occupational performance relative to cognitive, motor, or sensory skills. *The School Function Assessment* (Coster et al., 1998) is an excellent tool for analyzing children's functional performance in schools. It analyzes children's participation, need for task supports, and their activity performance relative to several areas important to using this frame of reference including functional communication, following social conventions, compliance with adult directives and school rules, positive interaction, and behavior regulation. The *Pediatric Evaluation of Disability Inventory* (Haley et al., 1992) also assesses social participation in addition to assessing functional and mobility skills. In addition to addressing functional motor skills important for occupational participation in early childhood, the *Miller Function and Participation Scales* (Miller, 2006), included home and school observation checklists for rating children's participation in daily routines, as well as their social skills and behavior and self-control.

When occupational therapists evaluate children's executive function, a rating inventory such as the *Behavior Rating Inventory of Executive Function* (BRIEF, Gioia et al., 2000) and the *Behavior Rating Scale of Executive Functioning–Preschool Version* (BRIEF-P, Gioia, Espy, & Esquith, 2003) provide important data relative to children's capacities for effortful control and emotional regulation including attention, flexibility, and emotional control. Executive function deficits are important to identify along with social skill deficits as the former may underlie social deficits (Kavale & Forness, 1996; Kiley-Brabeck & Sobin, 2006; Nigg et al., 1999).

The therapist should also directly observe how children interact in different small and large group activities as the social demands for interaction may be different. If assessing social participation in a school, a therapist might observe a child in a less structured activity time in the classroom as well as when the child needs to collaborate with peers on an art project, eat lunch in the cafeteria, or play a gross motor game with peers in physical education or on the playground. With age-appropriate or developmental expectations in mind, the following should be noted:

- Initiating and responding with peers
- Turn-taking, compromising, and negotiating in activities
- Aggression toward and from peers
- Incidences of helping and being helped by peers

When a therapist is assessing a young child, the opportunity to observe parent–child interaction in the context of a valued daily occupation is also helpful. It will help the therapist better understand some of the challenges faced by parent and child in their daily living activities as well as suggest the areas of intervention for social participation that may be most pressing. The quality and process of interaction should be noted along the following lines:

- Mutual engagement in activity
- Parent's or caregiver's and child's verbal and nonverbal expression of enjoyment, frustration, or anger
- The child's communication of needs and desires during the activity and the parents' subsequent response
- Structure set by the parent and the child's response to it
- Resolution of frustrations and problems during interaction

The *Early Coping Skills Inventory* (Zeitlin, Williamson, & Szezepanski, 1988) helps a therapist to analyze how young children from 4 to 36 months organize their behavior to initiate and respond to the demands of their physical and social world. *The Coping Inventory* (Zeitlin, 1985) guides a therapist in analyzing how actively, flexibly, and productively children from 4 through 16 years cope with environmental demands, as well as the demands of self. Both inventories are rating scales that a therapist may use after observing a child in a few activities. These tools are particularly helpful in that they guide a therapist in systematically identifying and reflecting on how a child manages everyday challenges and stressors in their daily occupations and the impact that the environment may have had on his or her responses. All children have some assets in one or more areas that can be used to foster adaptation; even children who have minimally effective coping skills have a few relative coping strengths that can be mobilized. A therapist is likely to discover this through a systematic analysis of a child's coping skills in activity.

After gathering all or some of these data, the therapist must integrate and interpret findings into an overall picture of the child's functional strengths and weaknesses relative to social participation. Although some children may exhibit pervasive deficits in social participation, it is important to identify relative strengths that can be maximized and the key deficits that present barriers to social participation. From a functional perspective, it can be anticipated that if intervention is directed toward the key problem areas, then problematic behavior will decrease overall and the child will experience greater success in his or her daily social activities.

As it has been described here, a full occupational therapy evaluation for social participation is difficult. In most settings, it is not possible. The therapist must identify what is relevant and critical to assess and what are feasible procedures for assessment in the particular practice environment.

POSTULATES REGARDING CHANGE

Occupational therapists are well suited to help parents and/or other primary caregivers create or modify daily household activities to increase the efficiency of daily routines, as well as to introduce, modify, adjust, or reframe some shared activities to promote parents' and children's engagement and enjoyment of one another.

When caregivers learn ways to modify the structure of children's physical environment and daily routines to support children optimally managing their temperamental capacities related to activity level, impulsivity, and intensity of mood children are more likely to be more successful in social participation. It is important that caregivers come to understand children's temperament so that they come to appreciate what is innate and then become open to considering adaptations to support children's capacity to participate in activities within their families and communities. Through repeated participation in meaningful routines such as mealtimes, bedtimes, social games with sensitive and responsive caregivers, children begin to internalize basic procedures for social interaction and develop strategies for emotional and behavioral regulation. Three postulates are listed to guide a therapist in helping parents understand their children's temperament so that they can develop effective routines for family living.

1. If a therapist assists care providers in understanding the discomfort of a child with a difficult temperament and how it can be managed in the child's and the family's

best interest, then the care providers and child will have more positive interactions.

2. If the therapist assists a child's care providers in establishing a routine for activities that are difficult or disorganizing for the child, then the child will become calmer, more cooperative, and organized around those activities.

3. If a therapist assists a child's caregiver to develop strategies to teach a child habits for social interaction that support the child's participation in daily family routines, then the child will be more available to learning to participate in daily family routines at his or her developmental or functional level.

To increase the likelihood of a parent providing the necessary physical and emotional support, it is important for the parent and child interaction to be viewed as primarily positive or rewarding. The child requires a sense of security to grow into a healthy, functioning adult. He or she needs to expect comfort and assistance when stressed or overwhelmed. Positive events that do not occur in some families create as much stress and are as damaging to a child's mental health as are negative interactions that do occur (Mash, 1984). An occupational therapist can create opportunities for a child and his or her caregiver to experience positive mutual interaction in activities where the parent is guided in providing assistance to the child. Four postulates regarding change are concerned with building a positive relationship between children and parents or care providers.

1. If a therapist provides a structured and supportive environment in which parent and child can enjoy mutual play, positive engagement between parent and child will be promoted.

2. If a therapist demonstrates ways that a parent or care provider can facilitate a child's positive engagement and functioning and provides an activity in which this can be practiced, then a parent or care provider will be more likely to promote the same behaviors in the child in the future.

3. If the therapist helps a parent identify what made an interaction between parent and child positive and successful in a therapy session and assists the parent in creating a positive environment, then a parent will more likely attempt to recreate similar positive interactions with their child outside of a therapy session.

4. If a therapist assists a parent in identifying and incorporating positive, pleasurable activities into their daily and weekly schedule with his or her child, the parent and child will develop rituals that enhance their relationship.

Learning to regulate emotion is a critical capacity for all social participation. When a person can manage and adjust the emotional states, he or she is more open to opportunities for social participation and flexible about how to work out differences with others.

1. If a therapist teaches a child to identify emotional states and recognize his or her own signals that the child's emotions are not modulated sufficiently for social participation, the child will begin to note his or her own signals over time.

2. If a therapist assists a child in recognizing the emotional signals of others through reading the nonverbal cues of others, then the child will begin to recognize the emotional cues of others over time.
3. If the therapist helps the child develop and use strategies to manage emotions and behavior in challenging events in their social occupations, the child will engage more successfully in the activities within that social occupation.
4. If a therapist teaches a child to use techniques to modulate emotion, including lessening anxiety in social situations and then provides opportunities for the child to practice those techniques in everyday occupations, then the child will begin to apply those techniques independently over time.

Occupational therapists have many opportunities to support children's social participation with peers (Figure 10.7). Therapists often work in school environments where they may work with children in small group settings within classrooms and in other school environments. They may also work in private practice or community settings where they may work with two children or a group of children. While one of the primary goals of therapy may frequently be related to the children's occupational functioning related to their sensory or motor capacities, it is important that therapists make use of the peer opportunities available to support children's development of capacities for social participation. At other times, therapists may lead or colead playgroups specifically

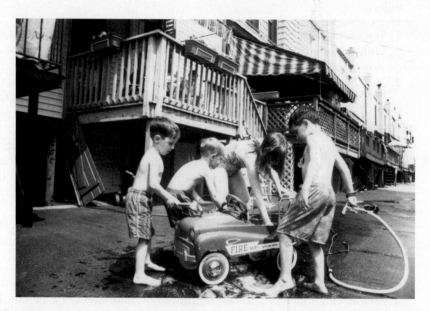

FIGURE 10.7 Working together requires emotional regulation as well as several social skills. These children are motivated to use all of these skills to work with each other on washing a miniature fire engine.

designed to develop children's skills related to social participation with their peers. Five postulates regarding change are concerned with peer interactions.

1. In a safe and accepting environment, if a child has the opportunity to participate in an enjoyable and intrinsically rewarding activity, then the child will more likely attempt to cooperate with peers in a group activity.
2. If a therapist teaches a child how to exhibit behaviors indicative of social orientation, the child will more likely be successful in engaging peers in social interaction.
3. If a child learns the basic social skills needed to play with other children, the child's positive peer interaction will likely increase and his or her interests and activity skills may also expand.
4. If a child learns to help peers or siblings and to accept help, then the child will be more likely to seek out and be sought by peers or siblings for mutual activity and friendship.
5. If a therapist assists a child working with other children to identify the rules necessary for group play, then the child is more likely to accept rules and limits. Furthermore, the child will be more likely to censor himself or herself and others within such a group.

APPLICATION TO PRACTICE

Consulting with Caregivers

If the helping professional assesses caregivers' readiness for change, it will guide them for intervention planning in a manner that supports caregivers' moving from recognizing a problem to taking action. If a therapist is not cognizant of a caregivers' readiness for change, the therapist may push the caregiver to implement an intervention plan only to face the caregiver's resistance to appropriately carrying out the plan and then to rejecting it as unworkable or unsuccessful.

Prochaska (1995) emphasized the importance of matching interventions to persons' particular stage within the change process. Occupational therapists can apply this work to their interventions with caregivers by recognizing caregivers' readiness to change how they interact and support children's social participation. Their intervention plans should be tailored to caregivers' present stage of readiness to promote caregivers' motivation to change.

Caregivers in the precontemplation stage may be optimally supported by engaging them in activities that increase their awareness of how they may influence the occurrence of children's problem behavior by their own habits and routines of social participation. Caregivers in the contemplation stage might benefit from reading books on how to support children in developing skills for successful social participation, or by planning and participating in activities in the presence of a therapist. Having the opportunity to reflect on what occurred afterward with a therapist is important.

In the preparation stage, therapists guide caregivers through exploring the interventions that would provide the caregiver with the skills to support children's social participation. Caregivers may collaborate with therapists in planning new activities or adapting familiar activities for children's increased social participation.

In the action stage, they may create new social opportunities for children in lieu of maintaining children's participation in environments that have not facilitated positive social participation or they may incorporate strategies for emotional or behavioral regulation into their preparation for daily occupational routines.

In early childhood, when dysfunction is evident in temperament, habits and routines, and social participation with caregivers and peers, the role of the therapist is to facilitate the relationship between the child and his or her caregivers. The therapist acts as a role model and advisor to caregivers. As an advisor, the therapist can enhance a parent's understanding of his or her child's temperament and make suggestions regarding the structure of daily routines that may help children respond more positively to family life. The therapist can help parents identify family priorities and develop clear behavioral goals for the child and strategies to achieve the goals. This can be particularly useful for a parent who must deal with a child who displays a difficult temperament. It helps the parent to provide a secure atmosphere with appropriate and consistent expectations that provide organization for such a child.

Role Modeling

In specific interactions, the therapist may serve as a role model by demonstrating effective ways of dealing with difficult behaviors or drawing the child into a positive interaction. The therapist may also coach a parent through an interaction or observe and then consult with the parent after the interaction. The therapist minimizes the degree to which he or she actively directs a situation to avoid becoming the sole authority figure. It is important that the therapist highlight parents' strengths in interaction after a parent–child session or during the session, if such a comment fits into the process. In this way, the therapist gives the parent authority, which promotes the child's confidence in the parent. It is critical that the child sees his or her parent as competent and someone to rely on. With some families who have experienced a great deal of negative interaction, it is important to remember that people are less likely to notice positive occurrences or behaviors when they have been immersed in negative interaction (Mash, 1984). The therapist can help family members begin to notice and enjoy positive moments even if they are brief. The goal is to serve as a consultant to the parents to enhance their everyday functioning with their children. The therapist works to increase the pleasure and the satisfaction that is experienced in parent–child interaction, and to assist parents in exploring and sharing activities with their children that will bring more frequent and consistent positive interaction.

The therapist sets up a reciprocal interaction in which the child learns that he or she can share concretely his or her interest in activity and depend on care providers for help and praise to foster positive parenting. The therapist should demonstrate an active respect for the child's feelings and growing autonomy. Through whatever activity chosen, the therapist can help the parent choose and provide gentle but firm behavioral limits and positive reinforcement for appropriate behavior. The therapist should have activity and behavioral plans that will likely accentuate the positive aspects of particular children, as opposed to their negative behavior that their parents may overly focus upon. Some parents have reported that they participated in parent–child activities with their child and the therapist because of their comfort level with the therapist. They stated that they only began to understand the value of parent–child activity and to enjoy it after they had experienced it over the course of time. Parents need to feel supported and accepted by the therapist to allow a therapist to intervene in a difficult parent–child relationship.

Occupational therapy can play a vital role in implementing change in the parent–child relationship by facilitating productive and pleasurable interaction through play and activity. This can be accomplished by working with individual families or leading a group of multiple parent–child dyads or triads. The former is most likely to occur when a family identifies a specific problem that it wishes to focus on solely, a group is not available or desirable to the parents, or difficulties in interaction are severe and are not likely to be resolved without the intensive teaching of skills. An occupational therapist may apply the Floortime approach advocated by Greenspan & Wieder (1998, 2006). This approach explicitly describes how developmental challenges related to sensory, motor, and cognitive processing and regulation impact children's emotional development and capacities for interactive play. It also articulates strategies for helping caregivers better engage and communicate with children nonverbally in play and ways to promote the emotional development of children with disabilities within play and daily living activities.

Therapists may choose to use group format in a school setting, hospital, or residential treatment center. In these environments, many families share similar concerns or difficulties and can provide a strong support network for each other. Olson (2007) describes a qualitative study of one parent–child group, and provides guidelines for developing a parent–child activity group (Figure 10.8). She provides a complete framework for setting up and leading such a group as well a rich description of one group that was set up on a child inpatient psychiatric unit over the course of several months. She examined what was observed to be helpful within the group design and process as well as what parents and children reported to be helpful to them. She also analyzed factors within the group environment and group process that appeared to limit parents and children engaging positively with one another.

Activity-Based Intervention When Parents Are I*ll*

Occupational therapists, in collaboration with other professionals, can help parents maintain a secure and supportive relationship with their children in spite of a parent's serious physical or emotional illness. When parents are ill and cannot physically take care of and interact with their children in their typical way, children may exhibit angry, anxious, avoidant, ambivalent, or solicitous behavior. Although other adults will most likely fill in and provide daily physical care for the children, it is critical that each child's

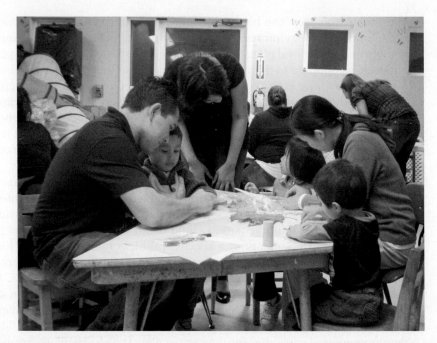

FIGURE 10.8 Parent–child occupation-based groups provide parents with the opportunity to explore activities that foster their children's development as well as provide a means for mutual engagement.

relationship with his or her parent who is ill be supported. Therapists should facilitate regular opportunities to communicate and interact. In this way, each child is assured that his or her parent is still available to him or her and that the child can still have a meaningful and positive relationship in spite of the parent's illness. It also gives children the opportunity to understand better their parent's condition by being able to observe the parent and be with him or her.

For the parent who is ill, the opportunity to engage with his or her children can have an equally positive emotional effect. Playful activity can soften a serious, unfamiliar, and adult-like environment (e.g., a hospital) into one wherein both child and parent experience the environment and situation as more comforting and supportive. It can give direction and a means for interaction when tension or emotion may be high. Besides being organizing and calming, it brings pleasure. This is especially true when an illness requires a long hospitalization or a long recuperation period. Activities should be organized and adapted to children's emotional and developmental needs, as well as to parents' level of physical stamina and emotional state. Olson (2006) describes specific guidelines about providing occupation-based intervention for promoting social participation between parents who are depressed and their young children. She applied cognitive behavioral therapy methods, useful for individuals with depression, to depressed parents engaged in cooccupation with their children. She fully describes the process of applying those guidelines in occupational therapy on a young mother diagnosed with depression and her baby over the course of an acute psychiatric hospitalization through facilitating this mother's interaction with her baby in everyday caregiving and play in her home.

Promoting Social Participation in Classroom Settings

Brown, Odom, & Conroy (2001) identified that high-quality appropriate play activities be organized in a way that promotes sharing, talking, assisting, and playing among children (Figure 10.9). The activities may be constructive, sociodramatic, or game play. Adult leaders may plan, arrange, introduce, and monitor the activities. If necessary, adults might suggest how children might play with one another. They might assign roles or ask children how they want to play with their friends. As play becomes organized, leaders partially withdraw from play and become monitors and supporters of the play. If children have difficulty talking, sharing, playing, or interacting, the leader encourages, prompts, or models appropriate behavior. Besides creating opportunities for children to play and interact in small groups, it is also important to consider strategically providing opportunities for children with disabilities to develop friendships (Buysse, Goldman, &

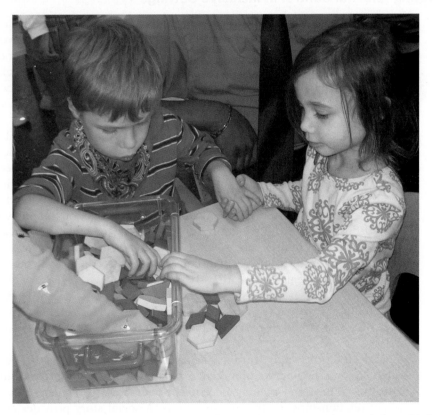

FIGURE 10.9 Children with disabilities are more likely to develop friendships with their able-bodied peers when they have the opportunity to participate mutually in activities.

Skinner, 2003). This includes setting up opportunities for children to play exclusively with particular peers so that they can learn to focus on the social cues and perspectives of a peer.

Teachers use interventions in their classrooms to promote emotional and social competence such as modeling, role play, and group discussion. They may instruct children on how to identify and label feelings and how to communicate with others about emotions and how to resolve disputes with peers. Occupational therapists can work with teachers in inclusive classrooms to engage children with disabilities not only in the lessons, but also in activities with individual peers to practice what is taught. Classroom-based programs have been more effective when they have targeted children's knowledge of emotions and children's emotional and behavioral self-control through classroom-based games that reward discipline and cooperation. In working with children with disabilities, it is also critical to consider creating opportunities where children can help others besides being a recipient of help from others.

Promoting Effortful Control in Inclusive Settings

To develop positive peer interactions, it is important for children to develop self-regulation skills and social thinking skills (understand the perspectives of others, have skills to negotiate differences in activity, and occupational goals with others). Interventions have been developed to support children's self-regulation and social thinking skills. Winner (2002) has well-described group strategies for promoting school-aged children's social thinking. She provides a clear description of the development of social thinking methods to assess it, as well as a series of intervention activities.

One of the most commonly used approaches for promoting children's behavioral regulation for social participation is Social Stories (Crozier & Tincani, 2007). Gray (1995) outlines social story guidelines that include descriptive, perspective, affirmative, and directive sentences. The key factual information about a situation is provided in the descriptive sentence, the likely thoughts and feelings about others in the situation are provided in the perspective sentence. Instructions about what the children should do based on the situation and perspective of others is provided in the directive sentences. Children are reassured with affirmative sentences that appropriate behavior will result in a positive consequence. Occupational therapists have developed special strategies for writing social stories related to sensory challenges in social situations. There is promising research that social stories are effective in helping some children with autism spectrum disorder manage social situations with the support of social stories (Crozier & Tincani, 2007; Sansosti, Powell-Smith, & Kincaid, 2004).

Social Stories apply learning theory along with a cognitive-behavioral approach to intervention. The intervention recognizes that some children have difficulty exhibiting effortful control and making decisions about how to regulate behavior to maintain social relationships in stressful situations. A social story provides cognitive cues that help a child think through the demands of the situation as well as to acknowledge how other participants in the social exchange might be thinking or how they are prosocially behaving. The Social Story then cues the child on what behavior should be chosen in the stressful situation so that they will be successful in the situation.

In reflecting on how to improve the effectiveness of Social Stories as an intervention, Crozier & Tincani (2007) identified the need to assess children's motivation to engage in social activities. Children who are uninterested in social activities are less likely to exhibit appropriate behavior even when behavioral expectations are clear. They highlight a need for possibly using a preference assessment to identify what is motivating for a particular child (Hagopian, Long, & Rush, 2004). They also suggest that practitioners and researchers should carefully consider the frequency with which children need to reread social stories to benefit from them over time and how to successfully fade the use of social stories so that gains from the use of them is maintained over time. They identify that some children appear to need social stories along with verbal prompts whereas other children may only need a social story to support their capacities relative to effortful control.

Executive functioning deficits may interfere with children's capacities to attend to joint activities. Children may have difficulty with inhibition, shifting topics or activities, initiating or planning activities, or controlling their emotional states. Addressing children's development of executive function supports their development of coping skills. Occupational therapists can help children and their caregivers learn strategies to support children's capacities to inhibit impulses, tolerate, and learn when it is important to shift topics and activities when working with others and use strategies to maintain their emotional control when strong emotions are aroused in activities. For example, therapists can apply Toglia's Multicontext Approach (Toglia, 2005) to teach children processing strategies for recognizing when and how to inhibit impulses or shift topics. Toglia's Multicontext Approach also guides a therapist in considering how to support generalization of strategy use through a sideways approach to activity analysis and grading (Figure 10.10). A therapist helps children first apply strategies to similar activities and gradually changes more of the features and conditions of the activities (Toglia, 2005).

Occupation-Based Groups to Increase Children's Social Participation with Peers

Occupational therapists lead groups to develop and support children's social participation in various settings including schools, after school programs, community centers, mental health facilities, children's hospitals, or private practices. Such groups are important for children experiencing challenges interacting and developing friendships with their peers. With the guidance of a group leader, occupation-based groups provide children with the opportunity to learn new skills, change behavior, and receive feedback from others within the context of peer group participation in a mutually valued activity. Children can learn and immediately apply strategies for emotional regulation as well as specific social skills to activity participation with a peer group. Over time, regular positive peer interaction within the context of shared occupation will support the development of friendship. Activity groups operate under the premise that children are intrinsically interested in play and peer acceptance. Unless children are severely

FIGURE 10.10 Children's games can be used to teach and provide opportunities to practice social skills.

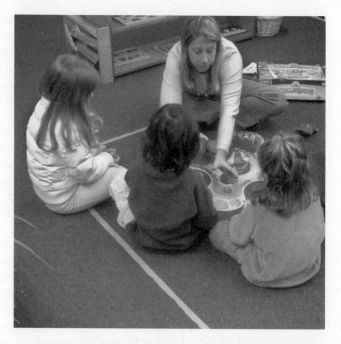

withdrawn or antisocial, they will be drawn into many activities if peers are involved. Their desire to be included in a peer group leads them to be open to the goals of others. In activity groups, the leader makes use of this natural desire to help children modify their behavior.

The chronological and developmental ages of the children and the particular goals that the children and their caregivers identify as important determine how groups are organized and focused. Successful groups for children of all ages typically employ behavior management techniques to help children control their impulses in support of a positive and organized social atmosphere. Individual and group contingencies are important. Individual contingencies refer to setting up reinforcements for individual children when they follow rules and work toward their social occupational goals. When a leader uses a group contingency, the leader reinforces the entire group when all members participate together and achieve a group goal in an activity. Therapists use cognitive-behavioral strategies for teaching children new skills related to emotional understanding, emotional regulation, and social skills.

Structuring an Activity Group

It is important that a leader of a children's activity group plan ahead and carefully identify the group's purpose, goals, and structure. In addition, a leader must carefully plan session activities to teach skills and to practice those skills. Critical elements in the design of successful groups are routine, rituals, and depersonalized controls in their group design. As in any human activity, functional routines allow people to complete necessary maintenance activities in the most efficient and effective manner with minimal stress and cognitive energy used. Rituals are important in the lives of all people. They also provide structure and highlight the uniqueness, importance, and stability of a social group. Rituals are calming and allow people to anticipate what will occur next. Depersonalized controls are rules about behavior that a group decides are necessary if a game or activity is going to be pleasurable or successful. They are not directed toward any person but toward the implementation of an activity. An authority figure is not passing judgment or holding the power. When a rule is broken, limits are set with the rule breaker because he or she interfered with the game or activity. The therapist should work toward cultivating interest contagion for the group activities (i.e., to spread enthusiasm for particular activities from one or a few children to the whole group) (Redl & Wineman, 1952). This will, of course, increase the positive atmosphere in the group; it will also facilitate greater group cohesion.

It is also important that therapists be aware of issues related to deviancy training in children's group. Deviancy training refers to the reinforcement that children receive from other children when they act in antisocial ways. When children who disrupt prosocial or constructive activity or act verbally or physically aggressive with others and are not appropriately redirected or censured by group leaders, they may gain status with the other children. Other children may identify with them and imitate their deviant behavior. Some studies have suggested that leaders can inadvertently create an environment that supports children learning to be more aggressive. It is critical that leaders use effective behavior management systems for groups, consider how they will effectively manage highly aggressive children within a group, and be attentive to the sometimes subtle peer reinforcement for negative behavior and curtail these interactions. All leaders of children's groups need to develop strong skills in engaging children in constructive activities as well as skills in addressing problematic behavior in groups (Dishion & Stormshak, 2007; Boxer et al., 2005; Lavallee, Bierman, & Nix, 2005).

Choosing Activities

Occupation-based groups may be developed around various play activities or tasks. The choice of activity depends upon the purpose and goals of the group, and the interests and developmental level of the children. Constructional activities provide opportunities to build task skills; they can also be organized to facilitate collaboration among children.

Feelings exert a powerful influence on choices, motivation, and continued engagement in occupation. Subjective experiences of occupational activities influence social participation. Individual emotional needs and preferences are reflected in one's occupational performance as much as one innate physical and cognitive capacities for activities. Children participate in building activities not just to develop fine motor skills but also out of an emotional need to create and to express their internal states (Olson, 1997). Different activities provide different outlets for expression and are satisfying at different times. If occupational therapists understand how a child's emotional state is affected by particular tasks and environments both human and nonhuman, the occupational therapist can create, modify, or adapt tasks and environmental conditions that satisfy emotional needs and transform negative or disorganized emotional states in support of positive social participation.

School-aged children are group-focused and game-focused; they have come to understand the importance of rules for the games or activities to be fun. Even children who are oppositional are more likely to abide by game rules. Through games, children can express competitive or aggressive feelings within a controlled, safe, and socially accepted structure. They can outwit and dominate each other or a leader momentarily and with pleasure because it is just a game. Effective games are emotionally engaging.

A therapist can teach or reinforce social skills or problem-solving strategies within games that the therapist or group creates or by modifying popular games. There are also several commercially available games that were specifically designed to address children's emotional regulation or social skills.

Another type of activity that children enjoy involves creating and sharing jokes, skits, and humorous pictures with each other. In the process, they ease frustration and disappointments of their everyday lives while entertaining and connecting with each other. They may parody authority figures in their plays or comic routines; parents and teachers laugh along with them and praise their creativity (Wolfenstein, 1954).

Winner (2002, 2005) articulated group plans and strategies for promoting children's and adolescents' abilities for perspective taking and self-awareness of their own behavior in groups. Sapon-Shevin (1986) describes a range of games that foster cooperation instead of competition. Jackson, Jackson, & Monroe (1983) developed a social skills curriculum that outlines sessions to teach 17 social skills. Elliott & Gresham (1991) designed lesson plans to address the social skills needs identified through the *Social Skills Rating System* (SSRS, Gresham & Elliott, 1989). Lane et al. (2005) described a step-by-step plan for implementing a social skills intervention based on the work of Gresham and Elliott. Although some may want to use social skill curriculums as written, they can also be valuable as resources when developing one's own group curriculum. They describe many group activities that are engaging to children in addition to fostering social skill development. The Center on Social and Emotional Foundations for Early Learning (http://www.vanderbilt.edu/csefel/modules.html) provides excellent resources for teaching young children socioemotional skills and how to manage social situations, as well as providing guidance for therapists working on behavior support plans for students.

Many resources for age-appropriate activities for children are available, and they may provide helpful ideas and direction, especially for the beginning therapist. The therapist should avoid presenting an activity as a lesson or to give an excessive amount of structure. This may inhibit the goal, to facilitate the emergence of natural play and the development of interactive patterns. Although step-by-step instructions may lessen a leader's anxiety about how successful children will be in completing an activity, it may limit children's exploration and discourage problem solving. Even when a therapist wants to teach a specific task or manipulative skill, after initial practice of the skill, the opportunity to use the skill by exploring and playing will enhance skill development. Most social skill curriculums recommend introducing a skill that is to be highlighted and learned in a session in a very structured manner, but these curriculums also suggest using play and activities in which children can spontaneously and naturally practice the skill as follow-up to the lesson.

Jackson (2002) identified good strategies that an occupational therapist may want to employ in engaging children in reflecting on learning activities in groups. He emphasizes that without a discussion, an activity may just be fun and not promote new learning. Discussion promotes the development of both cognitive and social skills. He summarizes the steps to a successful discussion with children as what, so what, now what, and summarization.

Dealing with Activity Group Process

In developing an activity group, it is important to remember that groups also have their own particular growth process over time. In the initial stages, group members are more dependent on the leader for structure and organization than they will be at later stages of group development. As they become accustomed to the group, members may resist the leader as they attempt to assert some control over the activities of the group. Members may appear disillusioned with the group; this is a normal part of group process. Helping members work through this leads to a more mature group stage where group norms are well respected and the group functions cohesively at its optimal developmental level. Although school-aged children require more structure and guidance from group leaders than groups of adolescents or adults do, they seek and need some control and responsibility within a group.

Throughout an activity group, a leader facilitates group and individual problem solving, encourages helping behaviors among children, participates in activity, and provides concrete task assistance as needed. Although the children may focus their conversation and interaction toward the leader, the therapist redirects interaction toward other group members whenever possible. In this way, the leader fosters positive peer interaction instead of rivalry among the children for the leader's attention. The leader may need to intervene in peer interaction within a group when difficulties arise that children cannot resolve on their own. One child may intimidate or bully other children into doing things his or her way. The group leader should work to redirect the group by appealing to all members' sense of fairness and guide the group toward negotiation. Clarification or interpretation of what the leader observes happening among the children may be helpful. This facilitates the children acquiring a greater understanding of their own behavior and that of their peers. It may reduce their anxiety about an uncomfortable situation, help clarify their own feelings, and lead to verbalizing their own concerns because it is clear that an adult is there to support and guide them. As a result of positive participation in an activity group over a period of time, children become more secure, related, self-reliant, confident, and socially skilled; behaviors that may have interfered with peer group functioning decrease significantly.

Grading the Amount of Frustration

When children have difficulty maintaining their composure in the face of challenges in activities, the therapist needs to grade the amount of frustration inherent in the activity. When an outburst or conflict occurs, a problem-oriented discussion helps children learn to identify their own emotional signals and then learn to resolve the situation adaptively. For example, if one child becomes angry during play, he or she may need to learn to remove himself or herself from the game to regain emotional control before the child can discuss his or her differences with his or her peers. Another child may burst into tears or destroy a project when he or she makes a mistake. With the therapist's and group's help, the child may explore how he or she can deal with frustration. The child learns that he or she can ask for help when he or she gets to a certain part of a project. Or, the child learns that he or she can ask for the therapist to help to fix a mistake before destroying his or her project.

Aggressive Behavior

The therapist may guide aggressive children in recognizing their developing anger and make connections between how their body feels, what they are thinking, and what they do. Once they can identify their own signs of developing anger, children can be taught relaxation or coping techniques. This may include specific physical relaxation techniques, learning to cope through stopping and talking oneself through a situation, or learning to take effective action such as removing oneself from a stressful situation. It is important when working with aggressive children to develop a positive and warm relationship with them. These children often feel that they are disliked by others. It is unlikely that a therapist will effectively influence any change in their behavior without the children feeling accepted and valued by the therapist.

Group Resistance

If a group meets over a length of time, sooner or later a therapist will be faced with resistance and his or her limits will be tested by group members. Although clear rules and consequences are important to enforce consistently with the help of the group members, it is also important not to fall into the trap of becoming a corrective, directive, and coercive authority figure. Children can provoke this and if the therapist is not reflective, a power struggle may ensue that may last over a period of groups. This may set a negative tone to the group's process and interfere with the therapist's ability to be an effective clinician. It is important to develop and maintain a positive and warm relationship with group members because this will help the children to see that they are accepted and valued by the therapist, which is a necessary prerequisite to promoting change.

When dealing with resistance or a challenge to one's limits, a therapist should first attempt to appeal to the group's sense of what is right and to engage members positively. Humor may also be helpful. At times, this will lead to children refocusing their energies positively; they may either reengage in the activity or share their issues. The group may need restructuring. Rules may not be working. An activity may be too challenging. At other times, children may need to be removed from the group for a time-out. Sometimes, it is necessary for the entire group to have a time-out within the group to reorganize. If particular children are removed, the leader should consider how he or she will reconnect with the children whom he or she removed from the group, and help them save face if necessary. Sometimes other members will decide that the children who are removed are bad and should not be in the group. The leader will need to reduce this type of scapegoating behavior. Other times, they may idolize the acting-out child who "told the leader off." The leader will need to set firm limits and shift the groups' values away from supporting deviant behavior Redl (1966).

The length of a group and the point at which the therapist intervenes in the process of play should be considered carefully so that the group can be refocused or the play can be terminated before the children's behavior becomes difficult to manage or aggressive. It is always better to end a group while the children feel invested in the activity and want to participate longer than to end when they cannot wait to get out of the group. This is not to say that an activity should be interrupted prematurely, but that the therapist should give the ending of the group as careful consideration as the beginning of the group. For a group to be successful, children need to have a desire to return to the group and to develop a strong interest in participation in the group.

Culture, Beliefs, and Values

Groups also reflect issues of the larger society of which they are embedded. It is important that therapists reflect on their own beliefs about culture, race, gender, and religion. Children and therapists come to a group experience with a belief system and a great deal of experience in dealing with these issues. Different subcultures within our society have varying practices related to gender, daily living, and religion that influence their approach to activities and to social interaction. These can have a significant impact on how persons participate in a group. For example, gender roles are more rigid and specific in some cultures than in others. Therefore, the choice of activity and expectations for interactions may have to be adjusted as the therapist learns about group members' culture.

At times, incidents occur in groups that reflect the prejudice and racism present in American society. Children may subtly or not so subtly exclude a child who has a different religion than other members or make racial slurs about another child. It is helpful to acknowledge these incidents and to help children understand them. Some children may have experienced themselves in similar situations as being less worthy, less competent, or less likeable instead of understanding that they were the target of racism or prejudice. Children from privileged backgrounds may have perceived themselves as better than their peers from less privileged backgrounds. The therapist may also subtly adjust the dynamics among members through the activity to promote more inclusive and accepting behaviors among members.

Sometimes children from minority backgrounds are initially guarded with or easily angered by having a therapist from a different background. They may be angry about how they have been treated by other persons in authority, from different cultures, and project that onto the therapist. Although limit setting is important, it is also important that the therapist not respond to the behavior as simply resistive behavior. The therapist's relationships with group members and the group members' relationships with each other can be dramatically altered if a therapist's hunches about prejudice or racism are sensitively explored. The therapist can listen to what may be behind anger and may ask for elaboration about similar experiences. The children can then be helped to gain control over anger that may be related to racism or prejudice and to use that anger adaptively.

The therapist should acknowledge and model interest and acceptance of multiple cultures through incorporating activities reflecting the cultures of the children involved in the group. In a supportive environment, children enjoy talking about activities that they have enjoyed with their families and in their communities; such a discussion can be a springboard for developing group activities. When children have had little experience with activities that reflect their cultural backgrounds, a therapist may share multicultural activity books with them through which they can learn about their own and different cultures by planning interesting group activities.

Termination

Dealing with either the last session of a group, or a member leaving a group, is as important as how the therapist initially organizes the group. Learning how to say goodbye and to appropriately mark transitions is a critical life skill. Just as most people find special events that mark most life transitions comforting and enjoyable, children enjoy planning a special activity to mark a group's ending. The therapist should guide the children in reflecting on and reveling in what they enjoyed about the group and what they accomplished or learned. Sharing feelings about saying goodbye and helping children make the transition toward other groups or community activities are important behaviors that the therapist should model.

Juan's Case Study: Helping a Child with Significant Disabilities Find Ways to Assist Peers

Creating opportunities for children with significant physical disabilities to help their peers in ways that their peers will value the assistance can be challenging. Occupational therapists can play an important role in creating or seizing opportunities for children with disabilities to help peers or siblings.

The occupational therapist working in an inclusive setting with Juan, a third-grade boy with cerebral palsy, observed that though Juan was participating in a class science activity of discovering what plants need to grow and how weeds suffocate or prevent plants from growing, his participation was minimal and not engaging for him. His classmates were using gardening tools to remove weeds that had grown around potted trees in the school's courtyard. Juan watched the other children effortlessly tug at the weeds, pull them out, and deposit them into a nearby trash bag. Juan was seated in his wheelchair and though an aide helped him put on a gardening glove and hold a tool, he could not reach the ground from his wheelchair or independently pull up weeds as he saw his friends do. He indicated to his therapist to deposit weeds.

There was a commotion as two children worked feverishly tugging at a particularly deep and large weed. They could not tear it from the ground. Two more children tried, and then three children tried to pull together. A teacher attempted. No one could remove the weed. Juan's therapist looked at Juan. "I bet we can tear that weed out, Juan. Do you want to try with me?" Juan used his augmentative device to communicate that he wanted to try.

Juan used his motorized chair to position himself next to the tree with the monster weed, still uncertain about what his role might be. His therapist took out some rope and tied it to the weed's base, and then tied the other end of the rope to Juan's chair. "OK, Juan! Reverse your chair and GET THAT WEED!!!" Juan smiled broadly, and with that command, Juan put his motorized wheelchair in reverse. Juan's entire class watched as the weed was wrenched from the earth. Cheers of "Yeah Juan!!" erupted amidst the fierce spontaneous clapping coming from his third-grade classmates. Juan was the unexpected hero of the hour.

Elena's Case Study: Finding an Activity that Promotes a Child's Social Participation

Elena is a fourth-grade girl who has cerebral palsy. She is wheelchair bound. Her ability to participate with her peers is limited as most activities require extensive modifications and teacher/therapist/peer support for successful participation. Given her physical limitations, Elena does not often experience leadership roles within her peer group. At times, she shares her original ideas and plans with peers, but a friend has to execute her plans. Typically, Elena does not initiate interaction or activity, and seems minimally connected and engaged in classroom activities with peers.

Elena's occupational therapist adapted some simple magic tricks that Elena would likely be able to execute with minimal/moderate assistance. She chose magic because Elena's parents told the therapist that Elena was intrigued by a magician that she had seen. Additionally, the activity is not just in the physical execution of the magic trick, the power is in knowing the secret about how the trick is accomplished and keeping the secret from one's audience. With the therapist, Elena explored books about magicians and simple magic tricks. Once she practiced a trick with the therapist serving as her assistant, she became focused on learning other tricks. Learning tricks and sharing her magic tricks with a peer or a teacher was incorporated into her therapy sessions. Elena now has an activity through which she can experience a sense of control, exert leadership, and gain the respect of her peers.

Tommy's Case Study: Creating Friendships

Tommy, a second grader diagnosed with Asperger syndrome, received occupational therapy services twice weekly to address sensory processing, fine motor and graphomotor dysfunction which interfered with his participation in academic tasks. Snack time and lunchtime presented significant social issues for him as he also exhibited feeding issues. He tended to chew food with his mouth open, frequently spilled his food on his clothes and on the table. Peers, as well as some teachers, expressed displeasure with his eating habits and he was often excluded in activities following a snack or lunch as peers said he was "disgusting." As an occupational therapist, it was important to address his sensory processing and oral motor issues, and to work with his mother and teacher around selecting appropriate foods that Tommy would be less likely to spill. It was also important to set up the snack and lunchtime environment in ways that promote Tommy's organization.

It was also important to directly address Tommy's difficulties related to social participation. Tommy expressed interest in interacting with other children, but he rarely focused on their cues or adjusted his behavior in response to their negative nonverbal or verbal communication. In conversation, he focused on topics that interested him and ignored topics that did not interest him. When he wanted a toy or an object, he grabbed it; he did not focus on his peers' reactions to his behavior or whether they might want the same toys or objects. Tommy intruded on the space of others if he was interested in an activity or object close to another child, while he became angry if others intruded on his personal space.

The occupational therapist started a lunch group to work on oral motor and mealtime habits, and on skills for successful social participation. She invited Robert, another child from Tommy's class. Robert often spent lunch in the nurse's office complaining of physical ailments as he hated the noise and mess of the crowded elementary school lunch room. Robert was an easygoing child who was initially not Tommy's identified friend, but he was open to eating and playing with Tommy in a quiet space during lunch and recess.

Tommy was enthusiastic about having the opportunity to eat lunch and play with Robert away from the other children. Tommy, Robert, and the therapist created procedures and rules for lunch that included how they would set up and clean up. They also discussed how the children would keep their food from spilling on the table and on themselves. A checklist was created so that the group could rate how successful they were in each group session. Similarly, Tommy and Robert helped the therapist develop rules for how to decide what activity the children would do after lunch. The therapist enforced the group structure created and guided the boys through negotiating mutual play. When disagreements occurred, the opportunity was used to focus both children on the emotional cues and perspective of the other. As Tommy and Robert found common interests and enjoyed their mutual play in the group, they developed a friendship that extended to their classroom and to after school play-dates.

Over lunch, Tommy and Robert talked about telling other boys about their special group. Two boys expressed interest in joining them. The two boys were added to the group. The rules and structure of the group were renegotiated to incorporate the viewpoints of the additional boys and to encourage play among the boys in pairs as well as in a group of four. Over play, the boys talked about how one classmate, Billy, bullied all of them some of the time, but particularly bullied Tommy. Tommy wanted to invite Billy to visit lunch club. The therapist used the opportunity of inviting Billy to the group to build a friendship between Billy and the other boys. The therapist guided the boys in working out their differences by identifying and sharing their desires and feelings. Over time, they also discussed how they experienced each other during activities in class and on the playground. When disagreements occurred, the therapist used the opportunity to introduce ways of managing anger and hurt feelings. Billy rarely bullied Tommy or the other boys within the group or outside of the group because he developed common interests and a friendship with them.

Over time, Tommy began to talk with bravado about wanting to bully other children who irritated him on the playground; he looked to Billy for approval. He identified with Billy's tendency toward aggressive behavior and saw Billy's bullying as a status that he desired. Within the group, the leader led the group members to discuss their experiences of being bullied and how that felt. The group leader also helped Billy to set limits with Tommy. This was important so that Tommy or other children were less likely to idealize the aggressive behavior that they observed and then to copy it to attempt to gain peer status and approval.

In the early phases of the group, children needed a point system to motivate them to control impulses, take turns and ask about the feelings of their peers. When children received a certain number of points for positive behaviors, they could trade in the points for special pencils, pads, or fidget toys. When children exhibited behavior indicative of limited emotional control or limited attention to the cues of others, they took brief time-outs to regain their composure. Over the course of a few months, group rewards were used. If group members were able to work together to negotiate play choices and to solve differences in the group, the group chose a special snack or activity.

Summary

In this frame of reference, the author summarized current literature on how children learn social participation skills and what commonly interferes with the social participation of children with disabilities. Current research and theory suggests that skills for social participation are critical for success in school and in adult life (Waterhouse, 2002; Zins et al., 2004). The behavioral (Skinner, 1974), social (Bandura, 1977; Dishion & Stormshak 2007; Guralnick et al., 2006; Prochaska, 1995), and social-cognitive (Vygotsky, 1978) learning theories provide the basis of the interventions discussed. Emotional engagement of children and caregivers with each other and in cooccupation are discussed as crucial supports in any intervention process. Occupational therapists' understanding caregivers' level of readiness for change and using this understanding to plan intervention is stressed as critical to the success of any intervention plan. It is essential that occupational therapists consider and explore children's social participation in their assessment process and at all levels of interventions. Pediatric occupational therapists in all practice environments can make a significant contribution to support children's social participation. It is a primary basis for children's satisfaction and success in their daily occupations.

REFERENCES

American Occupational Therapy Association. (2002). Occupational therapy practice framework: Domain and process. *American Journal of Occupational Therapy*, 56, 609–639.

Bandura, A. (1997). *Self-Efficacy: The Exercise of Control*. New York: Freeman.

Bandura, A. (1977). *Social Learning Theory*. New York: General Learning Press.

Boxer, P., Guerra, N. G., Huesmann, L. R., & Morales, J. (2005). Proximal peer-level effects of a small-group selected prevention on aggression in elementary school children: An investigation of the peer contagion hypothesis. *Journal of Abnormal Child Psychology*, 33(3), 325–338.

Brown, W. H., Odom, S. L., & Conroy, M. A. (2001). An intervention hierarchy for promoting young children's peer interaction in natural environments. *Topics in Early Childhood Special Education*, 21(3), 162–175.

Buysse, V., Goldman, B. D., & Skinner, M. L. (2002). Setting effects on friendship formation among young children with and without disabilities. *Exceptional Children*, 68(4), 503–517.

Buysse, V., Goldman, B. D., & Skinner, M. L. (2003). Friendship formation in inclusive early childhood classrooms: What is the teacher's role? *Early Childhood Research Quarterly*, 18, 485–501.

Chess, S., & Thomas, A. (1984). *Origins and Evolutions of Behavior Disorders: From Infancy to Early Adult Life*. New York: Brunner & Mazel Publishers.

Cole, P., Martin, S. E., & Dennis, T. A. (2004). Emotion regulation as a scientific contruct: methodological challenges and directions for child development research. *Child Development*, 75(2), 317–333.

Coolahan, K., Fantuzzo, J., Mendez, J., & McDermott, P. (2000). Preschool peer interactions and readiness to learn: Relationships between classroom peer play and learning behaviors and conduct. *Journal of Educational Psychology*, 92(3), 458–465.

Coster, W., Deeney, T., Haltiwanger, J., & Haley, S. (1998). *School Function Assessment*. San Antonio, TX: Psychological Corporation.

Crozier, S., & Tincani, M. (2007). Effects of social stories on prosocial behavior of preschool children with autism spectrum disorders. *Journal of Autism and Developmental Disorders*, 37(9), 1803–1814.

Denham, S. (1993). Maternal emotional responsiveness and toddlers' social-emotional competence. *Journal of Child Psychology and Psychiatry*, 34(5), 715–728.

Dishion, T. J., & Stormshak, E. A. (2007). *Intervening in Children's Lives: An Ecological, Family-Centered Approach to Mental Health Care*. Washington, DC: American Psychological Association.

Eisenberg, N., & Spinrad, T. L. (2004). Emotion-related regulation: Sharpening the definition. *Child Development*, 75(2), 334–339.

Eisenberg, N., Valiente, C., Morris, A. S., Fabes, R., Cumberland, A., Reiser, M., Gershoff, E. T., Shepard, S. A., & Losoya, S. (2003). Longitudinal relations among parental emotional expressivity, children's regulations and quality of socioemotional functioning. *Developmental Psychology*, 39(1), 3–19.

Elliott, S., & Gresham, F. M. (1991). *Social Skills Intervention Guide*. Circle Pines, MN: American Guidance Service.

Fantuzzo, J., & McWayne, C. (2002). The relationship between peer-play interactions in the family context and dimensions of school readiness for low-income preschool children. *Journal of Educational Psychology*, 94(1), 79–87.

Feldman, R., Greenbaum, C. W., & Yirmiya, N. (1999). Mother-infant affect synchrony as an antecedent of the emergence of self-control. *Developmental Psychology*, 35(1), 223–231.

Fiese, B. H. (2002). Routines of daily living and rituals in family life: A glimpse at stability and change during the early child-raising years. *Zero to Three*, 22(4), 10–13.

Fraser, M. W., Galinsky, M. J., Smokowski, P. R., Day, S. H., Terzian, M. A., Rose, R. A., & Guo, S. (2005). Social information-processing skills training to promote social competence and prevent aggression behavior in the third grades. *Journal of Consulting and Clinical Psychology*, 73(6), 1045–1055.

Gioia, G. A., Espy, K. A., & Esquith, P. K. (2003). *Behavior Rating Inventory of Executive Function-Preschool Version (BRIEF-P)*. Lutz, FL: Psychological Assessment Resources.

Gioia, G. A., Esquith, P. K., Guy, S. C., & Kenworthy, L. (2000). *Behavior Rating Inventory of Executive Functioning (BRIEF)*. Lutz, FL: Psychological Assessment Resources.

Gray, C. A. (1995). Teaching children with autism to read social situations. In: K. A. Quill (Ed). *Teaching Children with Autism* (pp. 219–241). New York: Delmar.

Greenspan, S. I., & Wieder, S. (1998). *The Child with Special Needs: Encouraging Intellectual and Emotional Growth*. Reading, MA: Perseus Books.

Greenspan, S. I., & Wieder, S. (2006). *Engaging Autism: Using the Floortime Approach to Help Children Relate, Communicate, and Think*. Cambridge, MA: Da Capo Lifelong Books.

Gresham, F. M., & Elliott, S. N. (1990). *Social Skills Rating System*. Circle Pines, MN: American Guidance Service.

Guralnick, M. J. (2006). Peer relationships and the mental health of young children with intellectual delays. *Journal of Policy and Practice in Intellectual Disabilities, 3*(1), 49–56.

Guralnick, M. J., Connor, R. T., Neville, B., & Hammond, M. A. (2006). Promoting the peer-related social development of young children with mild developmental delays: Effectiveness of a comprehensive intervention. *American Journal on Mental Retardation, 111*(5), 336–356.

Hagopian, L. P., Long, E. S., & Rush, K. S. (2004). Preference assessment procedures for individuals with developmental disabilities. *Behavior Modification, 28*(5), 668–677.

Haley, S. M., Coster, W. J., Ludlow, L. H., Haltiwanger, J. T., & Andrellos, P. J. (1992). *Pediatric Evaluation of Disability Inventory (PEDI): Development Standardization and Administration Manual*. Boston, MA: Boston University.

Henry, A. D. (2000). *Pediatric Interest Profiles: Surveys of Play for Children and Adolescents*. San Antonio, TX: Therapy Skill Builders.

Jackson, T. (2002). Why have a discussion? and four steps to a great discussion. In T. Jackson (Ed). *Conducting Group Discussions with Kids: A Leader's Guide for Making Activities Meaningful* (pp. 7–24). Cedar City, UT: Active Learning Center.

Jackson, N. F., Jackson, D. A., & Monroe, C. (1983). *Skill Lessons and Activities: Getting Along with Others*. Champaign, IL: Research Press.

Kavale, K. A., & Forness, S. R. (1996). Treating social skills deficits in children with learning disabilities: A meta-analysis of the research. *Learning Disabilities Quarterly, 19*(1), 2–13.

Keltner, B. (1990). Family characteristics of preschool social competence among black children in a Head Start program. *Child Psychiatry and Human Development, 21*(2), 95–108.

Kiley-Brabeck, K., & Sobin, C. (2006). Social skills and executive function deficits in children with the 22q11 deletion syndrome. *Applied Neuropsychology, 13*(4), 258–268.

King, G., Law, M., King, S., Hurley, P., Rosenbaum, P., Hanna, S., Kertoy, M., & Young, N. (2004). *CAPE/PAC: Children's Assessment of Participation and Enjoyment and Preferences for Activities of Children*. San Antonio, TX: Harcourt.

Kubicek, L. F. (2002). Fresh perspectives on young children and family routines. *Zero to Three, 22*(4), 4–9.

Lane, K. L., Menzies, H. M., Barton-Arwood, S. M., Doukas, G. L., & Munton, S. M. (2005). Designing, implementing, and evaluating social skills interventions for elementary students: Step-by-step procedures based on actual school-based investigations. *Preventing School Failure, 49*(5), 18–26. Educational Module,

Lavallee, K. L., Bierman, K. L., & Nix, R. L. (2005). The impact of first-grad "friendship group" experiences on child social outcomes in the Fast Track Program. *Journal of Abnormal Child Psychology, 33*(3), 307–324.

Lemerise, A., & Arsenio, W. F. (2000). An integrated model of emotional processes and cognition in social information. *Child Development, 71*, 7–18.

Maag, J. W. (2006). Social skills training for students with emotional and behavioral disorders: A review of reviews. *Behavioral Disorders, 32*(1), 5–17.

Mash, E. J. (1984). Families with problem children: children in families under stress. *New Directions for Child Development, 24*, 65–82.

Meyers, C., & Vipond, J. (2005). Play and social interactions between children with developmental disabilities and their siblings: A systematic literature review. *Physical and Occupational Therapy in Pediatrics, 25*(1/2), 81–103.

Miller, L. J. (2006). *Miller Function and Participation Scales*. San Antonio, TX: PsychCorp.

Nigg, J. T., Quamma, J. P., Greenberg, M. T., & Kusche, C. A. (1999). A two-year longitudinal study of neuropsychological and cognitive performance in relation to behavior problems and competence in elementary school children. *Journal of Abnormal Child Psychology, 27*(1), 51–63.

Norton, D. (1993). Diversity, early socialization, and temporal development: the dual perspective revisited. *Social Work, 38*(1), 82–90.

Odom, S. L., Li, S., Sandall, S., Zercher, C., Marquart, J. M., & Brown, W. H. (2006). Social acceptance and rejection of preschool children with disabilities: A mixed-method analysis. *Journal of Educational Psychology, 98*(4), 807–823.

Olson, L. J. (1997). Sublimations of the grade school child. In J. D. Noshpitz, P. F. Kernberg, & J. R. Bemporad (Eds). *Handbook of Child and Adolescent Psychiatry: Volume 2, The Grade School Child: Development and Syndromes* (pp. 107–113). NY: Juan Wiley & Sons.

Olson, L. J. (2006). When a mother is depressed: supporting her capacity to participate in co-occupation with her baby-A case study. *Occupational Therapy in Mental Health*, *22*(3/4), 135–152.

Olson, L. J. (2007). *Activity Group in Family-Centered Treatment: Psychiatric Occupational Therapy Approaches for Parents and Children*. Binghamton, NY: Haworth.

Olson, L., & O'Herron, E. (2004). Range of Human Activity: Leisure Activities. In J. Hinojosa, & M. L. Blount (Eds). *Texture of Life: Describing Purposeful Activity* (2nd ed., pp. 335–366). Bethesda, MD: American Occupational Therapy Association.

Prochaska, J. O. (1995). An eclectic and integrative approach: transtheoretical therapy. In A. S. Gurman, & S. B. Messer (Eds). *Essential Psychotherapies: Theory and Practice*. New York: Guilford Press.

Raver, C. C. (2002). Society for Research in Child Development. Emotions matter: making the case for the role of young children's emotional development for early school readiness. *Social Policy Report* *16*(3), 3–19.

Redl, F. (1966). *When We Deal with Children*. New York: Free Press.

Redl, F., & Wineman, D. (1952). *Children Who Hate*. New York: Free Press.

Redl, F., & Wineman, D. (1952). *Controls From Within-Techniques for the Treatment of the Aggressive Child*. New York: Free Press.

Richardson, P. K. (2002). The school as a social context: Social interaction patterns of children with physical disabilities. *American Journal of Occupational Therapy*, *56*, 296–304.

Rothbart, M. K., Ahadi, S. A., Hershey, K. L., & Fisher, P. (2001). Investigation of temperament at three to seven years: the children's behavior questionnaire. *Child Development*, *72*(5), 1394–1408.

Rothbart, M. K., & Bates, J. E. (1998). Temperament. In W. Damon (Series Ed.), & N. Eisenberg (Eds). *Handbook of Child Psychology, Social, Emotional, Personality Development*, Vol. 3 (pp 105–176). New York: Wiley.

Rubin, K. H., Daniels-Beirness, T., & Bream, L. (1984). Social isolation and social problem-solving: A longitudinal study. *Journal of Consulting and Clinical Psychology*, *52*(1), 17–25.

Sansosti, F. J., Powell-Smith, K. A., & Kincaid, D. (2004). A research synthesis of social story intervention for children with autism spectrum disorders. *Focus on Autism and Other Developmental Disabilities*, *19*(4), 194–204.

Sapon-Shevin, M. (1986). Teaching cooperation. In G. Cartledge, & J. F. Milburn (Eds). *Teaching Social Skills to Children* (pp. 270–302). New York: Pergamon Press.

Skinner, B. F. (1974). *About Behaviorism*. New York: Knopf.

Toglia, J. P. (2005). A dynamic interactional approach to cognitive rehabilitation. In N. Katz (Ed). *Cognition and Occupation Across the Lifespan: Models for Intervention in Occupational Therapy* (2nd ed., pp. 29–72). Baltimore, MD: American Occupational Therapy Association.

Townsend, S., Carey, P. D., Hollins, N. L., Helfrisch, C., Blondis, M., Hoffman, A., Collins, L., Knudson, J., & Blackwell, A. (1999). *Occupational Therapy Psychosocial Assessment of Learning (OTPAL), Version 2.0*. Chicago: Model of Human Occupation Clearinghouse, Department of Occupational Therapy, University of Illinois.

Vygotsky, L. S. (1978). *Mind in Society: The Development of Higher Psychological Processes*. Cambridge, MA: Harvard University Press.

Waterhouse, L. (2002). Social interaction impairments. *Developmental Variations in Learning* (pp. 57–79). Mahwah, NJ: Lawrence, Erlbaum Associates.

Winner, M. G. (2002). *Thinking about You, Thinking about Me*. San Jose, CA: Michelle Garcia Winner.

Winner, M. G. (2005). *Think Social! A Social Thinking Curriculum for School-Age Students: For Teaching Social Thinking and Related Social Skills to Students with High Functioning Autism, Asperger Syndrome, PDD-nos, ADHD, Nonverbal Learning Disability, and for all Others in the Murky Gray Area of Social Thinking*. San Jose, CA: Michelle Garcia Winner.

Wolfenstein, M. (1954). *Children's Humor: A Psychological Analysis*. Glencoe, IL: The Free Press.

Zeitlin, S. (1985). *Coping Inventory*. Bensonville, IL: Scholastic Testing Service.

Zeitlin, S., Williamson, G. G., & Szczepanski, M. (1988). *Early Coping Inventory*. Bensenville, IL: Scholastic Testing Service.

Zins, J. E., Weissberg, R. P., Wang, M. C., & Walberg., H. J. (Eds). (2004). *Building Academic Success on Social and Emotional Learning*. New York: Teachers College Press, Columbia University.

CHAPTER 11

A Frame of Reference
for Visual Perception

COLLEEN M. SCHNECK

Visual perception is the total process responsible for the reception and cognition of visual stimuli (Zaba, 1984). Some consider vision to be the most influential sense in humans. In fact, 70% of sensory receptors are allocated to vision, thus leaving 30% to the other senses. Vision is one of the distant senses that allow a person to understand what is occurring outside of his or her body or in extrapersonal space. Vision is a sensory receptor that feeds information to the individual, which allows us to plan and adapt to the world. It is important for learning and contributes to planning movement, as vision is needed as a guide until a motor plan is formed. "Seeing" involves input from all the other senses. Vision does not work in isolation but rather as a dynamic system of intersensory interactions. It is a process that requires interaction between the individual and his or her environment (Figure 11.1).

Skeffington (1963) was the first to propose a model that describes the visual process as the meshing of audition, proprioception, kinesthesia, and body sense with vision. He proposed that visual perception is not obtained by vision alone. It comes from combining visual skills with all other sensory modalities, including the proprioceptive and vestibular systems. Through extension of Skeffington's model, vision can be viewed as a dynamic blending of sensory information in which new visual and motor input are combined with previously stored data and then used to guide a reaction. Research demonstrates an expansive interconnectivity of sensory systems (Damasio, 1989; Thelen & Smith, 1994). Evidence of full brain activity when visualizing supports the concept that vision should be viewed within the totality of all sensory systems.

In a recent study, visual deficits were found in 68% of typical seventh grade participants (Goldstand, Koslowe, & Parush, 2005). Participants who passed a visual screening performed significantly better in visual perception than those who failed, thus supporting the need to include a vision assessment for those experiencing visual perceptual problems. In this study, the nonproficient readers had significantly poorer academic performance and vision screening scores than proficient readers, again emphasizing the need to attend to vision (Goldstand, Koslowe, & Parush). Because these visual perceptual problems can have serious ramification in limiting occupational participation well

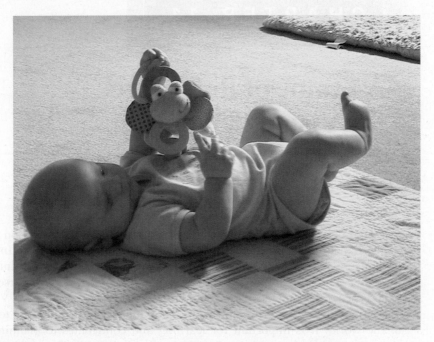

FIGURE 11.1 Infant using vision and touch to explore and learn about his toy.

beyond the school years (Brody, 1993; McLaughlin & Wehman, 1992), the importance of providing support services and intervention for children who are experiencing academic difficulties cannot be overstated. Occupational therapists (OTs) are often responsible for assessing and treating children to facilitate their learning at school when visual perceptual problems are interfering with their academic learning.

Perceptual function is the interpretation of visual sensory information. If a problem exists in this area, it can affect the child's performance in areas of occupation (Lee, 2006). One important occupation of the child is being a student. Students spend 30% to 60% of their school day on sustained reading, writing, and other desktop tasks utilizing vision (McHale & Cermak, 1992; Ritty, Solan, & Cool, 1993). Information processing in the visual perceptual domain has been identified as one of the major factors that can predict readiness for the first grade. Perceptual and perceptual motor skills are important aspects of academic performance such as reading and writing (Moore, 1979).

There are many other implications of visual perceptual problems on the occupations and life activities of children in addition to education, which include activities of daily living (ADL), work, play, leisure, and social participation. Functional problems that may result from visual perceptual issues in these areas include difficulties with eating, dressing, locating objects in their desk, batting a ball and driving, to name a few. Therefore, it is important for OTs to have a frame of reference to guide assessment and treatment in this area of practice.

THEORETICAL BASE

OTs have been influenced by cognitive and developmental psychology (Bandura, 1977; Gibson, 1969; Gibson, 1966; Piaget, 1952, 1964; Massaro & Cowan, 1993; Miller, 1988), education (Frostig & Horne, 1973; Kephart, 1971), neurology (Luria, 1980), and optometry (Getman, 1965; Scheiman, 2002; Skeffington, 1963) in developing a theoretical basis for understanding visual perceptual problems in children. Developmental and acquisitional theories can be used in guiding change by OTs for children with visual perception problems.

There are five basic assumptions made within the theoretical base of this frame of reference. These assumptions are believed to be true and are not tested. They are as follows:

- Visual perception is a developmental process.
- Visual perceptual processing is learned and increases with development, experience, and practice, and through stimulation from the environment (Figure 11.2).
- Children can learn by interacting with and observing adults and other children.
- Learning does not necessarily follow a developmental sequence. A deficit in one area does not predict a deficit or problem in another area.
- Difficulty with visual perception can interfere with daily occupations including the development of reading and writing skills.

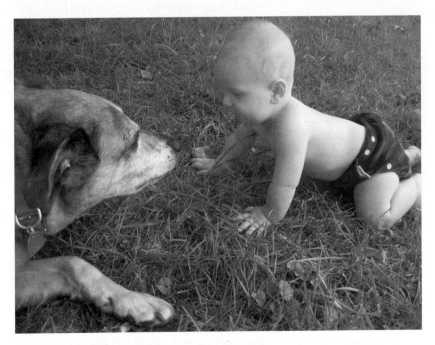

FIGURE 11.2 Baby exploring and learning about his environment.

Developmental Theories

Developmental theories view the development of skills as occurring along a continuum. Skill development is age dependent. See Table 11.1 for the developmental ages of visual perceptual skills.

Warren (1993a) presented a developmental hierarchy of visual perceptual skills using a bottom-up approach to evaluation and treatment (Figure 11.3). She suggests that with knowledge of where the deficit is located in the visual system, the therapist

TABLE 11.1 Developmental Ages for Emergence of Visual Perceptual Skills	
Perception	*Developmental Age*
Attention	Exhibits longer visual attention span to complete school assignments by 11–12 yr
Visual memory	Babies show significant visual memory ability by 6–7 mo (Rose, Feldman, & Jankowski, 2001). By 11–12 yr, expanded memory enables improved long-term recall
Object (form)	
Form constancy	Three-year-olds can sort objects on the basis of one dimension such as shape, size, or color. Dramatic improvement in the children aged 6 and 7 yr; less improvement from 8 to 9 yr of age (Williams, 1983)
Visual closure	At 4 mo, an infant is able to perceive partially hidden objects as unitary entities
Figure ground	Improves between 3 and 5 yr of age; growth stabilizes at 6–7 yr of age (Williams, 1983)
Spatial	
Position in space	Develops vertical to horizontal (3–4 yr) to oblique and diagonal (6 yr) (Cratty, 1986). Distinguish reversals (6 yr). Left–right concept: own body (6–7 yr) (Cratty). Directionality (8 yr). Development complete (7–9 yr) (Williams, 1983)
Spatial relations	Reaches accurately at 4–8 mo. Understanding of basic size by 3 yr. Understands concepts of space and time by 7 yr. Improves to approximately 10 yr of age (Williams, 1983)
Depth perception	Evident at 2 mo, developed by 4–8 mo. Shows fear of falling off high places like changing table
Topographic orientation	Improves to approximately 10 yr of age

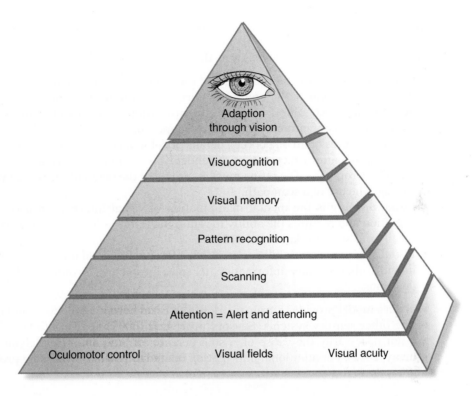

FIGURE 11.3 Hierarchy of visual perceptual skill development (Warren, 1993a).

could design appropriate evaluation and treatment strategies to remediate basic problems and improve perceptual function. To do this, it is necessary for the OT to have an understanding of the visual system, including both the visual receptive components and visual-cognitive components. Although Warren's model presents a hierarchy of skill development that is used to guide evaluation and treatment of visual perceptual dysfunction in adults with acquired brain injuries, it is useful for children with visual perceptual deficits as well. These levels develop not only with age but also in a hierarchy of influence. A hierarchy of visual perceptual skill development in the central nervous system (CNS) is presented in Figure 11.3. The definitions of components of each level are provided in the following list and are used in later descriptions of intervention.

Three primary visual skills, oculomotor control, visual fields, and visual acuity, form the foundation for all visual functions.

- *Oculomotor control* is the efficient eye movement, which ensures that the scan path is accomplished.
- *Visual fields* register the complete visual scene.
- *Visual acuity* ensures that the visual information sent to the CNS is accurate.

The next level on the hierarchy is visual attention, followed by scanning, pattern recognition, visual memory and lastly, visual cognition, with each building on the previous. Each level is listed below as they are represented in the hierarchy:

- *Visual attention* is the thoroughness of the scan path that depends on visual attention.
- *Pattern recognition* is the ability to store information in memory requiring pattern detection and recognition. This is the identification of the salient features of an object, including the configurable aspects (i.e., shape, contour, and general features) and the specific features of an object (i.e., details of color, shading, and texture).
- *Scanning* is pattern recognition dependent on organized, thorough scanning of the visual environment. The retina must record all of the detail of the scene systematically through the use of a scan path.
- *Visual memory* is the mental manipulation of visual information needed for visual cognition and requires the ability to retain the information in memory for immediate recall or to store for later retrieval.
- *Visual cognition* is the ability to mentally manipulate visual information and integrate it with other sensory information to solve problems, formulate plans, and make decisions.

Warren's model provides a framework for assessing vision alone without consideration of the other sensory systems. Sensory processing problems seem to be related to, but are not necessarily the cause of, visual perception problems (Henderson, Pehoski, & Murray, 2002). For additional information related to sensory processing problems, refer to Chapter 6.

Acquisitional Theories

Acquisitional theories focus on the learning of specific skills or subskills to function optimally within the environment (Figure 11.4). The developmental level of the child is not emphasized in acquisitional theories. The mastery of skills is the primary goal of this frame of reference. Behaviors are broken down into smaller subskills and built upon each other, resulting in complex skill development (Royeen & Duncan, 1999).

Age differences are expected within each age-group because of the maturational process as well as schooling influences. Visual perceptual performance is also influenced by our cultural and environmental experiences (Levine, 1987; Zimbardo, 1992). Some visual cognitive capacities are present at birth, and other higher level visual cognitive tasks are not fully developed until adolescence (Table 11.1). This development occurs through perceptual learning, the process of extracting information from the environment. Gibson (1969) noted, "Perceptual learning is defined as an increase in the ability of an organism to get information from its environments, as a result of practice with an array of stimulation provided by the environment" (p. 77). This increases with experience and practice and through stimulation from the environment. The child is active in investigating the world, and any environment may encourage perceptual development (Piaget, 1964). Behavior is viewed as a response to the environment either positively or negatively. Perceptual learning can be explained by the information processing model.

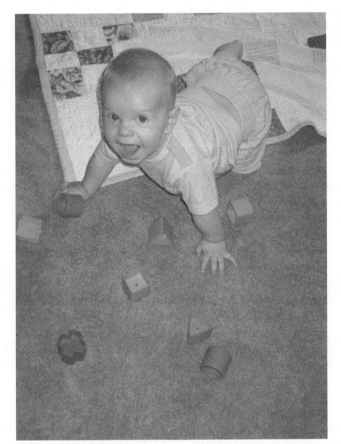

FIGURE 11.4 Environmental experiences help a baby to develop visual cognitive skills.

The term "visual information analysis," using an information processing approach, defines the ability to extract and organize information from the visual environment and to integrate it with other sensory information, previous experience, and higher cognitive functions (Scheiman, 2002; Tsurumi & Todd, 1998). The information processing model emphasizes the development of cognitive skills, particularly those related to attention, memory, thinking skills, and problem-solving abilities (Massaro & Cowan, 1993). It explains the flow of visual information processing through reception (input), organization and assimilation of visual information (processing) (Abreu & Toglia, 1987), and output (Figure 11.5). This model focuses on how the learner attends to, recognizes, transforms, stores, and retrieves information. The flow of information begins with the sensory input. Processing requires that the sensory input be attended to, compared with previously stored information, transformed into a cognitive/mental representation, and assigned meaning or acted upon. Output is the observable behavior that reflects whether learning has occurred, or it can be cognitive/mental information that is stored. Feedback to the system comes from the output, reinforcing observable behavior, and providing new input.

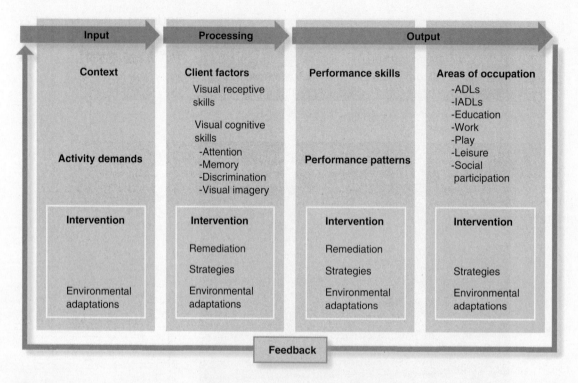

FIGURE 11.5 Visual processing model.

Input from the environment can be classified into form and space stimuli. Form stimuli include objects, two-dimensional pictures, and symbols (i.e., letters and numbers). Spatial stimuli include events and three-dimensional space. Input stimuli can be either sequential or simultaneous in nature (Levine, 1987). Sequential processing involves the integration of separate elements into groups wherein essential nature is temporal. Each element leads to another, enabling the child to perceive an ordered series of events. The order in which pieces of information are processed is critical to understanding. The information is usually language based. An example of sequential processing is the directions for building a model with Legos, a child following step-by-step pictures or a written direction. Simultaneous processing is when the visual information comes at one time. This type of information is usually visual and the concept of the whole is more important than the parts. For example, viewing a new toy at the store and then recalling it later to tell a friend.

Visual information processing can be conceptualized on a continuum from simple to complex (Abreu & Toglia, 1987). *Simple visual processing* involves little effort on the analytic ability to recognize objects, colors, and shapes and to make gross discriminations of size, position, and direction. Object processing, a subcategory of simple visual processing skills, is the ability to apprehend the meaning of objects through vision. *Complex visual processing* requires concentration, effort, and much analysis. It is the ability to accurately perceive detailed visual scenes, make subtle discrimination, and grasp the interrelationships among simultaneously presented visual stimuli.

Major Concepts

Visual perception involves a receptive component and a cognitive component. The visual receptive component is the process of extracting and organizing information from the environment. A person needs to have a good receptive component for the cognitive component to work efficiently. The oculomotor system enables the reception of visual stimuli and we need to consider the basic aspects of vision. The visual cognitive component is the ability to interpret and use what is seen.

Visual Receptive Functions

Visual receptive functions include acuity, accommodation, binocular fusion, convergence, oculomotor control including fixation pursuit and saccadic eye movements, stereopsis, and visual fields.

- *Acuity* is the ability to discriminate the fine details of objects in the visual field. A vision measurement of 20/20 means that a person can perceive at 20 ft.
- *Accommodation* is the ability of each eye to compensate for a blurred image. Accommodation refers to the process used to obtain clear vision (i.e., to focus on an object at varying distances). This occurs when the ocular muscle (the ciliary muscle) contracts and causes a change in the crystalline lens of the eye to adjust for objects at different distances. Focusing must take place efficiently at all distances, and the eyes must be able to make the transition from focusing at near point (a book or a piece of paper) to far point (the teacher and the blackboard) and *vice versa*. It should take only a split second for this process of accommodation to occur and this results in altering the focal distance of the eyes.
- *Binocular fusion* is the mental ability to combine the images from the two eyes into a single percept. There are two prerequisites for binocular fusion. First, the two eyes must be aligned on the object of regard; this is called "motor fusion," and it requires coordination of six extraocular muscles of each eye and precision between the two eyes. Second, the size and clarity of the two images must be compatible; this is known as "sensory fusion." Only when these two prerequisites have been met can the brain combine what the two eyes see into a single percept (Figure 11.6).
- *Convergence* is the turning of the eyes inward as the object of regard moves toward the observer.
- *Oculomotor skills* are efficient eye movements that ensure that the scan path is accomplished. There are three aspects to oculomotor skills: fixation, pursuit or tracking, and saccadic eye movement or scanning. *Fixation* is the coordinated aiming of the eyes while shifting rapidly from one object to another. This occurs when visual focus is on a stationary object. *Pursuit or tracking* refers to the continued fixation on a moving object. *Saccadic eye movements or scanning* is the rapid change of fixation from one point in the visual field to another.

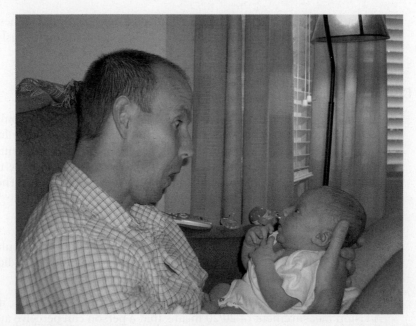

FIGURE 11.6 Newborns initially attend to faces, using the visual receptive skills that they have developed.

- *Stereopsis* refers to the monocular or binocular depth perception or three-dimensional vision.
- *Visual field* refers to the extent of physical space visible to an eye in a given position. Its average extent is approximately 65 degrees upward, 75 degrees downward, 60 degrees inward, and 95 degrees outward.

Visual Cognitive Functions

Visual cognitive functions include visual attention, visual memory, and visual discrimination.

- *Visual attention* is the ability to attend to visual stimuli. It involves alertness, selective attention, vigilance, and divided attention. A child develops long-term memory production that can be automatically executed without active attention, through practice and learning.
- *Visual memory* involves integrating visual processing information with past experience (both long term and short term). In short-term memory, the child uses a very small portion of his/her total knowledge base to recall visual information (Baddeley, 1986; Cowan, 1988). There are two general types of visual memory: domain-specific and procedural knowledge. Domain specific refers to memory of images, events, and facts. Procedural knowledge is a memory store for "how to" and includes strategies for accomplishing a task (Glover, Ronning, & Bruning, 1990). Encoding is the process of placing knowledge into memory.

- *Visual discrimination* is the ability to detect distinctive features of a visual stimulus and to distinguish whether the stimulus is different from or same as others. Visual discrimination involves recognition, matching, and sorting.

There are two main types of visual perception: object perception and spatial perception. Object perception is concerned with what things are. Object perception takes place in the temporal lobe of the brain. Object perception consists of form constancy, visual closure, and figure-ground perception. Spatial perception will be discussed after object perception.

- *Form constancy* is the recognition that forms and objects remain the same in various environments, positions, and sizes. It is the ability to see a form and being able to find it, even though the form may be smaller, larger, rotated, reversed, or hidden (Gardner, 1996). Form constancy helps a person develop stability and consistency in the visual world. It enables the person to recognize objects despite differences in orientation in detail. Form constancy enables a person to make assumptions regarding the size of an object, even though visual stimuli may vary under different circumstances. The visual image of an object in the distance is much smaller than the image of same object at close range, yet the person knows that the actual sizes are equivalent. For example, a school-aged child can identify the letter *A* whether it is typed, written in manuscript, written in cursive, written in upper or lower case letters, or italicized.
- *Visual closure* refers to the identification of forms or objects from incomplete presentations. This enables the child to recognize quickly objects, shapes, and forms by mentally completing the image or by matching it to information previously stored in memory. This allows the child to make assumptions regarding what the object is without having to see the complete presentation. For example, a child at his or her desk is able to distinguish a pencil from a pen, even though both are partly hidden under some papers.
- *Figure-ground perception* is the ability to perceive a form visually, and to find this form hidden in a conglomerated ground or model (Gardner, 1996); the differentiation between foreground or background, forms and objects. It is the ability to separate essential data from distracting surrounding information and the ability to attend to one aspect of a visual field while perceiving it in relation to the rest of the field. It is the ability to visually attend to what is important. For example, a child is visually able to find a favorite toy in a box filled with toys (Figure 11.7).

Spatial perception is being able to identify where things are in space. Spatial perception processing takes place in the parietal lobe. It involves position in space, spatial relations, depth perception, and topographic orientation (Figure 11.8).

- *Position in space* is the determination of the spatial relationship of figures and objects to oneself or other forms and objects. This provides the awareness of an object's position in relation to the observer or the perception of the direction in which it is turned. It is the discrimination of reversals and the rotations of figures (Hammill, Pearson, & Voress, 1993). The perceptual ability is important to understanding directional language concepts such as in, out, up, down, in front of, behind, between, left, and right. In addition, position in space perception provides the ability to differentiate

FIGURE 11.7 Toddler using figure-ground perception to find a toy in a toy box.

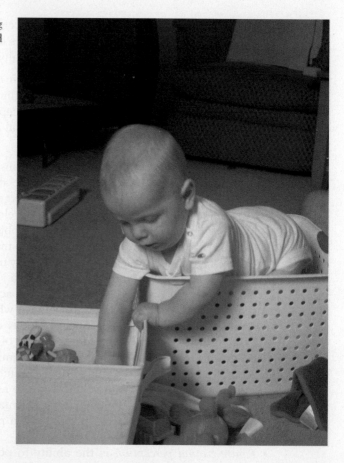

among letters and sequences of letters in a word or a sentence (Frostig, Lefever, & Whittlesey, 1966). For example, the child knows how to place letters equal spaces apart and touching the line; he or she is able to recognize letters that extend below the line, such as p, g, q, or y. Another aspect of spatial perception, now referred to as "object-focused spatial abilities," focuses on the spatial relations of objects irrespective of the individual (Voyer, Voyer, & Bryden, 1995). This includes skills evaluated by many formal assessments; however, poor performance of a formal test may or may not be linked to functional behavior.

- *Spatial relations* is the analysis of forms and patterns in relation to one's body and space and helps judge distances. There are two types: *categorical* which includes concepts of above/below, right/left, on/off and *coordinate* which specifies location in a way that can be used to guide precise movements.
- *Depth perception* refers to the determination of relative distance between objects, figures, or landmarks and the observer and changes in planes of surfaces. It is crucial to the child's ability to locate objects in the visual environment, to have accurate hand movements under visual guidance, and to function safely with tasks such as using

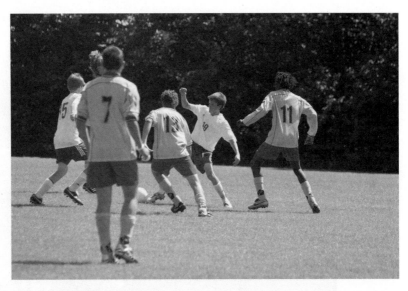

FIGURE 11.8 Teen using spatial perception to maneuver the soccer ball around opponents.

stairs or driving. This perceptual ability provides an awareness of how far something is, and it also helps move in space (e.g., walk down stairs).

* *Topographic orientation* is the determination and connection of the location of objects and settings and the route to the location. The ability to find one's way depends on a cognitive map of the environment. These maps include information about the destination, spatial information, instruction for execution of travel plans, recognition of places, keeping track of where one is while moving about, and anticipation of features. These are important means of monitoring one's movement from place to place (Dutton, 2002; Garling, Book, & Lindberg, 1984). In addition, the images that a person sees in the environment must be recognized and remembered if he or she is to make sense of what is viewed and if the individual is to find his or her way around (Dutton, 2002). For example, the child is able to leave the classroom for drinking water from the water fountain down the hall and return to his or her desk.

Visual Imagery/Visualization

Visual imagery/visualization is the necessary visual cognitive component that allows us to picture people, ideas, and objects in the mind's eye. It is important to reading comprehension and in planning, problem-solving, and organizational skills (Levine, 1994).

Eye–hand Coordination (Visual Motor Integration)

Eye–hand coordination (also called visual motor integration [VMI]) is the discrete motor skill that enables the coordination of the visual stimulus with the corresponding motor action (Law, Baum, & Dunn, 2005). Visual motor speed also depends on visual perception (Figure 11.9).

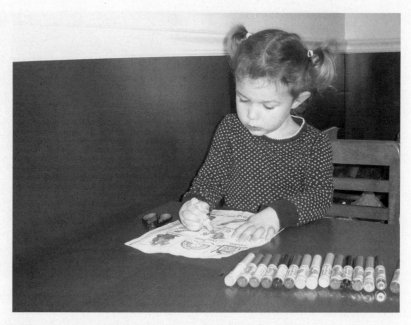

FIGURE 11.9 Toddle coloring using eye–hand coordination.

Dynamic Theory

Learning theories (Bandura, 1977; Rogers, 1951, 1957; Vygotsky, 1931) emphasize a child's development of visual analysis skills. The therapist provides a systematic method for identifying the pertinent, concrete features for form and spatial patterns, thereby enabling the child to recognize how new information relates to previously acquired knowledge based on similar and different attributes. The child learns to generalize to different tasks and therefore increasing occupational performance. Perceptual training programs use learning theories to remediate deficits.

In this frame of reference, the therapist uses the teaching–learning process and activity analysis and synthesis. The therapist first analyzes the skills that the child needs to learn. Then, the therapist models and shapes these behaviors through reinforcement until the child achieves mastery. Mastery of the skill provides its own reinforcement that allows the child to generalize that skill.

Task parameters should be considered which include environment, familiarity, directions, number of objects included, spatial arrangements, and response rate per object (Toglia, 1989). Parameters should initially be kept simple and then developed so that the child can handle multiple complex parameters. Task grading should also be considered through activity analysis. The environment can be structured in such a way as to provide the learner with the greatest likelihood of success. Practicing tasks in multiple environments helps increase generalization of the skill.

Modeling is the demonstration of a behavior or a skill (Figure 11.10). It is effective in promoting learning if the child is reinforced when the modeled behavior is imitated.

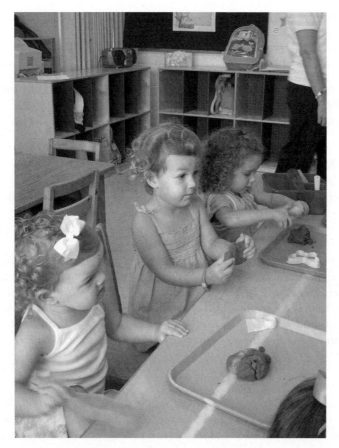

FIGURE 11.10 Children attending to a therapist modeling cutting shapes in play dough.

Modeling is used when the desired behavior or skill does not exist or when a complex skill does not yet exist in its entirety. From observing others, the child will form his or her idea of how response components must be combined and sequenced to the behavior. Later, this stored information will serve as the guideline for action. Modeling can have influence on learning primarily through formative function. Practicing the new behaviors can also help as a memory tool.

Learning can also be achieved through reinforcement. It serves as information and motivation in the learning process. Reinforcement for learning is essential and refers to the environmental stimulus that rewards or does not reward behavior. Reinforcement takes place through the environment, which includes the social and cultural context. It is used to encourage development of behaviors and skills and to shape them so that they will occur more frequently. Reinforcement that is given immediately following the desired behavior is a powerful method that can shape behavior automatically and unconsciously. It provides an effective means of regulating behaviors that have already been learned. The therapist can use words of praise or encouragement to foster skill development. Shaping means rewarding close approximations of a desired skill and is used when the skill does not exist. The therapist uses systematic cuing (Toglia, 1989) to guide the child during the teaching–learning process.

Three theoretical postulates underlie the dynamic theory of this frame of reference. They are as follows:

- Primary visual receptive skills form the foundation of all visual cognitive functions.
- Acquisition of skills is a result of reinforcement that results in learning.
- Behaviors result from environmental interaction.

FUNCTION–DYSFUNCTION CONTINUA

There are seven function–dysfunction continua found in this frame of reference.

Visual Reception Skills

Avoidance of visual work such as reading and visual fatigue are common problems seen when children have visual reception problems. When the child spends a lot of energy for visual motor activities, he or she may have little energy remaining for the visual cognitive piece of the activity. Visual reception skills are made up of two functions–dysfunction continua, oculomotor and visual reception skills. See Tables 11.2 and 11.3 for the function–dysfunction continua for oculomotor and visual reception skills.

Visual Attention

For visual perceptual skills, good visual attention is necessary so that the correct information can be attended to and then acted upon or stored in memory (Figure 11.11). Difficulty with attention can cause problems with spelling and letter formation. See Table 11.4 for indicators of visual attention dysfunction.

TABLE 11.2 Function–Dysfunction Continuum for Oculomotor Skills	
Proficient Oculomotor Skills	*Ineffective Oculomotor Skills*
FUNCTION: Efficient eye movements that ensure that the scan path is accomplished	*DYSFUNCTION*: Inefficient eye movements
Indicators of Function	**Indicators of Dysfunction**
Coordinated aiming of the eyes while shifting rapidly from one object to another (fixation)	Decreased ability to control and direct gaze
Able to visualize or focus on a stationary object (fixation)	
Visually fixate on a moving object (pursuit or tracking)	Turns head while reading across the page
	Loses place during reading
	Omits words
Able to change point of visual fixation from one point in the visual field to another rapidly (saccadic eye movements or scanning)	Overshoots or undershoots target
	Needs finger or marker to keep place

TABLE 11.3 Function–Dysfunction Continuum for Visual Reception	
Effective Visual Reception	*Difficulty with Visual Reception*
FUNCTION: Able to use vision accurately in terms of acuity, accommodation, binocularity, convergence, stereopsis, and visual field **Indicators of Function** Discriminates the fine details of objects in the visual field (acuity)	*DYSFUNCTION*: Unable to use vision accurately in terms of acuity, accommodation, binocularity, convergence, stereopsis, and visual field **Indicators of Dysfunction** Words blurry Holds book too closely Blinks frequently when engaging in visual work Squints to see chalkboard
Able to focus on an object at varying distances (accommodation) Combines the images from the two eyes into a single percept (binocularity)	Words blurry Lose place, missing important information Complains of seeing double Repeats letters within words Omits letters, numbers, or phrases Misaligns digits in number columns Squints, closes, or covers one eye Tilts head extremely while working at a desk Consistently show postural deviations at desk activities
Turns eyes inward as the object of regard moves toward the observer (convergence)	Excess—a condition in which the eyes have a tendency to turn inward rather than outward Insufficiency—a condition in which the eyes have a tendency to drift outward when being used for near work; the eyes work well at a far distance Eyestrain and discomfort
Monocular or binocular depth perception (stereopsis)	Difficulty with three-dimensional space
Awareness of visual physical space (visual field)	Runs into objects when walking Does not see a visual stimulus approaching

Visual Memory

Children with poor visual memory exhibit difficulty with spelling, mechanics of grammar, punctuation, capitalization, and the formulation of a sequential flow of ideas necessary for written communication. To write spontaneously one must be able to revisualize letters and words without visual cues; if visual memory problems exist, the child may have difficulty recalling the shape and formation of letters and numbers. There may be small and capital letters missing within a sentence, the same letter may be written in different ways on the same page, he or she may demonstrate the inability to print the alphabet from memory, legibility may be poor, and the child may need a model to write. Visual sequential memory was found to be one of the best predictors for handwriting speed and for children with handwriting dysfunction (Tseng & Chow, 2000). See Table 11.5 for indicators of function and dysfunction.

FIGURE 11.11 Toddler demonstrating good visual attention toward a picture book so that information can be stored in memory.

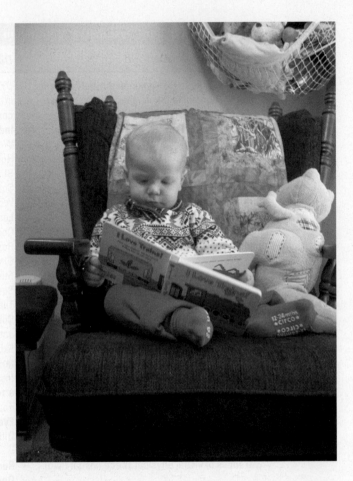

Visual Discrimination

There is a finite set of visual operations or routines used to extract shape properties and spatial relationships. Children usually orient to the top or bottom of an object to recognize it. Visual recognition is a breakdown of the active feature-by-feature analysis necessary for interpretation of a visual image. If a child demonstrates poor recognition of letters or numbers, then he or she may show poor letter formation in handwriting. Decoding ability, which utilizes form constancy, is the single best predictor of reading comprehension (Tui, Thompson, & Lewis, 2003). Reversals of letters and numbers occurring after age 7 often indicate poor visual discrimination especially in form constancy. An object recognition problem may indicate that the child is fixated on one portion of an object and not seeing the whole. For example, because of the difficulty in shifting visual attention to another aspect of the object or environmental scene, the child may miss essential features. In adults, visual agnosia is a disorder of recognition. The individual can identify objects by touch, but is unable to recognize objects visually

TABLE 11.4 Function–Dysfunction Continuum for Visual Attention

Visually Attends	*Difficulty Visually Attending*
FUNCTION: Visually attentive	*DYSFUNCTION*: Poor visual attention
Indicators of Function	**Indicators of Dysfunction**
Visually attentive to people and objects	Focus may be on irrelevant information
	Easily confused
	Difficulty screening out unimportant or irrelevant information
	Cannot see, recognize, or isolate salient features and therefore does not know how to focus attention
Explores and selects relevant visual information	Overattentiveness
Screens out irrelevant information	• Easily distracted
	• Does not attend long enough for memory
	• Overly focused on irrelevant information
	Underattention
	• Difficulty orienting to visual stimuli
	• May habituate quickly to a visual stimulus
	• Fatigues easily
	• Poor sustained attention
Concentrates on a visual stimulus (vigilance)	Reduced persistence at a task
	Difficulty maintaining visual attention
Focuses on two different stimuli at the same time (divided attention)	Can focus only on one task at a time

TABLE 11.5 Function–Dysfunction Continuum for Visual Memory

Remembers Visual Information	*Difficulty Remembering Visual Information*
FUNCTION: Ability to retain and use visual information	*DYSFUNCTION*: Difficulty retaining and retrieving visual information
Indicators of Function	**Indicators of Dysfunction**
Mentally manipulates visual information	Fails to attend adequately, which is needed for storage of visual memory
Retains information in memory for immediate recall or to store for later retrieval	Poor or reduced ability to recognize, match, or retrieve visual information
	Poor handwriting
	Prolonged response time
	Inconsistent recall abilities
	Letter reversals
Good memory for "how to" (domain-specific memory)	Poor memory of images, events, and facts
Good memory of images, events, and facts (procedural memory)	Poor memory for "how to"
Proficient visual sequential memory	Poor strategies for accomplishing a task
	Decreased handwriting speed
Stores visual information into memory (encoding)	Trouble storing visual information into memory
	Poor ability to use mnemonic strategies for storage

TABLE 11.6 Function–Dysfunction Continuum for Object (Form) Discrimination	
FUNCTION: Ability to percieve what things are	*DYSFUNCTION*: Unable to percieve what things are
Indicators of Function	**Indicators of Dysfunction**
Form constancy	Difficulty recognizing letter or words in different print, sizes, or in different environments
	May have difficulty copying from a different type of print or handwriting
	May not recognize errors in own handwriting and is not able to make corrections
	Letter and number reversals
Visual closure	May be unable to identify a form or object if an incomplete presentation is made
Figure ground	Difficulty perceiving an object that is not well defined, such as an object in a purse or drawer or visually confusing environments such as supermarkets
	May overattend to details and miss the big picture
	Overlook details and miss information
	Trouble attending to a word on a printed page because of inabiliy to block out the other words
	Poor visual search strategies
	Difficulty finding the sleeve on an all white shirt

despite normal visual acuity. This can occur in children as well. See Table 11.6 for indicators of function/dysfunction.

Visual Spatial

These skills are used to interact with and organize the environment. Visual spatial skills develop from an awareness of one's body concepts such as right/left, up/down, and front/back. The understanding of left/right is called "laterality," and directionality is the understanding of an external objects position in space in relation to himself or herself. This understanding allows the child to handle spatial phenomena in a visual manner. See Table 11.7 for the function–dysfunction continuum of visual spatial skills.

Visual Motor Integration

Motor skills of posture, mobility, and coordination may be affected by poor visual skills. Process skills of knowledge, temporal organization, organization of space and objects, and adaptation all can be affected by visual perception thus affecting VMI. Visual perceptual difficulties also affect the child's ability to use tools and relate materials to one another. The child may show problems with cutting with scissors, coloring, constructing with blocks or other construction toys, doing puzzles, using fasteners in dressing, and tying shoes (Figure 11.12). Of the seven subtests of the Test of Visual Perceptual Skills (TVPS), a common test used by OTs, deficits on the subtest of visual memory and visual spatial relationships seem to be most likely related to visual motor difficulties (O'Brien, Cermak, & Murray, 1988; Parush et al., 1998).

TABLE 11.7 Function–Dysfunction Continuum for Visual Spatial Skills

FUNCTION: Uses visual skills to interact with and organize the environment **Indicators of Function**	*DYSFUNCTION*: Does not use visual skills efficiently to interact with and organize the environment **Indicators of Dysfunction**
Position in space	Reversal of letters and numbers after 9 yr of age
	Reversal error in order of words and numbers
	Trouble discriminating among objects because of their placement in space
	Difficulty planning actions in relation to objects
	Letter reversals
	Writing and spacing letters and words on a page
	Difficult understanding directional language
Spatial relations	Left to right progression or writing words and sentences
	Overspacing or underspacing, trouble keeping in the margins
	Inconsistency in letter size and placement of letters on a line
	Inability to adapt letter sized to the space provided on the paper or worksheet
	Trouble orienting in the environment
Depth perception	Difficulty moving in space
	Difficulty recognizing the surface plane has changed
	Difficulty catching a ball
	Sorting and organizing personal belongings
Topographic orientation	Difficulty finding one's way in the environment
	Easily lost
	Difficulty determining the location of objects and settings

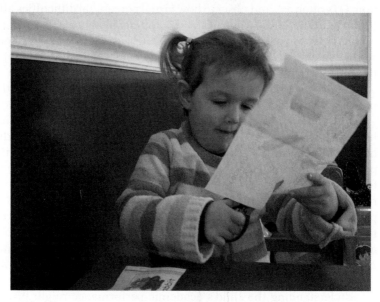

FIGURE 11.12 Preschooler showing oral motor overflow while using a tool in a visual motor task.

TABLE 11.8 Function–Dysfunction Continuum for Visual Motor Integration	
FUNCTION: Able to use vision to accurately perform motor tasks	*DYSFUNCTION*: Unable to use vision to perform motor tasks
Indicators of Function	**Indicators of Dysfunction**
Legible handwriting	Inability to copy letters and forms legibly
Skillfully build with blocks and Legos	Difficulty building with blocks and Legos
Adequate speed for visual motor activities	Decreased speed in visual motor activities

Handwriting is a VMI skill used by school-aged children. Factors associated with handwriting legibility are visual perception, eye–hand coordination, and VMI. Visual sequential memory was a significant predictor of handwriting speed (Feder et al., 2005). See Table 11.8 for indicators of function/dysfunction in VMI.

Visual perceptual problems can affect all aspects of the child's life and occupations. For instance, in ADL the child may have difficulty obtaining the supplies needed for grooming, such as using a brush and mirror to style hair, applying toothpaste to the toothbrush, fasteners, and matching clothes to name a few. Playing games with other children can be difficult because of the visual perception skills needed. Helping with the chores such as sorting and folding clothes may be impossible.

GUIDE FOR EVALUATION

To identify visual perceptual factors that limit occupational performance and participation, OTs often ask and observe how visual perceptual difficulties affect daily occupations (Chan & Chow, 2005), thus utilizing a top-down approach. Through the evaluation process, OTs try to determine the possible causes and types of visual perceptual dysfunction so that an effective intervention plan can be developed. It is helpful to start the evaluation process with a screening to determine the primary problem areas. Because of the complexity of visual perception, it is important to use various methods in the evaluation process including observation, review of history, and standardized tests.

One of the first steps in the screening process would be to review the child's medical history. It would be useful to determine if an ophthalmic or ophthalmologic evaluation has been done on the child and if there are any medical conditions that could affect performance in this area. Although a screening performed by the OT is not a substitute for a comprehensive examination by a vision professional, it can help establish the need for such an examination and also help the therapist to plan his or her therapy program, taking vision into consideration. Furthermore, if and when visual deficits have been properly diagnosed, the therapist could develop supportive, compensatory, and/or instructional strategies to help improve the child's performance within his visual capacities (Scheiman, 1997). Assessments that are used by OTs to assess visual reception skills are presented in Table 11.9.

Understanding the child's academic performance might provide some insight into the possibility of visual perceptual problems. Performing clinical observations of the

TABLE 11.9	Instruments to Assess Visual Reception		
Instrument	*Ages*	*Areas Assessed*	*Reliability and Validity*
Erhardt Development Vision Assessment (Erhardt, 1989)	Fetal—6 mo	Reflexive visual patterns; voluntary eye movements of localization, fixation, ocular pursuit, and gaze shift	Good interrater reliability; no test–retest reliability, construct and discriminate validity found
Visual Skills Appraisal (Richards & Oppenheim, 1987)	5–9 yr	Pursuit, scanning, alignment, and locating movements; hand–eye coordination; fixation unity	Information on reliability or validity not found
Pediatric Clinical Vision Screening for Occupational Therapists (Scheiman, 2002)	School age	Accommodation, acuity, binocular vision, ocular motility, refraction, visual field, visual information processing	Information on reliability or validity not found
Crane–Wick Test (Crane & Wick, 1987)	K-12 grades	Accommodation Saccadic eye movement Near point of convergence Eye teaming Pursuit of movement Visual processing Functional hearing	Information on reliability or validity not found

child's visual perceptual skills would also be useful. This can be done by watching a child engage in carefully selected play activities or functional tasks, such as creating block and pegboard designs, playing with Legos, drawing and writing, dressing activities, playing computer games, looking for hidden pictures in a confusing background, playing ball, and doing puzzles (Mulligan, 2003). Observations of procedural knowledge (strategies for accomplishing a task) and verbal-kinesthetic strategy (verbal, tactile, and motor strategies for accomplishing a task), to name a few, can also be observed (Figure 11.13). Cultural influences should always be considered in the evaluation process (Josman, Abdallah, & Engle-Yeger, 2006). It would also be helpful to observe the child in some academic tasks within a classroom setting, especially if the referral indicated that academic performance is a problem area. Interviews can also be used to determine where perceived problems are, or to find out how visual problems may be interfering with functional performance. Interviews should include the parents and/or care providers, and classroom teachers.

The second step in the evaluation process is to generate and test hypotheses to determine factors that support or hinder the child's ability to engage successfully in valued occupations (Mulligan, 2003). As the therapist proceeds with the evaluation process, a bottom-up approach following the developmental hierarchy of visual perception can be used to determine the types of deficits that are contributing to problems in occupations. Some norm-referenced tests are usually used in addition to interviews

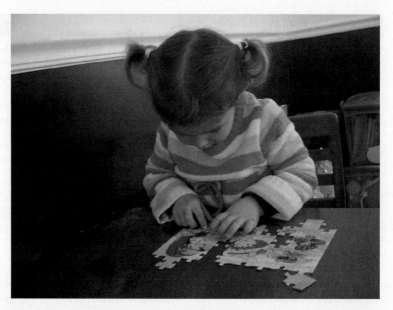

FIGURE 11.13 Observation of a child doing puzzles to assess procedural knowledge for accomplishing the task.

and clinical observations. There are various assessments developed to assist the OT. The visual perceptual instruments most frequently used by OTs are briefly reviewed in Table 11.10. This table provides assessments, the age ranges that they are appropriate for, and the specific areas assessed, so that the therapist can choose the most appropriate tool for use with the child.

Visual Spatial Assessment

Many of the instruments reviewed earlier also assess visual spatial skills. The assessments reviewed here only measure aspects of visual spatial skills. The Jordon Left–Right Reversal Test, Revised (Jordon, 1980) is a standardized test that can be administered individually or in a group. It is untimed and takes approximately 20 minutes to administer and score. The Reversals Frequency Test is a simple, easy-to-administer test devised to determine whether a child exhibits an abnormal number of letter or number reversals. See Table 11.11 for instruments to assess visual spatial skills.

Visual Motor Integration Assessments

The *Developmental Test of Visual Motor Integration* (VMI, Beery, Buktenica, & Beery, 2004), the Wide Range Assessment of Visual Motor Abilities (Adams & Sheslow, 1995), Test of Visual Motor Skills (TVMS, Gardner, 1995), the *Slosson Visual Motor Performance Test for Children and Adults* (Slosson & Nicholson, 1996), and the *Test of Visual Analysis*

TABLE 11.10 Instruments to Assess Visual Perception			
Instrument	*Ages*	*Areas Assessed*	*Reliability and Validity*
Developmental Test of Visual Perception, Second Edition (DTVP-2, Hammill, Pearson, & Voress, 1993)	4–10 yr	Eye–hand coordination Visual spatial relations Visual figure ground Visual motor speed Copying Position in space Visual closure Visual form constancy	Strong normative data Internal consistency for three composite scales were above 0.93 Test–retest reliability for a 2-wk interval 0.71–0.86 across subtests, 0.89–0.94 for composite scores Interrater reliability coefficients 0.87–0.94 across subtests, 0.95–0.97 for composite scores Concurrent validity between DTVP-2 motor items and VMI (0.89)
Motor-Free Visual Perception Test-Third Edition (MVPT-3, Colarusso & Hammill, 2003)	4–11 yr	Visual discrimination Visual memory Visual spatial relations Visual figure ground Visual closure	High test–retest reliability ($r = 0.81$) and internal validity ($r = 0.88$) Criterion validity determined relative to academic performance ($r = 0.38$) and intelligence ($r = 0.31$)
Test of Visual Perceptual Skills-Revised (TVPS-R, Gardner, 1997)	4–12.11 yr	Visual discrimination Visual memory Visual form constancy Visual spatial relationships Visual sequential memory Visual figure ground Visual closure	Test–retest reliability 0.33–0.78; 0.81 for total test (Brown, Rodger, & Davis, 2003) Content validity, test–retest reliability (Chan & Chow, 2005)
Test of Visual Perceptual Skills Upper Limits (TVPS-UL, Gardner, 1997)	12–18 yr	Visual discrimination Visual memory Visual form constancy Visual sequential memory Visual figure ground Visual closure	Cronbach's α coefficients 0.81–0.89 Reliability coefficient across all age levels was 0.86 Concurrent validity based on correlations with Bender Visual Motor Gestalt (0.31–0.81), DTVMI (0.46–0.64), TVMS-R (0.70)
Test of Pictures, Forms, Letters, Numbers, Spatial Orientation and Sequencing Skills (Gardner, 1997)	5–8 yr	Ability to perceive visual forms, letters, and numbers in the correct direction and sequence for words	Split-half reliability coefficients (0.10)–(0.95) Item validity ($rs = 0.14$–0.27)

(continued)

TABLE 11.10 (Continued)			
Instrument	*Ages*	*Areas Assessed*	*Reliability and Validity*
Sensory Integration and Praxis Tests (Ayres, 1989)	4–8.11 yr	Space visualization Figure ground Design copy construction Praxis	Interrater reliability (0.94–0.99) Content validity
Miller Assessment for Pre-schoolers (MAP, Miller, 1988)	2.9–5.8 yr	Figure ground Puzzle Eye–hand coordination Block design Object memory Draw a person	Interrater reliability (0.98) Test–retest reliability (0.81)

VMI, visual motor integration; TVMS-R, Test of Visual Motor Skills-Revised; DTVMI, Developmental Test of Visual Motor Integration.

Skills (Rosner & Fern, 1983) are used to assess VMI skills. These assessments will be briefly reviewed.

The *Developmental Test of Visual Motor Integration*, Fifth Edition, Revised (2004) (VMI) is a norm-referenced design copy test for ages 2 to 18 (full form) and 2 to 7 (short form). There are two additional optional subtests: (1) visual perception and (2) motor coordination. This test can be administered individually or in groups.

The *Wide Range Assessment of Visual Motor Abilities* (Adams & Sheslow, 1995) is an individually administered test taking approximately 15 to 25 minutes. Raw scores are converted to standard scores.

Test of Visual Motor Skills—Revised (TVMS, Gardner, 1995) is a norm-referenced design copy test. It is quick and easy to administer. The test is unique in that the types of errors are classified and scored to give qualitative information.

Test of Visual Analysis Skills (Rosner & Fern, 1983) is an untimed, individually administered, criterion reference test. The purpose is to assess if the child is able to determine the relationships necessary for integrating letter and word shapes. See Table 11.12 for age ranges, areas assessed, and psychometric information of these assessments.

TABLE 11.11 Instruments to Assess Visual Spatial Skills			
Instrument	*Ages*	*Areas Assessed*	*Reliability and Validity*
Jordon Left-Right Reversal Test, Third Revised Edition (Jordon, 1980)	5–12 yr	Reversals of letters, numbers, and words	Test–retest reliability (0.90)
Reversals Frequency Test (Gardner, 1978).	5–15 yr	Execution—write letters in lower case as dictated Recognition Matching	Information on reliability or validity not found

TABLE 11.12 Instruments to Assess Visual Motor Integration

Instrument	Ages	Areas Assessed	Reliability and Validity
The Developmental Test of Visual Motor Integration, Fifth Edition, Revised (VMI, Beery, Buktenica, & Beery, 2004)	2–18 yr	Three subtests	Test–retest (0.89), interrater (0.92), and internal ($r = 0.92$) reliability
Wide Range Assessment of Visual Motor Abilities (Adams & Sheslow, 1995)	3–17 yr	Drawing Matching Pegboard	Internal consistency (1.00–0.92) Test–retest correlation (0.86)
Test of Visual Motor Skills—Revised (TVMS-R, Gardner, 1995)	2–13 yr	Design copy	Reliability coefficients across all age levels was 0.86 Concurrent validity (0.23–0.48)
The Slosson Visual Motor Performance Test for Children and Adults (Slosson & Nicholson, 1996)	—	Screening test for perceptual organization and eye–hand coordination	Internal consistency (0.93) Test–retest reliability (0.97) Concurrent validity (0.59–0.64)
Test of Visual Analysis Skills (Rosner, 1983)	5–10 yr	Copying simple to complex geometric patterns	Validity (0.79–0.83)

POSTULATES REGARDING CHANGE

There are three general postulates regarding change in this frame of reference:

1. The therapist will create an environment that will facilitate the development of visual perceptual skills in accordance with the child's age and abilities.
2. Visual cognitive skills are facilitated through the use of teaching learning principles for remediation.
3. The therapist creates an environment that fosters the development of component parts of skills or specific skills.

There are six specific postulates regarding change for this frame of reference:

1. The development of visual receptive skills influences visual cognitive skills, which will result in the child's improved ability to engage in meaningful occupations.
2. Visual cognitive skills improve in an environment where there is modeling of a desired behavior and immediate reinforcement to the child regarding desired behavior.
3. The integration of lower level skills, such as visual attention, will develop higher level skills in visual reception and visual cognition, such as visual memory.
4. The integration of lower level skills, such as visual memory, will facilitate the development of higher level skills, such as visual discrimination.
5. The development of visual discrimination facilitates the development of visual spatial skills and VMI.

6. The therapist creates an environment that allows the child to use compensatory skills and environmental strategies to aid in visual cognitive skills and engaging in resulting occupations.

APPLICATION TO PRACTICE

Treatment planning requires an understanding of the underlying reasons for difficulty as well as a delineation of the conditions that influence performance (Toglia, 1989). A remedial approach focuses on the impairment underlying the vision problem, following the developmental process. An adaptive approach facilitates improved function through compensation using cognition. Compensation is any practical environmental adjustment such as assistance from others, training procedures that are activity or situation specific, and strategies and environmental adaptations (Zoltan, 1996). This approach provides training in the actual occupations meaningful to the child. Both approaches may be used in treatment.

Remediation, strategy use, and environmental adaptations are tools for treatment. With remediation, the goal is to improve deficit skills. It can involve intervention of underlying causes, or structured practice of specific skills so that these skills can develop and become more automatic (Gentile, 1997). Strategy use overlaps with remediation because certain deficits may be because of ineffective strategy use. Strategies for search, scanning, attention, monitoring work, and encoding information can be taught. While using strategies, environmental changes can be made to assist the individual to improve performance or function. Additionally, a therapist may change and make accommodations to the task so that success is possible. Sometimes, the child's performance is dependent on the environmental adaptations, and therefore the child's skills have not actually improved, as the accommodations are external to the child.

The child, his or her parents, teachers, and caregivers may need to be educated about the child's deficits and the intervention strategies. This can be very helpful throughout the intervention process. This education helps make those involved with the child aware of his or her limitations and the functional implications of the visual perceptual problems. Education also helps others to view the child in a different way. For example, rather than insisting that the child is lazy, they would recognize the problem and then could aid with cues or environmental adaptations.

Figure 11.5 earlier in the chapter presents the visual processing model and a guide to where these treatment approaches (remediation, strategies, and environmental adaptations) can be used. The following section presents treatment approaches following the visual processing model beginning with input.

Input: Environmental Adaptations

Visual input can be influenced by the context and the activity demands and should be considered in designing treatment activities. For example, the lighting should be adequate, but should not cause a glare on the workspace. When children are visually distracted in the classroom, one easy approach is to work with the teacher to make the classroom less busy visually, thereby increasing visual attention. The therapist might also suggest that child be positioned closer to the board so that objects on the sides of the classroom are not in his or her direct visual field. If a child has visual memory issues, the therapist can suggest to the teacher that drawers are labeled and that a cue card be made with directions for frequent tasks within the classroom. When a child has problems with topographical orientation, the therapist can suggest the use of landmarks to the child or suggest that signs with high color contrast be used in the environment.

Some suggestions for environmental adaptations to the activity demands include the following:

- Choosing activities that are motivating for the specific child
- Using manual activities that will encourage the child to view the movements; hand movements help educate the eye about object qualities
- Progressing the activity from simple to complex
- Variation of the task parameters to encourage variability of practice (Lesensky & Kaplan, 2000)
- Random and variable practice
- Part practice is more efficient for complex tasks such as dressing
- Whole practice is important for integrated timing in tasks such as handwriting.

Processing: Remediation of Visual Reception

The developmental model proposed by Warren (1993a,b) suggests that higher level skills evolve from integration of lower level skills. Remediation treatment would begin where the deficit is located lowest in the hierarchy (Figure 11.3). The therapist would design treatment strategies to remediate basic problems to improve perceptual function. If deficits occur at the foundational level, then activities to improve oculomotor skills would be incorporated into the treatment. Optometry and occupational therapy could collaborate on common goals related to the effects of vision on performance. Once oculomotor skills are efficient, treatment should proceed from attention to memory to visual discrimination. For example, general sensory stimulation or inhibition may be provided prior to visual activities to improve visual attention.

Processing: Remediation of Visual Cognition

The remedial approach utilizes repeated drills and exercises, in a teaching–learning environment, which are aimed at specific cognitive processes. It also assumes that occupations are composed of subcomponents which can be "remediated by a building block approach that emphasizes improvement in the hierarchical subcomponents to allow the structure of occupational performance to be reconstructed" (Zemke, 1994, p. 25).

The therapist uses specific techniques to promote remediation. These include setting task parameters, task grading, modeling, and reinforcement to encourage learning. Task parameters would involve using familiar objects, ensuring that directions are clear and structuring the environment to minimize distractions. The therapist can also consider limiting the number of objects used and the spatial arrangement of objects to help the child focus on the tasks at hand. The therapist might also limit the response rate per object (Toglia, 1989). The therapist would focus on simplifying the task until the child develops the skill to handle multiple parameters. Once the child develops more skill, the therapist can use activity analysis to grade the task to provide more challenges for the child. The environment for intervention should be structured to promote the greatest chance of success for the child. Once this occurs then similar tasks can be practiced in multiple environments to increase the potential for generalizing the skill.

Modeling and practice are remedial approaches that therapists use to develop visual cognition skills. Modeling involves demonstrating a behavior or a skill that the child can then imitate. Once the child imitates the behavior or skills, reinforcement will promote learning. This technique is used when a desired behavior or skill does not exist or when the therapist is trying to build a more complex skill from a rudimentary skill. The child will develop the ability to respond to various stimuli and situations based on the observation of therapist and other children who have already mastered these skills. The child can learn to combine and sequence skills and behaviors. Repetition helps the child to learn and store the information, so that it can be used later as a guide for action. Modeling provides the formative learning, whereas practicing new behaviors can reinforce the behaviors and serve as a memory tool.

Positive reinforcement is important in the learning process of visual cognitive skills. Reinforcement provides the child with feedback and serves as a motivation for the child. Positive reinforcement refers to the response that the therapist or the environment provides to reward positive responses. Such reinforcement may be made by the therapist, teacher, or vary depending on the social or cultural context. It encourages the development of behaviors and skills, and can be used to shape behaviors so that they occur more frequently or in a more appropriate manner. Reinforcement may be provided in various ways. If it is given immediately following the desired behavior, it can be very powerful and can have an automatic or unconscious effect on resultant behaviors. Reinforcement can also be a very effective way of regulating behaviors that have been previously learned. Words of praise can also foster skill development. Rewarding close approximations of a desired skill is called "shaping." This is also useful in developing skills and behaviors. Additionally, the therapist might use systematic cuing (Toglia, 1989) to assist the child during teaching–learning process. Different types of cues are presented in Table 11.13.

In the teaching–learning process, investigative questioning is another approach that can be used by the therapist to develop visual cognitive skills. After a correct response is obtained by the child, investigative questioning is used by the therapist to ask the child to explain his or her answer. The therapist should also consider when it is appropriate to permit a second try, prompt, demonstrate, extend or remove time limits, impose time limits, and change instruction and presentation (Gentile, 2005). Learning involves unobservable cognitive or mental processes such as memory and attention. Learning can be facilitated by the use of a multisensory approach. The child can benefit from using tactile input to learn shapes, letters, and numbers. By using textures, the child has additional sensory experiences. For example, letters can be formed with clay, sandpaper, beads, or pipe cleaners.

TABLE 11.13 Systematic Cueing (Toglia, 1989)	
Repetition cue	Child is asked to "look again" which indicates the child was incorrect. Observe if child can self-correct
Analysis cue	Therapist asks the child to describe further the form or object; assists the child to pay closer attention
Perceptual cue	Therapist emphasizes the critical feature of the form or object
Semantic cue	Therapist provides a choice of three categories

Additionally, there are many excellent educational computer programs that are highly motivating for children of all ages and can be used as part of an intervention approach. Computer programs have been designed to assess processing as well as increase reaction time, visual scanning, attention, speed of information, memory, and problem solving.

Processing: Visual Reception Strategies

Suggestions for visual reception strategy use include the following:

- Left to right searching
- Finger to follow lines in reading
- Ruler to keep place on a worksheet
- Close eyes frequently to rest to prevent visual fatigue
- Organized movement for scanning the environment to gather information

Processing: Visual Cognition: Strategies

Strategies are cognitive processes that support successful performance of visual cognition skills (Pressley et al., 1990). It has been shown that good strategy users are more successful with visual cognitive tasks. Children can be taught problem-solving strategies and then they are enabled to discover additional strategies that will support their skill acquisition. There are three types of strategies: domain-specific or goal-specific strategies that achieve a specific part of the task, monitoring strategies that evaluate the success of the strategy, and higher order or global strategies that are used to control and coordinate other strategies (Pressley et al., 1990).

Domain-specific or goal-specific strategies are often used for a short time and are often task or situation specific (Polatajko & Mandich, 2004). These are taught to the child by the therapist. They are used to solve specific performance issues as they arise. Situational strategies (Toglia, 1989) can be domain or goal specific. These could include the following:

- *Scanning*: Learning organized movement for scanning the environment to gather information.

- *Visual imagery*: Visualizing what one is looking for before initiating a visual search allows the child to have a visual image of what he or she is looking for.
- *Organization*: Organizing visual information in the environment whenever possible.
- *Visual analysis*: Silently verbalizing specific characteristics to help ascertain the meaning or function of the object (Toglia, 1989). This might include the shape, size, and thickness of an object. This process is similar to verbal mediation.

Todd (1999) suggested giving specific attention to the distinctive features of a visual stimulus (letters and numbers) through highlighting and verbal enabling to enhance visual discrimination learning. Verbal enabling involves emphasizing these characteristics of a visual stimulus through verbal, visual, kinesthetic, and tactical cues and referring to other familiar objects that have the same distinctive features. The child then uses the strategy of emphasizing distinctive features of letters and numbers and then memorizing them. Verbal labeling involves using speech to provide a name to a visual stimulus. This helps to also provide another type of input to be paired with the visual stimulus.

Strategies that can be used to increase visual attention include the following:

- Taking time-outs from a task
- Attending to the whole situation before attending to the parts
- Searching the whole scene before responding
- Monitoring the tendency to become distracted
- Devising time–pressure management strategies

The importance of getting the correct visual information for learning cannot be overemphasized. First the child needs to have good attention to the task, which allows the visual information to be stored in memory. Memory strategies are described in Table 11.14.

Monitoring strategies that can be taught to the child which can be used for self-monitoring a visual perceptual task are described by Toglia (1989). These strategies include the following:

- *Anticipation*: This is learning to predict potential difficulty in certain situations. The correct anticipation of problems leads to the ability to plan and initiate the use of strategies by the child.

TABLE 11.14 Memory Strategies

Chunking	Organizing information into smaller units, for example, cutting up worksheets and presenting one task at a time Information can be categorized or held together by some meaningful association to be stored in memory
Maintenance rehearsal	Repetition and practice
Elaborative rehearsal	New information is consciously related to knowledge already stored in long-term memory
Mnemonic devices	Helps organize information to enhance the retrievability through use of language cues such as songs, rhythms, and acronyms

- *Checking outcomes*: Interpretations are double-checked, which then allows the child to correct errors.
- *Pacing*: Learning when to slow down or speed up while doing tasks that require visual cognitive analysis.
- *Stimulus reduction*: Reducing the amount of visual information to be perceived at one time (Toglia, 1989).

Processing: Environmental Adaptations for Visual Reception

Modifications to the environment can be made to promote improved functioning and mitigate the child's limitations. Reducing glare can be useful for children with visual perceptual disorders. Some ways to limit glare are as follows:

- Change the lighting in the room, but ensure that the lighting is still good
- Modify the desk height or tilt the surface so that the child is properly positioned with limited glare
- Using pastel colored paper
- Recommend that the chalkboard be regularly cleaned

Other environmental adaptations to increase visual reception include the following:

- Providing visual stimuli that will assist the child to direct his or her attention
- Using a carrel to limit peripheral vision for a child who is distractible
- Limit the visual information that is presented at one time
- Using color-coded worksheets
- Placing a black mat under the worksheet to increase visual attention
- Using a "mask" that covers everything but the item on which the child needs to focus
- Moving closer to the board
- Columns for aligning numbers for math problems

Visual Cognition: Environmental Adaptations

Classroom materials or instructional materials and methods can be modified to accommodate the child's limitations and promote improved functioning. One of the primary modifications would be to promote increased visual attention through the reduction of potential visual distractions. Some examples of this would be as follows:

- Drawing lines on worksheets to group information to increase focusing
- Reorganizing worksheets using larger print or more space between areas requiring attention
- Cuing the child to important information by pointing, underlining with a marker, or verbalization
- Using the computer for specific activities

There are various adaptations that can be made to classroom and instructional materials to promote increased memory skills. Some examples are providing consistent experiences for the child; using consistent visualization activities as cues for encoding materials; and using various memory aids, such a notebooks, assignment pads, hand-help computers or calculators, tape recorders, etc.

Adaptations used in the classroom or with instructional materials that can be helpful in developing an understanding of spatial relations are as follows:

- Using graph paper for math examples, which help with spatially aligning numbers
- Placing visual cues on paper to indicate where a child should start and stop when writing
- Using a slant board at a desk to promote upright orientation may decrease directional confusion
- Pairing directional cues with verbal cues can decrease letter reversals
- Teaching the child to use his or her finger as a spacer between words

The following are some examples of classroom or instruction adaptations that can be used to promote shape, letter, and number recognition:

- Using a multisensory approach, where the child can employ a combination of sensory experiences including, but not limited to, feeling, tasting, and saying letters and numbers
- Forming letters with various tactile materials such as clay in sand with beads or with pudding
- Devising activities that move from simple to complex
- Using activities that include drawing, painting, and crafts to encourage exploration and manipulation of visual forms

Output: Remediations of Performance Skills

Vision is essential for integrating gross, fine, and oculomotor control. Gross motor components of balance, postural control are needed to support fine motor dexterity. Erhardt & Duckman (2005) suggest the following to improve visual motor skills:

- Selection of meaningful functional tasks
- Preparation of the therapeutic environment to encourage the child to initiate and explore materials and then structural tasks to ensure success
- Use of appropriate handling techniques
- Verbal and manual assistance
- Teach using the child's preferred sensory modes of learning
- Provide opportunities for practice and generalization

Motor skills such as posture, mobility, and eye–hand coordination or VMI should be addressed by the OT during intervention. Other frames of reference that appear in this text may be appropriate here. When working on remediation of performance skills, it is important to consider temporal organization and the energy for pacing and attending to visual tasks. Therapists must also consider the tools that are used during performance. A child must know the tool, its properties, and how it is used. Finally, the therapist must create an environment that supports performance by address and adapting the organization of the workspace and the objects within that environment.

Output: Strategies for Performance

The therapist works with the child to develop performance strategies that will help the child to be successful. One strategy is to give the child verbal step-by-step directions that describes how to complete the task. Included in these directions are motor and visual expectations of the task. It also includes organizing the workspace and the objects within to support performance. For example, when working on handwriting, the therapist designs the workspace, selects the writing implement, and gives the child verbal instructions on how to complete the task. The therapist should monitor the amount of energy needed to complete the task and should adjust the task demands accordingly. As the child progresses, therapist input decreases and the child should begin to self-evaluate his or her performance.

Output: Strategies for Occupation

Occupational therapy is concerned with performance in daily life and how performance affects engagement in occupations to support participation. Treatment is designed around what is important and meaningful to the child. Therefore, goals are created in collaboration with the child to address the targeted outcomes (Figure 11.14).

Practice of children's occupations with monitoring is important. Practice of an occupation progresses from the cognitive to the associative to autonomous stage following motor learning principles. The cognitive stage is the initial encoding of the instructions and cognitive attention is given to all aspects of the task. The associative stage shows improved performance with gradual detection and elimination of errors.

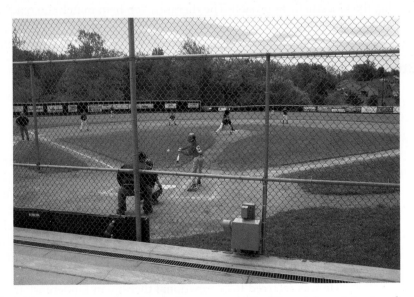

FIGURE 11.14 Participating in a baseball game, meaningful social participation for a child, involving visual perception.

During the autonomous stage, gradual improvement is seen. Practice in ADL, such as dressing and functional mobility, and instrumental activities of daily living (IADL), such as communication devices (computer and text messaging on the cell phone), community mobility, financial management, and meal preparation, will be needed at various stages of development. Work is begun in prevocational and vocational activities in school and at home. Often creative strategies to accomplish tasks are needed such as color coding of clothing, use of labels so that shirts are not put on backwards or inside out, various methods for tying shoes, sorting utensils, and grooming. Strategies can be used to help accomplish these tasks such as always putting keys in the same place so that one can find them.

Strategies may be used for education occupations such as mathematics (solving geometry problems), reading, and handwriting. For students who experience visual motor difficulties and therefore have poor handwriting ability, Chwirka, Gurney, & Burtner (2002) suggested that keyboarding may be a tool to assist individuals. Lee (2006) has developed a frame of reference for reversal errors in handwriting (Lee, 2006). In addition, specific handwriting programs can be utilized which offer strategies for children experiencing visual perceptual problems. For specific information about handwriting, see Chapter 13. For children with visual perception and reading problems, the therapist can help the teacher determine the best method for teaching the child to read and write. For reading, phonics approaches work well for children with visual perceptual problems because auditory and analytic strengths are used. The Orton-Gillingham method (Gillingham & Stillman, 1997) is another useful reading approach that utilizes multisensory input and reinforces learning through multiple senses. In the Fernald approach (Bingman, 1989), students trace over new words with their index finger utilizing the kinesthetic approach. The therapist can help match the reading program to each child's strengths.

Case Study Application

The following are two case studies to demonstrate examples of how to apply the visual perception frame of reference.

Case Study: Kyle, Aged 5 Years

Kyle, aged 5 years, is in kindergarten. He was born prematurely at 31 weeks' gestation. He remained in the neonatal intensive care unit (NICU) for 3 weeks with apnea of prematurity, hyaline membrane disease, and hyperbilirubinemia. At approximately 1 year, he was evaluated and seen by an early intervention program. His diagnosis included developmental delay and visual disorder including hyperopia, astigmatism, and right estotropia. He had surgery at 13 months for a resection of the right medial rectus muscle to correct the right estotropia. Glasses were prescribed for the hyperopia.

He was referred to occupational therapy in kindergarten because of poor fine motor skills and visual perceptual problems. Kyle was unable to complete the *TVPS* (Gardner, 1982) because of poor visual attention skills. He demonstrated head posturing, squinting, and blinking throughout the evaluation. Results of the evaluation indicated motor planning, visual perceptual, and visual motor problems. Occupational therapy screening of vision indicated vision problems and he was referred to a developmental optometrist. The findings of the optometrist included inadequate ocular mobility, reduced binocular skills, and amblyopia. Kyle received optometric therapy to increase oculomotor mobility, binocular skills, and eye patching. He was seen by the OT for fine motor, visual perceptual, and visual motor activities. Reevaluations at the end of the school year indicated significant improvement. He was able to complete and score age appropriately on the TVPS.

Case Study: Gene, Aged 8 years

Gene is an 8-year, 9-month-old student just entering third grade. He has been classified as being perceptually impaired. Most of Gene's day is spent in the regular third grade curriculum with his peers. Educational reports indicate that he is functioning at grade level in all areas of academics with the exception of reading and language arts. Gene receives supplemental instruction in these areas, daily, in the resource room.

An occupational therapy referral was generated because of the parental concern about the performance of fine motor skills and the team's outline of poor performance components, poor handwriting, and deficient auditory and visual perception.

Evaluation tools indicate that Gene's deficiencies lie primarily in the area of VMI and selective areas of visual perceptual weakness. An age-equivalent score on the *Test of Visual Motor Integration* is 6 years, 11 months. Although achieving a median perceptual age of 8 years, 2 months on the TVPS, areas of weakness were noted for visual spatial relations, visual figure ground, and visual sequential memory.

Evaluation of other foundational areas revealed deficiencies in processing movement sensation, mildly low tone, and reduced fine motor speed and dexterity. Classroom observations indicate that Gene transitions between four classrooms throughout the day as his program uses "team teaching." It is noted that Gene takes more time than the others "settling" into his desk and getting ready for the assignment. Each desk was observed to be of adequate size, and desk grouping varied from front, to back, to "desk grouping" in one class which required Gene to complete board copying from a side-view perspective. At the desk, Gene demonstrated poor placement and alignment of his work when writing.

A review of the curriculum and teaching styles revealed little or no opportunities for manipulative activities to reinforce concept development. There was a heavy focus on copying, worksheet completion, and drill repetition techniques.

Gene disliked change and became noticeably uncomfortable with the OT in the classroom. Given the findings, it was felt the OT could best provide for Gene's visual perceptual needs through integrated classroom programming and consultation with the family to focus on home strategies. Because of Gene's general discomfort with the OT coming into the mainstreamed classes, she worked directly with

Gene and his resource room teacher to set up strategies and materials that were then carried over into all classrooms.

Summary

The visual perception frame of reference is used for children who have difficulty interpreting and using visual sensory information. Such problems affect a child's performance in critical areas of occupation, including education, ADL, play, and social participation. The goals of the frame of reference are to aid the child in attending to and processing visual information so that it can be used for task performance.

The theoretical base of this frame of reference uses theories from cognition, developmental psychology, education, and optometry. It also uses Warren's (1993a) developmental hierarchy of visual perceptual skills, which presents a bottom-up approach to evaluation and intervention. The visual system is viewed as interacting with other systems for obtaining and processing information. Processing is seen as an ongoing and interactive approach involving input, processing, and output, followed by feedback which will bring about a change in behavior.

Application to practice follows this pattern involving input, processing, and output. Within input, the therapist can initiate various environmental adaptations, whereas in processing and output, the therapist employs techniques of remediation, strategies, and environmental adaptation. The ultimate goal of this frame of reference is to allow the child to engage in meaningful age-appropriate occupations.

REFERENCES

Abreu, B., & Toglia, J. (1987). Cognitive rehabilitation: A model for occupational therapy. *American Journal of Occupational Therapy, 41*(7), 439–448.

Adams, W., & Sheslow, D. (1995). *Wide Range Assessment of Visual Motor Abilities (WRAVMA)*. Wilmington, DE: Wide Range.

Ayres, A. J. (1989). *Sensory Integration and Praxis Tests*. Los Angeles, CA: Western Psychological Services.

Baddeley, A. D. (1986). *Working Memory*. Oxford, England: Clarendon Press.

Bandura, A. (1977). Self-efficacy: Toward a unifying theory of behavior change. *Psychological Review, 84*, 191–215.

Beery, K. E., Buktenica, N. A., & Beery, N. A. (2004). *Developmental Test of Visual-Motor Integration 5th Edition Revised*. Minneapolis, MN: Pearson Assessments.

Bingman, M. B. (1989). *Learning Differently: Meeting the Needs of Adults with Learning Disabilities*. Knoxville, TN: Tennessee University.

Brody, J. F. (1993). Vigilance for problems with a child's vision is vital. *New York Times*, C16.

Brown, G. T., Rodger, S., & Davis, A. (2003). Test of visual perceptual skills–revised: An overview and critique. *Scandinavian Journal of Occupational Therapy, 10*(1), 3–15.

Burpee, J. D. (1997). Sensory integration and visual functions. In M. Gentile (Ed.). *Functional Visual Behavior: A Therapist's Guide to Evaluation and Treatment Options*. Bethesda, MD: American Occupational Therapy Association.

Chan, P. L. C., & Chow, S. M. K. (2005). Reliability and validity of the test of visual-perceptual skills (non-motor)-revised for Chinese preschoolers. *American Journal of Occupational Therapy, 59*, 369–376.

Chwirka, B., Gurney, B., & Burtner, P. (2002). Keyboarding and visual-motor skills in elementary students: A pilot study. *Occupational Therapy in Health Care, 16*(2/3), 39–51.

Colarusso, R. P., & Hammill, D. D. (2003). *Motor-Free Visual Perception Test – Third Edition*. Novato, CA: Academic Therapy Publications.

Cowan, N. (1988). Evolving conception of memory storage, selective attention and their mutual constraints within the human information processing system. *Psychological Bulletin, 104,* 163–191.

Crane, A., & Wick, B. (1987). *Crane-Wick Test*. Houston, TX: Rapid Research Corporation.

Cratty, B. J. (1986). Visual – perceptual development. *Perceptual and Motor Development in Infants and Children* (pp. 292–313). Englewood Cliffs, NJ: Prentice Hall.

Damasio, A. R. (1989). Time-locked multiregional retroactivation: A systems level proposal for the neural substrates of recall and recognition. *Cognition, 33,* 25–62.

Dutton, G. (2002). Visual problems in children with damage to the brain. *Visual Impairment Research, 4,* 113–121.

Erhardt, R. P. (1989). Erhardt Developmental Vision Assessment (EDVA) (Rev. ed.). Tucson: Therapy Skill Builders.

Erhardt, R. P., & Duckman, R. H. (1997). Visual-perceptual-motor dysfunction: Effects on eye-hand coordination and skill development. In M. Gentile (Ed.), *Functional visual behavior: A therapist's guide to evaluation and treatment options* (pp. 133–195). Maryland: The American Occupational Therapy Association, Inc.

Erhardt, R. P., & Duckman, R. H. (2005). Visual-perceptual-motor dysfunction: Effects on eye-hand coordination and skill development. In: M. Gentile (Ed.), *Functional visual behavior in children: An occupational therapy guide to evaluation and treatment options* (2nd ed., pp. 171–229). Bethesda, MD: The American Occupational Therapy Association.

Feder, K. P., Majnemer, A., Bourbonnais, D., & Platt, R. (2005). Handwriting performance in preterm children compared with term peers at age 6 to 7 years. *Developmental Medicine and Child Neurology, 47,* 163–170.

Frostig, M. & Horne, D. (1973). *The Frostig Program for the Development of Visual Perception*. Hicago: Follett.

Frostig, M., Lefever, W., & Whittlesey, J. R. B. (1966). *Administration and Scoring Manual for the Marianne Frostig Developmental Test of Visual Perception*. Palo Alto, CA: Consulting Psychologists Press.

Gardner, R. A. (1978). Reversals frequency test. Cresskill, NJ: Creative Therapeutics.

Gardner, M. F. (1982). Test of visual-perceptual skills (non-motor). Burlingame, CA: Psychological and Educational Publications, Inc.

Gardner, M. F. (1995). *Test of Visual-Motor Skills – Revised Manual*. Los Angeles, CA: Western Psychological Services.

Gardner, M. F. (1996). *Test of Visual-Perceptual Skills (Non-Motor)- Revised*. Hydesville, CA: Psychological and Educational Publications.

Gardner, M. F. (1997). *Test of Visual Perceptual Skills Upper Limis (Non-Motor) Manual*. Los Angeles, CA: Western Psychological Services.

Garling, R., Book, A., & Lindberg, E. (1984). Cognitive mapping of large-scale environments: The interrelationship of action plans, acquisition, and orientation. *Environment and Behavior, 16,* 3–34.

Gentile, M. (Ed.). (1997). *Functional Visual Behavior*. Bethesda, MD: American Occupational Therapy Association.

Gentile, M. (2005). *Functional Visual Behavior in Children: An Occupational Therapy Guide to Evaluation And Treatment Options* (2nd ed.). Bethesda, MD: The American Occupational Therapy Association. pp. 171–229.

Getman, G. N. (1965). The visuomotor complex in the acquisition of learning skills. In J. Helmuth (Ed.). *Learning Disorders*, Vol. 1(of 3) (pp 49–76). Washington, DC: Special Child Publications.

Gibson, J. J. (1966). *The Senses Considered as Perceptual Systems*. Boston, MA: Houghton Mifflin.

Gibson, E. J. (1969). *Problems of Perceptual Learning and Development*. New York: Appleton, Century, Crofts.

Gillingham, A., & Stillman, B. W. (1997). *The Gillingham Manual: Remedial Training for Children with Specific Disability in Reading, Spelling, and Penmanship* (8th ed.). Cambridge, MA: Educators Publishing Service.

Glover, J. A., Ronning, R. R., & Bruning, R. H. (1990). *Cognitive Psychology for Teachers*. New York: MacMillan.

Goldstand, S., Koslowe, K., & Parush, S. (2005). Vision, visual-information procession, and academic performance among seventh-grade school children: A more significant relationship than we thought? *American Journal of Occupational Therapy, 59,* 377–389.

Hammill, D. D., Pearson, N. A., & Voress, J. K. (1993). *Developmental Test of Visual Perception* (2nd ed.). Austin, TX: PRO-ED.

Henderson, A., Pehoski, C., & Murray, E. (2002). Visual-spatial abilities. In A. C. Bundy, S. J. Lane, & E. A. Murray (Eds). *Sensory Integration: Theory and Practice* (2nd ed., pp.124–140). Philadelphia, PA: FA Davis Co.

Jordon, B. A. (1980). *Jordon Left-Right Reversal Test* (2nd ed.). Los Angeles, CA: Western Psychological Corporation.

Josman, N., Abdallah, T. M., & Engel-Yeger, B. (2006). A comparison of visual-perceptual and visual-motor skills between Palestinian and Israeli children. *American Journal of Occupational Therapy, 60,* 215–225.

Kephart, N. C. (1971). *The Slow Learner in the Classroom* (2nd ed.). Columbus, OH: Charles C. Merrill.

Law, M., Baum, C., & Dunn, W. (Eds). (2005). *Measuring Occupational Performance* (2nd ed.). Thorofare, NJ: Slack.

Lee, S. (2006). A frame of reference for reversal errors in handwriting: A historical review of visual-perceptual theory. *School System Special Interest Section Quarterly, 13*(1), 1–4.

Lesensky, S., & Kaplan, L. (2000). Occupational therapy and motor learning: Putting theory into practice, OT Practice, 13 -16.

Levine, R. E. (1987). Culture: A factor influencing the outcomes of occupational therapy. *Occupational Therapy in Health Care, 4,* 3–16.

Levine, M. (1987). *Developmental Variation and Learning Disorders.* Cambridge, MA: Educators Publishing Service.

Levine, M. D. (1994). *Educational Care: A System for Understanding and Helping Children with learning Problems at Home and in School.* Cambridge, MA: Educators Publishing Service.

Luria, A. R. (1980). *Higher Cortical Functions in Man.* New York: Basic Books.

Massaro, D. W., & Cowan, N. (1993). Information processing models: Microscopes of mind. *Annual Review of Psychology, 34,* 383–425.

McHale, K., & Cermak, S. A. (1992). Fine motor activities in elementary school: Preliminary findings and provisional implications for children with fine motor problems. *American Journal of Occupational Therapy, 46,* 898–903.

McLaughlin, P. J., & Wehman, P. (Eds). (1992). *Developmental Disabilities: A Handbook for Best Practices.* Stoneham, MA: Butterworth-Heineman.

Miller, L. J. (1988). *Miller Assessment of Preschoolers.* San Antonio, TX: Psychological Corporation.

Moore, R. S. (1979). *School Can Wait.* Provo, UT: Brigham Young University Press.

Mulligan, S. (2003). *Occupational Therapy Evaluation for Children: A Pocket Guide.* Philadelphia, PA: Lippincott Williams & Wilkins.

O'Brien, V., Cermak, S. A., & Murray, E. (1988). The relationship between visual-perceptual motor abilities and clumsiness in children with and without learning disabilities. *American Journal of Occupational Therapy, 42,* 359–363.

Parush, S., Yochman, A., Cohen, D., & Gerson, E. (1998). Relation of visual perception and visual-motor integration for clumsy children. *Perceptual and Motor Skills, 86,* 291–295.

Piaget, J. (1952). *The Origins of Intelligence in Children* translated by Margaret Cook. New York: International Universities Press.

Piaget, J. (1964). Development and learning. Ithaca. NY: Cornell University Press.

Polatajko, H. J., & Mandich, A. (2004). *Enabling Occupation in Children: The Cognitive Orientation to Daily Occupational Performance (CO-OP) Approach.* Ottowa: CAOT Publications ACE.

Pressley, M., Woloshyn, V., Lysynchuk, L. M., & Martin, L. M. et al. (1990). A primer of research on cognitive strategy instruction: The important issues and how to address them. *Educational Psychology Review, 2,* 1–58.

Richards, R. G. & Oppenheim, G. S. (1984). Visual Skills Appraisal. Novato, CA: Academic therapy Publications.

Ritty, J. M., Solan, H., & Cool, S. J. (1993). Visual and sensory-motor functioning in the classroom: A preliminary report of ergonomic demands. *Journal of the American Optometric Association, 64*(4), 238–244.

Rogers, C. R. (1951). *Client Centered Therapy.* Boston, MA: Houghton Mifflin.

Rogers, C. R. (1957). The necessary and sufficient conditions of therapeutic personality change. *Journal of Consulting Psychology, 21,* 95–103.

Rose, S. A., Feldman, F. F., & Jankowski, J. J. (2001). Attention and recognition memory in the first year of life: A longitudinal study of preterm and full-term infants. *Developmental Psychology, 37,* 135–151.

Rosner, J., & Fern, K. (1983). A new version of the TVAS: A validation report. *Journal of the American Optometric Association, 54*(7), 603–606.

Royeen, C. B., & Duncan, M. (1999). Acquisition frame of reference. In P. Kramer, & J. Hinojosa (Eds). *Frames of Reference for Pediatric Occupational Therapy* (2nd ed.). Philadelphia, PA: Lippincott Williams & Wilkins.

Scheiman, M. (1997). The efficacy of vision therapy for convergence excess. *Journal of the American Optometric Association, 68*(2), 81–86.

Scheiman, M. (2002). *Understanding and Managing Vision Deficits: A Guide for Occupational Therapists* (2nd ed.). Thorofare, NJ: Slack.

Skeffington, A. N. (1963). *The Skeffington Papers* (Series 36, No. 2, p. 11). Santa Ana, CA: Optometric Extension Program.

Slosson, R. L., & Nicholson, C. L. (1996). *Manual: Slosson Visual Motor Performance Test for Children and Adults*. East Aurora, NY: Slosson Educational Publications.

Thelen, D., & Smith, L. B. (1994). *A Dynamic Systems Approach to the Development of Cognitions and Action*. Cambridge, MA: MIT Press.

Todd, V. R. (1999). Visual information analysis: Frame of reference for visual perception. In P. Kramer, & J. Hinojosa. (Eds). *Frames of Reference for Pediatric Occupational Therapy* (2nd ed., pp. 205–256). Philadelphia, PA: Lippincott Williams & Wilkins.

Toglia, J. P. (1989). Visual perception of objects: An approach to assessment and intervention. *American Journal of Occupational Therapy, 43*, 587–595.

Tseng, M. H., & Chow, S. M. K. (2000). Perceptual-motor function of school-age children with slow handwriting speed. *American Journal of Occupational Therapy, 54*, 83–88.

Tsurumi, K., & Todd, V. (1998). Tests of visual perception: What do they tell us? *School System Special Interest Section Quarterly, 5*(4), 1–4.

Tui, R. D., Thompson, L. A., & Lewis, B. A. (2003). The role of IQ in a component model of reading. *Journal of Learning Disabilities, 36*, 424–436.

Voyer, D., Voyer, S., & Bryden, M. P. (1995). Magnitude of sex differences in spatial abilities: A meta-analysis and consideration of critical variables. *Psychological Bulletin, 117*, 250–270.

Vygotsky, L. S. (1931). Development of higher mental functions. In *Psychological Research in the U.S.R.R.* Moscow: Progress Publishers.

Warren, M. (1993a). A hierarchical model for evaluation and treatment of visual perceptual dysfunction in adult acquired brain injury I. *American Journal of Occupational Therapy, 44*, 391–399.

Warren, M. (1993b). A hierarchical model for evaluation and treatment of visual perceptual dysfunction in adult acquired brain injury II. *American Journal of Occupational Therapy, 47*, 55–66.

Williams, H. (1983). *Perceptual and Motor Development*. Englewood Cliffs, NJ: Prentice Hall.

Zaba, J. (1984). Visual perception versus visual function. *Journal of Learning Disabilities, 17*, 182–185.

Zemke, R. (1994). Task skills, problem solving, and social interaction. In C. Royeen (Ed.). *AOTA Self Study Series: Cognitive Rehabilitation*. Rockville, MD: American Occupational Therapy Association.

Zimbardo, P. G. (1992). *Psychology and Life* (13th ed.). New York: HarperCollins.

Zoltan, B. (1996). *Vision, Perception, & Cognition: A Manual for the Evaluation and Treatment of the Neurologically Impaired Adult* (3rd ed.). Thorofare, NJ: Slack.

CHAPTER 12

A Frame of Reference for Motor Skill Acquisition

MARGARET KAPLAN

A child's ability to learn, interact with the environment, and develop increasingly complex skill depends on many factors. This chapter focuses on motor skill acquisition in children with developmental disabilities and/or delays. Difficulty with the motor aspects of daily living tasks, play and educational activities, communication, and social interaction can result from many underlying diagnoses and impairments. Because movement arises from the interaction of multiple processes, including those related to sensory/perception, cognitive, and motor systems, pathology in any of these systems can result in impairments that may potentially constrain functional movement.

Several authors and clinicians have attempted to illustrate the application of concepts from the movement sciences to occupational and physical therapy practice (Carr & Shepherd, 1992, 1998; Duff & Charles, 2004; Goodgold-Edwards & Cermak, 1989; Mathowietz & Bass-Haugen, 2008; Schmidt & Lee, 2005; Valvano, 2004; Westcott & Burtner, 2004). These reflect individual perspectives on a developing information base and different clinical experiences related to various client populations.

THEORETICAL BASE

Gentile (1987, 1992) developed a model of skill acquisition based on knowledge from the movement sciences. Elements of this model have been adapted for practice by several authors (Duff & Charles, 2004; Goodgold-Edwards & Cermak, 1989; Valvano, 2004; Westcott & Burtner, 2004). The movement sciences draw on theory and research from motor learning and control, human ecology, cognitive and developmental psychology, biomechanics, muscle physiology, and neurophysiology. This chapter presents an evidence-based model of skill acquisition based on a systems approach to motor control and a review of current evidence on motor control and motor learning in children. This model is particularly applicable to occupational therapy because of the emphasis on person-task-environment and the active role of the learner.

Motor Control, Motor Learning, and Motor Development

Motor control is the ability to regulate or direct the mechanisms essential to movement. These mechanisms are found in the person, in the task demands, and in the environment. The major question addressed in this field is: How do the body systems interact with the environmental conditions and the task demands to produce effective solutions to movement problems? Specific issues are usually investigated with controlled experimental research involving specific aspects of postural and movement control.

Motor learning is the study of the movement processes associated with practice, such as experience, motivation, reinforcement, motor skill, and developmental progress, that lead to a relatively permanent change in a person's capability for skilled action (Schmidt & Lee, 2005). Current issues in this field include the role of feedback and types of practice in learning new skills and factors that influence generalization of learning among different skills and environments. The role of motivation and meaningfulness of the action goal to the person have been investigated by researchers in motor learning and motor control. There is substantial evidence that control mechanisms used are different and learning is improved when a person is involved in a purposeful, functional activity as opposed to being involved in a repetitive, nonpurposeful activity or being passively moved by another person (Gliner, 1985; van der Weel, van der Meer & Lee, 1991; Thelen et al., 1993; Carr & Shepherd, 1992).

Motor development is the study of how motor behavior changes over the lifespan. Current issues address age-related differences in motor performance as a result of development and maturation as well as the influences on motor development resulting from factors such as genetics, body dimensions, environment, motivation, experience, practice, and expectations. The contemporary view of motor development recognizes that change in motor skill results from the interaction of these factors. In addition, children develop motor skills in varied ways that are influenced by personal and environmental characteristics. These characteristics interact as the child searches for solutions to motor problems. This can explain why children use various strategies to perform activities and explore the environment. This is in contrast to traditional views that describe motor development as following a rigid sequence that is based on the maturation of the central nervous system. Recent work in motor development has documented the emergence of anticipatory reach very early in infancy and demonstrated the role of practice in the development of early prehensile behavior and control (Claxton, 2003; Duff & Charles, 2004; von Hofsten, 1997; Thelen, 1998). In addition, study of the development of postural control in typically developing young children has described the reactive postural control which occurs initially in upright positions. As the child practices in these positions and reacts to shifts in the center of gravity associated with body movement, the child learns to anticipate or use feedforward mechanisms to prepare for reaching, for instance, to the side for a toy. With practice, these anticipatory adjustments, in combination with the action (e.g., reaching for a toy) become preferred movement patterns with decreasing variability. Children with neurological and developmental problems do not learn to use these anticipatory postural adjustments in the same way as typically developing children (Bly, 1996; Eliasson,

Gordon, & Forssberg, 1992; Gordon & Duff, 1999; Valvano, 2004). These children do not develop preferred movement patterns; instead, they show increased degree of variability in movement patterns used during the same action (e.g., reaching to the side for a toy). In addition, children with developmental and neurological problems have more difficulty with attending to a conversation or a task and maintaining postural control than do typically developing children (Huang & Mercer, 2001; Huang, Mercer, & Thorpe, 2003).

Dynamic Systems Theory

There has been a shift away from the traditional reflex hierarchical view of motor behavior to principles based on dynamic systems theory (Mathiowetz & Bass-Haugen, 2008). The traditional view of motor behavior and development assumes that motor control difficulties are caused by problems in the central nervous system. Problems in the central nervous system cause abnormal tone, which is, in turn, the cause of motor control difficulties. The developmental sequence is seen as necessary for normal development, and the central nervous system is viewed as hierarchical with "higher" centers controlling "lower" centers. A newer way of thinking about motor behavior is the dynamic systems theory, which has had an important effect on the current view of how movement is acquired and organized. (Bernstein, 1967; Kamm, Thelen, & Jensen, 1990; Mathiowetz & Bass-Haugen, 2008). This theory views movement as emerging from the interaction of many systems. The three general systems are the person, the task, and the environment. Subsystems within the person can include emotional, cognitive, perceptual, sensory, motor, and other physical systems such as cardiovascular, musculoskeletal, and neurological. Systems outside of the person that influence motor performance and skill acquisition (e.g., the characteristics and complexity of the task and the environment in which it must be performed) are also considered.

All systems interact at one point in time to accomplish a particular goal. In this view, no one system has logical priority for directing or influencing the others. The subsystems "in charge" will vary with specific task requirements and environmental demands. The resulting movement is a solution to a particular problem that emerges from this interaction. The emergent motor behavior is usually the most efficient one available given the condition of each individual system. Each individual develops preferred movement patterns for common functional tasks through active experimentation, experience, and practice. This view of how movement is organized implies that the interaction of multiple systems can be affected by change in any one of them. The subsystems within the person, task, and environment that have a potential for change are often referred to as "control parameters" (Mathiowetz & Bass-Haugen, 2008). Control parameters are viewed as the subsystems that constrain task performance. If these subsystems are modified or changed, a new movement pattern may emerge. Therapists should therefore consider the child's preferred and most efficient patterns of moving and all of the person-task-environment subsystems (control parameters) affecting the child's task performance when planning intervention.

Principles of Learning Theory

This frame of reference employs several principles from learning theories (Levine, 1987; Thorndike, 1932, 1935; Travers, 1977; Vygotsky, 1978). They involve practice, experimentation, variation, developmentally appropriate support, and feedback.

Practice and experimentation with various strategies provide the child with opportunities to acquire skills. One of the most important factors in acquiring new motor skills is the amount of practice (Gentile, 1992). Practice is when the child has the occasion to repeatedly try to produce motor behaviors that are challenging or just beyond his or her current level (Schmidt & Lee, 2005). Through practice, the child can experiment with different types of solutions for motor problems. Random practice with varied tasks appears to be more effective for long-term learning (Schmidt & Lee, 2005). Practice is most effective when the child is challenged, while, at the same time, keeping the goals attainable.

Variation in the context of practice promotes the development of flexible strategies and generalization of learning. Optimally, practice should occur during typical, functional, routines throughout the day (Palisano, Snider, & Orlin, 2004). Evidence is beginning to be published that supports the anecdotal observation and common belief that young children learn best through practice that is occurring over time and not during a massed practice session (McDonnell, 1996; Seabrook, Brown, & Solity, 2005). Through this process, the child can generalize the learned strategy from one task to another and from one setting to another (Lee, Swanson, & Hall, 1991; VanSant, 1991). This is critical if the child is to use skills acquired in the therapy session in other settings. If practice can continue, or can occur primarily, in the home and other of the child's natural environments (i.e., during functional and daily tasks), then learning will improve (Hadders-Algra, 2000; von Vliet & Henegan, 2006).

Developmentally, appropriate support is needed to assist children to master new skills. The zone of proximal development (Vygotsky, 1978) is a useful concept for designing activities and tasks with achievable goals. This zone refers to the distance between the actual developmental level of the child, what the child can achieve through independent problem solving, and the level of the child's potential for achieving the tasks with adult assistance. The concept of "scaffolding" describes the adult support and instruction that is necessary to assist children to master skills that are just beyond their current capabilities (Vygotsky, 1978). An adult who is attuned to the current abilities of a child, his/her interests, and the possibilities of task accomplishment with assistance, can provide this support to enable the child to reach a new level of skill. Occupational therapists can assist parents, caregivers, teachers, and others in recognizing the child's zone of proximal development (what is developmentally within the child's reach at this time) and a way to provide the scaffolding the child needs to help him or her attain and practice the new skill. These concepts have been applied in the area of cognitive development in the past but seem to be just as applicable in the promotion of motor skill acquisition.

Feedback assists the child in understanding the results of his or her movements (Levine, 1987; Thorndike, 1932, 1935; Travers, 1977). Feedback, although frequently verbal, can consist of gestures, facial expressions, auditory and tactile cues, and, when necessary, manual guidance. Whenever feedback is used, it should be focused, succinct, and appropriate to the child's cognitive, language, and sensory abilities. Motor learning and skill acquisition is enhanced by feedback given after performance. One research study (Winstein & Schmidt, 1990) has shown that frequent, consistent feedback is not effective for long-term learning. Therefore, it was proposed that feedback should be given after 50% of the movement attempts. Feedback should decrease as learning progresses. Feedback should be given when the child's performance has more inaccuracy than is acceptable. Further, after the child has made several attempts at a task, it is quite effective to give summary feedback of performance, rather than feedback after every try (Schmidt & Lee, 2005). As the child moves toward mastery of a task, he or she begins to use feedback from his or her own body to get information. This helps the child to better understand the outcome of movements, anticipate upcoming events, and plan alternative strategies (Brooks, 1986). As the child develops more skill, he or she is encouraged to rely more on internal feedback and self-evaluation of performance rather than external feedback.

Concepts

This section will describe important concepts for developing an understanding of this frame of reference. These include the child, task, skill, environment, and regulatory conditions.

The child's abilities are in relation to all subsystems. Subsystems within the child include emotional, cognitive, perceptual, sensory, motor, and other physical systems such as cardiovascular, musculoskeletal, and neurological. Understanding the child's complexity will guide the evaluation process as the therapist develops an understanding of the child in the context of his or her life, abilities, and limitations.

A task is a sequence of activities or movements that share a purpose and goal. Tasks have characteristics related to their complexity, degree of structure, and purpose. They are also influenced by the social and physical demands of the environment (Mathiowetz & Bass-Haugen, 2008). The impact of the environment on tasks is seen in the later discussion of regulatory conditions. By nature, tasks lend themselves to analysis so that the therapist can identify their component parts. It is of critical importance to identify those aspects of the task that present a challenge to the child. A child will choose to engage in a specific task because it has meaning and purpose. A child will practice and repeat attempts to perform a task that is motivating to her. Therefore, it is crucial for the therapist to focus on tasks that are important and meaningful to the family and child. Functional tasks, which are goal directed and important to the child and family, are the focus of intervention in this frame of reference. For young children, the meaning of a particular task may be inferred by their level of interest and self-selection. Caregivers and older children can be asked which activities are meaningful to them. Once important and motivating tasks are selected, a task analysis can determine the child-task-environment match. This is the congruence of the child's abilities, the task demands and the barriers or facilitating aspects presented by the environment. At that point, the therapist can, in collaboration with family, teacher, and others, consider whether it will be most effective to try to teach the child a new strategy, develop a higher level of motor control, modify the task demands, or modify characteristics of the environment.

Skill is consistency in achieving a motor goal with economy of effort (Gentile, 1992). The therapist facilitates the child's search for a solution to what he or she wants to do. We can manipulate such factors as task demands, characteristics of the environment, the child's goal, preparation for movement, and the level of support provided. Skill in performing a motor task does not imply that one specific motor pattern is used. There are many possible movement patterns and strategies that could be used to accomplish a specified task. For example, it cannot be assumed that children who have demonstrated skill in feeding themselves with a spoon are all using the same neuromotor organization in their movement strategies, even if their movements look very similar to each other. In fact, as skill increases, the child should be developing variable movement strategies that emerge as a factor of changing task demands and environment characteristics.

The environment in which a child performs a task is considered a major factor in task performance according to this frame of reference. Occupational therapists consider the physical, social, personal, temporal, and cultural aspects of the environment when designing their evaluations and interventions (AOTA, 2002). All aspects of the environment have the potential to influence the child's motor control of task performance. It is the therapist's responsibility to identify aspects of the environment that may facilitate or increase the challenge a particular task presents and to decide whether to enhance or modify these factors. Certainly, an environment that has multiple sensory features such as noise, visual stimulation, textures, and movement can be an overwhelming situation to a child with a sensory processing disorder. Another child, who needs added sensory stimulation in order to maintain an alert, focused state, may find this environment facilitating to skilled movement. The therapist balances environmental characteristics with child abilities to present a challenge to the child that is not totally beyond the child's potential.

Regulatory conditions are aspects of the environment that determine movement specifics such as force, timing, and distance or magnitude for successful task outcome (Gentile, 1987). Gentile (1987) classifies tasks on two dimensions based on regulatory conditions: whether the environment is stationary or in motion during the task and whether the environment varies each time the task is performed (intertrial variability). This system describes a continuum between open and closed tasks as defined in Figure 12.1.

Closed tasks are those in which the environment is stationary during task performance. Some closed tasks have little variability during each performance (e.g., brushing teeth, washing hands, and toileting) (Figure 12.2A). Other closed tasks have more variability (e.g., self-feeding where variability is present from meal to meal with different foods, utensils, and set-up positions) (Figure 12.2B). Greater intertrial variability places more demands on a child, and movement strategies must be more flexible than they need be in tasks with lesser intertrial variability.

Open tasks are those in which the environment is in motion and include some intertrial variability (Figure 12.3). These tasks place the most demands on a child. In addition to force and distance, movement strategies must take into account the

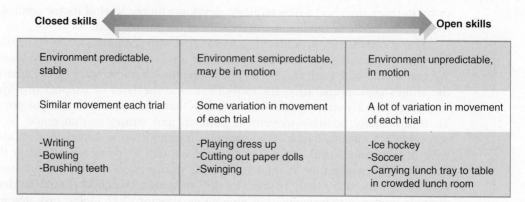

Closed skills ←		→ Open skills
Environment predictable, stable	Environment semipredictable, may be in motion	Environment unpredictable, in motion
Similar movement each trial	Some variation in movement of each trial	A lot of variation in movement of each trial
-Writing -Bowling -Brushing teeth	-Playing dress up -Cutting out paper dolls -Swinging	-Ice hockey -Soccer -Carrying lunch tray to table in crowded lunch room

FIGURE 12.1 The open/closed task continuum for motor behavior.

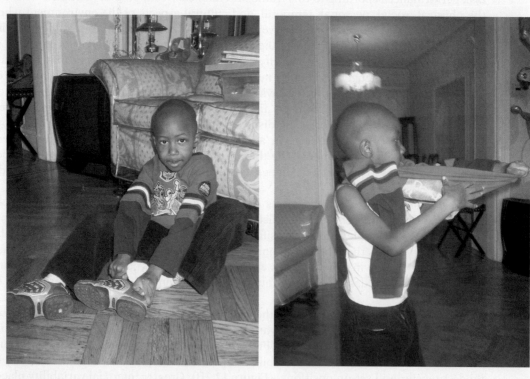

FIGURE 12.2 A., Closed task with little variability (same shoes each time). B., Closed task with greater variability (different shirts each time).

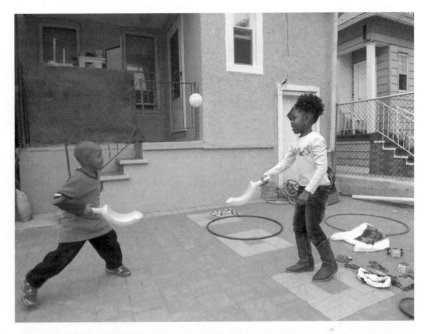

FIGURE 12.3 Open task with different demands on the child.

regulatory condition of timing. Children with developmental and motor delays and disorders often have difficulty when timing becomes important to task completion.

When a child is in the early stages of learning a motor skill, Gentile's (1987) classification scheme suggests that a child should be given a closed task with lower demands before progressing to open tasks with higher demands. The type of practice needed to develop a motor skill in a closed task will entail repetitions in a less variable environment. Skill in an open task will require practice in an environment that includes variability in movement, timing, force, and magnitude.

Child-Task-Environment Match

A motor skill acquisition frame of reference is concerned with the child's ability to solve movement problems to accomplish everyday functional tasks, participate in self-care, school, play, mobility, and social interaction. Tasks chosen to be addressed in occupational therapy must be important, meaningful, and achievable to the child based on his or her functional levels within the context of his or her family. It is important that there be a match between the capabilities of the child, the task demands, and the environmental characteristics in which the task is to be performed (Figure 12.4).

The characteristics of the task and environment can be modified to encourage the child to use different movement strategies (Kaplan, 1994). For example, a desired toy can be placed near the arm and hand that is not used as often or positioned higher in space to require increased use of shoulder extension. Hip adduction can be promoted by

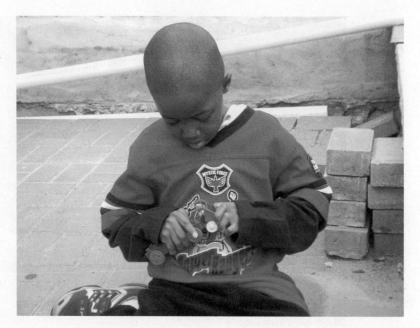

FIGURE 12.4 Very attentive child playing favorite train building game.

having the child creep between two cushions placed close together. Toys or objects can be used that require the use of both hands or a specific type of manipulation.

Physical and sensory characteristics of the task or the environment can be important to a child's success and are often systematically manipulated during intervention (Figure 12.5). For example, a child may initially practice a task in an environment with low noise levels, subdued lighting, and little distraction from other children. The task could be adapted to include only tactile characteristics that are acceptable to the child. These sensory variables could be systematically changed as tolerated to represent more closely the natural environment in which a child must perform the task. Other

FIGURE 12.5   Child-task-environment match.

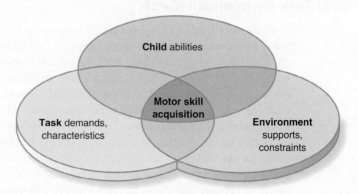

characteristics of the task can also be modified (e.g., the size, shape, texture, pliability, and amount of visual contrast and detail). Cognitive aspects of the task (e.g., several steps, whether problem solving is required, and information processing demands) are also commonly analyzed and manipulated during intervention. The psychosocial demands of a specific task and environment may also be important to a child's ability to develop skill in that task. For example, if children feel that their movement attempts may be successful and will meet with positive attention, they may be motivated to try harder and try more often than if there is little hope of positive feedback from others or if they are convinced that they will not be successful.

Stages of Learning

The acquisition of a motor skill is a process, and the requirements for practice, feedback, the role of the therapist, and the involvement of the learner should vary based on the level of skill in a particular task for a particular learner. Gentile (1992) has described early and late stages of learning. During early stages of learning, the learner must find movement strategies to match the particular features of the task and environment to achieve the goal. To accomplish this, the child must engage in active problem solving, plan a movement, and evaluate the plan based on the outcome of the movement actually produced. This requires that the child focus on those conditions in the environment that will determine the successful movement strategy (Figure 12.6). The learner must retain the goal and plan in memory. Then the actual movement and outcome must be compared with the information retained in memory. This process places substantial cognitive and attentional demands on the child and can present difficulty for many children with developmental delays and disorders.

At this stage, the environment needs to be structured to encourage the child to actively plan and experiment with movement strategies. One element of the environment is the adults who relate to the child. These adults can help the child to remember the goal and movement outcome and provide feedback on the outcome without focusing on the movement strategy used. Important conditions in the environment can be highlighted for the learner and he or she can be encouraged to try alternative strategies. Any movement pattern generated by the child at this early stage is acceptable. The specific movement pattern chosen by the child is considered less important than the child's active involvement and problem solving in the situation. Movement strategies that may limit future or more complex movement and tasks can be modified by changing environmental conditions. For example, a child who prefers using only one hand and arm to reach for and manipulate toys or objects can be given motivating, exciting tasks or toys, for which the manipulation requires both hands.

During any movement, there are multiple joints and muscles to control, all of which can move in multiple directions. When first learning a new movement, it can be difficult to understand the most efficient way in which to control all of these possible movement options. This is sometimes called the "degrees of freedom" problem (Bernstein, 1967). In early stages of learning, the therapist should expect movements that involve cocontraction of opposing muscle groups (sometimes referred to as "fixing")

FIGURE 12.6 The child focuses on the characteristics of the pink circle and its distance from her.

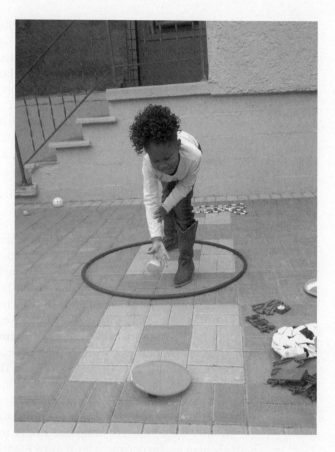

and appear inefficient or awkward. These movements may be effective preliminary strategies for attempting a new motor skill when the child is experimenting with balance, coordination, and motor planning. The movement will not be smooth and flowing until the child has learned to coordinate multiple joints, muscles, and limbs and account for forces such as gravity (Gentile, 1992).

During later stages of learning, skill is developed in a particular task. Different tasks have different requirements based on the context and function of the action. At this stage, a person can structure the conditions for practice and promote self-evaluation of the performance and outcome by the child. The child should be encouraged to rely less on others for informational feedback. For certain tasks, the emphasis will change from evaluating the outcome (successful or not) to more specifically monitoring and evaluating the performance and movement strategies used.

Practice

Practice and experimentation with varied strategies is essential to skill acquisition. In addition, the focus of practice should be on "actions" and not on patterns of movement (von Hofsten, 2004). Action refers to the intent of the child when he or she acts on the environment. Evidence from neuroscience shows that the brain represents movement in terms of actions even at the level of neural processes. A specific set of neurons, mirror neurons, are activated when perceiving as well as when performing an action. These neurons are specific to the goal of actions and not to the mechanics of executing them (Gallese et al., 1996; Rizzolatti & Luppino, 2001). Infants will adjust their hand position differently if their purpose is to grasp the toy and throw it than to grasp the toy and put it in a tube (Claxton, 2003). Therefore, practice should focus on the goal of the action, not on the specifics of the movement pattern. This approach is consistent with a model that provides therapy services in the context of functional tasks and play activities where the action of the play or game or school task is the focus of the therapy.

Another important factor in motor skill acquisition is the amount and type of practice (Gentile, 1992). Ericsson, Krampe, & Tesch-Romer (1993) have defined deliberate practice as "activities that have been specially designed to improve the current level of performance" (p. 365). The goal of deliberate practice is for the child to experiment with generating solutions to motor problems. Practice may be structured by a therapist in such a way that one task is practiced repeatedly before moving on to practice a different task. This is referred to as "massed practice." Random or discrete trial practice, where a person practices varied tasks in a random order, is another way to structure practice. Schmidt and Lee's (2005) review of recent research in motor learning has suggested that using random practice of varied tasks is better for long-term learning than massed practice. Performance during the random practice session may initially appear worse than when using a blocked practice approach, but retention of learning is improved when random practice is used. However, research on types of practice is usually performed with adults and usually in clinical settings. The effects of other types of practice with children, especially in natural settings, has not been systematically evaluated. One important aspect of most therapy programs is to integrate practice into existing routines in order to expand the child's opportunities to practice skills throughout the day rather than only with a professional in a specified session.

For practice to be effective, one should strive to provide as much challenge as possible while keeping the goal achievable. Vygotsky's (1978) concept of the zone of proximal development is helpful in developing achievable goals, activities, and tasks. The zone of proximal development refers to the distance between those tasks that the child can perform completely by himself or herself and those tasks that the child has the potential to perform with some assistance. With effective support and teaching, children can master the skills in their zone before they can master skills that are beyond it. Although this concept has been applied to cognitive development in the past, it may be useful in promoting learning of motor skills as well.

Variation in the context of practice can promote the learning of flexible strategies, which will be important for tasks in which there is more intertrial variability. This will aid in the child's ability to more easily generalize a strategy from one context to another and may help to transfer a strategy from a therapy setting to a more natural setting in the community, school, or home (Lee, Swanson, & Hall, 1991; Schmidt & Lee, 2005; VanSant, 1991). By analyzing the contexts in which the tasks are to be used, conditions that commonly vary can be considered when promoting skill acquisition. Practice in natural environments such as the home, classroom, and playground is optimal. If this is not possible, certain conditions may be simulated during practice.

The effectiveness of practicing a whole task versus separate parts of a task in isolation of the whole task has also been studied. Tasks that cannot easily be broken down into steps (e.g., riding a bicycle or throwing a ball) should be practiced as whole tasks. Some more complex tasks (e.g., cleaning a room) can be more easily broken down into steps and practiced as parts. However, attempting to practice balance separately from the manipulation aspect of reaching and grasping a toy or object will likely be less effective than practicing balance within the context of a functional activity such as reach and grasp of a cup for drinking or a toy for playing (Winstein, 1991).

A technique often used in therapy with children is manual guidance, where the child is physically guided through the task. A therapist usually does this at the very beginning stages of learning if the child does not seem to have an idea of what do. Research has explored the use of guided learning versus discovery (trial and error learning) and found little benefit of guided experiences over nonguided and only in the beginning stages of learning, getting the "idea" (Schmidt & Lee, 2005). This implies that manual guidance, or hand over hand guidance, should only be used when the child cannot generate attempts on their own that are "in the ballpark" of the intended movement. It should be discontinued as soon as possible so that the child can engage in the trial and error learning process.

Feedback

Feedback given after performance can affect motor learning and skill acquisition (Bly, 1996). Extrinsic feedback is feedback given by others to help the child understand the outcome of his or her movement and is often verbal but can also consist of gestures, facial expressions, auditory and tactile cues, and, when necessary, manual guidance. With increasing skill, the child will use intrinsic feedback from his or her own body to get information about the outcome and to help plan alternative strategies. As time progresses, the child should be encouraged to become less dependent on feedback from others and encouraged to evaluate his or her own performance. In early stages of learning, general feedback about performance, referred to as "summary" feedback, is thought to be more helpful than feedback that is more specific and detailed (Gentile, 1992; Schmidt & Lee, 2005).

It has been demonstrated that even in early stages of learning, constant feedback or feedback after every attempt can impede retention of learning. Recent research studies suggest several strategies that may improve retention of skills (Winstein, 1991; Winstein & Schmidt, 1990). On the basis of this research, feedback should be given after approximately 50% of the movement attempts. As learning progresses, there should be a decrease or fading of feedback. For instance, a child who is learning to feed himself or herself is not given feedback about performance after each spoonful although some inaccuracy and spillage is observed. If the child spills the entire contents or misses the bowl, then feedback is given to help the child evaluate his or her performance and try another way to scoop and bring the spoon to his or her mouth. In this case, the therapist must decide on the error range that is acceptable before feedback is given. Summary feedback would be given after several spoon-to-mouth attempts and may take the form of comments like, "you are getting most of the food in your mouth" or "you are spilling much less that you did last week."

The content of feedback used should be brief and appropriate to the child's cognitive, language, and sensory abilities. For example, a child who has very limited receptive language abilities, or a very young child, may be given a series of hand claps, an exaggerated smile, or a pat on the back after several successful attempts. A child with limited visual abilities should be given feedback in an auditory or tactile form.

Feedback should focus on the goal of the movement or the task, not on a specific movement strategy. This is sometimes referred to as "knowledge of results" (KR) or "giving information feedback about the outcome" (Gentile, 1992, p.32). The feedback given would comment on the outcome, for example, "you spilled very little" or "you did it!."

Informational feedback and suggestions can be given in different ways. The most common method is verbal, but a person can also model a different way of moving or can physically move the child using manual guidance to have him or her feel an alternative way of moving. Physical positioning or manual guidance is used only after other methods have been unsuccessful because it is the child who must generate the movement solution for learning to occur most efficiently (Figure 12.7). These methods

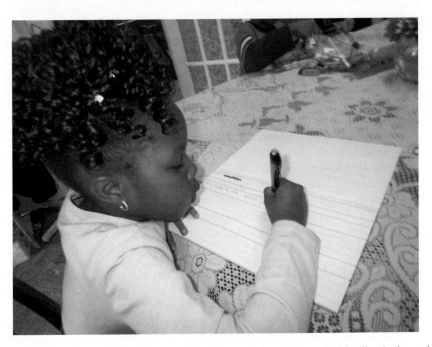

FIGURE 12.7 The therapist provides manual guidance followed by verbal feedback about the goal of the movement: "You stayed within the lines!"

can be used to encourage a child to try another movement strategy if the one he or she is using is unsuccessful or inefficient. They may also be used to redirect a child to the task, remind him or her of the goals, or motivate the child to continue trying. Children often require help remembering the goal and attending to the characteristics in the environment, which are important to a successful outcome. The therapist may direct the child's attention to the object by using contrasting colors; by limiting extraneous sensory stimuli; or by using verbal, visual, or manual prompts to point out salient characteristics. It may also be helpful to give feedback after a brief interval that allows the child to process his or her own feedback about the action first (Gentile, 1992).

However, the therapist should encourage the child to become less reliant on feedback from the therapist and increase the ability to assess his or her own movement and performance. The content of feedback can include questions for the child to help engage in this problem solving (e.g., "What do you think about what you did? What seemed to work well and not so well? What are some other ways you could try?").

Assumptions

There are a few basic assumptions that distinguish a motor skill acquisition frame of reference based on motor learning, control, and development principles from other frames of reference that focus on the development of motor skills. These assumptions have consequences for evaluation and intervention.

- The most important assumption is that functional tasks help organize behavior. The focus of evaluation and treatment is the person's ability to engage in those tasks that are meaningful. A related assumption is that successful performance of meaningful tasks emerges from the interaction of multiple personal and environmental systems. Therefore, evaluation and intervention must consider these multiple systems.
- Another assumption is that the motor problems observed are the result of all the systems interacting and compensating for some damage or problem in one or more of those systems. Evaluation and intervention would seek to identify which subsystems can be changed or affected to enable a new or more efficient skilled motor behavior to emerge. This is quite different from the assumption found in other frames of reference related to motor development (i.e., motor problems observed are the direct result of neurological damage). In those frames of reference, intervention must directly influence the neurological system, which is not the case with the motor skill acquisition frame of reference.

A thorough understanding of the movement sciences is still emerging. The information presented was based on a review of available studies that are limited in the range of ages, populations, contexts, tasks, and motor skills studied. More information is needed to fully understand how children acquire more efficient motor skills. However, there is beginning support for the emphasis on functional tasks and consideration of the person, task, and environment as they interact and have an impact on emergent motor skills.

FUNCTION–DYSFUNCTION CONTINUA

The motor skill acquisition frame of reference is somewhat unique from other frames of reference in that continua of function and dysfunction are defined by the performance in the specific skill to be acquired. The child's abilities related to performing a task reflect the functional end of the continuum, whereas the child's inabilities or difficulties related to performing a task reflect the dysfunctional end of the continuum. That is, the child can either perform a skill needed to function in the environment, or cannot. Therefore, there are no specific continua defined for function and dysfunction within this acquisitional frame of reference. A criterion-referenced dichotomous measure (i.e., yes, the child can perform the specific skill; or no, the child cannot perform the skill) can be used when generating a specific function–dysfunction continua for a child. Also, the task can be analyzed and the task components that the child is able to do and unable to do can be identified. Function and dysfunction is determined by the environment within which the skill must be performed. The environments in which the task will be used can be analyzed to identify the supports and constraints to performance that are present. Furthermore, a child's developmental status provides only a background for this frame of reference and is considered when determining if the skill to be acquired is reasonable to expect of the child. For example, it would be unreasonable to expect a 3-year-old child to learn to write sentences, whereas it is reasonable to expect a 3-year-old child to be learning to dress himself.

Function–dysfunction continua can be identified for any task that is necessary for the child to perform within the environment. It can range from simply the ability to grasp and release a desired toy, to independence in activities of daily living (ADL) skills, to the ability to interact in a socially appropriate manner. Skills in the motor skill acquisition frame of reference are always environmentally specific. Within the frame of reference, each prioritized task that is important or essential to the child is observed. Relative to each observed task, there is one function–dysfunction continuum—the child is either able to perform the task or unable to perform the task.

Indicators of Function and Dysfunction

The indicators of function are those aspects of the task that the child is able to perform (Table 12.1). These indicators identify the child's abilities and strengths related to task performance and are reflective of motor skill acquisition. For example, the child may be able to push his or her arms through the jacket sleeves once it has been positioned and pull up the zipper once it has been engaged by an adult.

The indicators of dysfunction are those aspects of the task that the child is unable to perform and reflect difficulties in motor skill acquisition. These indicators identify the child's inabilities and needs related to task performance. Using the example mentioned earlier, the child may be unable to pull the jacket sleeve from behind his or her back and engage the zipper. Indicators of dysfunction in this frame of reference direct one's attention to possible deficits that could be remediated and characteristics of the task or environment that are too demanding and require modification (i.e., child-task-environment do not match). For example, the child may have decreased active

TABLE 12.1 Indicators of Function and Dysfunction for Motor Task Performance	
FUNCTION: **Indicators of Function**	*DYSFUNCTION:* **Indicators of Dysfunction**
Child is able to perform a motor task	Child is unable to perform a motor task
Child's environment supports task performance	Child's environment does not support task performance
Task requirements are within a child's capabilities with or without environmental support	Task requirements are beyond the child's capabilities with environmental support
Child-task-environment match	Child-task-environment do not match

range of motion at the shoulder girdle and have limited manual dexterity and bilateral coordination to engage the zipper. The task and environment could then be modified by encouraging an overhead versus behind-the-back approach to putting on the jacket or substituting Velcro fasteners for the zipper. Or the child may benefit from preparation of the shoulder muscles to relax and lengthen before being asked to complete the task, remediation activities to promote manual dexterity and bilateral coordination. The demands of the task and environment need to match the developmental level and capabilities of the child.

GUIDE FOR EVALUATION

It is important to note that evaluation is a dynamic process and does not necessarily follow a specific order. The following is a general guideline for evaluation. It is important for each occupational therapist to learn to observe and organize this information in a way that is efficient and effective for himself or herself. Factors related to the child, task, and environment, as well as the interaction of all three, must be evaluated so the intervention can address all three of these important areas.

The process consists of the following steps: focusing first on the child, then the task, then the environment, and finally, the interaction of all three areas:

Child

1. Discussion with child, family, teacher, and other care providers:
   - Identify the tasks that are most important for the child to perform effectively at home, school, and in the community. For younger children, this information may be inferred by observing the child's level of interest and self-selection of tasks.
   - From these tasks, identify the tasks with which the child is reportedly having difficulty. Prioritize the tasks related to home, school, or community life on which occupational therapy intervention will focus (e.g., self-feeding, dressing, handwriting, activating computer keyboard or switch, engaging in play activities, handling money, using public transportation, maintaining one's daily living space).
   - Identify whether the motor skills to perform these tasks are within the child's capabilities or are reasonable to expect the child to perform based on the child's age and sociocultural contexts.

2. Observe the child doing each prioritized task in the environment where it is naturally performed. If this is not possible, find out about these environments and attempt to simulate them if this is feasible. Assess the task characteristics, environmental demands, and child's capabilities and stage of learning as these relate to motor skill acquisition for each specific task. In addition, standardized functional evaluations such as the *Pediatric Evaluation of Disability Inventory* (PEDI) (Haley et al., 1992), the *School Function Assessment* (SFA) (Coster et al., 1998), and the *School Assessment of Motor and Process Skills* (AMPS) (Fisher et al., 2005) can be used to assist with the identification, prioritization, and documentation of the child's current level of abilities.

3. Evaluate the motor and process skills or factors within the child that are most likely to influence motor skill acquisition in this task. For example, if a child's skill in feeding seems to be limited by the child's ability to grasp the spoon and bring it to the mouth, it would be reasonable to further evaluate the child's grasp, range of motion, muscle tone, and strength as well as postural control. Only skills and factors that have a high likelihood of or are observed to be limiting task performance should be evaluated. To evaluate factors such as muscle tone, strength, range of motion, memory, problem solving, sensory regulation, visual discrimination, and coping skills, the occupational therapist can use specific assessments that examine these areas in more detail.

Task

4. Analyze the requirements and characteristics of each prioritized task. Explore the components of the task, see where the child is having difficulties and which aspects of the task he or she can do well. This process of task analysis is critical in identifying whether aspects of the task are influencing performance and if so, which aspects may be influencing performance. The information gained can assist with decisions about the feasibility of task modification or the use of alternate tasks.

Environment

5. Analyze the demands and characteristics of the environment in which each task will be performed. Consider the physical characteristics (space, furniture, objects, work and support surface, lighting, glare, noise, distractions, and overall organization), the regulatory conditions (which affect the necessary timing, force, and magnitude of movement), and the sociocultural contexts (demands, expectations, instructions, and presentation of task). Environmental analysis is critical in identifying whether and which aspects of the environment are influencing performance. The information gained can assist with decisions about whether environmental modification is feasible or with a determination of which factors are interfering with task performance. Observation in the actual environment where the task is performed is also helpful in identifying child skills or client factors that may be interfering with performance.

The next few steps of the evaluation process involve looking at the interaction of the child, task, and environment.

6. Regulatory conditions are aspects of the environment which determine movement specifics that impact on the task. Tasks need to be analyzed from the perspective of Gentile's closed and open task taxonomy; several steps; sensory motor, cognitive, and psychosocial demands; degree of structure; and characteristics of materials: size, shape, texture, weight, pliability, and inherent visual cues and contrast.

7. Examine the following questions relative to the child's performance of tasks in relation to environment:

   • What is the child able to do? In what environments? (indicators of function)
   • What is the child unable to do? In what environments? (indicators of dysfunction)
   • What is interfering with motor skill acquisition that is reflected in task performance? Describe task and environmental constraints and child skill deficits.
   • What is supporting motor skill acquisition that is reflected in task performance? Describe task and environmental supports and child skill capabilities.
   • What can improve the child's motor skill acquisition or task performance? Consider feedback, practice, and task or environmental modification. The information gained from asking this question and from performing the next step in this evaluation process can be directly applied to intervention (refer to postulates regarding change).

8. Explore possible modifications of the task and environment. Modify the task and/or environmental conditions, allow the child to practice the task under the new conditions, and provide feedback about motor skill performance and outcome.

9. Reassess motor skill acquisition by observing the child's task performance with preliminary modifications, feedback, and practice provided.

10. The final step is the interpretation of evaluation and recommendations for intervention: Information about motor skill acquisition and factors that support and constrain task performance and skill acquisition is described for each prioritized task. On the basis of this information, goals and objectives are developed pertaining to motor skill acquisition of each task and an intervention plan is developed among the team members.

Evaluation is a dynamic process (McCaffrey-Easley, 1996). The primary focus is on the child-task-environment interaction, which is an assessment of the child while performing each prioritized task in specific environments. Observation shifts back and forth among the child's capabilities, the task characteristics, and environmental demands. The evaluation interpretation and recommendations focus on interaction between all three of these areas.

POSTULATES REGARDING CHANGE

On the basis of the emerging research in motor control, motor learning, and motor development, the following postulates regarding change guide intervention directed at motor skill acquisition. There are four general postulates, as follows:

1. If there is a match among the task requirements, environmental demands, and the child's abilities, then it is more likely that motor skill acquisition will be improved.

2. If the child understands what is to be achieved and is provided with clear information about the expected motor skill performance and outcome, then it is more likely that motor skill acquisition will be improved.
3. If the child is encouraged to independently problem solve to find his or her own optimal movement strategies to perform tasks in a safe environment that can support error, then it is more likely that motor skill acquisition will be improved.
4. If the child is provided with a task that is challenging (i.e., possible at the child's upper limit of capabilities or zone of proximal development) and motivating, it is more likely that motor skill acquisition will be improved.

There are seven specific postulates, as follows:

1. In earlier stages of learning, if feedback is focused on movement outcome and the critical features of the task and environment (not on movement performance), then it is more likely that motor skill acquisition will be improved.
2. In later stages of learning, if feedback is summarized (rather than detailed) and provided when movement performance demonstrates a greater than acceptable level of error (error range), then it is more likely that motor skill acquisition will be improved.
3. If the child is encouraged to self-evaluate his or her own movement performance and outcome by focusing on inherent body and perceived environmental feedback, then it is more likely that motor skill performance will be improved.
4. If the child is provided with randomized practice of tasks in the situations in which they typically occur, then it is more likely that motor skill acquisition and long-term retention will be improved. (However, the child with severe cognitive disabilities may benefit from massed practice especially in the early stages of learning.)
5. For open tasks, if the child is provided with variability and unpredictability during practice, then it is more likely that motor skill acquisition will be improved for open tasks.
6. If the child practices and is provided feedback about motor skill performance and outcome in natural settings for that task, then it is more likely that motor skill acquisition will be improved in those settings.
7. If the motor skill is practiced in various contexts and daily routines, then it is more likely that the motor skill will be generalized, transferred to, or used in other contexts and daily routines.

APPLICATION TO PRACTICE

The motor skill acquisition frame of reference described in this chapter incorporates child-task-environment match with the concepts of practice and feedback combined with task and environmental modification to improve motor skill acquisition. The focus of this section will be to describe in more depth how to apply the general and specific postulates regarding change to improve motor skill acquisition. Intervention is directed toward improving motor skill acquisition related to each task as specified in the goals and objectives developed from the evaluation. However, to use this frame of reference, the therapist will need to integrate his or her knowledge and skills in task/environmental analysis and modifications. This process is foundational to occupational therapy practice and has been described consistently in occupational therapy literature (Law et al., 2005; Mathiowetz & Bass-Haugen, 2008; Phipps & Roberts, 2006).

This frame of reference can be used with children who have a wide variety of underlying problems that may be contributing to their ability to learn motor skills. Information relevant to the type of problem must be considered when designing and implementing intervention. The specific methods used in this frame of reference may be different for the child with sensory regulation/processing problems as compared with the child with hypertonicity. For example, for a child with hypertonicity, a therapist may use the motor skill acquisition frame of reference alone or in conjunction with another frame of reference like Neuro-Developmental Treatment; however, the therapist must always consider theories and knowledge about spasticity. The motor skill acquisition frame of reference can be used with other approaches or by itself, but the therapist always considers available knowledge relevant to the specific problems of the child.

In this frame of reference, task performance reflects motor skill acquisition. Through observation of the child's task performance, the occupational therapist obtains important information about the task, environment, and child who is supporting or constraining task performance. The goal of intervention is to obtain a child-task-environment match to improve task performance. To do this, the therapist modifies the task and environment or addresses the performance skills or capabilities that have the potential to improve task performance.

The child needs to understand what is expected of him or her and may need to be reminded of the expected movement outcome or goal of the task to be performed. The therapist provides information feedback about critical features of the environment and the movement outcome that was performed by the child. The child can be shown how his or her movement outcome was similar to and different from the expected outcome. The therapist can provide the child with a visual model of the expected outcome, such as a completed drawing or a completed dressing task with the garment positioned and oriented in the expected fashion. The child can then be encouraged to compare his or her own outcome with the visual model. For children with visual impairments, verbal and tactile information can be provided for the child to make this comparison. It is important that the expected outcome be achievable and reasonable given age, ability level, and sociocultural expectations. This information can be obtained from caregivers, chart review, or criterion-referenced testing.

At times, particularly with young children or children who have difficulty learning, it may be necessary to use manual guidance to help the child understand the movement that is required for the task. In this case, the therapist would move the child through a task once or several times until the child begins to initiate the movement on his or her own. The intent of manual guidance is to use it only until the child has the idea of the movement and then to withdraw it as soon as possible. The intent is not to facilitate or inhibit particular muscle groups or movement patterns. It is important in this approach that the child develops his or her own movement strategy and not have a strategy imposed by the therapist.

Some children with cognitive impairments or who learn more slowly may need more extensive periods of repetition or massed practice to learn or retain new skills than others. It may be necessary to practice a task in each of the contexts in which it will be used because of the difficulty with generalization of skills and long-term retention of learning in many people with more severe learning problems. Each child should be encouraged to independently problem solve to the best of his or her ability using various movement strategies to achieve the goal. This will allow the child to find his or her own strategies for movement. Once the child develops personalized strategies for movement, then he or she is more likely to improve motor skill acquisition. After the child has performed the task, it is important to wait a few seconds to allow the child to process or make use of his or her own body and perceived environmental feedback before providing additional therapist feedback. This time period can vary for each child and should be monitored accordingly.

To promote motor skill acquisition in the early stages of learning, the tasks need to be challenging, motivating, and relevant to the child's life experiences. To do this effectively, the therapist needs to understand the child's skills and limitations and adapt or devise tasks that are challenging but not beyond the child's capabilities with necessary support. The therapist may use the understanding of the zone of proximal development to structure tasks that the child can do now only with some assistance but are within the child's potential range for achieving independently. Furthermore, based on the therapist's understanding of the child's environment, tasks are structured to be meaningful and relevant to the child's life.

During the early stages of learning, the therapist attempts to match the child's capabilities with the task requirements and environmental demands. This may involve the use of adaptive equipment, positioning devices, and assistive technology; modifying the task or the environment; or providing feedback to make it easier for the child to process and use critical features of the task. Once the child understands the expected movement outcome, it is important to reduce therapist feedback and encourage the child to make use of his or her inherent body and perceived environmental feedback. The therapist should provide a summary or general versus detailed feedback and after the child's movement performance falls outside a given or preset error range instead of immediately after each attempt. However, some children may require more immediate or frequent feedback in the early stages of learning because of their unique learning and psychosocial preferences and needs. The therapist must weigh these factors along with the information provided from research in the movement sciences when deciding on when to provide feedback.

During the later stages of learning, the child is reminded to self-evaluate movement performance and outcome by focusing on his or her inherent body and perceived environmental feedback. Rather than describe to the child the difference between his or her movement outcome and the expected outcome or the specific movement strategies that were inefficient or ineffective, the therapist will ask the child questions to help him or her generate his or her own ideas and solutions about movement performance and outcome. Potential questions could be: "What do you think about what you did?," "What seemed to work well and not so well?," and "What are some other ways you could try?" When the child is unable to generate his or her own ideas or solutions, the therapist can engage in this process with the child and provide more feedback about movement performance and outcome. The therapist can demonstrate to the child how he or she moved and explain why particular movement strategies may not have been effective. The therapist should suggest, demonstrate, or instruct the child in other movement strategies only if and when the child has difficulty generating alternate movement strategies on his or her own. However, therapist-generated movement strategies may not be efficient or effective in achieving the movement outcome because the therapist does not have full access to the child's inherent body and perceived environmental feedback. There is no one "normal" or "best" movement strategy to use to accomplish a particular task. The most efficient strategy for a person depends on the state of all the systems interacting in and around the person at a particular time.

The child should practice whole tasks. The child should not practice one isolated part of a task without the experience of doing the whole task (e.g., practicing putting the arm in the shirt sleeve without practicing putting on the whole shirt). The child may be able to do parts of the task independently and require physical assistance and more feedback from the therapist for the other parts of the task. Practicing whole tasks is important because the task, environmental conditions, and information that the child has to attend to and manage are incorporated into the practice sessions and completing a task is intrinsically rewarding. These conditions are not addressed when practicing isolated parts of tasks, especially the timing and sequencing demands that need to be managed while performing whole tasks.

Therapists often structure treatment sessions to allow the child to practice basic skills that are important to many tasks (e.g., balance). If at all possible, balance should be practiced as part of a task, not separately, on therapy equipment such as a therapy ball or bolster. Many children have difficulty transferring skills (e.g., balance) learned on equipment (e.g., on a ball) to those tasks in which they need to use balance (e.g., dressing or reaching for and manipulating toys or eating utensils).

The therapist must structure practice conditions to include variability and unpredictability of movement, while the child practices open tasks because these are inherent characteristics of these tasks. The child can be encouraged to develop a repertoire of strategies to deal with the unpredictability of the regulatory conditions and the quickness in movements that are necessary to perform many motor skills.

Various tasks should be provided and practiced as soon as the child understands the specific task performance and outcome. This will allow for randomized practice, which will improve the potential for skill acquisition and long-term retention. Some children take longer to understand this and may require more massed practice until they have demonstrated that they understand expected task performance and outcome. Other factors (e.g., the child's information processing abilities and learning preferences) have to be considered when deciding when to transition from massed to random practice. In addition, children with more severe cognitive disabilities or children who may need more time to understand the expected movement outcome or goal may need more massed practice. Massed practice may need to be provided in each of the settings where the movement skill will be used because children with severe cognitive disabilities may have great difficulty in generalizing the movement skills learned in one setting or for one daily routine to another.

During early and later phases of learning, the child should be encouraged to practice the movement skills in various contexts, with different materials, and for different daily routines. This can provide the child with a larger repertoire and more flexible strategies in dealing with a greater number of tasks and environmental demands. This can improve long-term retention and generalization of the movement skills acquired. Some children with cognitive impairments may need to practice in the environment where the task is to be used with the same materials that will be used on a daily basis. In addition, some children may not benefit from simulated environments or tasks.

In the motor skill acquisition frame of reference, the goals and objectives are directed at functional task performance. The goal identifies the task performance in which effort will be directed by the child and selected caregivers. The objectives are the smaller aims that indicate whether the child is making progress toward this goal (Mager, 1975). Objectives need to be measurable and include the task performance (e.g., donning jacket and engaging and pulling up zipper), the expected level or criterion of performance (e.g., able to do three times in a week, with or without certain conditions), the necessary conditions of task performance (i.e., task modification and verbal reminder, verbal and tactile feedback, and practice), and the contexts where task performance occurs (e.g., home and classroom).

Intervention is task oriented and context specific because motor skill acquisition is contingent on the child's capabilities, task requirements, and environmental demands. What works for one child in one task or in one environment may not work for or in others. Therefore, it is important to carefully monitor the effectiveness of this intervention by reviewing and updating behavioral objectives and documenting observable behaviors that can indicate progress in motor skill acquisition. This is important because there is still much that is unknown about the effectiveness of the postulates regarding change that have been described earlier in this chapter.

Other frames of reference presented in this book may be used in combination with this frame of reference. In particular, the occupational therapist may use the biomechanical, Neuro-Developmental Treatment, sensory integration, and visual perception processing frames of reference. Specifically, the biomechanical frame of reference can assist with motor skill acquisition in seating, positioning, work-surface design, and set up of task-related materials. The visual information processing frame of reference also can assist with task and environmental modification. The therapist should be aware of possible conflicts arising from differences in the theoretical bases of other frames of reference, particularly assumptions; ideas about the role of the therapist, child, and family; and priorities in goals.

The application of this frame of reference will be demonstrated using a case of a 6-year-old child who is receiving occupational therapy services. The name and any identifying characteristics have been changed to protect confidentiality. The pictures are used for illustration and are in simulated environments.

Natalie's Case Study

Natalie is a 6-year-old girl who lives at home with her parents, her maternal grandmother, a 12-year-old brother, and a 4-year-old sister. The family lives in a three-bedroom apartment in an urban area and both parents work full time during the day. Natalie attends a public school within walking distance of her home. She attended preschool at age 3 years and received occupational, physical, and speech therapy as well as special education services. Since starting kindergarten at age 5 years, she receives occupational therapy and physical therapy each two times per week. She is currently in a first grade, regular education classroom with services from a special educator who consults with the regular education teacher. Natalie has recently been diagnosed with a learning disability and developmental coordination disorder (DCD). She has some postural weakness and tires easily. Fine motor and bilateral tasks are difficult for her.

Occupational Therapy Evaluation

Information about Natalie was initially obtained by reviewing her educational file and talking to Natalie, her teachers, and parents. The focus was on analyzing the child-task-environment match. There were several strengths and needs that were identified from the educational file review and informal discussions with the teacher and parents. In addition, the PEDI was administered and scores indicate an age delay in accomplishing dressing using fasteners only. Scores in all other areas on the PEDI were within age level. The SFA was administered to delineate specific difficulties in school participation. The scores on the SFA indicate that Natalie has some difficulty in participation during transitions between classroom and other school areas. She uses the wall in the hall for support and often waits for most of the class to go ahead of her. She does not participate fully on the playground and likes to watch others performing physical activities such as kickball. She has some difficulty completing some classroom tasks that require handwriting and fine motor manipulation activities such as art projects and copying homework from the board. Natalie's strengths include that she is ambulatory and independent, but somewhat slow, in all aspects of self-care except zippers, snaps, small buttons, and tying shoes (with occasional reminders needed for quality and thoroughness). Additionally, she has very supportive and resourceful parents. She also is very social, articulate, and has good persistence and frustration tolerance for tasks that she enjoys doing such as art activities, cooking activities, and games such as freeze tag, musical chairs, and concentration card game.

Natalie has difficulty with most tasks that require fine controlled movements of her hands; bilateral coordination; and increased strength, endurance, and balance. Natalie's parents are very pleased with her progress in reading and in performing self-care tasks. They are most concerned about her handwriting skills and want to help with her school performance as much as they can. The tasks that Natalie and Natalie's teacher report as most problematic and which will be addressed in the evaluation are as follows:

• Handwriting
• Fine motor tasks that require bilateral coordination, such as scissor use, for art and classroom activities
• Carrying her lunch tray and opening food containers in the lunchroom while other children are moving about

- Balance, running, and ball activities during physical education (PE) and on the playground

The last three tasks are open tasks because aspects of the environment are in motion and the task requirements and environmental demands vary each time the task is attempted. Handwriting can be considered to be further on the continuum toward a closed task as the environment is not in motion and only some aspects of the task change each time a person is writing.

Observation of Task Performance

The tasks identified were observed in the contexts where, and at the time when, Natalie typically performed them during the school day. While all of the tasks mentioned earlier were observed, one task, art activities requiring scissors and other bimanual abilities, will be described in-depth to demonstrate the process of evaluation when using a motor skill acquisition frame of reference. This task will also be discussed later to demonstrate intervention using this frame of reference.

Art Project

The class was engaged in making a card for Mother's Day. Materials were distributed to small group cluster tables (six children's desks pushed together). The materials were large pieces of paper of different colors, markers, crayons, glitter in small cups, glue sticks, scissors, magazines (for pictures), and cups with small decorative items to stick onto the cards with glue. The children were instructed to fold the large paper into a smaller sized card and to write "Dear Mom, Happy Mother's Day" and their name. They were free to add other touches to their cards. Natalie appeared to understand the goal of the activity and was able to lean over to the middle of the table and choose a piece of paper for the card, a marker, and a glue stick. She had difficulty folding the paper evenly and had to try it several times to get the edges even. When the card was better, but not even, she proceeded to write on the front of the card, "Dear Mom." She wrote the first three letters very large and ran out of room, regarded her work, and put the paper aside. She started over with a new paper. This time, she did not write on the front of the card, but used the glue stick and glitter and just made a design on the front. Inside the card, she wrote "Love, Natalie." The letters were not all legible, were of unequal size, and the spacing was uneven. With prompting from the teacher, she then took a scissor and tried to cut out a picture of a flower from a magazine. It was difficult for her to simultaneously manipulate the magazine and the scissors in order to cut out the object. However, when the page was ripped out from the magazine and a line was drawn around the flower, she was able to follow the line successfully. At this point, most other children were finished, and Natalie said she was finished although she said later that she would have liked to put more decorations on the card but that she was tired of working. She leaned over and rested on her desk often during this activity and wrapped her legs around the legs of the chair. She often held her head up with one arm and hand which then created difficulty in manipulating the materials.

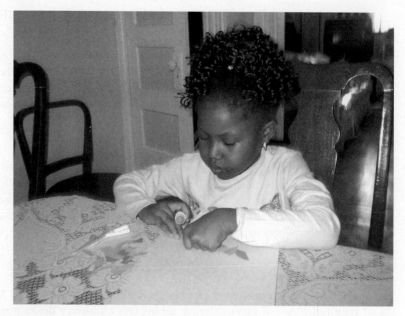

FIGURE 12.8 Natalie manipulates paper and scissors during an art activity.

During this task, Natalie demonstrated the ability to problem solve when something was difficult for her (Figure 12.8). She also evaluated her own performance without feedback. Her performance was affected by poor hand and finger dexterity, awkward and immature grasp of scissors and marker, poor bilateral coordination, and limited endurance. Some of the task demands were clearly above her present capabilities such as cutting something directly out of a magazine and writing letters on a blank page without lines. The environment did not seem distracting to Natalie, but she did not ask for help from other children or the teacher. The prompts she received from the teacher were helpful to her performance. The teacher gave her the extra visual cue of a line around the flower in the magazine and this improved Natalie's performance. Natalie might have benefited from increased cueing from an adult to try a different method or cueing from a template of letters to refer to for letter formation (as she uses during handwriting activities). She was able to share objects during the task but did not appear to be aware of other children's work or presence.

It is important to note that Natalie's performance improved when she was given a visual cue to follow for cutting with the scissors. She also responded positively to the teacher's prompt to try a task that was difficult for her (cutting with the scissors). Because these methods appeared to be effective, they will also be incorporated into Natalie's intervention (which will be described in more detail later). It was evident during the evaluation that Natalie clearly understood the desired goal and many of the movements required. She had more difficulty with some of the movement components and needs to refine them to perform these tasks more accurately and

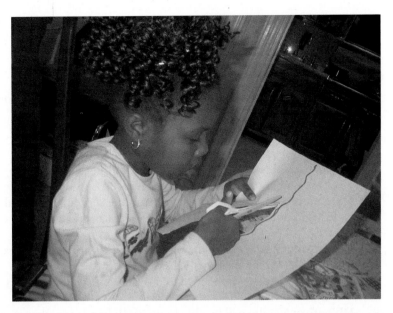

FIGURE 12.9 Natalie manipulates paper and scissors during an art activity with enhanced visual cues.

efficiently. This indicates that, for these tasks, Natalie is not in the earliest stages of learning but is transitioning from early to later stages. Consequently, based on the specific postulates regarding change, feedback can begin to be focused on some of the movement performance issues rather than solely on the movement outcome. In addition, Natalie can be encouraged to use more self-evaluation of her own movement performance and outcome (Figure 12.9).

The observation indicated that Natalie had some difficulty with grasp, manipulation of objects, and postural control. Therefore, an assessment was conducted of grasp of different sized and shaped objects, in-hand manipulation skills, hand strength, and dexterity. In addition, postural control was evaluated by assessing balance reactions, anticipatory postural control, and visual motor coordination with ball activities and motor planning. This assessment revealed immature grasp of the pencil, weakness resulting in fatigue with hand use (e.g., handwriting) of more than 1 minute, and poor in-hand manipulation. Scores in the *Test of In-Hand Manipulation* reveal difficulty with translation, shift, and rotation components. Postural reactions were within normal limits (WNL), but anticipatory postural adjustments were delayed or absent resulting in clumsy movements and difficulty in executing voluntary movements, especially gross motor action sequences. During motor planning activities, Natalie has ideation of, but has difficulty with execution of the movement. When trying to catch or kick a ball, Natalie has difficulty with balance and with timing. She is much more successful with a ball task in which the ball is stationary and she can kick it in her own time. The *Bruininks Oseretsky Test of Motor Proficiency* (Bruininks & Bruininks, 2005) was given 6 months ago.

Natalie's scores are below the −2 standard deviation level compared to her age peers in the area of body coordination, and at the −1.5 standard deviation level in the areas of fine manual control and strength and agility.

Goals and Objectives

These are examples of possible functional goals for two of the problem areas identified for Natalie:

Goal: Natalie will be able to complete in-class writing assignments in manuscript (printing) legibly within the time allotted.

Objective: kal Natalie will be able to print one sentence with enhanced visual cues of top and bottom darkened lines with 80% of the letters legible.

Objective: Natalie will be able to print one sentence with enhanced visual cues of top and bottom darkened lines with 80% of the letters on the line and the same size.

Goal: Natalie will be able to complete her art projects in the classroom within the time allotted for these activities.

Objective: Natalie will be able to use the scissors to cut out a circular object given enhanced visual cues.

Objective: Natalie will be able to use both hands together to stabilize, manipulate, and fold a piece of paper to instructions during an art project.

Goal: Natalie will be able to kick the ball during her PE class activity of "kickball" when it is her turn, and be able to run to the first base.

Objective: Natalie will be able to kick a stationary ball toward an intended direction and maintain her balance.

Objective: Natalie will be able to kick a slowly moving ball in any direction and maintain her balance.

Objective: Natalie will be able to kick a slowly moving ball in a desired direction and maintain her balance.

Intervention

It is important when applying the motor skill acquisition frame of reference to use the postulates regarding change to guide intervention. One general postulate states that if the child clearly understands the goal and what is to be achieved, then motor skill acquisition will be improved. By having Natalie identify the tasks that are both important and challenging for her and describe how she would like to be able to perform these tasks, it is more likely that she will be clear about the goals of intervention. It is also more likely that she will be engaged in tasks that are important, motivating, and challenging, which is another general postulate in this frame of reference. The teachers both agreed to ask Natalie what she would like her final art product to look like. When possible they will offer her a visual model of letters or a product for a comparison. By choosing activities that Natalie is motivated to engage in, there is increased likelihood that she will persist, and problem solve by trying other methods. She will be supported by the teacher or therapist to challenge herself by attempting activities that are difficult. The team agreed to prompt Natalie to use her problem-solving abilities by asking her to think of another way to do it instead of giving her specific directions. Since Natalie is beginning to be able to self-evaluate, we want everyone to encourage this. We can ask Natalie things such as, "how did that work out?," or "did that come out the way you wanted?"

All of these strategies flow from the general postulate stating that if there is a match among the task requirements, environmental demands, and the child's capabilities, then it is more likely that motor skill acquisition will be improved. The cues and prompts used by adults in the environment can change task requirements and context to support Natalie's performance. The therapist will work on integrating practice opportunities during the school day for grasp, in-hand manipulation, finger dexterity, and strength.

Natalie continued to work on her handwriting daily in the classroom, with weekly monitoring from the occupational therapist related to writing speed, letter spacing, and alignment. She also was provided with a writing slant board positioned on her desk, which appeared to offer her a greater biomechanical and visual advantage when writing. The occupational therapist, Natalie, and the teacher agreed to experiment with sitting on a therapy ball or an inflatable disc on her chair to see if the movement afforded by inflatables might improve her ability to maintain an upright posture while engaged in seated activities. Because visual cueing seemed to improve performance, Natalie practices handwriting in the classroom using paper with very dark lines on it. She also uses a finger spacing strategy to produce equal spacing between words. The teacher encourages Natalie to evaluate each word she writes and to circle it if it is legible and within the lines. When Natalie gets 10 circles, she brings her work to the teacher and gets a big star sticker on her work.

Natalie was concerned about being able to use the scissors, so the therapist worked with her and used some massed practice sessions, first cutting angles and circular lines and then, in later sessions, cutting around shapes or pictures without lines (Figure 12.10). The therapist monitored Natalie's classroom performance during and after these sessions of massed practice to evaluate the effects during naturally occurring scissor use in the classroom. As Natalie's ability with scissors improved, massed practice was discontinued.

For several weeks, the therapist worked with Natalie in the classroom during art and handwriting activities to make sure that the visual cue strategies were effective and to reinforce Natalie's self-evaluation and problem solving. This program of integrating occupational therapy into the child's school day is consistent with the postulates regarding change in this frame of reference. Motor performance and generalization to other tasks will improve if practice and feedback occur during daily routines and in natural contexts and involves variability. As Natalie developed a habit of self-evaluation and her fine motor abilities were improving, the therapist began to work with Natalie during other types of school tasks such as during recess on the playground and during PE.

Physical Education

Natalie enjoyed kickball in the park with her father and siblings. She was motivated to try to join in at this game during PE at school. However, when she played the

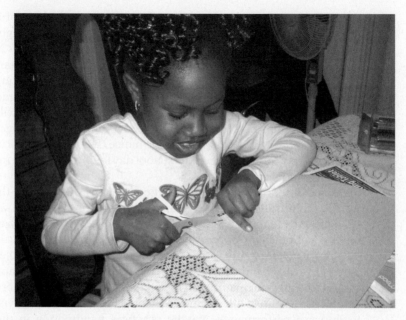

FIGURE 12.10 Massed practice of scissor use during an individual occupational therapy session.

game with her family, they made some adjustments to the task demands. They rolled the ball very slowly to her and she let it stop before actually kicking it. Then, they let her have a moment before she had to run to the base. These adjustments to the task demands allowed Natalie to engage in an activity that was challenging but possible with the adjustments (Figure 12.11). This is a nice example of "scaffolding" by a family to support the child's practice of a challenging activity that may help her to move to the next developmental level in skill.

However, when playing kickball in school, Natalie often just watched the activity as the task demands were not adjusted for her level of ability. Natalie did not want to have special rules just for her; she wanted to be able to play with the rest of the class. During the evaluation, the therapist had observed that Natalie had difficulty with anticipatory postural control and with timing in a moving environment and felt that these were the major underlying factors in Natalie's problems with kickball. The PE teacher, who was not aware that Natalie really did want to participate, was willing to modify the task by rolling the ball very slowly to Natalie and giving her more time before she had to run to the base, but Natalie did not want this modification. Instead, the PE teacher worked with the occupational therapist and developed some new games for the class that used a balloon for kicking as that moved more slowly. The children all had to freeze and spell WAIT out loud with the teacher before they could move after someone kicked the ball. This was actually positive for many of the children who had difficulty in waiting.

In addition, the therapist increased Natalie's practice time by asking her family to play catching, throwing, hitting, and kicking games with a balloon or nerf ball

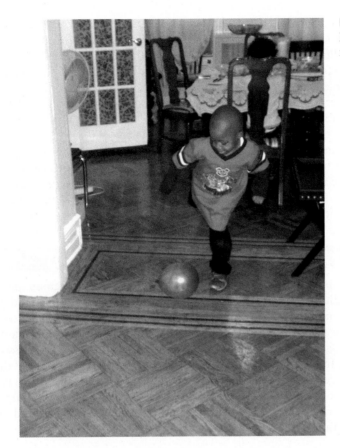

FIGURE 12.11 A child playing kickball at home, with some adjustments to the task demands.

that could be used in the apartment. The therapist instituted a preparation activity for the class at the beginning of the gym period, which the PE teacher carried out after a few weeks. This preparation involved clapping in front, above head, to each side, and behind while standing first on one foot then the other. Anyone who wanted to stand near the wall could do so. The children thought making all this noise was quite fun and it gave Natalie some opportunity to practice anticipatory postural control. The therapist practiced this activity with Natalie in occupational therapy sessions using massed practice. In addition, the occupational therapist practiced strategies with Natalie to develop anticipatory postural control. Natalie described to the occupational therapist what she was going to do before she did it. For example, Natalie described that she was going to kick the balloon with her right foot as hard as she could. Then, the occupational therapist asked Natalie to close her eyes and visualize herself doing this. Then Natalie tried the kick. The occupational therapist waited a few moments for Natalie to process the movement information feedback from her own body and look at the effects of her action. Then the occupational therapist provided summary feedback such as "look, you kicked the balloon, but then you fell down." The occupational therapist then encouraged

Natalie to think how to do it a little differently next time. The occupational therapist found that she had to use manual guidance for a few sessions as Natalie was getting frustrated at falling each time she tried to kick the balloon. After giving Natalie some postural stabilization during kicking for a few sessions, the occupational therapist was able to give less and less input and then withdrew it altogether within 3 weeks. By practicing the entire activity and using these strategies, Natalie did develop better ability to maintain an upright position while kicking the balloon. Her timing also improved as she learned to watch the balloon carefully. Grading the task by first using a stationary object, then a very slowly moving one, gradually moving up to a faster moving object, was helpful to Natalie's learning. Natalie's teacher liked the new "waiting" version of kickball and instituted variations of this game for recess and free play, thereby increasing Natalie's practice time during naturally occurring activities during her school day.

Summary

The motor skill acquisition frame of reference described in this chapter proposes a major shift in the traditional roles and responsibilities of both the therapist and the child during the intervention process. The child is seen as an active learner and as responsible for his or her own learning. The therapist is seen as a partner with the child, family, and others in the problem-solving process—a facilitator of the child's acquiring new or more efficient motor skills. Instead of supplying specific strategies that are "done to" the child, this frame of reference requires the therapist to be an analyst of the child, task, and environment and to be creative in structuring a learning situation that will improve the child's ability to perform specific tasks. The emphasis on functional tasks and on active learning fits easily with traditional occupational therapy, philosophy, and practice.

ACKNOWLEDGMENTS

The author thanks the Alleyne/Ligon family for allowing her to take photographs illustrating the concepts of motor skill acquisition.

REFERENCES

American Occupational Therapy Association. (2002). Occupational therapy framework: Domain and process. *American Journal of Occupational Therapy*, 56, 609–639.

Bernstein, N. (1967). *Coordination and Regulation of Movements*. New York: Pergamon Press.

Bly, L. (1996). *What is the Role of Sensation in Motor Learning? What is the Role of Feedback and Feedforward?* NDTA Network, 1–7.

Brooks, V. B. (1986). *The Neural Basis of Motor Control*. New York: Oxford University Press.

Bruininks, R., & Bruininks, B. (2005). *Bruininks-Oseretsky Test of Motor Proficiency* (2nd ed.). Minneapolis, MN: NCS Pearson.

Carr, J. H., & Shepherd, R. B. (1992). *Motor Relearning Program for Stroke* (2nd ed.). Rockville, MD: Aspen.

Carr, J. H., & Shepherd, R. B. (1998). *Neurologic Rehabilitation: Optimizing Motor Performance*. Oxford: Butterworth-Heinemann.

Claxton, L. J. (2003). Evidence of motor planning in infant reaching behavior. *Psychological Science, 14,* 354–356.

Coster, W., Deeney, T., Haltiwanger, J., & Haley, S. (1998). *School Function Assessment.* San Antonio, TX: Psychological Corporation.

Duff, S. V., & Charles, J. (2004). Enhancing prehension in infants and children: Fostering neuromotor strategies. *Physical and Occupational Therapy in Pediatrics, 24*(1/2), 129–172.

Eliasson, A. C., Gordon, A. M., & Forssberg, H. (1992). Impaired anticipatory control of isometric forces during grasping by children with cerebral palsy. *Developmental Medicine and Child Neurology, 34,* 216–225.

Ericsson, K. A., Krampe, R. Th., & Tesch-Romer, C. (1993). The role of deliberate practice in the acquisition of expert performance. *Psychological Review, 100,* 363–406.

Fisher, A., Bryze, K., Hume, V., & Griswold, L. (2005). *School AMPS.* Fort Collins, CO: Three Star Press.

Gallese, V., Fadiga, L., Fogassi, L., & Rizzolatti, G. (1996). Action recognition in the premotor cortex. *Brain, 119,* 593–609.

Gentile, A. M. (1987). Skill acquisition: action, movement and neuromotor processes. In J. H. Carr, R. B. Shepherd, J. Gordon, A. M. Gentile, & J. M. Held (Eds). *Movement Science: Foundations for Physical Therapy in Rehabilitation* (pp. 93–154). Gaithersburg, MD: Aspen.

Gentile, A. M. (1992). The nature of skill acquisition: therapeutic implications for children with movement disorders. In H. Forssberg, & H. Hirschfeld (Eds). *Movement Disorders in Children, Medicine and Sports Sciences,* Vol. 36 (pp. 31–40). Basel: Karger.

Gliner, J. A. (1985). Purposeful activity in motor learning theory: an event approach to motor skill acquisition. *American Journal of Occupational Therapy, 39,* 28–34.

Goodgold-Edwards, S. A., & Cermak, S. A. (1989). Integrating motor control and motor learning concepts with neuropsychological perspectives on apraxia and developmental dyspraxia. *American Journal of Occupational Therapy, 44,* 431–439.

Gordon, A. M., & Duff, S. V. (1999). Fingertip forces during object manipulation in children with hemiplegic cerebral palsy: anticipatory scaling. *Developmental Medicine and Child Neurology, 41,* 166–175.

Hadders-Algra, M. (2000). The neuronal group selection theory: Promising principles for understanding and treating developmental motor disorders. *Developmental Medicine and Child Neurology, 42,* 707–715.

Haley, S. M., Coster, W. J., Ludlow, L. H., & Haltiwanger, J. T. (1992). *Pediatric Evaluation of Disability Inventory: Development, Standardization and Administration Manual.* San Antonio, TX: Psychological Corporation.

von Hofsten, C. (1997). On the early development of predictive abilities. In C. Dent-Read, & P. Zukow-Goldring (Eds). *Evolving Explanations of Development* (pp. 163–194). Washington, DC: American Psychological Association.

von Hofsten, C. (2004). An action perspective on motor development. *Trends in Cognitive Sciences, 8*(6), 266–272.

Huang, H., & Mercer, V. (2001). Dual task methodology: Application in studies of cognitive and motor performance in adults and children. *Pediatric Physical Therapy, 13,* 133–140.

Huang, H., Mercer, V., & Thorpe, D. (2003). Effects of different concurrent cognitive tasks on temporal-distance gait variables in children. *Pediatric Physical Therapy, 15,* 105–113.

Kamm, K., Thelen, E., & Jensen, J. I. (1990). A dynamical systems approach to motor development. *Physical Therapy, 70,* 763–775.

Kaplan, M. (1994). Motor learning: Implications for occupational therapy and neurodevelopmental treatment. *Developmental Disabilities Special Interest Section Newsletter, 17*(3), 1–4.

Law, M., Missiuna, C., Pollack, N., & Stewart, D. (2005). Foundations for occupational therapy practice with children. In J. Case-Smith (Ed). *Occupational Therapy for Children* (5th ed., pp.53–87). St. Louis, MO: Mosby, Elsevier Science.

Lee, T., Swanson, L., & Hall, A. (1991). What is repeated in a repetition? Effects of practice conditions on motor skill acquisition. *Physical Therapy, 71,* 150–156.

Levine, M. (1987). *Developmental Variation and Learning Disorders.* Cambridge, MA: Educators Publishing Service.

Mager, R. F. (1975). *Preparing Instructional Objectives.* Belmont, CA: Pearson.

Mathiowetz, V., & Bass-Haugen, J. (2008). Assessing abilities and capacities: motor behavior. In M. V. Radomski, & C. Trombly (Eds). *Occupational Therapy for Physical Dysfunction* (6th ed., pp. 186–211). Philadelphia, PA: Lippincott Williams & Wilkins.

McCaffrey-Easley, A. (1996). Dynamic assessment for infants and toddlers: The relationship between assessment and the environment. *Pediatric Physical Therapy, 8,* 62–69.

McDonnell, A. P. (1996). The acquisition, transfer, and generalization of requests by young children with severe disabilities. *Education and Training in Mental Retardation and Developmental Disabilities, 31*(3), 213–234.

Palisano, R. J., Snider, L. M., & Orlin, M. N. (2004). Recent advances in physical and occupational therapy for children with cerebral palsy. *Seminars in Pediatric Neurology, 11*(1), 66–77.

Phipps, S. C., & Roberts, P. S. (2006). Motor learning. In H. M. Pendleton, & W. Schultz-Krohn (Eds). *Pedretti's Occupational Therapy* (6th ed., pp. 791–800). St. Louis, MO: Mosby, Elsevier Science.

Rizzolatti, G., & Luppino, G. (2001). The cortical motor system. *Neuron, 31,* 889–901.

Schmidt, R. A., & Lee, T. D. (2005). *Motor Control and Learning: A Behavioral Emphasis* (4th ed.). Champaign, IL: Human Kinetics.

Seabrook, R., Brown, G. D., & Solity, J. E. (2005). Distributed and massed practice: From laboratory to classroom. *Applied Cognitive Psychology, 19*(1), 107–122.

Thelen, E. (1998). Bernstein's legacy for motor development: how infants learn to reach. In: M. Latash (Ed). *Progress in Motor Control: Bernstein's Traditions in Movement Studies,* Vol. 1 (pp. 267–288). Champaign, IL: Human Kinetics.

Thelen, E., Corbetta, D., Kamm, K., & Spencer, J. P. (1993). The transition to reaching: Mapping intention and intrinsic dynamics. *Child Development, 64,* 1058–1098.

Thorndike, E. L. (1932). *Fundamentals of Learning.* New York: Teachers College, Columbia University.

Thorndike, E. L. (1935). *The Psychology of Wants, Interests, and Attitudes.* New York: Appleton-Century-Crofts.

Travers, R. M. W. (1977). *Essentials of Learning* (4th ed.). New York: Macmillan.

Valvano, J. (2004). Activity-focused motor interventions for children with neurological conditions. *Physical and Occupational Therapy in Pediatrics, 24*(1/2), 79–107.

VanSant, A. (1991). Motor control, motor learning, and motor development. In P. C. Montgomery, & B. H. Connolly (Eds). *Motor Control and Physical Therapy: Theoretical Framework and Practical Applications* (pp. 13–28). Hixson, TN: Chattanooga Group.

van Vliet, P. M., & Henegan, N. R. (2006). Motor control and the management of musculoskeletal dysfunction. *Manual Therapy, 11,* 208–213.

Vygotsky, L. S. (1978). *Mind in Society: The Development of Higher Psychological Processes.* Cambridge, MA: Harvard University Press.

van der Weel, F. R., van der Meer, A. L., & Lee, D. N. (1991). Effect of task on movement control in cerebral palsy: Implications for assessment and therapy. *Developmental Medicine and Child Neurology, 33,* 419–426.

Westcott, S. L., & Burtner, P. (2004). Postural control in children: Implications for pediatric practice. *Physical and Occupational Therapy in Pediatrics, 24*(1/2), 5–55.

Winstein, C. J. (1991). Knowledge of results and motor learning—implications for physical therapy. *Physical Therapy, 71,* 140–149.

Winstein, C. J., & Schmidt, R. A. (1990). Reduced frequency of knowledge of results enhances motor skill learning. *Journal of Experimental Psychology: Learning, Memory, Cognition, 16,* 677–691.

CHAPTER 13

A Frame of Reference for the Development of Handwriting Skills

KAREN ROSTON

Handwriting is a major component of elementary school education. Teachers require students to write down their assignments, take notes during a lesson from the board, and to write homework assignments. This frame of reference (FOR) for the development of handwriting skills is designed for elementary school students who have difficulties transcribing their written assignments onto paper to communicate their ideas to others, including teachers, parents, and peers. After instruction by a teacher, these students find the graphomotor task arduous and do not develop automaticity with so-called "lower level" skills (like transcription and spelling) that are needed to progress efficiently and successfully in the written school curriculum. Occupational therapists, although not teachers of handwriting, can provide varied practice for students, as well as sharing their knowledge of fine motor, visual motor, visual perceptual, motor planning, bodily kinesthetic, and attentional delays that might have an impact on the activity demands of the skill of making letters and words on a page. They can use a student's strengths to compensate for his or her weaknesses, discover the strongest mode of intelligence and learning, provide adaptations to the environment, and use his or her knowledge of technology as a possible final compensation and adaptation in occupational performance.

Occupational therapists find that many elementary school-aged children who have Individualized Education Plans (IEPs) are initially referred from teachers or parents who believe that a child has difficulties with handwriting in the areas of legibility and/or speed in transcribing written work. Occupational therapists who evaluate children often hear from parents and teachers that students have so much to say but are not able to write it all down. Parents and/or teachers report that a student finds it difficult to translate his or her thoughts and/or learned information into legible written text. Written homework assignments may necessitate a family member acting as a scribe. Students report that they cannot read notes they take in class, negatively impacting their learning. The ability to accurately, legibly, and swiftly take notes during a lecture can result in an increased ability to review and retain academic information (Graham, Harris, & Fink, 2000). Teachers also report that they are often unable to read written work produced in class or for homework assignments. Students with legible handwriting receive better grades, have better spelling, are able to express themselves in writing more easily and fluently, and can complete homework and schoolwork in less time and with more grade-appropriate content. Teachers give better grades to legible work, which may affect an individual student's ability to continue to the next grade (Hammerschmidt & Sudsawad, 2004; Weintraub & Graham, 1998). Transcribing written work legibly during a final draft is important to success in school (Laszlo & Broderick, 1991; Weintraub & Graham, 1998; Sudsawad et al., 2002).

There is no current research that supports that any one handwriting program is better than any other. The requirements necessary for learning handwriting are: teachers demonstrating letter formation, using directional arrows as reminders, working with models, continually practicing in the classroom and at home, giving students accurate feedback on results, embedding lessons in meaningful written activities, and so on. These can be applied to any or all programs to make them more effective. Handwriting is most successfully taught when a school system or school uses a unified curriculum. In that way the students will have consistency by hearing the same language again and again when learning the task, as well as when receiving feedback and when becoming familiar with the practice requirements (Figure 13.1). They will also understand the advantages and purposes of continued practice as their legibility and/or speed increases.

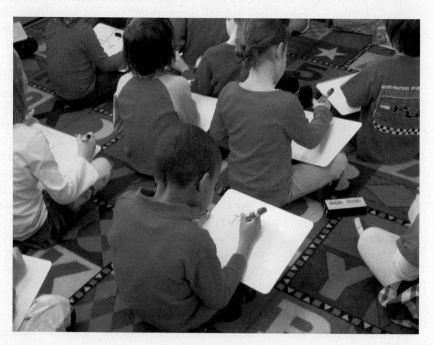

FIGURE 13.1 A kindergarten class practices "word wall" words on the rug, using markers on white boards. The class is making up sentences using the words before writing them down.

THEORETICAL BASE

This theoretical base is developed primarily from Gardner's *Theory of Multiple Intelligences* (Gardner, 1991, 1993, 1999, 2006), Schmidt's *Schema Theory of Discrete Motor Skill Learning* (1974), and Guadagnoli and Lee's *Theory of the Optimal Challenge Point* (2004).

Theory of Multiple Intelligences

Gardner's *Theory of Multiple Intelligences* is both a neurobiological and acquisitional theory, based on the progression of streams of development that promote changes in a child. It describes how a child acquires knowledge both as his or her neurobiological processes develop and as he or she acquires knowledge by using multiple kinds of intelligence. It promotes using a child's strongest, most proficient modes of intelligence to offset any difficulties he or she may have with learning.

According to Gardner (1993), there are many views or definitions of intelligence, one being what is tested on an intelligence test (referred to as the "g"). He believes that these standardized, traditional tests only test linguistic and logical–mathematical intelligence and that there are several other kinds of intelligence that must be addressed so that more students can learn effectively. Gardner states that every person is good at learning through a combination of different intelligences. When students have learning difficulties, the teacher and the occupational therapist could work together so that the students can find their strengths in whichever array of intelligences in which they are most proficient. The goal is being able to aid a particular student in learning the information he or she needs to know to succeed in the academic environment.

Gardner (1999) defines intelligence as:

> a biopsychological potential to process information that can be activated in a cultural setting to solve problems or create products that are of value in a culture ... , (intelligences) are potentials-presumably, neural ones-that will or will not be activated, depending upon the values of a particular culture, the opportunities available in that culture, and the personal decisions made by individuals and/or their families, schoolteachers, and others (pp. 33–34).

The first two intelligences (the g) that Gardner addresses are the ones typically tested in the school setting: linguistic and logical–mathematical (1993, 1999, 2006). Linguistic intelligence is the ability to understand spoken and written language, including syntax and pragmatics, as well as having the skill to learn the meanings of words and to use language(s) to communicate, write, and remember information. Logical–mathematical intelligence is the ability to analyze problems and mathematical operations, do research, detect patterns, use deductive reasoning, and think logically.

Gardner (1991, 1993, 1999, 2006) has criteria for the following additional intelligences, one of which is its "susceptibility to encoding in a symbol system" (1999, p. 37). Symbols are developed by a culture to methodically and exactly communicate relevant information. Intelligences are not "good" or "bad" but can add to and enhance a person's learning to participate in his or her society and culture. Other intelligences include:

- *Musical intelligence*: Skill in the performance, composition, and appreciation of musical patterns, as well as the ability to recognize pitches, tones, and rhythms.
- *Bodily kinesthetic intelligence*: The capability to use one's body or parts of the body to coordinate movement, solve problems, and make things.
- *Spatial intelligence*: The ability to solve problems by distinguishing the patterns of both large and small spaces.
- *Interpersonal intelligence*: The ability to understand the intentions, wishes, and aspirations of other people; to be able to work well with a group.
- *Intrapersonal intelligence*: Self-understanding; the ability to recognize one's own feelings, fears, motivations, and so on, and to use this information to manage one's life.

Gardner suggests that we teach—give feedback to—the intelligences that compromise a student's strongest mode of learning. The therapist can combine bodily kinesthetic and/or spatial intelligence, for example, to facilitate learning in a student who has strengths in these areas.

The ability to relate one symbol to another is a needed developmental step that is used in the educational environment so that students can learn (Gardner, 1993). To teach the values of a society, a culture develops symbols and symbol systems. For example, numbers are the concrete 1:1 representation of a single item or a group of items. The number conveys, in a specific manner, how many items are being referred to (you have 1 apple, 54 peas, etc). Letters are not complete symbols by themselves in the same way. This may be the reason they are initially difficult to learn for some students. They have meaning only when they are part of a word or words. Learning letters needs to be embedded in the context of words to have meaning for the young learner. Written language is part of linguistic intelligence, with the implication that written expression and language development are intertwined.

School-aged children have already learned symbol use during early play. For example, dolls are babies. Toy trucks are "real" trucks. Tricycles are motorcycles. Small stoves are "real" stoves. Blocks are houses or cities or roads, and so on. Children also symbolize when they draw (Figure 13.2). A square with a triangle on top is a house, for example. A series of circles may be "my mother" and so forth. Children can pretend with more abstracted ideas and activities as well without props, like "flying" with paper planes or with only their hands, making things and people with clay, pretending to be doctors, garbage collectors, delivery people, "driving" vehicles such as cars, planes, tractors, and so on.

One reason why play is important is that it encourages flexible symbol development as well as social interactions when symbolic play occurs with peers. Play is the work of children, their primary occupation (Reilly, 1974). In pretend play, a child has to be aware that he or she is using symbols and that others can pretend also so that they can participate in the pretend premise together: playing "house," going on a "trip," dressing up as "cats," and so forth. The premise is "I believe you. You believe me. And we participate in the pretend environment together"(Gardner, 2006).

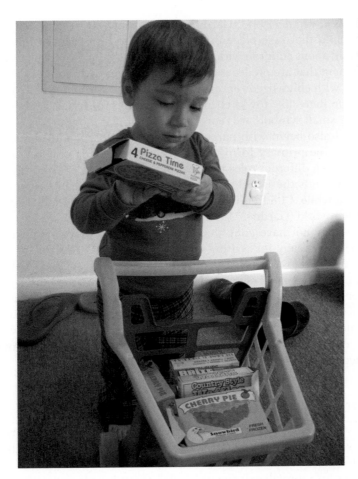

FIGURE 13.2 This boy is pretending to "shop" with his little cart. He is using toys to "pretend" an adult activity.

By around 5 years of age, a student is ready to learn symbols and symbol systems like letters and words. Children initially consider a symbol as any entity that represents or refers to another entity. The entity can be abstract or material. A major task for a young child is learning to interpret symbols as he or she learns to read and write (Gardner, 2004).

Handwriting can be defined as a codified system of a finite number of standard symbols that exist in a specific language. To be used functionally, letters in combinations become the graphic written representation of a word and of the sounds in that word. Letters provide meaning when they are grouped into words and sentences, then paragraphs, essays, stories, poems, biographies, letters, and so on. Indeed, handwriting is still required for all the assignments students need to be able to produce while in school, after graduation, and in the work environment. Symbols are more effectively taught when embedded in meaning and should not be taught in isolation for the most effective learning to take place (Gardner, 1991).

In *The Unschooled Mind* (1991), Gardner talks about the streams and waves of development in a child that take place during the first to fifth years of life. Although nowhere does he talk about children with special needs, he does give focus to the stages of symbol development that are predecessors to writing letters/symbols. At first, pretend play happens alone with child-sized representations of adult "props," which are smaller versions of grown-up items like toy kitchens, bikes, tea sets, or trains. A child needs to recognize that these small symbols are representations of real things.

Interactions will also begin with parents, siblings, and peers with the same small "props." This play is the primary form of symbol use for young children and allows them to experiment with different roles in social dyads or groups. Pretend play requires that the child understands the inherent nature of an object but can assign it another temporary role for a while. Children imagine and use their imagination to learn about and understand their world (Gardner, 1991).

Some students may not have gone through these stages, which might mean they are not developmentally ready for writing alphabetic symbols. It might be part of an occupational therapist's role to work in consultation with a teacher to help identify where students are in the streams of symbol development and on these precursor skills before actual letter symbols are learned. I have heard many occupational therapists state that if a child does not cognitively know a letter(s), "He or she is not writing but drawing the letters." Gardner's theory appears to bear this out. If one does not know what the letter symbolizes, or that it is part of a written language system, what meaning does it have, even if someone learns the motor plan (Figure 13.3)?

Theory of Discrete Motor Skill Learning

Remember the saying "practice makes perfect"? A learner can achieve accuracy with a new motor skill by varying the conditions of each practice and by knowing the specific results: the knowledge of the results (KR) (Schmidt, 1975). When learning a new motor skill, a person forms an internalized, general "rule" about how to correctly perform it. The *abstraction*, or idea, of the results of the practice is the *schema*. More practice will update and expand the schema so that the next time the same motor task is performed, it will be done more accurately and successfully. To make the motor act more accurate, one needs to practice it in varied conditions, with varied sensory input, to enlarge the schema. Each time the act is practiced, the sensory input from vision, the position of the body (kinesthesia), the sounds in the environment, and so forth are slightly or definitely different. This variability allows the schema to enlarge (Schmidt, 1975).

When performing a motor act, the person decides what outcome he or she wants: the goal or action plan. After the act, the results can be assessed to see if the action is more or less accurate than the last time it was performed. These experiences allow the idea, or schema, about how to accurately perform the motor skill to expand. Every time the skill is practiced and the results are assessed for accuracy, one's schema (or *motor understanding*) gets better and more comprehensive and can be used more automatically. To correctly assess the outcome of the motor act, one must be able to compare the actual feedback to the expected feedback through the KR. The goal of the motor act should be

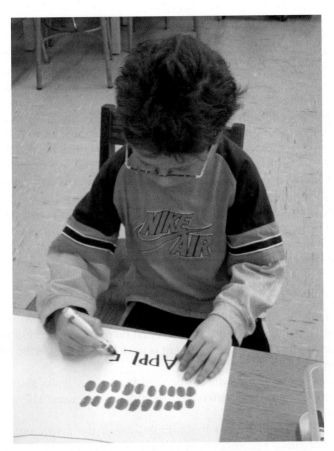

FIGURE 13.3 Handwriting practice combined with a math lesson: He made two groups of 10 apples.

clear, and the plan that is developed through practice should incorporate the sensory information in the environment in which the motor act takes place.

For example, let us examine the skill of pitching a ball. When you first learn to pitch, there are many skills to master, such as how to hold/grasp the ball, how to shift the weight in your legs, how to move your arms, where to look, and so on. Each time you throw the ball (either at a target [stationary or moving] or at a person's "strike zone"), you judge if you have thrown accurately enough to achieve your goal. If you have not, you might make adjustments in your stance, the force of your pitch, or your arm movements. You evaluate the results of each pitch and see which one was the most accurate. This is how a schema develops.

With more practice under varied sensory conditions (i.e., a windy day, a noisy crowd, bright sun, etc.), a person would not have to think of each part of the motor act, as it would become automatic. As the schema expands by abstracting all this accurate information, the new goal could be refining the accuracy of the pitch or changing the speed or placement of the ball. People who are extremely skilled at a motor skill continue to practice it throughout their lives to achieve their goals of proficiency. An example of someone with this kind of expertise would be an Olympic athlete, a professional dancer, a golfer, a calligrapher, or a major league baseball player.

Of course, this is an oversimplification of Schmidt's theory. Schmidt hypothesizes that we all have *generalized motor programs*, each of which is a general memory representation of an action. With practice, a learner develops a *motor response schema*, which is responsible for providing the rules for a specific action in a specific sequence and situation (i.e., throwing a small or big ball outdoors, indoors, etc.). The *recall schema* adds the characteristics of specific response instructions to the motor program and initiates the execution of a motor goal (the action plan). It is the recall schema that enlarges with the KR and allows for the production of the more accurate movement. During the performance of a discrete motor skill, the *recognition schema* allows the learner to evaluate the correctness of the action by comparing the actual sensory feedback against the expected sensory feedback and make movement corrections to the original action plan. The learner can recognize if the movement was correct by using the recognition schema. Schmidt also talks about the *initial conditions* in learning a motor skill, which consist of body and limb positions, the environment, and sensory input prior to the response.

There is specific information stored after each movement:

- *Response specifications*: Specific requirements of the actions to be performed, such as direction, speed, force, height, and so on. These must be part of the action plan *before the action can be carried out*. After the movement is performed, the specific results that are needed are stored.
- *Sensory consequences of skill performance*: Received from the sensory systems during and after the movement, providing actual feedback from the senses. The specifics are stored after the movement.
- *Response outcome*: Information about the comparison of the actual outcome (KR) with the intended outcome. The success of the actual outcome response compared to the expected outcome in the initial action plan is stored in the schema after the movement;

So, a schema becomes *a set of internalized rules* that abstracts information during practice sessions from the response specifications, the sensory information received during and after the movement, and the knowledge of the outcome results. This information will be abstracted and stored in the motor response and recall schemas so that a more accurate outcome can be produced the next time a specific motor act is performed. The strength of a schema is based on having a variety of initial conditions, response specifications, and sensory feedback along with the response outcome of prior motor experiences.

Optimal Challenge Point

Guadagnoli and Lee's (2004) Theory of Optimal Challenge Point proposes that practice is the single most important factor when it comes to learning a new skill. Further, they hypothesize that "skill improvement is generally considered to be positively related to the amount of practice" (p. 212).

Guadagnoli and Lee's theory defines when and for what tasks blocked or random practice should take place to best achieve efficacy in learning a motor skill. *Blocked practice* is when one discrete motor skill is being repeatedly practiced before moving on to another discrete motor skill. *Random practice* occurs when there is no specific order to the practice and/or when several discrete motor skills are practiced at the same time. The theory also describes the *optimal challenge point,* which is the point where the most learning takes place or the point where the best possible amount of information is available to be interpreted by the learner. When the learner reaches the optimal challenge point, inefficiency and uncertainty in performance are reduced, and the benefits of the practice are maximized.

The difficulty of a motor task is divided into two categories:

- *Nominal task difficulty*: Defined as the characteristics of a task, the "constant amount of task difficulty, regardless of who is performing the task and under what conditions it is being performed" (p. 213). The nominal task difficulty is the name of the task, for example "write the letter 'a'." This is a task of low nominal difficulty. A handwriting task with high nominal difficulty might be the completion of a five-paragraph essay in legible cursive writing during a specific time frame. Another task of high nominal difficulty might be producing a person's name using calligraphy. (Calligraphy is defined as specialized, formalized letters made with "old-fashioned" writing instruments, such as a fountain pen or a pen one dips into a jar of ink. It is often used in writing on diplomas, awards, or wedding invitations. This is the "art" of handwriting and is not often used now.) The degree of nominal difficulty of a task is defined by the motor and perceptual requirements of its performance.
- *Functional task difficulty*: Is defined as "how challenging the task is relative to the skill level of the individual performing the task and to the (practice) conditions under which it is being performed" (p. 213). If a beginning learner is asked to write letters in a noisy or crowded classroom, the functional difficulty of the task increases. Random practice, with increased contextual interference, increases the functional difficulty of a task.

The task variables in practice are the accurate KR, the sensory consequences of the motor act, and contextual interference. KR adds potential information to the schema of the motor skill. *Contextual interference* refers to the "interference that results from practicing various tasks or skills within the context of practice" (Magill, 2001, p. 289). Contextual interference is a factor the first time a motor act is performed. It adds to the functional difficulty of a task and adds to the information available to the learner. The contextual interference is inherent in the motor task. With each practice of the task in blocked practice, the contractual interference is less of a factor, and the task gets easier, smoother, or better; the amount of information added to the schema during each practice is less; the uncertainty is less; and the potential for the schema to enlarge is less.

During random practice trials, the contextual interference is always part of the motor performance, and the schema enlarges and retains the new information. The high variability in the performance leads to better retention of the motor skill. The result is that when presented with a novel letter, there will be more information on how to transcribe it in the schema. Handwriting acquisition by motor learning proposes that high contextual interference conditions are effective because the child has the opportunity to make comparisons among the various movements that he or she has in memory (Ste-Marie et al., 2004). Ste-Marie and her colleagues state that

> Individual letter handwriting will most likely be transferred to the task of handwriting words. Handwriting a word is more akin to a random structure of presentation than to a blocked structure of presentation. That is, handwriting the individual letters A, B, and C could easily transfer to the task of handwriting the word CAB.... Practicing the handwriting of letters in a random presentation, then, might more closely match the demands of handwriting words, which can be considered the real-life transfer task of handwriting skill (Ste-Marie et al., 2004, p. 116).

Random practice produces learners who had a greater speed of transcribing words and a greater accuracy than the learners who were part of a blocked practice group. A random acquisition schedule is recommended for teaching handwriting skills.

The Theory of the Optimal Challenge Point describes how to use KR and contextual interference effectively in relation to the skill level of the student and the task. Information about the task is given to the student, or, more effectively, the student defines it himself/herself via an *action plan* (a goal). With the sensory input during and after task completion, contextual interference, and by accurate feedback (KR), the resultant information enlarges the schema of the discrete motor plan. One of the objects of giving accurate KR is to reduce the *uncertainty* inherent in a task. As the functional difficulty of a task increases, there is more uncertainty as to the outcome of the action plan that can be reduced by accurate KR. With more practice and an enlarged schema, a student will become more proficient in a task. There is less uncertainty, and the initial action plan will be more accurate. The outcome is that KR will have a reduced amount of information to be processed. As the task gets harder (e.g., with combining letters into words in cursive), there is less certainty over the outcome of one's movements—the action plan—and about the outcome before KR.

Practice conditions may also affect the difficulty of a task through the amount of sensory information available during task completion. In a classroom, increased noise or other forms of sensory input (many classrooms have considerable visual distractions) may result in a student not hearing and/or understanding instructions. This could increase the functional difficulty of the writing task. Because of this, it is important to practice the task in the environment in which the writing practice has to take place. The motor plan will become more accurate, and the sensory consequences will become part of the motor plan.

Learning is *assumed* to have taken place when a change in the motor outcome is observed. Motor learning is the direct result of the amount of information available that can be interpreted during performance by the learner through his or her skill level. These variables are related to the functional difficulty of the task. The amount of information available influences learning. First, learning cannot occur when there is inadequate or missing information. Second, too much information impedes learning. Finally, learning depends on the optimal amount of information given at the child's skill level (Guadagnoli & Lee, 2004).

The *optimal challenge point* is the degree of functional task difficulty a student needs to optimize the learning of a specific discrete motor skill. It is the best possible amount of potential information that can be interpreted and used accurately by the learner. When the optimal challenge point is approached, there will be more information (less uncertainty) that can be used to increase the accuracy of the schema for that motor skill. After the optimal challenge point is reached, there may be too much information—an overload—so that the student would not be able to process it. The skill would not improve and could, in fact, degrade. When this occurs, the occupational therapist could increase the functional difficulty of a task by using more complex tasks in random practice (which increases the contextual interference) for more accurate learning to be incorporated into the schema.

The ability to achieve successful task performance is different with the student's skill level and the level of the nominal difficulty of the task, meaning the characteristics of the task—the task name. When the nominal difficulty increases, one can expect that the performance will not be as accurate until the uncertainty is reduced and new information is incorporated into the schema. For example, a task with the lowest nominal difficulty that concerns us in the FOR is writing a single letter with vertical and/or horizontal lines, such as a "T." If we were asking a fifth grader to write the same single letter, the functional difficulty would be easy although the nominal difficulty would remain the same. If we were asking a new kindergarten student to write the same letter, the functional difficulty would be harder as the student has to first incorporate the contextual interference and the sensory information inherent in the classroom environment to learn the schema of a new motor task. The nominal difficulty of the task is still the same. The first grader, who has had a year of practice, should be able to achieve some success with this skill. We could predict this outcome because of the low nominal difficulty inherent in the task. The functional difficulty of writing in the classroom, which is harder than writing in a quiet separate space, makes the task harder. Hopefully, the motor plan of that letter would already have been incorporated into the schema of the use of that letter in a word. For schema development, enlargement, and accuracy to take place, one needs an action plan (a goal), the conditions of practice, which includes the sensory elements, contextual interference, and accurate feedback (KR) to learn to perform a new motor skill.

Our job as occupational therapists is to help the teacher and the child discover what that optimal challenge point is and when it is reached so that performance does not degrade. The optimal challenge point changes along with the requirements of the task and where it is performed—learning all the letters of the alphabet and then forming them into words, sentences, paragraphs, and so on (Table 13.1). We want the motor plan of the letters to be information that is stored in the schema so that transcribing the letters in the words used when composing is automatic and can be used as an adjunct to language development and reading.

Practice variables influence performance and learning. They make a skill easier or harder and define its functional difficulty. Random practice with experienced learners leads to better retention than blocked practice in tasks with lower nominal difficulty because it has to incorporate contextual interference. Random practice will produce less motor learning for tasks with higher nominal difficulty. Random practice increases the functional difficulty of a task.

TABLE 13.1 Management of Practice Variables to Reach the Optimal Challenge Point

	Random Practice with Contextual Interference = (No Specific Order in Practice of a Motor Skill)	Blocked Practice without Contextual Interference = (One Motor Skill is Repeatedly Practiced)	Knowledge of Results
Low Nominal Difficulty	Better retention of learning for experienced learners who can incorporate more information into schema Largest learning potential	For new learners: more effective early in practice, until schema development has begun Blocked practice has low contextual interference	Less frequent, shorter, more random, less immediate knowledge of results = most learning
High Nominal Difficulty	For skilled learners: can incorporate more information into schema	Best for tasks with complex knowledge of results	Blocked presentation of knowledge of result, more frequent, and/or immediate knowledge of results or both = largest learning effect
Low Functional Difficulty	—	More effective early in practice	—
High Functional Difficulty	Increases task functional difficulty For skilled learners: can incorporate more information into schema Leads to more retention/enlarging of schema		Less frequent or immediate knowledge of results = higher functional difficulty Blocked complex knowledge of results = more retention of learning

Blocked practice in tasks with lower functional difficulty is most effective early in the practice. Retention of information by new learners is better under blocked practice conditions. For beginning learners, the low levels of contextual interference in blocked practice produces better learning when beginning a new motor task, while random practice (with high contextual interference) is better for retention of a new task for a skilled student. The student will incorporate more information into his or her schema, and it will become more accurate.

When a student is writing in cursive (which has a higher nominal level of difficulty), the knowledge of the results of the practice should be more frequent and/or immediate to have the largest learning effect. The increased frequency or the immediate presentation of KR increases performance but decreases retention. Decreased frequency or delayed KR presentation increases the functional difficulty of the task. The optimal length and amount of KR is task dependent. Tasks of different nominal difficulty need different KR. Learning nominally difficult tasks is related to the size of the KR summary. That is, larger summaries produce larger learning effects. Blocked KR will produce better learning than a random schedule of KR.

With tasks of low nominal difficulty, the largest learning effect will take place with less frequent or less immediate KR given in a random schedule. A task of higher functional difficulty with more complex KR allows for the retention of more information with a blocked schedule. To increase the efficient processing of the optimal amount of information into the schema, early learners would benefit from having information presented in small amounts in blocked schedules and with a shorter KR summary or less variability in practice until the schema of a movement pattern is developed.

Later learners have improved processing efficiency and should be able to acquire the learning of the motor skill more efficiently, depending on the functional difficulty or complexity of the task and the learner's accumulated schema development. Modeled demonstrations during the acquisition of a motor skill will have a positive effect on learning and make a task easier to perform. With tasks of high nominal difficulty and random practice, modeling increased motor performance secondary to the degree of functional difficulty of the task. With tasks of low nominal difficulty, modeling negatively affected learning as it did not allow for the learner to generate his or her own action plan.

Teaching Writing

How do we teach learning of the alphabet? We need a cognitive learning theory (Gardner, 1991, 1993, 2004) that the teacher uses and the occupational therapist understands. This is in addition to motor learning/skill acquisition theories (Schmidt, 1975; Guadagnoli & Lee, 2004) (see Chapter 12) that use varied practice with the explicit knowledge of the results of the practice (KR) and the understanding of the effectiveness of either blocked or random practice. This practice can be provided by the teacher or adapted for students with difficulties in this area by an occupational therapist. The occupational therapist can consult with a teacher about possible adverse sensory information in the classroom environment and suggest adaptations.

The idea of an accurate, efficient motor plan facilitates learning of a new skill and the transfer of that learning to another new skill with the same generalized motor plan. As we have learned, *drill* (also known as *"rote practice"*) may not be the most effective mode of retaining learning. Physically guiding a learner's hand when transcribing a letter would prevent the learner from generating his or her own action plan and, in fact, may degrade it. When the learner uses random practice conditions, such as using the letter in a word, the task becomes more demanding in its motor performance as it has greater uncertainty. Although this is more effortful (greater contextual interference), it results in better retention and the transfer of learning to new words. The more "a"s a student writes at the beginning, middle, and end of various words with various letter combinations, the more random practice takes place with increased contextual interference. This is what we want to happen to increase retention and transfer of learning so that we can smoothly reproduce the motor skill in a novel situation.

In summary, Gardner (2004) has posited that a 5- to 7-year-old child is ready to learn and understand codified symbols (known as the "alphabet") of our language, but that he or she needs to be taught in the context of words, which are the symbols that have meaning. Motor learning theory tells us that to develop an accurate schema for the discrete motor plan of each letter we need to practice it in practice sessions with the optimal amount of information. This will produce automaticity in handwriting as well as in spelling. These are the skills needed so that higher level composing skills can be used more effectively to express and communicate a learner's ideas through transcription in the academic environment.

Assumptions

Assumptions in this FOR are as follows:

- Students have been taught the basic skills of handwriting by their teacher(s) and that teacher(s) provides ongoing support for the production of legible, efficiently produced letters and numbers in manuscript (print) in the lower grades and in cursive (script) starting at the end of the second grade or beginning of the third grade.
- Functional visual perceptual skills are assumed to be prerequisite skills for good handwriting (see Chapter 11). In this FOR, we are concerned with the ability to perceive "the set of letters of our alphabet (each of which) is characterized by a set of distinct features, which in different combinations permits a unique characterization of each one" (Gibson, 1971).
- A student needs good posture to have legible handwriting (i.e., feet flat on the floor, knees and hips at 90 degrees, elbows flexed, wrists slightly extended). A good position places the body and arms in relationship to the writing task so that it can be efficiently performed. Posture is the stabilizing and aligning of a child's body while he or she performs an activity. A child stabilizes by maintaining trunk control and balance when writing without evidence of transient (i.e., quickly passing) propping or loss of balance. A child's alignment refers to maintaining an upright sitting or standing position without the need to be propped during task performance (AOTA, 2002).
- Good proximal control leads to functional and effective distal control of a writing tool. It has been observed in the classroom that students do not always have the optimal size chair or table that occupational therapists assume is necessary for good posture, which is usually identified as when a student's feet are flat on the floor, the trunk in an upright neutral position with the elbows flexed to a certain degree and the arms in a certain position on the desktop. The head should optimally be maintained in midline with the chin tucked and the shoulders should be generally of equal height for ergonomic posture. The pelvis should also be in neutral, neither anteriorly nor posteriorly tilted. The dominant upper extremity should be able to be used effectively during task performance; this requires fluent, effortless, and automatic movement patterns. The wrist should be used for writing while in slight extension.
- The slope of the letters in the handwriting, as long as it is consistently demonstrated, does not aid or detract from legibility.

FUNCTION–DYSFUNCTION CONTINUA

This FOR has four function–dysfunction continua.

Writing Posture

Function is the ability to maintain an upright posture without fatigue, which might result in propping momentarily on the surface of the desk, or continually leaning onto the desk with the trunk (Table 13.2). The dominant upper extremity should have the ability to use fluid and effective movements during the writing task and the student should be able to easily and unconsciously make necessary postural adjustments. Dysfunction is the inability to perform the writing task while displaying the above postural ergonomics and/or adjustments, and/or using increased physical effort, including moving the upper extremity fluidly and easily across the page, or displaying a loss of balance or weight bearing on the writing surface.

Students who have automaticity in the skill of handwriting have been observed to produce a legible product in many positions, whether seated cross legged on the floor, on a bench, or with a writing notebook on their laps, and so on. It is when using the alternate, less-stabilized positions that a student with difficulties in task performance secondary to poor automaticity in the handwriting task has more problems producing a legible product.

TABLE 13.2 Indicators of Function and Dysfunction for Posture for Writing

Excessive Postural Responses	*Typical Postural Responses*	*Inadequate Postural Responses*
DYSFUNCTION: Excessive postural stability during writing tasks **Indicators of Dysfunction**	*FUNCTION*: Effective writing posture **Indicators of Function**	*DYSFUNCTION*: Lack of postural stability during writing tasks **Indicators of Dysfunction**
Propping momentarily with an upper extremity on the writing surface	Maintains an upright posture with feet on a support surface	Loss of balance or maintaining weight bearing on the writing surface
Elbow at an awkward angle, student is too far from the writing surface or too close to the writing surface	The upper extremity is used effectively and with fluent movement patterns during task performance	Student needs help moving upper extremity across the page
—	Able to make postural adjustments during the writing task	Unable to make postural adjustments during the writing task
Head held flexed to the right/left	Head is maintained in midline with chin tuck	Hyperextension of the neck—no chin tuck
Shoulders hiked to the right or the left	Shoulders are equal	Adducted or abducted scapula(e)
More than slight extension	Wrist in slight extension	>45 degrees flexion
Thoracic extension or kyphosis	Trunk in neutral	Lateral flexion to the right or left or more significant kyphosis or thoracic extension
Asymmetrical pelvis	Pelvis neutral	Increased anterior or posterior pelvic tilt

TABLE 13.3 Indicators of Function and Dysfunction for Components	
Supportive Components	*Unsupportive Components*
FUNCTION: Components support handwriting	*DYSFUNCTION*: Components do not support handwriting
Eyes follow what is being transcribed without head movement	Eyes within 6 in. of paper and/or entire head movement is needed to maintain visual regard
Attends to task demands	Frequently distracted from writing task
Able to repeat directions	Unable to repeat directions
Copies an unfamiliar sentence by groups of words	Copies an unfamiliar sentence by letter (or by word in upper grades)
Does not vocalize while writing	Subvocalizes each letter before he or she writes it

Components

The internal factors that influence writing efficiency might include a student's ocular-motor skills, attention, and memory (Marr, Windsor, & Cermak, 2001; Weintraub & Graham, 1998). Function in the area of components is when a student can separate eye movement from head movement during transcription tasks, copy an entire sentence and/or homework assignment from near or far point, and be able to write without his or her eyes being too close to the page, defined as within 6 in. (Table 13.3). In addition, a student must be able to attend to the task demands so that the student finishes with a product that is the same as the rest of the class. A student must do all this using functional ergonomic posture.

Dysfunction is when a student does not keep an upright posture because of difficulties in the area of functional ocular-motor skills; keeping his or her head close to the paper, leaning the head on the hand or arm when it is on the desk surface, copying from a near or far point sample, letter by letter, or word by word in the upper grades and/or subvocalizing the letters and/or words before they can be written.

Use of Writing Tools

Prerequisite skills for legible handwriting reported in the literature are tool manipulation, dominant hand use, and crossing the midline of the body with the dominant hand. For functional use, the writing paper should be positioned at the midline of the body. A student should be able to turn the pencil, or other writing tool, over to erase with the same hand that is used for writing (Table 13.4). The nondominant hand should stabilize the paper. The student should exhibit dynamic movement of the fingers and should not be holding the tool too tightly, displaying whitening of the DIPs and/or PIPs. The tool should be able to be used with fluidity on both sides of the page; the side of the dominant hand and across the midline on the contralateral side. It should also be used fluidly from the top to the bottom of the paper. Dysfunction is not being able to write fluidly and easily while using a pencil, pen, or other tool.

TABLE 13.4 **Indicators of Function and Dysfunction for Writing**	
Writes	*Difficulty Writing*
FUNCTION: Effective writing tool use	*DYSFUNCTION*: Ineffective writing tool use
Indicators of Function	**Indicators of Dysfunction**
Positions paper in midline	Slants paper to the right or left
Does not erase	Excessive erasing
Erases easily	Excessive erasing/holes in paper
—	Transfers pencil to nondominant hand to erase
Nondominant hand stabilizes the paper	Nondominant hand does not stabilize paper

Grasp

Occupational therapy literature focuses on a component and/or developmental model of grasp development (Burton & Dancisak, 1999; Koziatek & Powell, 2003; Summers, 2001; Windsor, 2000; Yakimishyn & Magill-Evans, 2000). Table 13.5 is based on Schoen's (2001) classification of grasp patterns as used in the *Handwriting Checklist* (Roston, Hinojosa, & Kaplan, in press).

It has long been assumed by occupational therapists working in this area that a student needs to use a dynamic tripod grasp to write legibly and that a dynamic tripod grasp is necessary to prevent fatigue in longer assignments. However, research has not found this assumption to be accurate (Dennis & Swinth, 2001). Function in the area of grasp requires that a student has the ability to securely grasp the writing instrument and manipulate it to easily make erasures, without experiencing fatigue or pain in the hand or wrist while completing the assigned academic task (Table 13.6). The student must be able to calibrate the right amount of force and speed needed to easily complete the task at the same rate as his or her peers. Dynamic smooth movements of the fingers are necessary and should be able to be performed with automaticity, part of the motor

TABLE 13.5 **Classification of Grasp Patterns As Used in the *Handwriting Checklist***		
Mature Grasp	*Transitional Pencil Grasp*	*Primitive Pencil Grasp*
Writing instrument stabilized against the radial side of the third digit by the thumb with the index finger on top of the shaft Thumb to index finger in full opposition Fourth and fifth digits slightly flexed	Writing instrument stabilized between thumb and fingers in one of two ways: 1. Finger–thumb position characterized by an open web space and one to four fingers in opposition to the thumb 2. Writing instrument held against index finger with thumb crossed over toward index finger	Writing instrument stabilized in palm of hand Finger–thumb position characterized by a closed web space

TABLE 13.6 Indicators of Function and Dysfunction for Grasp	
Efficient Grasp	**Ineffective Grasp**
FUNCTION: Ability to manipulate writing tools effectively	*DYSFUNCTION*: Unable to manipulate writing tools effectively
Indicators of Function	**Indicators of Dysfunction**
Securely grasps the writing instrument	Drops the writing instrument
—	Exhibits whitening of the DIPs and/or PIPs
Manipulates the writing instrument to erase	Transfers the writing instrument to the other hand to erase
Does not experience fatigue or pain in the hand or wrist during the writing task	Fatigue or pain in the hand or wrist during the writing task
Calibrate the right amount of speed to finish the writing task	Writing is too slow
—	Cannot finish the task at the same rate as his or her peers
Exhibits dynamic, smooth movements with the digits	Exhibits rigid, jerky, movements with the upper extremity
—	Uses the entire upper extremity as a unit to move the writing instrument across the paper

schema of transcription, to incorporate the skills of transcribing into the swift and legible completion of written work.

Writing Legibility

The burden of attending to letter formation, size, line regard (alignment), and spacing does not allow a student to utilize his or her higher level work skills that clearly displays his or her knowledge of the subject (Amundson, 2001). Rosenblum, Chevion, & Weiss (2006) found significant differences in students who produced proficient versus nonproficient handwriting in the areas of letter width, height, how high the writing instrument was held from the paper, and how many times a student lifted the writing instrument from the paper. They found that "poor handwriters maintained the pen above the writing surface (in-air time/length) for significantly larger percentages of the writing time.... Moreover, [there was] a considerable movement of the pen above the writing surface" (p. 405).

There are many different kinds of handwriting necessary in life: legible writing for a final draft of a school assignment, writing in answers on a test, or signing one's name on an official document like a loan agreement, for instance. Students in elementary school use handwriting for everything from transcribing dictated notes, copying from the board or a near-point sample, taking notes during a lecture, writing drafts of an assignment, keeping a personal journal, passing notes to a classmate, and/or answering a short answer test, to name a few. All these may or may not meet legibility requirements for work turned in to the teacher, but they must be legible to the student to provide

TABLE 13.7 Indicators of Function and Dysfunction for Legibility	
Legible Handwriting	*Illegible Handwriting*
FUNCTION: Handwriting is easily readable	*DYSFUNCTION*: Handwriting is hard or impossible to read
Indicators of Function	**Indicators of Dysfunction**
Letters/words sit on the line; not above or below	Letters/words above or below the baseline
	Letters float between the lines
Size of letters is uniform	Unevenly sized letters
	Most letters too big, too small, or a combination
Letters/words formed with consistently smooth marks onto the paper	"Wobbly" lines
	Vertical marks far from the vertical
	Horizontal parts of letters far from horizontal
	Circular forms not circular and/or smooth
	Unrecognizable as a specific letter
Spacing between letters is even	Letters touching, crowded so that they cannot be distinguished from each other
Letters do not touch	Not enough space to distinguish words from each other
Space between words allows reader to distinguish the word as a separate distinct unit	Too much space between words
Speed of writing is same as peers	Writing is slower than peers
	Cannot finish assignments in time allotted

information for review or retrieval. The ability to accurately, legibly, and swiftly take notes during a lecture can result in an increased ability to review and retain academic information (Graham, Harris, & Fink, 2000).

It should be noted that writing fast and writing legibly are two different tasks and may be inversely related (Van Doorn & Keuss, 1991; Weintraub & Graham, 1998). Fluid, legible handwriting is a basic skill that is part of a student's ability to learn through writing. Despite advances in technology, handwriting remains an important skill that should be taught as part of an integrated educational curriculum to assure students' success in academic programs (Table 13.7).

GUIDE TO EVALUATION

Before performing any evaluation, it is necessary for an occupational therapist to get informed consent from a child's parents. During this process, the therapist should consider discussing school academic functioning with both the teacher and the parent. A checklist can be effectively used for this. Then the therapist can compare the two checklists, and may discover two different sets of problems. The parents and teacher might be interviewed to find out their perspectives on the student's area(s) of difficulty. As more than 40% of the referrals that occupational therapists receive are for difficulties in the area of handwriting, the checklist should include questions about handwriting legibility, speed, and tool use, as well as questions about functional visual skills, sensory processing, attentional issues, and learning issues in general.

When the referral is received, an in-class observation should be scheduled during a writing task with the teacher so that the therapist can observe how the student forms letters (i.e., whether the child is economical and proficient in producing the letters, or if his or her formation is random and arduous, or if he or she demonstrates motor plans). Most importantly, therapists should also consider reviewing the student's written academic work performed both in class and as homework. Therapists then look at the overall legibility as well as the subskills of alignment, spacing, and size (Figure 13.4). Therapists also may discuss with the teacher on what prereferral strategies he or she has tried and found either successful or unsuccessful. These might include changing where a student sits in class, encouraging use of a different pencil or paper, or giving the student frequent movement breaks. At the beginning of each school year, in some school systems, therapists might consider giving an in-service and present a list of interventions and adaptations to all the teachers, with explanations of why and when to use them.

If several related service professionals are evaluating a student, such as physical therapists, speech and language pathologists, and/or special educators support services (resource room), the *School Functional Assessment* (SFA, Coster et al., 1998) may be used by the team. Another assessment tool an OT might use is the *School Assessment of Motor and Processing Skills* (AMPS) (Fisher et al., 2005). If this is not possible (or if the teacher and/or parents feel it is "just" handwriting, and the referral is only for occupational therapy services), the occupational therapist does

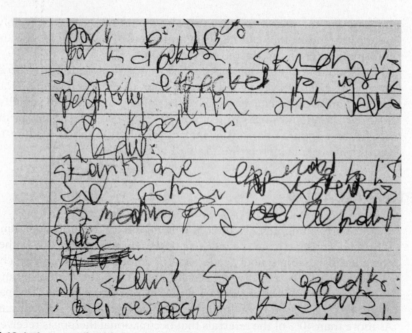

FIGURE 13.4 The most illegible handwriting I ever saw. An eighth grade girl.

his or her independent evaluation. After observations in the classroom, therapists usually see the child individually to give one or more standardized tests. For first and second graders, this might include a test of handwriting, such as the *Minnesota Handwriting Assessment* (MHA, Reisman, 1999), a tool with good psychometric properties that tests overall legibility and speed of manuscript writing. It has a standard manuscript form as well as a D'Nealian form (a form of printing that is somewhat of a hybrid between standard manuscript form and script). If students are in the third to fifth grades, therapists might administer the cursive version of the *Evaluation Tool of Children's Handwriting* (Amundson, 1995) or another criterion-referenced test.

Overall, the occupational therapist is evaluating how a student is performing compared to his or her peers. Is the student in the middle of the class or at the low end? Where does the difficulty lie? Ask the student. Students can often pinpoint their own problem areas. It is important that a student understands what you are looking for and why, as well as how the occupational therapist can help. One fourth grade student, for example, felt it was "unfair" that the teachers could not read what he wrote. He did not want to use a word processor or any test adaptations. I showed him a research article confirming that teachers give better grades to students with good handwriting. He understood the potential ramifications of his poor handwriting, but still did not want to be a willing participant in the therapeutic process. He also understood that he needed a scribe as a test modification, as his own teachers would not be grading the tests. Again, he thought this was "unfair." I ended up as a consultant to the teacher and to his parents and made a recommendation for further counseling.

To pinpoint the specific underlying problematic area(s), occupational therapists may also give a test of visual–perceptual and/or fine motor skills, such as:

- The *Wide Range Assessment of Visual Motor Abilities* (WRAVMA, Adams & Sheslow, 1995), which has a fine motor section along with a section on matching (visual spatial) and drawing (visual motor) skills. The WRAVMA is a norm-referenced test that gives percentile scores and standard scores. Students usually like it and it can be readily administered in one or two sessions, depending on the age and attention span of the child. It is easy and fast to score, the test directions are clear, and results in a lot of information. It is for students from 3 to 17 years of age.
- The *Beery-Buktenica Developmental Test of Visual Motor Integration-5*, (VMI, Beery, Buktenica, & Beery, 2004), which has a visual motor section and a visual perceptual section as well as a motor coordination section. This norm-referenced assessment is easy to administer in a timely fashion and also gives standard scores and percentile scores.
- The *Developmental Test of Visual Perception-2* (DTVP-2 Hammill, Pearson, & Voress, 1993), which tests several specific visual perceptual and fine motor skills, tends to take more time than either of the above tests, but gives you more specific information as to which visual perceptual and/or motor skill is giving the student the most difficulty. It is also a norm-referenced test. As it is much longer than the other two tests mentioned above, it will take longer to administer. There is also an adolescent/adult version available.

There are many other assessments available. It is important that the therapist chooses assessment tools carefully and makes sure that it has good psychometric properties. Read the manual. Give the test to several students to gain familiarity with giving it as part of an evaluation. Although no one test can recommend a student receives occupational therapy services, these tools, combined with classroom performance, teacher and parent interviews, and clinical observations, can provide a framework for the results of the evaluation. In all school systems, a standardized, norm-referenced test is a required part of the evaluation.

If the student does not get instruction in handwriting, it is usually recommended that the teacher implement a program in the classroom. This is often not a popular option, as the teachers have much mandated material to cover during the course of the day. Therapists might give the teacher research that supports the importance of instruction in handwriting. Teachers ultimately determine whether they have the time, resources, or ability to integrate handwriting instruction in their classroom. Some schools/districts have remedial time after school during which a teacher or assistant teacher can provide this instruction.

Once occupational therapy services are mandated for a child, the therapist's treatment plan should include various interventions. These include working in the classroom with the child and consulting with the teacher on environmental and/or curricular adaptations. In this manner, learning the motor skill(s) of letter formation can occur in the environment in which the student will have to perform, with naturally occurring sensory consequences.

Motor skill practice should continue in all elementary grades, especially when cursive writing is introduced. Cursive writing has higher nominal demands than manuscript, as every joining of two letters may need a different motor plan. This makes the nominal difficulty of writing in cursive harder than writing in unjoined manuscript letters. Also, students in third grade and up are expected to produce a higher quality and quantity of written work while learning the motor plans for new letter formations. This involves higher nominal and functional difficulty.

POSTULATES REGARDING CHANGE

- If a student has varied practice with the specific knowledge of the results, then his or her schema will enlarge, become more accurate, and the child will be able to form letters accurately, especially when they are embedded in words (Figure 13.5).
- If the student uses good alignment of the trunk and maintains trunk control and balance when interacting with a writing tool such as a pencil, pen, marker, and/or crayon, then the student will be more likely to use efficient arm movements during task performance.
- If the therapist provides varied practice and feedback with the knowledge of the results during the student's performance when practicing handwriting tasks, then the student will improve the quality of his or her task performance in the classroom.
- When a schema has become established, the student can produce novel movements because of the newly acquired ability to interpolate from past practices of the same

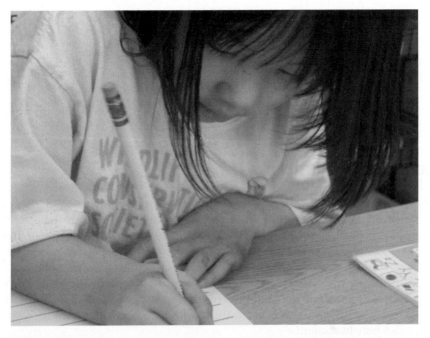

FIGURE 13.5 A first grade girl practicing handwriting. This girl has worked hard, has legible writing, and helps her peers by demonstrating accurate letter formation.

motor skill. This allows the student to determine what response specifications are necessary to achieve the desired outcome.

- Random practice provides the ability to accurately enlarge the schema of the motor act with a task of low nominal difficulty, such as making a letter.
- For the acquisition of a motor skill in the classroom to take place, low levels of contextual interference, using blocked practice, will aid in the motor skill acquisition for beginning skill levels. Once a schema has been formed, higher levels of contextual interference using random practice will provide information that can be incorporated into the enlarged, more accurate schema of the discrete motor skill.
- When learning tasks with high nominal difficulty, such as those that might present themselves when learning cursive, more frequent or immediate presentation of the accurate knowledge of the results (KR), or both, will produce a larger learning effect, but less retention.
- For tasks of low nominal difficulty, such as writing the individual letters of the alphabet, a random and delayed presentation of the KR or a larger summary feedback will produce the largest learning effect.
- When a symbol, like a letter, is being taught, it needs to be embedded in meaning in a word, for the student to learn the motor skill to transcribe it accurately while in the academic environment.

- When producing a task with high nominal difficulty, such as writing an essay in the classroom with a lot of conversations with classmates, blocked feedback will produce better learning than random feedback.
- Complex skill learning will be enhanced and a reasonably stable movement pattern will be acquired when the student is provided with a practice environment that facilitates performance.
- If practice is provided in a student's strongest types of intelligences, the child will be able to learn the lesson more easily and retain the information longer.

APPLICATION TO PRACTICE

Occupational therapists work in different environments in the school system. While we might understand that optimal best practice occurs in the classroom, this may be impractical or impossible because of many factors. One factor is that teachers are the "boss" of the classroom. Some teachers do not like to have occupational therapists (or anyone) in their room. The teacher may see you as a person who can "relieve" her from the presence of a difficult student. Therapy sessions may be scheduled during a time that is not appropriate for treatment (during reading, for instance). In these cases, one might consider giving in-services to the staff on how occupational therapy in the classroom can benefit students.

Although there may be a variety of reasons to remove a learner from the classroom for therapy, one reason may be the need for blocked practice. Some students need more time for blocked practice of skills to begin accurate schema development that needs a separate environment.

The examples that are provided here show different methods of service delivery for handwriting remediation.

Jane's Case Study: Working in a Classroom

It should be noted that while students in first grade do not necessarily have a mature grasp, most have a transitional grasp pattern and several, including Jane, the student I am working with, have a primitive grasp pattern. Jane has a diagnosis of apraxia. To learn any gross or fine motor skill requires large amounts of practice, both blocked to begin with, and random practice with contextual interference, to reinforce her schema of the task and to make it more accurate. We have not as yet discovered her optimal challenge point; therefore more detailed and specific information is required in the modeling of letter formation. She has developed strategies for spacing using a "space buddy" (a wide tongue depressor that she has decorated) or her left finger. Lately, the idea of spaces between words has become more automatic and she can gauge the distance as part of the motor plan.

Jane also has difficulty with oral motor tasks, and before she started kindergarten last year, could only speak about 20 words. Her intelligibility has increased slightly, and her vocabulary has increased to grade level. The teacher and I have tried to have her dictate her work but this is distracting to the other students and is often unintelligible, so the task is difficult for the girl and for the person recording her sentences. This adaptation does not add to her graphomotor schema and is generally frustrating for all concerned—Jane and the person recording her work.

Jane can produce most of the upper case letters of the alphabet in a size larger than her peers, in a manner that is awkward and effortful with a grasp on the pencil that causes her DIPs and PIPs to whiten. Her wrist is flexed and fixed. This produces upper case letters that are large and ill formed. She has uneven spacing between the letters of the words. The alignment is poor and the rate of transcription is slow and effortful.

In general, any written task is so arduous that Jane never finishes any written work and we are currently making curricular modifications in the amount of work she needs to produce. She has been refusing to write the lower case letters of the alphabet as she does not have the beginnings of a schema for most of the lower case versions of the letters. She needs to copy every word letter by letter although she can verbally spell the word. If she erases, or crosses letters out, which happens frequently, Jane is unable to calibrate the force necessary to complete the task demands. This results in tears and holes in the paper. Most of her work is crumpled and torn. She is insecure as to her performance and exhibits anxiety and resultant stubbornness when asked to practice. Jane's participation in any written task is therefore very limited.

We have started having additional handwriting practice outside of the classroom environment. This strategy has proved to have limited efficacy in carryover to her in-class academic work, perhaps because it is outside of the environment in which it needs to take place. In addition, during all seated writing activities, Jane needs constant verbal cues to maintain an upright posture. Without these reminders, she would lean over the desk to keep her eyes close to the page. Last year she wore glasses, but her pediatrician told her that she did not have to wear them anymore. She does not dissociate her eye movement from her head movement, and displays frequent distractions from the work at hand. In general, she maintains weight bearing on the desk with both arms, which reduces the fluidity and effectiveness of her upper extremity movements during writing tasks. Jane finds making postural adjustments difficult, and sometimes needs physical as well as verbal assistance.

It appears that Jane will not develop an accurate motor schema for transcription skills until the task is somehow made less effortful in all areas. Her chair and desk are at a good height, and she can maintain her feet on the floor. She is in a good position to watch the lesson. We have tried various adapted paper, with little success until recently. She had used a 3-in ring binder on its side, slanted like an old-fashioned desktop, which was efficacious for a while, but she did not want to use it, as no one else in the room had one. After several were made available to other students, she has been more willing to use it. All the students in her class have been given access to various pencil grips, so Jane is not the only one using one. Hers is a triangular grip, which gives her more control over the movements of the paper. We have tried dictation, but, again, it is difficult and most importantly, she would like to perform the activity herself.

Gregory's Case Study: Individualized Treatment in the Therapy Room

Gregory has a diagnosis of attention deficit hyperactivity disorder. He is a twin and was born prematurely. He presents with a double cleft lip and palate repair and has constant colds with a runny nose. Gregory is smart, and can do the work. The quality of his work overall is poor. He knows how to form letters and make the word endings into words (for example, <u>b</u>at, <u>c</u>at, <u>s</u>at). However, he is quick to write down his answers, and then proceeds to write them over and over, in different "styles" of writing, until the paper is covered with words and the results are illegible. Some of his "styles" are robot writing (typically rounded letters are made with box-like letters), "clown" writing (all letters have big "smiles" at the ends of them), and bubble writing (all letters are doubled so they look "fat" and "bubbly").

Although this may sound like a very dissimilar problem, it appears that Gregory also does not have a consistent transcription schema that he can use in academic work. He is unable to judge if his work is legible. He thinks if he writes enough, then it must be okay. His teacher feels that Gregory is just "playing around" and is annoyed at his inability to follow directions.

In the therapy room, Gregory was given the Minnesota Handwriting Assessment (MHA). His scores were "performing well below his peers" in the areas of size, alignment, and form. His rate and spacing were "performing like peers." He is a visual–spatial and kinesthetic learner who has not developed a dominant motor schema for classroom transcription work. His teacher requires conformity to her classroom rules, and the parents agree, so we have recommended occupational therapy services to promote the development of a dominant manuscript motor schema.

Gregory is being helped by a behavioral intervention plan. In the therapy room, he is encouraged to do his work slowly so that he will receive a smiley face. All his service providers throughout the day use the "smiley face intervention." He is trying to set a record of receiving smiley faces for 5 weeks. Because of this intervention, we are able to see more attention focused on producing acceptable academic tasks, and increasing his participation in classroom activities. His *slow* handwriting is becoming easier to read, as his motor schema to write at a decreased rate of speed develops, incorporates and he becomes able to produce more accurate transcription skills.

Peer Support

Jane was offered help and encouragement by two typically developing peers. Jane continues to have handwriting and writing practice every day, either in the classroom or in the therapy room. In the separate environment of the therapy room, we warm up our hands with an activity, such as making letters out of play doh, making drawings of her choice on a vertical surface, making bead jewelry: typical/traditional sensory motor activities. We then continue with blocked practice on raised line paper and a slant board, and then continue with random practice. Jane has achieved some success in the quiet environment, but it is not transferring to the classroom. The only adaptation she has accepted is the raised line paper, which helps her make letters that are slightly smaller than before. The concern exists that having no accurate schema formation will prevent her from being an active participant in the curriculum and may prevent her from progressing to the next grade. Her frustration level is increasing and negative behavioral changes are starting to occur, which are also detracting from her learning.

Both Jane and Gregory can be effective participants in the curriculum, but a high level of random practice will be required for accurate motor learning. Additionally, carryover in all areas of academic function will be necessary to achieve success. Although Gregory has been motivated by a behavioral plan to continue with varied random practice, Jane has not accepted the fact that she will need continual practice, as every motor act needs a separate and often practiced component. It is critical to engage students in varied random practice activities, preferably in the natural environment, with the optimal challenge point being identified, so that their motor learning schemas are accurate and automatic and the act of writing is about conveying their thoughts, opinions and knowledge thereby making them the most effective learners that they can be.

Tiffany's Case Study: Individual and In-class Instruction

Tiffany started a general education kindergarten class at a public school in New York City at 4.10 years of age. She has a diagnosis of right hemispheric fetal stroke, which resulted in left-sided hemiplegia (Figure 13.6). This functionally impacts

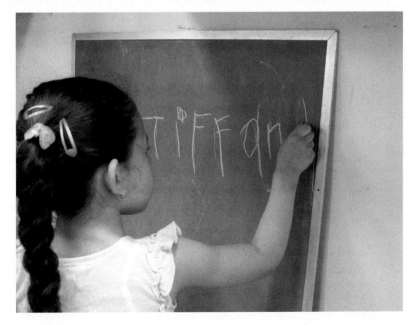

FIGURE 13.6 Tiffany doing one of her favorite activities: rainbow writing. She used different colors of chalk to go over the practice letters in her name.

her left side in her upper extremity, trunk, and lower extremity. She also has concomitant left visual neglect. She started the year with a splint on her left hand, but it was becoming too small for her and we discontinued its use.

Tiffany is a fiercely independent girl, with a terrific sense of herself and what she wants to accomplish. One of the goals in the kindergarten curriculum is for all children to be able to write their first and last names, using upper and lower case letters, by the end of the year. Tiffany was excited about pursuing this goal and was an active participant in all activities.

She had other goals, of course, that occupational therapy could address in treatment:

- Tiffany's teacher wanted her to stop "bumping into things" and "being so messy" when performing a classroom routine and or activity.
- She needed to be able to cross the midline of her body with her unaffected right arm to perform functional classroom work.
- She needed to learn to "look to the left" to learn academic tasks, produce written work, and complete activities in the Mathematics curriculum.

These treatment goals were approached with the same motor learning principles that we were applying to the discrete motor skill of forming individual letters for handwriting tasks, developing the schema for the task by varied practice. As she became more able to accurately perform crossing the midline with her unaffected (right) upper extremity and looking to the left, her teacher had commented that she was able to negotiate the classroom environment more easily. We also began every school day by using kinesiotape to tape her left hand in a functional position so that she could use it more effectively as an aid in performing her occupation as a student.

Tiffany had learned to write the "T I F F" in her name from her preschool occupational therapist. The "T" and the "I" were legible, but the "F" had a series of seemingly random horizontal lines running down the vertical stroke.

I evaluated her using Fisher, Bryze, Hume & Griswold (2005) School AMPS to see her function in the classroom, and the WRAVMA in the therapy room. Tiffany showed moderately inefficient schoolwork task performance, and she needed frequent assistance to complete the classroom tasks assigned by the teacher. She had difficulty with manipulating tools, such as markers, pencils, and scissors, difficulty coordinating all bilateral tasks, although she could use her left hand to stabilize the paper when writing or drawing or stabilizing the cap of a marker. She had a difficult time calibrating the necessary amount of force and the extent of movement when interacting with tools. Her attention to task demands was intermittent and she needed to look at what the other children were doing to continue the activity and complete the job. She needed frequent cueing by the teacher or aide to clean up and to use task objects in a more efficient manner. She had particular difficulty noticing or responding to the placement of objects/tools that she needed to use. She often knocked over her glue or paint onto another's desk and did not seem to know the boundaries of her workspace. She had difficulty anticipating problems and often did not have enough of whatever supplies she needed. She also did not prevent problems from reoccurring the next time the task was performed.

On the School AMPS, her motor percentile rank was less than 1%, below age expectations, and her process score was 15%, which is within age expectations, although in the low average range.

Tiffany's functional visual skills were assessed using *Pediatric Clinical Vision Screening for Occupational Therapists* (PCVS-OT, Scheiman, 2002) for saccades (looking from one static object to another static object) and pursuits (tracking a moving object). As she appeared to have a significant left neglect, as well as some neglect in both superior visual fields, a recommendation to be evaluated by a developmental optometrist was made.

In the schoolroom, a curricular writing task was part of the "Name of the Day" or "Star Name" curriculum. One child would be chosen and the teacher would write his or her name on the board. She would show them how to make the letters and, after the name was written, she would draw a line around the name to show them the shape. Tiffany had "tall letters" T, f, f; "short letters" i and a; and a "long letter" y. On her day, Tiffany would be in the special chair in the front of the room and her classmates would ask her questions as part of an interview process. Then they all got "story" paper, with a box at the top, and three widely spaced lines underneath. Their writing job was to write their name and the date at the top of the paper, make a picture of something about Tiffany, and "write" three things about her pets, favorite color, and eye color—whatever they had learned in the "interview." Spelling or legibility did not count. The class also had a "word wall" that filled up with classmates' names and favorite words. Each child also had a manuscript alphabet strip taped onto the desk and his or her name written on wide-lined paper with a dotted line in the middle.

Formal handwriting instruction was usually started in January of kindergarten, as the teacher said that little hands were not ready for the hard job of handwriting at least until then. She had the students do a lot of drawing, connect the dots work, mazes and other pencil (or marker) and paper games. She demonstrated how to use all the available writing tools with control and accuracy. The occupational therapist provided adaptations for Tiffany to use if she wanted them: a nonslip mat for under her paper and adaptive scissors. But Tiffany wanted to do everything by herself—just like everybody else. She worked hard on holding down the paper with her left hand as well as functionally using the spasticity to maintain a firm grip on the marker top so she could open it independently.

In January, the teacher had the students participate in a more structured handwriting program. They had to practice how to write their name at their desks on paper or on white boards with various media: markers, pencils, and crayons. Occasionally they wrote while sitting on the floor in "circle time," or kneeling on the floor, using their chairs as writing surfaces, providing differing sensory input. She also used blocked and random practice for this skill with low nominal and functional difficulty. Writing her name was a meaningful task for Tiffany and she was very enthusiastic whenever she had some success.

I worked with Tiffany whenever possible in class, which provided random practice, higher contextual interference, and summary KR and in the therapy room when she needed blocked practice. We worked in blocked practice sessions with immediate and summary feedback (KR) to develop the schema for the letters in her name. The optimal challenge point was often hard to determine as Tiffany was an enthusiastic learner ("I did it!") and she was not an accurate judge of when the task became too hard for her, possibly causing a degradation of performance that could negatively impact accurate schema development. The letters we used were all in her name, providing meaning for the activity, as well as increasing her ability to meet curricular demands.

Some of the materials we used:

- On vertical surfaces
  - Chalkboard
  - Magnadoodle held on the wall with Velcro
  - White board
- On slanted surfaces
  - Adapted slant boards that had paper, chalkboards, and white boards on them
  - 3-in notebook
- On the desk surface
  - A small chalkboard with lines
  - Story paper (both horizontal and vertical)
  - Paper with different types of lines and visual cues, including raised lines
  - Different colored paper
- Writing tools
  - Pencils: large diameter, regular no. 2 pencils, triangular pencils (short and long), "golf" (short) pencils, and short pencils with very soft lead that made darker lines while using less pressure, and rainbow pencils
  - Crayons: standard, triangular, round balls, rectangular, rainbow stubby crayons
  - Pens: roller ball, gel, felt-tip with big and small diameters and heights
  - Chalk: typical white and yellow as well as colored, round chalk, egg-shaped chalk, "sidewalk" chalk, and animal-shaped chalk
- Other surfaces
  - We wrote over carpet squares with our fingers
  - We wrote over "bumpy boards" with crayons
- Other activities
  - Drawing letters in the air
  - Drawing letters on each other's backs (mystery letters)
  - Writing while in quadruped on the floor
  - Writing in shaving cream
  - Writing in finger paint

Tiffany needed blocked practice for the "f," the "a" and especially, the "y." We used various combinations of the above media to find the ones she liked the best and produced the best results, reaching the optimal challenge point. Our sessions would begin with this selection and then we would first demonstrate how to form the letter, and then practice. There was always a model with directional arrows she could refer to, even when she had an action plan of her own. During blocked practice, she received immediate feedback (KR), and also evaluated each group of the same letter as to which one was the best: summary feedback. When she achieved success, we would change one parameter, which she would again choose (stand at the big chalkboard, sit and write on the bumpy board, etc.). Again, practice with different sensory information and varying feedback was provided. At the end of the practice, she could put a sticker on the "best" letters.

Tiffany had difficulties with the retention of the motor plan for some letters, especially the lower case "a" and the "y." We kept on practicing these two letters; the "a" became more and more accurate, but the "y," with its diagonal lines, was more difficult for her (Figure 13.7).

We continued to play games. Tiffany loved "tic-tac-toe," so she was motivated to learn to make the grid herself (horizontal and vertical lines) and she could pick any letter in her name to be used as her mark, although she was encouraged to pick "y" (Figure 13.8). I could pick any letter in my name for my mark. We would teach each other how to make the letter and then play several games. What fun we had! One of the rules was to tell each other if we could not read the letter. I gave continuing summary feedback (KR) during this activity that provided random practice to increase retention of the motor plan.

An activity Tiffany especially loved was "making pictures" (drawing), following the "directions" in *Ed Emberley's Drawing Book of Animals* (Emberely, 2006). There are no words in the books. They graphically display the kinds of lines (often letters)

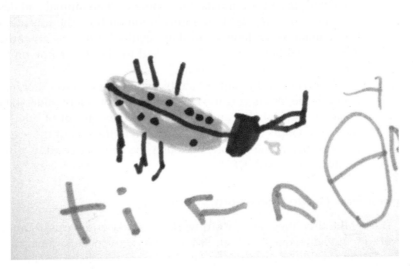

FIGURE 13.7 Tiffany had just started making lower case letters. Notice the "a." She knew that a circle and a line were both involved, but did not have the schema of the motor plan of the entire letter.

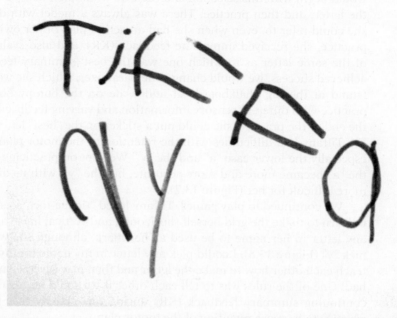

FIGURE 13.8 In this picture, Tiffany made the "a" and the "y" legibly, with good formation. It was formed on a 4 in. × 5 in. piece of paper. The lower case 'n' is reversed. Her name did not fit on the 4 in. × 5 in. paper.

needed to make the animals. She would pick an animal and describe how she was making it. In this way, I got information on how she was adding self-feedback to her schema of the letters and dots required. She was an enthusiastic participant and admired her pictures. Tiffany had to sign her name on the front or back of every picture "like real artists do."

At first, Tiffany had difficulty with the graphic differences and similarities between the letters (Figure 13.9). She did not really understand the symbols that make up the alphabet and did not have the concept of how to begin to combine them into words beyond her name, even at the end of the year. She did learn how to write her name legibly, although the schema continued to need intermittent reinforcement with KR.

Working in a First Grade Classroom

During the time they have "word work" in a first grade classroom, I work with a table of four students, one of whom has a mandate for occupational therapy, one of whom was being evaluated for services (and has subsequently been mandated for occupational therapy), and two who are typically developing learners. The lesson plan concerns word groups or endings; "it," and "an," for instance, and how many words a student can think of to write down with these word endings.

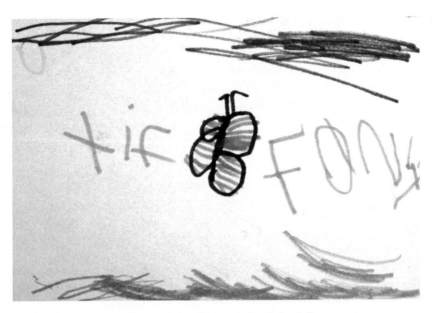

FIGURE 13.9 Tiffany developing her schema for the "a" and the "y."

During a typical lesson, the teacher and I demonstrate how to form the letters in the air, using verbal cues, and the entire class repeats what we did, both motorically and orally, which aids the implementation of their action plan and aids in accurate schema development. The students then write down the ending pair and try and guess the words they can make by adding a letter in front of it. Therefore, varied random practice is provided in the context of the lesson, with the use of words embedding the letters in meaning for more accurate symbol development.

The teacher has given them the strategy of going through the alphabet to come up with new words, for example: **it**-bit-fit-hit-kit-lit-pit-sit-wit, or: **an**-can-fan-man-pan-ran-tan. We then model, demonstrate, and give them verbal directions on how to make each letter, and again repeat the sequence of letter formation of the word in the air. We talk about the meanings of the words and how to use them in sentences. The learners, with the letters and endings embedded in the meaning of the words, use this random practice, and have multiple opportunities to initiate their own action plans. They form the words on the page in their notebooks. Summary feedback is given after each word group by the teacher, the occupational therapist, or one of their fellow students. They are asked to circle the most legible words they wrote and show them to the other students at the table. This work takes between 30 and 45 minutes every day and every student must participate.

This lesson uses the students' kinesthetic, visual spatial, and linguistic intelligences to reinforce the spelling and transcription of the words and also increases the enlargement of a more accurate schema (Figure 13.10). The two students, who have difficulties with transcription tasks, as well as the typically developing students work, are observed

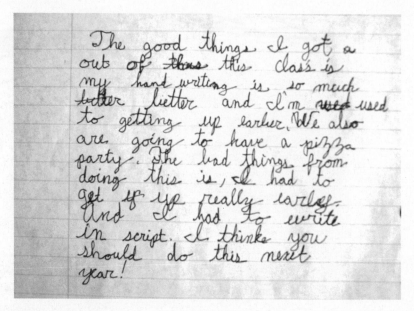

FIGURE 13.10 Student's report on the results of a fifth grade group cursive handwriting intervention.

by the occupational therapist, so that letter reversals, misspellings, or malformations are corrected immediately. In this way, inaccurate information about forming individual graphemes does not become part of their schema.

 Summary

This FOR for the development of handwriting skills is based on a systematic approach to establishing schema and motor skills necessary for the formation of letters. The therapist provides the child with opportunities to develop and practice these skills and the child is an active learner in this process. The development of schema allows for the acquisition of basic motor skills necessary for writing. Once these basic motor skills have been established, the child is able to generalize these skills to more complex fine motor acts, which are necessary for functional handwriting within a classroom setting.

REFERENCES

Adams, W., & Sheslow, D. (1995). *Wide Range Assessment of Visual Motor Abilities (WRAVMA)*. Wilmington, DE: Wide Range, Inc.

American Occupational Therapy Association. (2002). Occupational therapy: Domain and process. *American Journal of Occupational Therapy, 56,* 609–639.

Amundson, S. J. (1995). *ETCH Examiner's Manual Evaluation Tool of Children's Handwriting*. Homer, AK: O.T. Kids Inc.

Amundson, S. J. (2001). Prewriting and handwriting skills. In J. Case-Smith (Ed.), *Occupational therapy for children*. (pp. 545–570). St. Louis, MI: Misby-Year Book.

Beery, K. E., Buktenica, N. A., & Beery, N. A. (2004). *Beery-Buktenica Developmental Test of Visual-Motor Integration* (5th ed.). Austin, TX: Pro-Ed.

Burton, W. A., & Dancisak, J. M. (1999). Grip form and graphomotor control in preschool children. *American Journal of Occupational Therapy*, 54(1), 9–17.

Coster, W. J., Deeney, T. A., Haltiwanger, J. T., & Haley, S. M. (1998). *School Function Assessment (SFA)*, Standardized version. Boston, MA: Boston University.

Dennis, J. L., & Swinth, Y. (2001). Pencil grasp and children's handwriting legibility during different-length writing tasks. *American Journal of Occupational Therapy*, 55, 175–183.

Emberely, A. (Ed). (2006). *Editor Emberele's Drawing Book of Animals*. New York: Little, Brown and Company.

Fisher, A., Bryze, K., Hume, V., & Griswold, L. (2005). *School AMPS*. Fort Collins, CO: Three Star Press.

Gardner, H. (1991). *The Unschooled Mind: How Children Think and How Schools Should Teach*. New York: Basic Books.

Gardner, H. (1993). *Frames of Mind: The Theory of Multiple Intelligences*. New York: Basic Books.

Gardner, H. (1999). *Intelligence Reframed. Multiple Intelligences for the 21st Century*. New York: Basic Books.

Gardner, H. (2004). *The unschooled mind: How children think and how schools should teach*. New York: Basic Books.

Gardner, H. (2006). *Multiple Intelligences*. New York: Basic Books.

Gibson, E. J. (1971). Perceptual learning and the theory of word perception. *Cognitive Psychology*, 2, 351–368.

Graham, S., Harris, R. K., & Fink, B. (2000). Is handwriting causally related to learning to write? Treatment of handwriting problems in beginning writers. *Journal of Educational Psychology*, 92(4), 620–633.

Guadagnoli, M. A., & Lee, T. D. (2004). Challenge point: A framework for conceptualizing the effects of various practice conditions in motor learning. *Journal of Motor Behavior*, 36(2), 212–224.

Hammerschmidt, L. S., & Sudsawad, P. (2004). Teachers' survey on problems with handwriting: Referral, evaluation, and outcomes. *American Journal of Occupational Therapy*, 58(2), 185–192.

Hammill, D. D., Pearson, N. A., & Voress, J. K. (1993). *Developmental Test of Visual Perception* (2nd ed.). Austin, TX: Pro-Ed.

Koziatek, M. S., & Powell, J. N. (2003). Pencil grips, legibility, and speed of fourth-graders' writing in cursive. *American Journal of Occupational Therapy*, 57(3), 284–288.

Laszlo, J. K., & Broderick, P. (1991). Drawing and handwriting difficulties: reasons for and remediation of dysfunction. In J. Wann, A. M. Wing, & N. Sovik (Eds). *Development of Graphic Skills: Research Perspectives and Educational Implications* (pp. 259–281). London: Academic Press.

Magill, R. A. (2001). *Motor Learning: Concepts and Applications* (6th ed.). Dubuque, IA: Brown and Benchmark.

Marr, M., Windsor, M. M., & Cermak, S. (2001). Handwriting readiness: Locatives and visuomotor skills in the kindergarten year. *Early Childhood Research & Practice: An Internet Journal on the Development, Care, and Education of Young Children* 3(1), electronic version.

Reilly, M. (Ed). (1974). *Play as Exploratory Learning*. Beverly Hills, CA: Sage Publications.

Reisman, J. (1999). *Minnesota Handwriting Assessment*. San Antonio, TX: Harcourt Assessment.

Rosenblum, S., Chevion, D., & Weiss, P. L. (2006). Using data visualization and signal processing to characterize the handwriting process. *Pediatric Rehabilitation*, 9(4), 404–417.

Roston, K., Hinojosa, J., & Kaplan, H. Using the minnesota handwriting assessment and handwriting checklist in screening first and second grader's handwriting legibility. *Journal of Occupational Therapy, Schools, & Early Intervention*, 1(1), 100–115.

Scheiman, M. (2002). *Understanding and Managing Vision Deficits: A Guide for Occupational Therapists* (2nd ed.). Thorofare, NJ: Slack Inc.

Schmidt, R. A. (1975). A schema theory of discrete motor skill learning. *Psychological Review*, 82, 225–260.

Schoen, S. (2001). The effectiveness of the pencil grasp to promote acquisition of a mature pencil grasp in school-aged children. Unpublished doctoral dissertation, New York University.

Ste-Marie, D. M., Clark, S. E., Findlay, L. C., & Latimer, A. E. (2004). High levels of contextual interference enhance handwriting skill acquisition. *Journal of Motor Behavior*, 36(1), 115–126. Retrieved from the internet, 8/27/04.

Sudsawad, P., Trombly, A. C., Henderson, A., & Tickle-Degnen, L. (2002). Testing the effect of kinesthetic training on handwriting performance in first-grade students. *American Journal of Occupational Therapy, 56*(1), 26–33.

Summers, J. (2001). Joint laxity in the index finger and thumb and its relationship to pencil grasps used by children. *Australian Occupational Therapy Journal, 48*(3), 132–141.

Van Doorn, R. R. A, & Keuss, P. J. G. (1991). Dysfluency in children's handwriting. In J. R. Wann, A. M. Wing, & N. Sovik (Eds.). *Development of Graphic Skills: Research Perspectives and Educational Implications* (pp. 239–247). London: Academic Press.

Weintraub, N., & Graham., S. (1998). Writing legibly and quickly: A study of children's ability to adjust their handwriting to meet common classroom demands. *Learning Disabilities Research and Practice, 13*(3), 146–152.

Windsor, M. M. (2000). Clinical interpretation of "grip form and graphomotor control in preschool children". *American Journal of Occupational Therapy, 54*(1), 18–19.

Yakimishyn, E. J., & Magill-Evans, J. (2000). Comparisons among tools, surface orientation, and pencil grasp for children 23 months of age. *American Journal of Occupational Therapy, 54*(5), 565–572.

CHAPTER 14

An Acquisitional Frame of Reference

AIMEE J. LUEBBEN • CHARLOTTE BRASIC ROYEEN

The purpose of this chapter is to provide a basic understanding of a frame of reference for skill acquisition, theories that form the basis for this frame of reference, and corresponding practice applications. After providing an introduction that offers a historical perspective, this chapter presents the theoretical base with concepts and definitions, assumptions, and theoretical postulates. The acquisitional frame of reference is further delineated into function–dysfunction continua with indicators of function and dysfunction, a guide for evaluation, postulates regarding change, and application to practice. In the acquisitional frame of reference, occupational therapists use two important legitimate tools of the profession: the teaching–learning process and activities, especially activity analysis and synthesis. At a fundamental level, the acquisitional frame of reference is synonymous with the teaching–learning process.

INTRODUCTION

A frame of reference for skill acquisition focuses on the acquisition of specific skills required for the optimal performance within an environment. With this focus in mind, occupational therapists plan intervention and provide activities solely for the purpose of acquiring specific skills. The primary goal of an acquisitional frame of reference is learning: mastering each skill or subskill required of an activity (Mosey, 1986).

In the occupational therapy profession, the acquisitional frame of reference is a conglomeration of learning theory concepts. For the most part, learning theories are based on the hypotheses and experimental research of prominent scientists in three areas: behaviorism, cognitive science, and neuroscience.

At the beginning of the 20th century, behavioral scientists (primarily psychologists) lay the groundwork for acquisitional learning theories. Edward Lee Thorndike, Ivan Petrovich Pavlov, and John B. Watson were three prominent psychological theorists studying stimulus response. Thorndike's (1932) connectionism theory viewed learning as trial and error. Pavlov (1941), known for his experiments based on classical conditioning, showed the influence of reinforcement. Watson (1917) was among the first to use the term "behaviorism" to show how humans develop through conditioning and learning. Other behavioral theorists applying stimulus–response principles were Hull (1951, 1952), Guthrie (1935), and Tolman (1932, 1958).

Although many early behaviorists worked with more simple experimental systems such as dogs or rats, theorists in the middle of the 20th century were starting to apply behavioral principles to humans. B. F. Skinner began with animal research models, but became interested in programmed learning and teaching machines. His theory of operant conditioning (Skinner, 1953, 1954, 1971, 1974) with reinforcement (or reward) as a central focus has been widely applied to education and parenting.

Two other psychologists made contributions to learning theory, starting in the 1960s. Albert Bandura expanded the role of observation and modeling in learned behavior in his social learning theory (Bandura, 1965, 1977). Carl Rogers' work on the use of unconditional positive regard, client-centered therapy, and the role of therapists in the treatment setting has provided basic theoretical information on how the therapist approaches intervention (Rogers, 1951, 1957; Rogers & Freiberg, 1994).

Cognitive science, the second area that provided a basis for learning theories, came from a melding of interdisciplinary researchers interested in attention, perception, communication, and information processing (Gardner, 1985). Early cognitive scientists were from separate disciplines such as psychology, communications, mathematics, and engineering. Cognitive scientists, particularly the cognitive psychologists according to Eric Kandel, "were interested in investigating the mechanisms in the brain that intervene between a stimulus and a response—the mechanisms that convert a sensory stimulus into an action" (2006, p. 296). Kandel explained that cognitive psychology emerged in response to limitations of behaviorism that tended to simplify behaviors whereas cognitive psychologists were more interested in complexity.

While behaviorism was becoming increasingly important in learning in the 1960s and cognitive science was gaining speed, there were other scientists studying higher brain function. Behaviorists and cognitive scientists started collaborating with these researchers working in neuroscience (the third area that provided a foundation for learning theories) in the 1970s and 1980s. The result of the collaboration is what Kandel (2006) calls "the new science of mind": the merging of biological science (concerned with brain processes) with behavioral and cognitive psychology (concerned with mental processes).

Kandel's (2006) neuroscience research has shown that learning and memory are formed in stages and based on synaptic connections. Short-term memory, created by strengthening existing synapses, lasts minutes. Long-term memory, which requires creation of new synapses, lasts days or longer. New synaptic connections involve rewriting the genetic code to form new proteins, the basis for improved connectivity. His experiments propose that short-term memory grades naturally into long-term memory through repetition. According to Kandel, "practice does make perfect" (Kandel, 2006, p. 206).

Rapid advancements in imagining sciences and the emphasis on evidence-based practice have also helped drive scientific thinking around learning, memory, and behavior. There is a currently strong movement toward collecting and analyzing patterns (Viamontes & Beitman, 2006), comparing traditional and systems approaches (Aleksandrov, 2006), and investigating the role of other brain regions, such as the cerebellum (Rapoport, van Reekum, & Mayberg, 2000), in cognition and behavior. To provide client-centered care, scientists are also beginning to use advanced brain diagnostics to match brain patterns with interventions (Moras, 2006).

In the occupational therapy profession, principles from learning theories form the theoretical base of the acquisitional frame of reference. The acquisitional frame of reference flourished in occupational therapy in the late 1960s and early 1970s (Hollis, 1974; Norman, 1976; Rugel et al., 1971; Sieg, 1974; Smith & Tempone, 1968; Trombly, 1966; Wanderer, 1974). Currently, practitioners continue to use the acquisitional frame of reference prominently. Each time a therapist uses the teaching–learning process as a legitimate tool, the practitioner has applied the acquisitional approach in providing therapeutic services.

Describing the acquisitional frame of reference as the linking of learning theories, Mosey (1986) indicated that the acquisitional frame of reference may at first resemble the developmental frame of reference in that the therapist works on skill development. While there appear to be many similarities between the developmental frame of reference and acquisitional frame of reference, there are several key concepts that distinguish the two theoretical approaches. The developmental frame of reference views the development of skills as occurring along a continuum: skill development is age dependent. Children learn new skills when they have reached the developmental level necessary to support the skill. There is a hierarchy of skills in the developmental frame of reference: skills must be learned at a certain stage of development before other skills can be acquired. In a developmental frame of reference, learning is viewed as predictable, stage specific, sequential, and cumulative.

In the acquisitional frame of reference, learning is not stage specific, sequential, or cumulative. Although the developmental level of the child may be acknowledged in an acquisitional frame of reference, there is no particular emphasis made during practice. Behaviors, in an acquisitional frame of reference, are simply broken down into smaller component steps and built upon each other, resulting in acquisition of complex skills (Figure 14.1).

THEORETICAL BASE

Behavior, in an acquisitional frame of reference, is viewed as a response to the environment. The environment either reinforces and strengthens a behavior (positive reinforcement) or fails to provide a positive reinforcement by giving no reinforcement or ignoring behaviors (negative reinforcement). The role of the environment in eliciting adaptive responses is of primary importance in the acquisitional frame of reference. Because humans acquire new skills—they learn—by interacting with a reinforcing environment, working in authentic and naturalistic environments is central to using an acquisitional frame of reference.

Concepts and Definitions

Learning (skill acquisition) in an acquisitional frame of reference is influenced by interaction between the environment and a person's behavior. Emphasis is placed on (1) the context of the environment, (2) functional behaviors, and (3) learned skills. Each of these concepts is explored in greater detail.

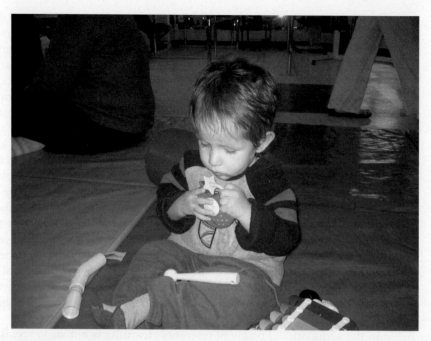

FIGURE 14.1 Child working on basic grasping skills.

Context of the Environment

The *context of the environment* is the primary determinant of behavior in an acquisitional frame of reference. The environmental context encompasses everything that is external to the individual (including human and nonhuman elements) and provides reinforcement for behavior. If the environmental context does not afford or elicit certain behaviors, the behaviors will not emerge. An example of environmental context is the cultural or ethnic background of the family. Environmental reinforcers refer to the positive or negative stimuli that occur in the child's external environment (Figure 14.2).

Initially, the environment helps with acquisition of a skill. Across time, repetition and practice help reinforce the skill, allowing the child to generalize that skill to new contexts. Over time, the reinforcer from the environment changes. For example, when a parent is trying to develop independence in grooming skills, the parent may reinforce every positive step the child takes toward independence. As the child gets older, the parent no longer needs to provide reinforcement for each independent act, but the peer group reinforces the child when he or she is clean, groomed, and dressed in a similar way as other children. Through this, the child is able to generalize the intrinsic importance of independence in self-care skills; the child bathes and performs grooming tasks appropriately without external (extrinsic) reinforcement. Therefore, a broad scope of experiences within the environment is essential for the acquisition of a wide array of skills.

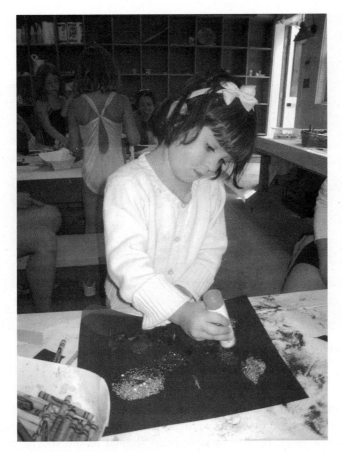

FIGURE 14.2 Environmental stimuli for positive behaviors.

Functional Behaviors

The term "functional behaviors" refers to specific behaviors a child needs to attain to succeed in the environment. To become a more permanent part of the child's repertoire, these behaviors need reinforcement. From an occupational therapy perspective, the therapist looks at the components or steps that will lead to the specific behaviors the child needs to acquire. The therapist shapes or provides reinforcement for any behaviors that contribute to skill acquisition: the goal of the intervention. A set of behaviors is acquired, which ultimately assists the child in achieving the skill. For example, to acquire the skill of brushing hair, the therapist will have the child begin working on grasping skills to acquire the ability to pick up small objects. As this intervention progresses, the child refines grasping skills to hold a hairbrush in a hook grasp. Next, a therapist teaches the child to use the brush to groom his or her hair. The therapist approximates the skills that are needed to perform the final task (i.e., brushing hair) through the use of other activities, which leads to functional behavior. Functional behavior is dependent on context. The context is predominant in determining what is functional and what is truly necessary.

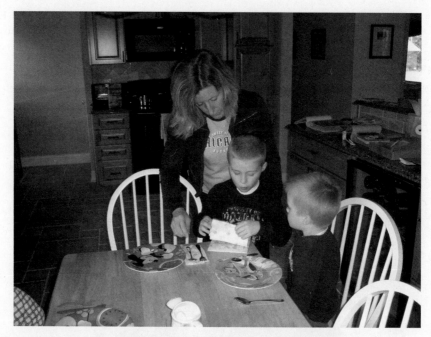

FIGURE 14.3 Child working on acquiring learned skills.

Learned Skills

Learned skills focus on the skills that need to be acquired for performance in the specific environment. Integrating the context of the environment and functional behaviors results in learned skills (Figure 14.3). Behaviors have been shaped to the specific skills that are needed as well as the environment focuses on that need. To identify learned skills that are essential for the child, the therapist must consider the environmental context, the functional behaviors that are present, and new skills that must be acquired and generalized through strategies such as reinforcement and shaping.

Reinforcement refers to the environmental stimulus that rewards or does not reward behavior. Reinforcement takes place through the environment, which includes the social and cultural context. Skill development and its subsequent adaptive responses to environmental stimuli are contingent or dependent on positive (rewards) and negative (does not reward) reinforcement. In an acquisitional frame of reference, higher level skill development begins with the simple and progresses to the complex. Additionally, the environment is structured in such a way as to provide the learner with the greatest likelihood for success (Skinner, 1953). Reinforcement is used to encourage the acquisition of behaviors and skills and the more frequent occurrence of behaviors and skills.

As stated earlier, *positive reinforcement* strengthens behavior by rewarding the desired behavioral response. Skill development is thus contingent on positive reinforcement. Reinforcement can be intrinsic or extrinsic. Intrinsic reinforcement includes

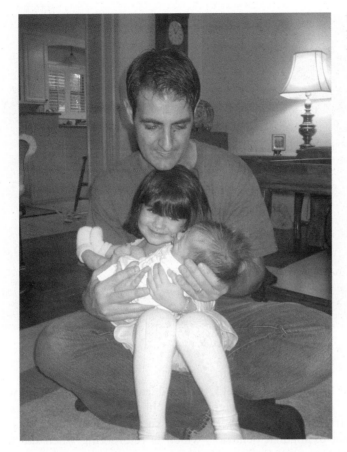

FIGURE 14.4 Parent providing positive reinforcement for the acquisition of caring skills.

feeling pride for a job well done and knowing something has been completed to high quality level. Extrinsic reinforcement can be tangible (e.g., food, money, stickers, tokens, small toys, earning time, or special events) or nontangible (e.g., words of encouragement, praise, and hugs) (Figures 14.4 and 14.5). For children, reinforcement that incorporates a physical and emotional human response can be extremely powerful. While the use of positive reinforcement is the cornerstone of the development of skills and adaptive responses, the extinction of nonadaptive behaviors is dependent on the use of negative reinforcement.

Negative reinforcement is used to extinguish nonadaptive behaviors. Examples of nonadaptive behavior are the inability to make eye contact when appropriate, leaving a bathroom without washing hands, or twirling a toothbrush in a toilet. When ignored, a behavior is negatively reinforced.

Punishment is the use of physical or verbal acts to extinguish behaviors that are perceived as not being valuable or appropriate. It is important not to categorize punishment solely as a negative reinforcement. For some children, punishment is a positive reinforcement that results in the acquisition of nonadaptive behaviors. To illustrate, if a

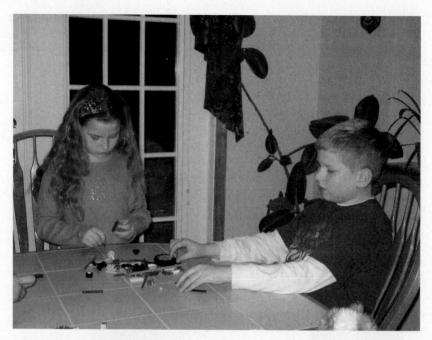

FIGURE 14.5 Modeling a desired skill.

child is punished for hitting another child, the child learns that punishment will follow if someone sees him or her hit another child. The child may then pursue nonadaptive behavior such as hitting when no teacher or other student is around. In this example, punishment does not extinguish behavior, which is reinforcing when the individual receives attention (Skinner, 1954). For other children, punishment can serve as a negative reinforcer. When one child hits another and is then sent to "time-out" as punishment, he or she may stop hitting behaviors.

Vicarious reinforcement is used to describe learning that occurs through observation. Vicarious reinforcement occurs when a child has observed the positive or negative reinforcement of behavior in other children (Bandura, 1965). Bandura proposed that learning takes place not only through direct experience; children can learn or acquire new behaviors simply by observing the reinforced or nonreinforced behaviors of others, hence the term "modeling" (Bandura, 1965, 1977). Children learn and develop skills by observing children and other models such as teachers, parents, or therapists who are performing the desired skill (Figure 14.6). This human ability to learn and acquire new behaviors through observation of others has been substantiated through neuroscience by the discovery of mirror neurons (Rizzolatti et al., 1996).

Shaping is rewarding close approximations of a desired skill. For occupational therapists, shaping draws heavily on the understanding of activity analysis and synthesis. The therapist can analyze the activity and understand the component steps. From that understanding, the therapist can shape a desired skill by building on each component

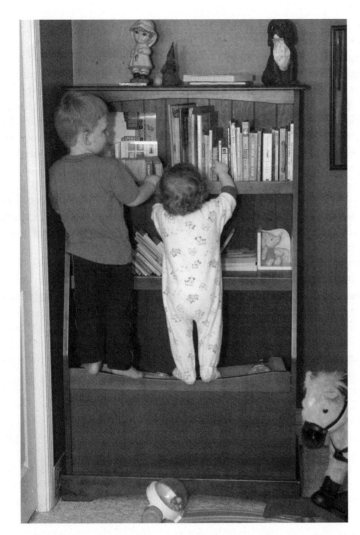

FIGURE 14.6   Modeling   of skills.

of the task. In this situation, it is important to understand the components of the task in addition to the whole activity. Shaping of skills is accomplished in small increments with close approximations of the desired behavior rewarded. For example, if a child was learning to dress independently and put his or her pants on all by himself or herself, it would not matter if the pants were on backward (at first), as long as the child did it independently. Thus, dressing is being "shaped."

Schedules of reinforcement are the ways, time intervals, and methods of organizing reinforcement to promote the acquisition (i.e., increasing or decreasing) of particular behaviors or skills. There are three main types of reinforcement schedules: (1) continuous, (2) partial, and (3) intermittent. With a continuous reinforcement schedule, sometimes referred to as a "contingency reinforcement" or "management schedule," the reward is given every time the behavior occurs. Every response is reinforced. A continuous reinforcement schedule is thought to lead to a rapid acquisition of the behavior (Kaplan & Saddock, 1998), though this may not be the most effective reinforcement schedule for permanency of acquisition. In a partial reinforcement schedule, reinforcement is only given some of the time that the behavior occurs, and there is no discernible pattern regarding when the reinforcement will take place. Partial reinforcement is thought to be the strongest form of reinforcement in shaping behaviors (Hergenhahn, 1988). With this form of reinforcement, the individual does not know when the reward will occur and, therefore, tends to exhibit the desired behaviors more frequently. Behaviors shaped in this manner are also the hardest to extinguish. An intermittent reinforcement schedule refers to reinforcement that is based on intervals either fixed or variable. In a fixed ratio intermittent schedule, reinforcement occurs at regular intervals, such as every fifth response. A variable ratio intermittent schedule is when reinforcement occurs at varying intervals, such as every third time, then after the fifth time, and then every second time.

Once a behavior or skill is firmly established (often through extrinsic reinforcement), the ability to maintain the skill becomes intrinsically reinforced. In other words, performing the behavior or skill correctly (performance results is the desired goal) in and by itself becomes self-reinforcing (Bandura, 1977). It is suggested that self-reinforcing behaviors provide some level of meaning to the person. Although some believe that it is ultimately an intrapsychic event that underlies response to reinforcement, intrapsychic events are not a major component of reinforcing responses that shape behavior.

Generalization occurs when a skill or behavior learned in one environment can be applied in a similar, yet different situation or in another environment. Examples of generalization include a child who can flush a toilet independently by using a manual handle designed for hand use on a home toilet, pushing a foot-based handle on an institutional toilet at school, or using an automatic flush mechanism that relies on motion detection. Generalization also occurs when a person is able to adapt by adding extra steps for success. For instance, someone who requires a secondary flush on a toilet with automatic flush mechanism can activate the mechanical button or handle provided or can replicate the same motion that activated the automatic flush.

According to learning theorists, all behavior is shaped by the environment (Norman, 1976). Although not readily apparent, the environment provides positive and negative reinforcements. It is the role of the therapist to observe and identify what stimuli in the environment are shaping a child's behavior and how. In addition to the positive and negative reinforcing value the environment holds, experience and exposure to environmental stimuli provide children with the opportunity to acquire new skills.

One critical aspect of the environment is the therapist. The therapist creates the environment and sets the tone for the intervention. In this acquisitional frame of reference, the works of Rogers (1951, 1957) contribute an important element: unconditional positive regard. Unconditional positive regard is used as a platform for all interventions. The therapist creates an atmosphere of acceptance and accepts the child for who he or she is. This does not mean that all behaviors are accepted, but that child is accepted unconditionally. Children behave in ways that will gain positive reinforcement from others and, therefore, act accordingly. This type of environment is a powerful tool for reinforcement. According to Rogers (1995), change is more likely to occur when the therapist accepts the client at his or her current level of functioning.

Assumptions

The acquisitional frame of reference has five major assumptions. Together, these five assumptions constitute the core beliefs underpinning the acquisitional frame of reference.

The first major assumption is that intrapsychic dimensions are irrelevant to the behavior shaped by the environment. Considering the age-old debate between "nature" and "nurture," this assumption states that "nurture" is more important, that all behavior is determined by the past and current environment. Essentially, neuroscience has demonstrated that the "nurture" aspect in turn influences "nature." Kandel (2006) has shown that learning acquired through environmental interaction (nurture) can ultimately result in changes in the "nature" of the organism. The nature of the organism changes with the formation of long-term memory that requires new synaptic connections developed by forming new proteins through genetic code rewriting. Consequently, there is little room for "meaning" or for intrapsychic dimensions that a person may bring to the behavior. Environment, as used here, refers to the physical, social, and cultural dimensions external to the body.

The second major assumption is that the therapist accepts the child unconditionally and without judgment. This creates the environment that is conducive to learning and the development of functional skills. Children can learn by interacting and observing other children and adults. They behave in ways that will gain them positive reinforcement from others, especially people important to them such as mothers, fathers, and teachers. This assumption is a platform on which intervention is based.

The third major assumption is that competence, or the belief that a person can act and have influence over the environment, results from learning skills. In the acquisitional frame of reference, acquiring skills (hence the name *acquisitional* frame of reference) is of paramount importance to mastery and self-competence—not intrapsychic processes.

The fourth major assumption is that a skill is a skill is a skill. No skill is more important than another or serves as a foundation for another skill. In an acquisitional frame of reference, learning may not follow a developmental sequence. It stands to reason that according to this frame of reference, a deficit in one performance area does not predict, predicate, or necessarily correlate with a deficit or problem in another performance area. Unlike a developmental perspective, acquisition of skills does not require reconstructing, reexperiencing, or mastering previous developmental stages. Functioning in a particular environment is of particular importance in an acquisitional frame of reference.

The fifth major assumption is that practice makes perfect. Neuroscience (Kandel, 2006) has shown that through repetition and practice organisms learn by interacting with a reinforcing environment. Humans acquire skills through repetition and practice of those specific new skills with appropriate reinforcement within a particular environment.

THEORETICAL POSTULATES

Theoretical postulates state the relationship between concepts in the theoretical base. There are three main theoretical postulates in the acquisitional frame of reference.

- Acquisition of skills, which results in learning, is a result of reinforcement.
- Function is not stage specific.
- Behaviors result from environmental interaction.

Acquisition of skills, which results in learning, is a result of reinforcement. The term "acquisition of skills" refers to the idea that behavior, or observable human activity, is predominately influenced or primarily impacted by the environment through negative and positive reinforcement. Positive reinforcement results in a learned behavior. Negative reinforcement results in getting rid of unwanted behaviors or nonadaptive behaviors. To teach a skill, therefore, behavior must be (1) reinforced directly or (2) reinforced through seeing someone else being positively or negatively reinforced. Each time a child performs a newly learned skill correctly, positive reinforcement needs to occur. During skill acquisition, different schedules of reinforcement, which were introduced in an earlier section, may be used successfully. For some children, some reinforcers are stronger than others.

Function is not stage specific. For a person, the environment and events are more important in determining the behavior than the individual's developmental stage. The acquisitional frame of reference assumes that function is more important than any identifiable stages of development. Further, the specific stages of development bear no relevance to this frame of reference. Rather, the most important determinant of behavior is the environment and what the environment elicits in terms of behavior or function. Thus, function is considered in quantitative terms (i.e., the child can do a specific task or cannot do that task). Quality, initially secondary to the ability to perform a function, may become more important during other times of skill acquisition. In the acquisitional frame of reference, the goal is function, not achievement of a specific developmental task. Function can be acquired in any order based on the unique needs of the child within the environment.

Behaviors result from environmental interaction. If overall behavior is a result of environmental demand, then adaptive behavior results from interaction with an environment that has been or is designed for learning a particular skill. Adaptive behavior, as used here, refers to changes in behavior to accommodate new challenges in the environment.

FUNCTION–DYSFUNCTION CONTINUUM

The acquisitional frame of reference is somewhat unique compared to other frames of reference because each continuum of function and dysfunction is defined by the specific behavior to be acquired. In the acquisitional frame of reference, a child can either perform a skill needed to function in the environment or the child cannot. When generating a specific function–dysfunction continuum for a particular child, a criterion-referenced dichotomous measure is used: (1) yes, the child can perform the specific skill or (2) no, the child cannot perform the skill. Function and dysfunction can also be determined by the environment where the skill must be performed. A child, for example, may be independent in washing hands at home, but not at school.

Furthermore, a child's developmental status can provide background for this frame of reference. Not of major importance, developmental status can be considered when determining if the specific skill to be acquired is appropriate at that developmental stage. For example, a 2-year-old child developmentally would not be learning to tie shoelaces so tying shoes would not be an optimal skill to have a 2-year-old child learn. Deciding to have this 2-year-old child work on undressing skills, however, would be appropriate because a child of this age should be removing clothing.

Once a task or activity has been determined necessary for a child to function in his or her environment, then the therapist performs an activity analysis to divide the task into components or steps that consist of skills, behaviors, or both. These component steps are often further subdivided to provide a true representation of a task. After activity analysis, an occupational therapist designs a task-specific function–dysfunction continuum that lists the required component steps to complete the skill. Dysfunction is when any task needed for the environment cannot be performed independently. At times, a child may be able to demonstrate a particular skill, but the skill may need to be shaped to increase the frequency of occurrence or to improve the quality.

A function–dysfunction continuum can be identified for any task necessary for the child to perform within a particular environment. A task or skill forming the basis of a function–dysfunction continuum can range from the ability to make eye contact, to independence in self-care skills, to the ability to interact in a socially appropriate manner. Skills in the acquisitional frame of reference are always environmentally specific. A child may be able to demonstrate appropriate behaviors and skills to perform a specific task in one environment, but may be working on a similar task in another environment. At first, it is important whether a child can perform a specific skill, not how well a child can do that specific skill. After acquisition of a basic skill, determining how well a child performs (the quality of the skill) may be important.

Indicators of Function–Dysfunction

Within the acquisitional frame of reference, it may be impossible to discuss function and dysfunction in a general manner because the behavior of a person is so specific to a particular environment. For a child, behavior must be at an appropriate level and linked to the specific context of the environment. Additionally, the environment is an important determinant of behaviors to be learned. A child may operate at a higher functional level in a specific skill at home or in a familiar classroom than if expected to function in an unfamiliar environment such as a new school.

In the first example, a child is using his or her own fork at home, working on self-feeding (Figure 14.7). Within the acquisitional frame of reference, any attempt during initial skill acquisition, such as self-feeding, is acceptable as a starting point.

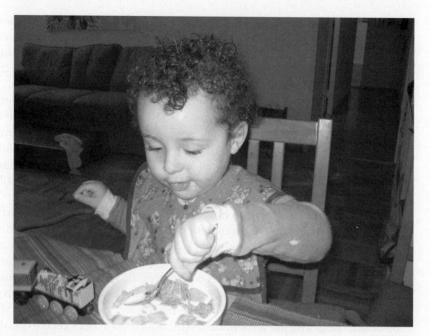

FIGURE 14.7 Grasping a utensil to begin self-feeding.

In Table 14.1, the indicators of self-feeding function include grasping the fork, stabbing food with the fork, moving the fork to the mouth, taking food from the fork into the mouth, and swallowing food. At first, it would not matter if the child gets most of the food on his or her face or clothes as long as the child attempts to self-feed. Further, it would not matter if self-feeding is done with much protest, as long as the child makes an attempt at self-feeding. Indicators of self-feeding dysfunction include the opposite: not grasping the fork, not stabbing food with the fork, not moving the fork to the mouth, not taking food from the fork into the mouth, and not swallowing the food. All attempts at self-feeding or any component of self-feeding would be reinforced so that behaviors could be shaped to develop strong functional skills.

TABLE 14.1 Indicators of Function and Dysfunction for Self-Feeding (With a Fork)

Self-Feeds with a Fork	*Does Not Self-Feed with a Fork*
FUNCTION: Able to self-feed with a fork	*DYSFUNCTION*: Unable to self-feed with a fork
Indicators of Function	**Indicators of Dysfunction**
Grasps the fork	Does not grasp the fork
Stabs food with the fork	Does not stab food with the fork
Moves the fork to the mouth	Does not move the fork to the mouth
Takes food from the fork into the mouth	Does not take food from the fork into the mouth
Swallows food	Does not swallow food

In the acquisitional frame of reference, environment is paramount. A child who is independent in self-feeding at home may go with his parents to a restaurant that has different utensils than at home. In the restaurant, the child may have difficulty with a basic indicator of function: grasping the fork. The parents may need to feed the child. This child might be able to generalize independence in self-feeding to other environments if his or her parents had packed an extra fork from home or had the child practice self-feeding at home with various different types of utensils found in everyday places outside the home.

For the same child at home, another example is washing hands. At the beginning of skill acquisition, the ability to wash hands is the issue, not how well a child can do this task. In Table 14.2, indicators of hand washing function include moving to the sink, turning on the faucet to wet hands, accessing soap (in a dispenser or as a bar), rubbing hands together to distribute the soap, rinsing hands, turning off the faucet, getting the towel, drying hands, returning the towel, and leaving the sink area. Indicators of hand washing dysfunction are the opposite: not moving to the sink, not turning on the faucet to wet hands, not accessing soap, not rubbing hands together, not rinsing hands, not turning off the faucet, not getting the towel, not drying hands, not returning the towel, and not leaving the sink area.

Depending on the child and environment, the listing of indicators of hand washing function and dysfunction can be shortened, expanded, or customized. The listing could be shortened for a child beginning to acquire hand washing skills. This child might have four indicators of hand washing function: turning on the faucet to wet hands, using soap, rinsing hands, and drying hands. At the start of skill acquisition, there might be a focus on prioritized indicators of function with less emphasis placed on aspects such as moving to and from the sink, turning off faucets, and final disposition of towels.

The listing of hand washing function and dysfunction indicators could be customized for a child who is independent in every aspect of hand washing at home, but encounters dysfunction in a new environment such as public restroom with automatic

TABLE 14.2 Indicators of Function and Dysfunction for Washing Hands

Washes Hands	*Does Not Wash Hands*
FUNCTION: Able to wash hands	*DYSFUNCTION*: Unable to wash hands
Indicators of Function	**Indicators of Dysfunction**
Moves to sink	Does not move to sink.
Turns on faucet to wet hands	Does not turn on faucet to wet hands
Accesses soap	Does not access soap
Rubs hands together	Does not rub hands together
Rinses hands	Does not rinse hands
Turns off faucet	Does not turn off faucet
Gets towel	Does not get towel
Dries hands	Does not dry hands
Returns towel	Does not return towel
Leaves sink area	Does not leave sink area

faucets, soap dispensers, and towel machines. At first, the child might show some indicators of dysfunction that include not turning on the faucet, not accessing soap, and not getting the towel. Learning how to operate several types of bathroom equipment in multiple restroom environments often takes practice before successful skill acquisition can take place.

GUIDE FOR EVALUATION

Occupational therapists using an acquisitional frame of reference have many choices for evaluation. The choices range from standardized assessment instruments to nonstandardized assessment tools. An optimal method of collecting information about a child's function may be a combination of standardized assessment devices and nonstandardized assessment tools in an integrated approach.

Typically, standardized assessments involve administration and scoring procedures, comparisons for performance, and appropriate psychometric properties (validity, reliability, and sensitivity). There are two basic types of standardized assessments: (1) criterion-referenced instruments allow comparison to a standard and (b) norm-referenced tools permit comparison to a group. Some standardized assessment instruments are developed to be either criterion referenced or norm referenced; other instruments are designed to be both, while still other tools have criterion-referenced aspects differentiated from norm-referenced parts. The manual for a particular standardized assessment manual is a primary source for determining how to use information gathered by a certain tool. Standardized assessment tools should form the core of the information gathering process.

Although a purist would consider some of the standardized assessment tools (especially the norm-referenced instruments) to be developmental, these tools often provide checklists of tasks, skills, behaviors, functions, and performance that can be used by therapists operating under an acquisitional frame of reference. Additionally, standardized assessments are increasingly being required by reimbursement sources to determine need for therapy.

Self-care is a primary area of concern for pediatric occupational therapists. Two of many standardized assessments available are the *Inventory of Early Development–II* (IED–II; Brigance, 2004) and the *Scales of Independent Behavior–Revised* (SIB–R; Bruininks et al., 1996). The IED–II, standardized for children from birth to 7 years, includes as one of 12 criterion-referenced skill areas a self-help section that consists of eight skills areas: feeding and eating, undressing, dressing, unfastening, fastening, toileting, bathing, and grooming. Each of the individual items for the areas is designed to operate as a mini function–dysfunction continuum. A child is either able to perform the skill or not. The SIB–R is a norm-referenced (infancy to 80+ years) and criterion-referenced instrument that uses evaluator observation or client/caregiver report to provide information for four skill clusters including personal living which consists of five subscales: eating, toileting, dressing, self-care, and domestic skills. Individual items of the SIB–R are scored, depending on a child's level of performance, on a four-point scale with function at one end and dysfunction at the other (and two points in between). Using standardized assessment during the initial evaluation and subsequent reevaluations permits comparison of a child's performance to a standard or other group, allowing occupational therapists the ability to leave evidence of occupational therapy effectiveness.

Although therapists can take advantage of a standardized instrument's strong external validity (ability to generalize) by comparing a person's function to a group (norm referenced) or to a standard (criterion referenced), this type of assessment may not address the uniqueness of a person within an environment. To assess the uniqueness of a child within a particular environment, many occupational therapists rely on nonstandardized assessment tools, particularly observation. In fact, most therapists using an acquisitional approach begin with general observation. The therapist observes the child within the environment and identifies the demands of the environment to determine the required skills. The therapist combines knowledge of the age-appropriate levels of tasks with an understanding of the child and the environment and its demands. Therefore, classic observation is a powerful and appropriate guide for evaluation available for use in the acquisitional frame of reference.

Within a specific environmental setting, the therapist begins by observing to see whether a required skill can be performed. The decision is black-and-white: the skill can be performed or the skill cannot be performed. The following series of questions can assist the therapist in determining the presence of function or dysfunction.

- What are the observable skills of the individual within the environment?
- What are the physical characteristics of the environment in which the individual needs to perform?
- What are the sociocultural characteristics of the environment in which the individual needs to perform?
- What additional skills, if any, are required in the current environment?

Because the acquisitional frame of reference is accordingly individuated to a person, using this approach requires considerable skill on the part of the therapist. Each particular question should be addressed. For the acquisitional frame of reference, there are no established evaluation protocols. Each assessment tool used should be specific to the child receiving intervention. The therapist must determine what skills need to be acquired by the child for the child to be successful within the environment.

After the demands of the environment and the child's ability to perform the tasks have been identified, the therapist completes a more focused observation. A focused observation provides additional information about the component steps of the skills in addition to what aspects of the environment are encouraging or interfering with the child's performance. Observation at this level also requires classic activity analysis and synthesis skills of the therapist. The therapist needs strong abilities to analyze the activity and understand the component steps to determine if and how these components are interfering with the performance of the task. Additionally, the therapist must identify potential positive and negative reinforcement. Activity analysis and synthesis helps the therapist determine more specific areas that require intervention and what reinforcers will be effective within a particular setting. During more focused observation, a therapist determines:

- What are the specific component steps of the tasks?
- Which of these component steps can the child do well, and which require intervention?
- Which skills need to be shaped?
- What are identifiable positive and negative reinforcements?
- What constitutes a positive reinforcer and what constitutes a negative reinforcer for the child?
- Within this environment, which would be the most powerful positive reinforcers?

In summary, for most therapists operating under an acquisitional approach, evaluation consists of a nonstandardized assessment tool: observation of performance of the skill in the context of the environment. This type of assessment involves the identification of the tasks required by the environment, the component steps of the tasks, and the positive and negative reinforcers present in the environment that influence skill development.

POSTULATES REGARDING CHANGE

Postulates regarding change define the therapeutic environment that needs to be created and suggest methods used by the therapist to facilitate change. When the results of evaluation indicate dysfunction, intervention focuses on the acquisition of component parts of skills or specific skills. These learned skills are necessary to be successful within the environment. For the acquisitional frame of reference, eight postulates regarding change have been identified.

The first two postulates are general postulates regarding change for the acquisitional frame of reference.

1. If the therapist provides positive reinforcement specific to the child and the environment, then the child will be more likely to acquire component steps of skills or specified skills.
2. If the therapist provides negative reinforcement specific to the child and the environment, then nonadaptive behaviors will be more likely to be extinguished.

Once a dysfunction or deficit has been identified, the next six postulates regarding change relate more specifically to occupational therapy intervention.

1. If the therapist provides reinforcement specific to the child and the environment, then the child will be more likely to acquire component steps of skills or specified skills.
2. If the therapist uses various schedules of reinforcement specific to the child and the environment, then the child will be more likely to acquire component parts of skills or specified skills.
3. If the therapist provides reinforcement for any attempt at a behavior, then the child is more likely to acquire the behavior.
4. If the therapist reinforces component parts of a skill, then behavior will be shaped so the child can acquire the skill.

5. If a child acquires specific skills and those skills are reinforced, then the skill has the potential of being self-reinforcing and generalized to other settings.
6. If reinforcement is consistent across settings, then skills are more likely to be acquired.

APPLICATION TO PRACTICE

The acquisitional frame of reference is often used in occupational therapy. This approach is so much a part of occupational therapy practice that therapists frequently are not aware that they are using the acquisitional frame of reference. Yet a behavior or skill that is viewed as beneficial to the child is rewarded with positive reinforcement, and a behavior or skill that is viewed as negative meets with negative reinforcement and attempts to extinguish that behavior. The acquisitional frame of reference can function alone as a frame of reference or can be used in conjunction with other frames of reference that are consistent with learning theories.

To use an acquisitional approach, the occupational therapist needs to identify the specific skill or behavior that he or she wants to develop. That skill or behavior should be one that is compatible with and necessary for optimal (or at least improved) functioning within the environment. If it is a complex skill, then the therapist must use activity analysis and synthesis, beginning with activity analysis: breaking down the skill into components. Once that skill, behavior, or necessary components have been identified, the therapist needs to identify a reinforcer that is valuable to the child and the environment. It may be praise, a token, or a sticker, but it has to be something that the child wants and is compatible with the environment (Figure 14.8). The therapist then provides this reinforcement whenever the child makes an attempt at the desired behavior. At first, the quality of the attempt is not important—the emphasis is on the attempt itself. This exemplifies the first postulate regarding change: if the therapist provides positive reinforcement specific to the child and the environment, then the child will be more likely to acquire component parts of skills or specified skills.

The same approach is used with negative or nonadaptive behaviors. The therapist would need to identify the behavior that is nonadaptive. The therapist would identify a negative reinforcer that is specific and has relevance to the child and is compatible with the environment. It can be anything that the child does not want to occur, such as being put in "time-out," being sent to a room alone, or having a favorite food or dessert withheld. A negative reinforcer is used when the behavior appears; with repeated use, the negative reinforcer is likely to extinguish that behavior. It is critical that the positive or negative reinforcer be specific and meaningful to the child and the environment for effectiveness. The child works harder for something that he or she values highly and modifies behavior to avoid something that he or she does not like. With the acquisitional frame of reference, the therapist must match the reinforcers, both positive and negative, with the child and the environment to achieve maximum success.

When using the acquisitional frame of reference, the schedules of reinforcement presented in an earlier section are important. A child is more likely to acquire a skill or behavior if various reinforcement schedules are used. The child may come to expect praise for each attempt if it is offered every time, yet the child may work harder when

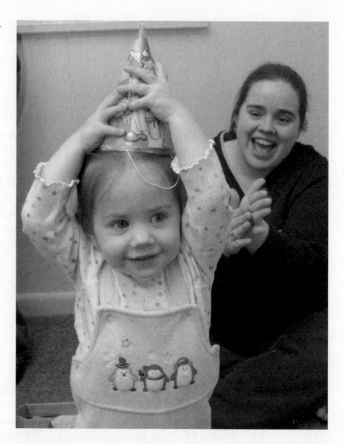

FIGURE 14.8 Clapping as a reward for a desired act.

that reinforcement is less predictable and comes at random intervals. The therapist needs to match the reinforcement schedule with the child and often must try different schedules to see which one works better.

The quality of performance is usually not initially important in this frame of reference. The child gets reinforcement for all or most attempts at a task. This includes the component parts of that skill. If the child is rewarded when attempting something, then he or she is more likely to make additional attempts at the task. The focus on quality does not come until much later, if at all. At the beginning, it is more important to reward the child for continued work on a skill or behavior—positive reinforcement will provide the reward. This provides the basis for the acquisition of more complex skills (Figure 14.9). With each component rewarded, the desired behavior or skill gradually becomes integrated into the child's repertoire. As the skill acquisition progresses, the therapist shapes the behavior by requiring more complex skills or behaviors before a reward is given. The therapist may also use a varied schedule of reinforcement.

A child learning to self-feed, for example, initially eats with fingers. This tends to be messy, yet the therapist ignores the mess and provides positive reinforcement for attempts at self-feeding. When the child moves to using a fork, the therapist may give

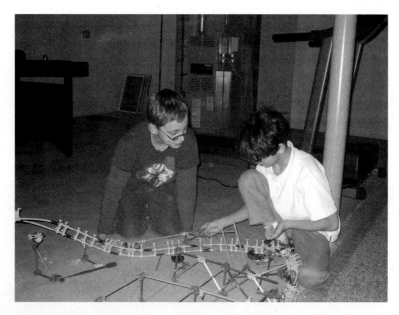

FIGURE 14.9 Social interaction supports skill development.

positive reinforcement for just stabbing the food with the fork, which is a component part of eating with a fork. This is shaping the behavior. The therapist is letting the child know this is a valued act and is part of the skill of self-feeding (Figure 14.10). Then when the child brings the fork with some food on it to his or her mouth, the child is rewarded again, continuing the shaping of the skill. Yet when the child flings the fork and the food onto the floor, the therapist gives negative reinforcement in the hope of extinguishing that behavior. At the beginning, the emphasis is on rewarding positive attempts, ignoring quality of performance, and using negative reinforcement to extinguish unwanted behaviors. Further, as the child is able to self-feed, the behavior itself becomes rewarding, reinforcing itself. This reinforcement allows the child to begin to generalize. Self-feeding is seen as important, and the child begins to understand its importance, not just during the time of the intervention but at any time.

Once a child has been referred for an evaluation, the first step in the process is to use the nonstandardized assessment tool: observation of the child in his or her natural environment. This may be the home setting, school, or playground or at a social gathering. The therapist is observing the child's behavior and is simultaneously observing the physical and social environment and the interaction between the child and the environment (Figure 14.11). It is critical to identify what constitutes positive reinforcers and negative reinforcers (as well as potential reinforcers) within the setting.

To show how to use an acquisitional approach to provide evidence of the effectiveness of occupational therapy intervention, consider the example of Julio, who is working on washing his hands independently at school. In this example, the

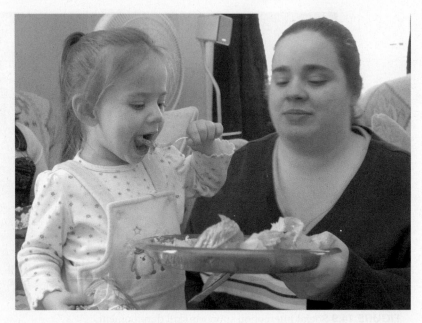

FIGURE 14.10 The valued skill of self-feeding.

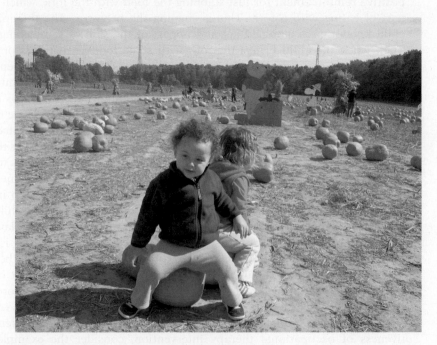

FIGURE 14.11 Observing children interacting in the natural environment.

occupational therapist has already performed an initial evaluation (using nonstandardized assessment: observation) and designed an intervention program that is being carried out by classroom personnel. The intervention program includes a partial schedule of reinforcement based on a token system. Julio is working to earn time on his favorite thing: the classroom computer. In this example, the therapist checks Julio's progress twice a month, adding to his intervention as needed. Of course, the example is specific to Julio in a single environment: his current classroom. But the example allows for application of the same ideas for Julio in a different school or a completely different environment such as the movie theatre. The example also provides some ideas for generalizing the concept of acquisition of any skill to another child in different environment.

Because of the uniqueness of the acquisitional approach, therapists can easily convert a listing of indicators for function–dysfunction for a particular skill into an operational checklist to be used for evaluation and intervention purposes. As an example, Table 14.3 provides a checklist for the skill acquisition of hand washing. In the checklist,

TABLE 14.3 Hand Washing Checklist										
Name:			*Skill: Washing Hands*							
		Date Added				Date Checked				
Number	Step Description									
10	Leaves sink area									
9	Returns towel									
8	Dries hands									
7	Gets towel									
6	Turns off faucet									
5	Rinses hands									
4	Rubs hands together									
3	Accesses soap									
2	Turns on faucet to wet hands									
1	Moves to sink									
	Total score (date)									

each indicator of function becomes a step for a skill. Notice that the checklist shows a reverse ordering compared with Table 14.2, which shows the indicators of function and dysfunction for washing hands. The item, move to sink, is the top indicator of function and the bottom step (step 1) of the skill checklist.

In the checklist, each row shows the level of skill acquisition for one step across dates. A row begins with a step number, a description of the step, and the date a particular step (and description) was added to the listing. The remaining cells in the row show a child's acquisitional level of performance for a particular date the skill was checked. The column, date added, allows for flexibility: the steps of a skill can be added at later dates instead of being deployed all at once.

In school, Julio is working on washing his hands independently. On January 3, following initial evaluation of Julio's hand washing skills, his occupational therapist designed a checklist. Tables 14.4 and 14.5 show two versions of a checklist. Table 14.4 is a simple version that uses a simple criterion-referenced dichotomous measure (X is yes: able to perform and blank cell is no: unable to perform).

Julio's initial checklist (both versions) contains six steps (moving to the sink, turning on the faucet to wet hands, accessing soap, rubbing hands together to distribute the soap, rinsing hands, and turning off the faucet). With Julio's steady progress in skill acquisition of hand washing, steps 7 and 8 (getting the towel and drying hands) were added on January 14. Two additional steps, returning the towel (9) and leaving the sink area (10) were added on February 1. The therapist checked Julio's hand washing skills seven times: January 14, January 28, February, 1, February 28, March 1, March 28, and April 1. According to the simple version of the checklist (Table 14.4), Julio was independent for the first step on January 14 and two steps (step 1 and 2) on January 28. Julio was independent on 9 of 10 steps (all except step 7) on March 28 and independent for all 10 steps of hand washing on April 1. The total score (e.g., Julio performed 9 of 10 steps on March 28) for the date can be used for the purpose of showing improvement of skill acquisition across time.

Table 14.5 adds a level of complexity to the checklist by allowing for scoring of the quality of skill acquisition. At times, determination of how well a child performs a skill or component step may be of importance. Rather than using a simple dichotomous scale (indicating X for skill step attainment), this version uses the following ordinal scale: 4 for independent, 3 for requires verbal cue, 2 for requires gesture, 1 for requires physical assist, and 0 for resistance/refusal.

In Table 14.5, the quality (not just presence or absence) of Julio's hand washing skills was assessed on the same seven dates. The design of the more complex version of this checklist works at two levels. First, the table can be viewed as a line graph with the bold line around a cell indicating total number of items scored as 4 (independent) on a particular date. (The bold line outlining a cell uses the first column, step number, of the checklist for a secondary purpose: to show the total number of steps performed independently.) For example, when checked on February 1, Julio performed three steps independently (1. move to the sink, 2. turn on the faucet, and 6. turn off the faucet). The bold outline of the cell at the level of the third step indicates at a glance that Julio acquired three steps of hand washing at an independent level on February 1.

TABLE 14.4 Julio's Hand Washing Checklist (Simple Version)

Name: Julio			Skill: Washing Hands						
			Date Checked						
Number	Step Description	Date Added	1-14	1-28	2-1	2-28	3-1	3-28	4-1
10	Leaves sink area	2-1						X	X
9	Returns towel	2-1						X	X
8	Dries hands	1-14						X	X
7	Gets towel	1-14							X
6	Turns off faucet	1-3			X	X	X	X	X
5	Rinses hands	1-3				X	X	X	X
4	Rubs hands together	1-3					X	X	X
3	Accesses soap	1-3					X	X	X
2	Turns on faucet to wet hands	1-3		X	X	X	X	X	X
1	Moves to sink	1-3	X	X	X	X	X	X	X
	Total score (date)		1	2	3	4	6	9	10

TABLE 14.5	Julio's Hand Washing Checklist (Complex Version)									
Name: Julio			*Skill: Washing Hands*							
			Date Checked							
Number	Step Description	Date Added	1-14	1-28	2-1	2-28	3-1	3-28	4-1	
10	Leaves sink area	2-1				3	3	4	4	
9	Returns towel	2-1				1	2	4	4	
8	Dries hands	1-14		1	2	3	3	4	4	
7	Gets towel	1-14		1	1	2	3	3	4	
6	Turns off faucet	1-3	2	3	4	4	4	4	4	
5	Rinses hands	1-3	1	2	3	4	4	4	4	
4	Rubs hands together	1-3	1	1	2	3	4	4	4	
3	Accesses soap	1-3	0	1	2	3	4	4	4	
2	Turns on faucet to wet hands	1-3	3	4	4	4	4	4	4	
1	Moves to sink	1-3	4	4	4	4	4	4	4	
	Total Score (date)		11	17	22	31	35	39	40	
	Average Score		1.8	2.1	2.7	3.1	3.5	3.9	4.0	

Scale: 4 = Independent, 3 = verbal cue, 2 = gesture, 1 = physical assist, and 0 = resistance/refusal.

Table 14.5, the more complex version, also works at a second level. Below the double line (under the steps), there are two additional rows: a total score for the date (adding Julio's performance based on the ordinal scale for each checked day) and an average score (adding Julio's performance based on the ordinal scale for each checked day and then dividing by the number of skill steps at that particular date). Although the simple version of the checklist provides a total score for the date that consists of the count or frequency of steps performed independently for a specific date, the complex version provides a more sensitive scale that may pick up smaller changes of performance over time.

Julio's average score, for example, changed slightly (3.9 to 4.0) from March 28 to April 1, respectively. On April 1, Julio was able to perform all steps of hand washing independently compared with being checked 2 weeks earlier when he needed verbal cueing to get the towel (step 7). For a child working on the acquisition of more than one skill, the average performance score for the column would be a better choice because one skill (such as hand washing used in this example) might have 10 steps and second skill might have 12 steps. Using the average performance score for the column would allow acquisition across more than one skill to be compared even though the number of steps for a particular skill might be different.

Using the acquisitional frame of reference, Julio's therapist developed a listing of indicators of function that she customized for Julio within his environment. She then converted the function indicator listing into a checklist, which she used to show change across time. By using a nonstandardized assessment approach—the conversion of function indicators into a checklist—the therapist was able to show Julio's progress in skill acquisition across time. With the checklist, the therapist was able to leave evidence of effectiveness of occupational therapy intervention.

Julio's progress toward hand washing skill acquisition is just one example of a single skill for one child. Consider the possibilities available because of the uniqueness of the acquisitional frame of reference that allows individualization to one skill for a single person in his or her environment. Following observation, a function indicator listing could be designed and converted into a skill checklist—for any skill, any person, and any environment. The possibilities are endless.

Summary

The acquisitional frame of reference focuses on the acquisition—learning—of specific skills or subskills required to function optimally within the environment. Mastery of skills or appropriate behaviors is the primary goal of the frame of reference. The theoretical base of acquisitional frame of reference is drawn from principles and assumptions based on learning theories. In the acquisitional frame of reference, the therapist uses two important legitimate tools of the profession: the teaching–learning process and activities, especially activity analysis and synthesis. Through the analysis of the skill or behavior to be acquired, the therapist identifies component steps a child needs to learn. The therapist then shapes skills or behaviors through the reinforcement of these component steps until the child achieves mastery of the behavior or skill. Mastery of the skill, which provides intrinsic reinforcement, allows the child to generalize that skill or behavior.

REFERENCES

Aleksandrov, Y. I. (2006). Learning and memory: Traditional and systems approaches. *Neuroscience and Behavioral Physiology, 35*(9), 969–985.

Bandura, A. (1965). Influence of a model's reinforcement contingencies on the acquisition of imitative responses. *Journal of Personality and Social Psychology, 11*, 589–595.

Bandura, A. (1977). *Social Learning Theory*. Englewood Cliffs, NJ: Prentice-Hall.

Brigance, A. H. (2004). *BRIGANCE® Inventory of Early Development–II (IED–II)*. North Billerica, MA: Curriculum Associates.

Bruininks, R. H., Woodcock, R. W., Weatherman, R. F., & Hill, B. K. (1996). *Scales of Independent Behavior—Revised (SIB-R)*. Rolling Meadows, IL: Riverside Publishing.

Gardner, H. (1985). *The Mind's New Science: A History of the Cognitive Revolution*. New York: Basic Books.

Guthrie, E. R. (1935). *The Psychology of Learning*. New York: Harper & Brothers.

Hergenhahn, B. R. (1988). *An Introduction to Theories of Learning* (3rd ed.). Englewood Cliffs, NJ: Prentice-Hall.

Hollis, L. I. (1974). Skinnerian occupational therapy. *American Journal of Occupational Therapy, 28*(4), 208–212.

Hull, C. L. (1951). *Essentials of Behavior*. New Haven, CT: Yale University Press.

Hull, C. L. (1952). *A Behavior System: An Introduction to Behavior Theory Concerning the Individual Organism*. New Haven, CT: Yale University Press.

Kandel, E. (2006). *In Search of Memory: The Emergence of a New Science of Mind*. New York: W. W. Norton & Company.

Kaplan, H. I., & Saddock, B. J. (1998). *Synopsis of Psychiatry* (8th ed.). Baltimore, MD: Williams & Wilkins.

Moras, K. (2006). The value of neuroscience strategies to accelerate progress in psychological treatment research. *Canadian Journal of Psychiatry, 51*(13), 810–822.

Mosey, A. C. (1986). *Psychosocial Components of Occupational Therapy*. New York: Raven Press.

Norman, C. W. (1976). Behavior modification: A perspective. *American Journal of Occupational Therapy, 30*(8), 491–494.

Pavlov, I. P. (1941). *Conditioned Reflexes and Psychiatry*. New York: International Press.

Rapoport, M., van Reekum, R., & Mayberg, H. (2000). The role of the cerebellum in cognition and behavior: A selective review. *Journal of Neuropsychiatry and Clinical Neurosciences, 12*(2), 193–198.

Rizzolatti, G., Fadiga, L., Gallese, V., & Fogassi, L. (1996). Premotor cortex and the recognition of motor actions. *Cognitive Brain Research, 3*, 131–141.

Rogers, C. R. (1951). *Client Centered Therapy*. Boston, MA: Houghton Mifflin.

Rogers, C. R. (1957). The necessary and sufficient conditions of therapeutic personality change. *Journal of Consulting Psychology, 21*, 95–103.

Rogers, C. R. (1995). *On Becoming a Person: A Therapist's View of Psychotherapy*. Boston, MA: Houghton Mifflin.

Rogers, C. R., & Freiberg, H. J. (1994). *Freedom to Learn* (3rd ed.). New York: Merrill.

Rugel, R. P., Mattingly, J., Eichinger, M., & May, J., Jr. (1971). The use of operant conditioning with a physically disabled child. *American Journal of Occupational Therapy, 25*(5), 247–249.

Sieg, K. W. (1974). Applying the behavior model to the occupational therapy model. *American Journal of Occupational Therapy, 28*(7), 421–428.

Skinner, B. F. (1953). The science of learning and the art of teaching. *Harvard Educational Review, 24*, 86–97.

Skinner, B. F. (1954). *About Behavioralism*. New York: Knopf.

Skinner, B. F. (1971). *Science and Human Behavior*. New York: Macmillan.

Skinner, B. F. (1974). *Beyond Freedom and Dignity*. New York: Knopf.

Smith, A. R., & Tempone, V. J. (1968). Psychiatric occupational therapy within a learning context. *American Journal of Occupational Therapy, 22*, 415–420.

Thorndike, E. L. (1932). *Fundamentals of Learning*. New York: Teachers College, Columbia University.

Tolman, E. C. (1932). *Purposive Behavior in Animals and Men*. New York: The Century Co.

Tolman, E. C. (1958). *Behavior and Psychological Man: Essays in Motivation and Learning*. Berkeley, CA: University of California Press.

Trombly, C. A. (1966). Principles of operant conditioning related to orthotic training of quadriplegic patients. *American Journal of Occupational Therapy, 20*, 217–220.

Viamontes, G. I., & Beitman, B. D. (2006). Neural substrates of psychotherapeutic change. Part I: The default brain. *Psychiatric Annals, 36*(4), 225–236.

Wanderer, Z. W. (1974). Therapy as learning: Behavior therapy. *American Journal of Occupational Therapy, 28*(4), 207–208.

Watson, J. B. (1917). Psychology as the behaviorist views it. *Psychological Bulletin, 20*(2), 158–177.

CHAPTER 15

A Biomechanical Frame of Reference for Positioning Children for Functioning

CHERYL ANN COLANGELO • MARY SHEA

The biomechanical frame of reference for positioning children for functioning is applied when a person cannot maintain posture through appropriate automatic muscle activity because of neuromuscular or musculoskeletal dysfunction. Consequently, artificial supports are provided, temporarily or permanently, to substitute for lack of postural control and to provide the most efficient positions of the body for participation in meaningful activity.

Every time a person moves in relation to another person or object, the person must first move in relation to a greater force (i.e., gravity). This movement is done in a subtle way. Each time a person eats a sandwich, embraces a child, or reaches for a book, he or she must always relate first to the earth's gravitational pull. For controlled movement, the human body must provide a stable center from which the head and limbs can move. Every peripheral movement creates a shift in the center of gravity that requires a compensatory postural reaction to prevent falling in the direction of the movement.

Gravity affects the human body on physical, mechanical, and physiological levels. Physically, gravity pulls the body toward the earth. It makes a person tend to fall down. It also makes the movement of limbs away from the earth's surface more difficult to execute. Mechanically, each time a person extends a limb away from the center of the body (e.g., when reaching), a lever arm is created that tends to topple the body by pulling the trunk in the direction of the limb. Fortunately, there are mechanical and physiological mechanisms that help the body to adapt to the forces of gravity. Receptors, triggered by changes in speed, direction, and joint position, stimulate an equilibrium reaction that activates stabilizing musculature and allows the body to remain upright or balanced. Through interaction of these receptors with a healthy nervous system and responsive muscles, the human body reacts to the forces of gravity in a predictable and functional way. Thus the term "biomechanical," this is the interaction of physical forces with the responses of a living being.

The general goals of the biomechanical frame of reference for positioning children for functioning are twofold. The first goal is to enhance the development of postural reactions by reducing the demands of gravity and by aligning the body. The second goal more directly addresses performance skills by providing external support for proximal stability to improve distal function and skilled activity. This reduces the need for, or the demands on, postural reactions and compensatory techniques. By providing proximal external support, we can assist the child in accomplishing a task that is important to him or her.

The biomechanical frame of reference for positioning children for functioning is frequently used as a primary approach with children who have severe physical disabilities. In addition, this frame of reference is used in combination with other frames of reference to maximize a child's potential for movement and function. For example, often it is used in conjunction with dynamic therapeutic handling (e.g., Neuro-Developmental Treatment, Brunnstrom, or proprioceptive neuromuscular facilitation). When applied in this way, it allows for a carryover of goals throughout the day in the absence of constant physical handling.

THEORETICAL BASE

The biomechanical frame of reference for positioning children for functioning draws from theories in physics and physiology, as well as those addressing motor development. It addresses the implications of physical and physiological principles on motor development. Two assumptions are accepted by the biomechanical frame of reference for positioning children for functioning in terms of normal development: (1) motor patterns develop from sensory stimulation and (2) automatic motor responses, which maintain posture, develop in a predictable way. This frame of reference also contains the assumption that impairment of musculoskeletal or neuromuscular functions can interfere with effective postural reactions and that motor control emerges not only from neuromuscular functions, but also from their interaction with factors such as motivation, personal attitudes and coping styles, and the social, physical, and cultural environment.

Motor Patterns Develop from Sensory Stimulation

Motor behaviors most often are reflexive in infancy. Reflexes are stereotypical reactions which occur in response to specific stimuli that generally are tactile, proprioceptive, or vestibular in nature. These motor patterns, once executed, provide additional sensory input, which contributes to the modification of reflexes and development of motor control. One example of a stereotypical reflexive reaction is the asymmetrical tonic neck reflex. The asymmetrical tonic neck reflex is elicited by turning the head, producing extension and abduction of the arm on the face side with flexion, and by adduction of the arm on the skull side. When a baby extends an arm as part of this reflex and comes in contact with an object, then the baby receives simultaneous sensations from proprioceptors in the shoulder related to reaching, tactile receptors in the hand, and visual awareness of the hand and object. The baby ultimately associates these sensations with the experience of touching an object, and, by reproducing the "feeling" of shoulder and arm movements, may reach successfully and touch the object again. The implication is that motor patterns are elicited by and develop from sensation.

Automatic Motor Responses That Maintain Posture Develop Predictably

The most sophisticated postural responses, righting and equilibrium reactions, are well developed by the second year of life. Righting reactions are movements that maintain alignment of the head in space and of the trunk in relation to the head. For example, if a seated child leans forward to rest his or her arms on a desk, neck extension is the righting reaction used to maintain his or her head in an upright position despite the forward tilt of his or her trunk. Equilibrium reactions are movements that help to maintain balance when the child's center of gravity is disturbed by an external force. Examples of external forces that provoke equilibrium reactions are when a child is pushed and when a child is carrying or manipulating a heavy object. Equilibrium reactions are manifested by movements of the trunk and extremities in the direction opposite to the displacing force to reestablish the center of gravity. If a seated child is pushed backward, his or her trunk curves forward, accompanied by forward thrusting movements of the limbs. This may involve shoulder flexion with elbow extension or hip flexion with knee extension. If the child is pushed toward the left, the equilibrium reaction is demonstrated when the child's trunk curves against the force to the right. This reaction may also involve abduction and extension of the right arm and leg.

Equilibrium reactions often can be accompanied by protective reactions. Protective reactions are limb movements that occur in the same direction as the displacing force. The primary purpose of these reactions is to protect the body from harm by breaking a potential fall. When the seated child is pushed to the left, the equilibrium response causes the right limbs to extend to regain the center of gravity. Concurrently, the left limbs may extend and abduct protectively. Equilibrium reactions also may be seen alone. This occurs more frequently with slow or gentle displacement. Equilibrium reactions may be replaced entirely by protective reactions when the displacement is more vigorous. In the example mentioned earlier, if the seated child had been pushed hard to the left, then the left limbs would have extended and abducted to protect the head in the event of a fall.

Righting and equilibrium reactions form the foundation for movements from one position to another. They assist in the maintenance of body position when the center of gravity is changed by moving or by engaging the limbs with objects. Before these reactions can develop, the child must integrate specific lower level reflexive responses, which are primarily for survival such as flexor withdrawal or rooting (e.g., turning the head in the direction of a stimulus to the mouth or cheek). Higher level reflexive responses, such as the asymmetrical tonic neck reflex and positive supporting reactions, which provide movement and proprioceptive input, must also be integrated into functional movement. Development is overlapping, so that as one level approaches completion, the next has already begun to develop. These levels continue to develop sequentially, within the body in a cephalocaudal fashion and in space from a horizontal to vertical position.

Another developmental sequence that is relevant to the biomechanical frame of reference for positioning children for functioning has been described as motor patterns, which were investigated by Margaret Rood (Stockmeyer, 1967). Along with cephalocaudal and horizontal–vertical sequences, postural reactions can be viewed within this third category.

Motor patterns include sequences of motor development that go from unorganized movement to skilled movement (skilled movement includes the maintaining of posture and the ability to reestablish a center of gravity). Skilled motor patterns depend on the ability to bear weight without collapsing and the ability to shift weight from one part of the body to another.

The process of motor development begins with mobility during infancy. Initially there is a good deal of phasic movement, the lowest level of muscular control, which consists of large undirected movements (e.g., spontaneous kicking, waving, and banging). Muscles that primarily perform phasic movements tend to be superficial and distal members of the flexor group and often cross over more than one joint. They are used more for "light" work (i.e., movement of distal parts) than for "heavy" work (i.e., prolonged contractions needed for posture). Later in development, phasic movements are under more voluntary control and therefore are incorporated into skilled movements.

After the child has acquired mobility of these larger movements, he or she begins to develop stability. Stability refers to the child's ability to maintain a weight-bearing position by the cocontraction of agonist and antagonist muscles around a joint. Muscles that primarily perform tonic contractions tend to lie more deeply and proximally and generally are extensors that cross over only one joint. They are responsible for sustained tonic contractions around a joint. These muscles are under greater reflex control than phasic muscles.

Once a child has developed stability, he or she is able to bear weight (i.e., to maintain a posture). From there, he or she begins to play with movement in that position. For example, take the prone on elbows position. At first the child supports himself or herself on his or her arms, but if the child begins to move, he or she may collapse. Soon the child can rock from side to side on his or her elbows without falling over. This grading of movement indicates that the child can create movement (mobility) in a joint without losing the joint's capacity to support (stability); this is referred to as "mobility superimposed on stability." Functionally, this appears as weight shifting (i.e., the ability to transfer some or all of the weight-bearing load to another joint or to maintain support in one joint as the body's center of gravity changes slightly). When the baby rocks laterally in a prone position, the weight is partially shifted back and forth between the two shoulders. A complete shift of weight to one shoulder frees the other side for reaching. Even then, the weight-bearing shoulder must engage in weight-shifting activity because movements of the freed arm cause the body's weight to shift slightly over the weight-bearing shoulder.

The ability to superimpose mobility on stability can be demonstrated in two ways when a baby in the prone position is observed while propped on a bed: (1) if an adult sits alongside the baby, the adult's weight depresses the mattress; the baby must shift weight away from the mattress depression to avoid rolling over (Figure 15.1) and (2) when this same baby reaches for a toy in the prone on elbows position, he or she must readjust his or her center of gravity toward one shoulder for weight bearing. These movements free the baby's other arm to reach for the toy.

This reaching out action demonstrates the baby's transition to another level of motor development (i.e., the acquisition of skilled movement). Skill is the highest level of motor function. In the example mentioned earlier, the distal portion of the baby's arm is free, and this serves as the basis for volitional, coordinated movement. The ability of the shoulder to hold the arm out in space and yet direct placement of the hand reflects the development of stability on mobility. Phasic movements have been refined into skill through their interaction with tonic movement, weight bearing, and weight shifting.

Components of Postural Control and Skill Development in Developmental Positions

The biomechanical frame of reference for positioning children for functioning focuses on function within a relatively static position rather than on transitional movements. It is essential, therefore, to examine the developmental sequence of motor behaviors characteristic of various positions. Children with neuromuscular dysfunction often have immature motor patterns; an understanding of this sequence contributes to a therapist's ability to facilitate change.

Supine Position

Although flexor tone predominates in the newborn, it is modified by the influence of the tonic labyrinthine reflex, which causes an increase of extensor tone in the supine position. Gravity also strongly influences the movements of the newborn; the head is held to the side and the scapulae are retracted and accompanied by shoulder elevation and external rotation. Despite increased extensor tone in the supine position, the hips are flexed. Yet, gravity pulls them into abduction and external rotation. Because of the influence of the asymmetrical tonic neck reflex, the newborn experiences more extensor tone on the face side and more flexor tone on the skull side of the body. The flexor pattern on the skull side causes shoulder retraction and lateral trunk flexion, which moves the infant's center of gravity over to the extended face side. This provides the initial sensation of weight shifting and weight bearing on the extended side. Each time the infant turns his or her head, he or she shifts weight slightly to the other side.

Flexor activity contributes to emerging midline control as the baby manages to center his or her head. Eventually, the baby is able to flex his or her neck against gravity enough to achieve a chin tuck, at which point the chin comes in contact with the chest. Later, this controlled flexion, when combined with neck extension, provides head control in an upright posture.

In the supine position, the infant develops the ability to bring his or her hands to the chest and then reach upward by using a succession of movements. This is first accomplished using internal rotation, then shoulder flexion, and, finally, protraction against gravity (Figure 15.1). The ability to reach out in the supine position in a directed and controlled fashion, which is a skilled movement, begins at the same time that the infant masters weight bearing in the prone on elbows position (i.e., mastery of mobility superimposed on stability in the shoulders). As the infant reaches upward and outward, a stable base of support is needed to keep from flipping over. Initially, abdominal support is low, and the legs are held off the floor because of the flexed, abducted, and externally rotated hips. The development of the abdominal musculature in conjunction with a decrease in hip flexor tone allows the infant to plant the soles of his or her feet

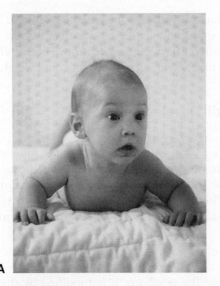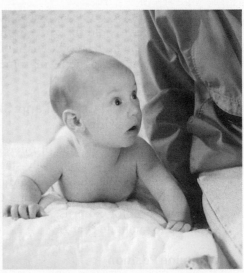

A   **B**

FIGURE 15.1 The infant is in prone position (A), and shifts his weight toward his left side to keep from rolling into the depression when his mother sits on the bed (B).

firmly on the supporting surface, contributing to trunk stability during reaching. It is important to be aware that directed reaching in the supine position can be mastered with limited demands on head and trunk control because the child is supported fully, whereas reaching in the upright position requires additional control of the head and trunk to maintain a vertical position.

During infancy, eye movements are not separated from head movements. Visual fixation and tracking are influenced by the development of head control. Oral motor control is influenced by the force of gravity on the jaw and tongue and the development of postural tone. Initially, in the supine position, the infant's tongue goes toward the back of his or her mouth and the lips and jaw are slightly open. As the ability to flex against gravity develops in the neck, a similar development occurs orally: the jaw closes, the lips come together more easily, and the tongue can come forward. A more mature sucking pattern is now possible.

Prone Position

Following several crowded months of flexion in the womb with resulting physiological flexor hypertonus, the effects of the tonic labyrinthine reflex in the prone position increase flexor tone even further in the newborn. This results in a little ball of a person in the prone position. Hip flexion places the buttocks high in the air, so that body weight is distributed over the chest and face area. The newborn's head is turned to the side for breathing. The infant must hyperextend his or her neck to raise the head or turn it from side to side because the spine is descending from the pelvis toward the neck. Maintaining the head in a righted position using hyperextension requires a great deal of energy. Head righting in the prone position does not develop until the hips begin to extend, the pelvis approaches the supporting surface, and the spine becomes more horizontal with weight distributed along the trunk and pelvis. This postural change decreases the amount of neck extension needed to right the head. At first, head righting is accompanied by unopposed extension of the upper trunk. This prepares the neck and back extensors for additional heavy work in any upright position.

When infants prop on their arms, flexor muscles work in conjunction with extensor muscles. The chest muscles bring the arms forward and down, so that elbows that were previously behind the shoulders now come directly beneath the shoulders in a tonic, weight-bearing position. Once the upper trunk can be supported on the forearms and back extension is modulated by interaction with flexors, graded movements of the neck can be accomplished by the interplay of flexion and extension (Figure 15.2). This provides for ease of volitional head movement. From this maturational base of neck mobility and stability, directed head movements and skilled eye and oral movements can develop in upright positions.

Once the infant has developed stability in the shoulders, he or she begins to weight shift. Weight shifting requires the infant to move his or her chest over the weight-bearing

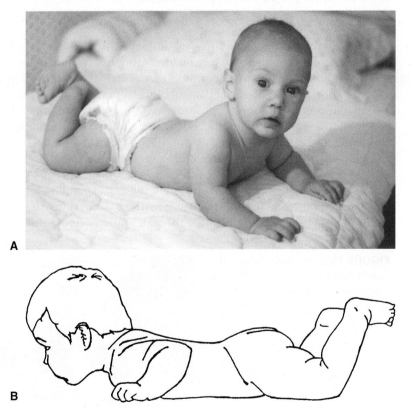

A

B

FIGURE 15.2 Before protraction develops in the prone position (**A**), elbows are behind shoulders, trunk is horizontal, and neck hyperextension is necessary to right the head (**B**).

arm to change his or her center of gravity. This allows the infant to maintain balance on an unstable surface or to reach out with the opposite arm. This action curves the spine, thereby elongating the weight-bearing side of the body and shortening the non–weight-bearing side. The pattern of extension on the weight-bearing side and flexion on the mobile side can be seen during weight-shifting activities in all positions as the child matures.

Although the focus of this section has been on movements of the head and upper extremities because of their relevance to functional activity in a static posture, the biomechanical frame of reference for positioning children for functioning also recognizes the critical role of the pelvis in the maintenance of stability. This is different from the frequent concentration on the development of pelvic movements in relation to end-goal ambulation.

Lower trunk and pelvic stability in the supine position allows for controlled head and arm movements, preventing the child's body from rolling whenever the head is turned or an arm reaches out. In the prone position, balanced interaction of neck flexion with extension for head control, and placement of shoulders and elbows for weight bearing, depends on the position of the pelvis and legs.

Side Lying Position

The tonic labyrinthine reflex has no influence in the side lying position; therefore, asymmetrical movements can be executed more easily. Side lying provides dramatically different sensory input to either side of the baby's body to help develop a sense of laterality or the awareness and control of the separate sides of the body (Figure 15.3).

In the prone and supine positions, the infant coordinates dorsal extensors with ventral flexors for trunk stability. Side lying requires more sophisticated control because the flexors and extensors on one side of the body must work together and in opposition to the coordination of flexors and extensors on the other side. Lateral head righting in side lying is a good example: the neck flexes to the upside through the activation of upside flexors and extensors against relaxation of the corresponding muscles on the downside.

The lateral neck flexion against gravity that develops in side lying as the child rights his or her head contributes to neck stability and head control in the upright

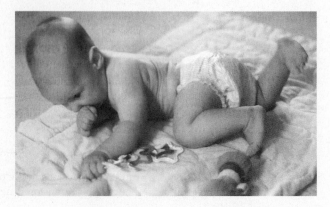

FIGURE 15.3 In side lying, the weight-bearing leg is extended and supporting and the non–weight-bearing leg is flexed and mobile.

posture. For example, in sitting or standing, every shift in weight to one side of the body necessitates lateral neck flexion to maintain the head in a righted position. The repeated movement of the head against gravity in the side lying position helps this movement become effortless in the upright position. The same principle applies to the lateral trunk flexion that appears later in side lying as the child begins to prop on one arm.

The interaction between dorsal trunk extensors and ventral flexors bilaterally is also essential in side lying. Too much extension pulls the child onto his or her back; too much flexion causes him or her to roll forward. This interaction is particularly important as the infant experiments with head and arm movements because each of these movements shifts the infant's center of gravity.

Once stable in side lying, the infant has an excellent opportunity to try out skilled arm and hand movements of the upside arm. This horizontal position demands less trunk control than sitting, reducing the stress of controlling posture and skilled movements simultaneously. No weight-bearing demands are made on the shoulder of the arm that is not reaching (as opposed to the prone position) nor does the infant have to work against gravity to use his or her hand in front of his or her face, as in the supine position. When the infant reaches out toward an object on the floor with his or her upside hand, it naturally falls toward the midline and into the visual field.

Sitting Position

Sitting is the infant's first independent upright position. Head and shoulders have become stable in the horizontal positions, and, although the demands of gravity on neck extension decrease when upright, the infant still must master the interaction of muscle groups in the neck to produce controlled head movements in the new position. Until that point, the infant often uses elevated shoulders to nestle the head to help steady it. This shoulder elevation frequently limits arm mobility.

Infants use ring sitting (i.e., hips abducted and externally rotated, knees flexed), which provides a wide base of support and a low center of gravity. The back is rounded and lower back extension has yet to develop. The shoulders and arms provide postural stability in one of two ways: (1) shoulders can be retracted to assist upper back extension to compensate for the rounded lower back or (2) arms can be extended and used as props in front of the infant to keep him or her from tumbling forward (Figure 15.4). In the latter sitting posture, known as "tripod sitting," neck hyperextension is required to right the head and often is accompanied by an open jaw. In either scenario, the hands are not free to engage in play. Muscle activation for postural adjustments is initially largely variable and direction specific. In normal development, in the latter part of the first year, muscle activation patterns for postural control become less variable and more refined (Hadders-Algra, Brogren, & Forssbreg, 1996, 1996a). As head and trunk control develop, the back straightens and shoulders, which had been elevated and retracted, come down and forward. As the pelvis becomes stable, the wide base is no longer necessary and long sitting is possible. In long sitting, the legs come together, putting the hip joints in a more neutral position than in ring sit. This makes weight shifting to the side easier because one hip can move into extension and external rotation, while the other flexes and rotates internally.

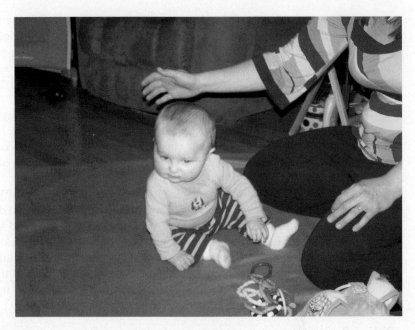

FIGURE 15.4 The infant must use his arms to prop in early unsupported sitting. His hands are not free for exploration, and the pelvis is forward for stability.

The ability to weight shift over the hips has implications for midline crossing with the arms, allowing for more functional activity with the arms. As the child rotates the trunk and reaches toward the contralateral side, he or she must weight shift over the contralateral side. The mature sitter can reach with a fully extended arm in all planes and still maintain posture and equilibrium.

Standing Position

In the biomechanical frame of reference, standing is viewed as an alternate postural base for skilled movements of the head and arms rather than as a dynamic prerequisite for walking. It is particularly important for those children who are least likely to stand or walk independently.

The standing position is unique because of the amount of extensor activity required to maintain the posture. As in sitting, when the child begins to stand, he or she uses scapular retraction to assist with upper back extension and to compensate for the lordosis created as the lower back is pulled forward by the weight of the abdominal cavity. As abdominal control develops, the pelvis tilts posterior into a neutral position, the spine becomes straighter, and the arms are liberated for skilled use.

When the standing posture is fully developed, a child can maintain a resting position of erect spine, neutral or slightly posterior pelvic tilt, and hips extended with neutral rotation. The knees are extended but not hyperextended. "Locking" of the knees may be used in the absence of muscular stability to provide mechanical stability. Ankles are at 90 degrees of flexion and in neutral alignment laterally. If irregularities occur in the distal parts of the lower extremities during standing, proximal stability is influenced.

It should be noted that mobility in and out of positions has not been discussed. Although an understanding of these concepts is critical to the knowledge base of the occupational therapist, these are not used in the biomechanical frame of reference. In this frame of reference, posture is looked at in a relatively static way, emphasizing those components that contribute to a stable, relatively immobile trunk as a basis for distal movements.

Interference with Postural Reactions That Result from Damage or Dysfunction

Dysfunction of the musculoskeletal system has serious implications for postural control. As discussed in the previous section, mobility of all major joints is essential to weight shifting and equilibrium reactions. Fixed bony deformities and muscle contractures clearly would interfere with this freedom of movement. Lack of proper bone formation similarly can affect the balanced interaction of the movements needed for a child to keep himself or herself righted in space. For example, incomplete development of the spinous processes on one side can result in a fixed lateral flexion of the spine. The fixed lateral flexion of the spine interferes with weight shifting onto the affected side in sitting. Without lateral movements to the opposite side, the child is unable to reestablish his or her center of gravity and is likely to fall to the affected side.

A compensatory movement or posture is the body's attempt to correct an error. In the previous example with fixed lateral flexion of the spine, compensatory positions are necessary in the neck and hips. Two possible compensations are (1) the child flexes the neck or nonaffected part of the spine in the opposite direction, creating an S curve while keeping himself or herself upright or (2) the child uses one arm as a prop to support the tipping trunk. In the first situation, neck mobility is limited with possible negative effects on visual and oral motor function and soft tissue shortening with increased tendency for scoliosis. In the second situation, bimanual activity is impossible. Compensations often decrease mobility in joints that are not affected directly by the initial deforming process, because the compensatory positions must be maintained to provide a stable posture. They may occur in the presence of bony deformities and in any situation in which normal movement patterns are compromised.

Motor problems that result from the neuromuscular dysfunction caused by central nervous system (CNS) deficits (e.g., cerebral palsy or static encephalopathy) are extremely diverse and complex. Motor problems are more diverse because such neuromuscular dysfunction is more global and is rarely isolated to one specific site in the body. Similarly, motor dysfunctions are more complex because the manifestations of these deficits can fluctuate in relation to many factors, including changes in the child's position in space, effort in activities, affect, and stimulation in the environment. Hadders-Algra, Brogren & Forssberg (1996) found that children with spastic diplegia had difficulty with the coactivation of muscles and recruitment order of the muscles for postural adjustments. While basic direction specificity for postural control is preserved in most children, Hadders-Algra et al. (1999) found two children with spastic tetraplegia were unable to sit independently because of a loss of direction specificity.

Neuromuscular dysfunction often affects muscle tone. Within this frame of reference, muscle tone refers to the muscle's responsiveness to stretch. A common error is to confuse high tone with strength and low tone with weakness. Normal tone gives muscles the ability to contract on command and to maintain or cease activation as necessary. Normal tone depends on the integrity of motor neurons and muscle fibers, and the ability of the CNS to receive and respond to proprioceptive cues with the simultaneous excitation of certain muscles and inhibition of others. Normal muscle tone allows the muscle to react immediately with enough tension for weight shifting and support yet still have enough "give" to allow for quick changes in movement (Scherzer & Tscharnuter, 1982, 1990).

Muscles characterized by low tone, or hypotonia, produce delayed responses. Children who have hypotonic musculature are "floppy." Their ability to sit upright and function is completely affected by gravity. Their shoulders and backs often are rounded and their hips generally are abducted and externally rotated. Their joints are very mobile. However, they may develop compensations for inadequate antigravity responses in the upright position (e.g., shoulder retraction and lumbar hyperextension). Despite low muscle tone, the compensatory muscle groups may be shortened or contracted because they often are used to maintain posture. Owing to this compensation, prolonged shortening or contraction of the muscle groups because of such compensation may result in decreased range of motion and deformity.

Muscles that exhibit high tone or hypertonus often are described as "spastic." They exhibit a hyperactive stretch reflex. Clinically, this means that the muscle shows increased resistance to passive stretch. Functionally, these muscles generally respond to activation with full, rapid contractions. Antagonist muscles may be relatively inactive or they may cocontract with less force. This results in ungraded movements that are maintained with the muscle in a shortened state and decreased joint mobility. Hypertonicity appears primarily in antigravity muscle groups; however, all muscles in the group may not be hypertonic, even though it may appear otherwise. When the muscles work together as a group, the hypertonic muscles influence those muscles that have normal tone to produce atypical postural patterns. Two atypical postural patterns are (1) a flexion pattern of flexion, abduction, and external rotation in the upper extremities and (2) an extension pattern of extension, internal rotation, and adduction in the lower extremities. Children who show hypertonicity resist gravity and do not succumb to its force. They also have limited range of motion because of the overactivity of certain muscle groups. In addition, it is important to note that muscles which may not be hypertonic can become shortened because they are part of a pattern of movement initiated and maintained by hypertonic muscles.

It is also possible to have fluctuating muscle tone. This condition is commonly referred to as "athetosis." In this case, antagonistic muscle groups contract and reflex almost in turn rather than interactively. This causes exaggerated movements with little control in the midranges.

In addition to muscle tone, it is important to consider the effects of the action of the muscles on the joints. One example of this is the multiarthrodial muscles (i.e., those muscles that cross over more than one joint). The control of such joints may be particularly affected when children have high tone or shortening, and this has implications for postural control. For example, the hamstrings, which run across both hips and knees, often are shortened in children who have tone irregularities. It is difficult for these children to elongate those muscles over both joints simultaneously, making it difficult for them to combine hip flexion with knee extension. It is hard for these children to sit for long periods of time, especially in a wheelchair with their feet out in front of them. This is because the knee extension is too great for the length in the hamstring musculature. This in turn compromises hip flexion and the pelvis is pulled into a posterior tilt. To stay upright, these children develop a compensatory forward curve the trunk. A solution to this is presented in the "Application to Practice" section of this chapter.

When children have intact CNSs, their movements and postures are affected by touch, proprioception, sight, sound, smell, health, and attitude. The influences of these factors are exaggerated in children who have tone problems. Postural stability in children who have CNS dysfunction may be influenced by movement, position in space, position of the head, tactile stimulation, stress or effort, temperature, surface support, intensity of environmental stimulation, and affect.

Movement includes active and passive movement and movement of individual joints or of the body through space. Efforts to initiate active movement and rapid passive movement of a joint in a hypertonic child may increase tone. Rapid changes in speed can increase tone, particularly when unexpected. Slow, gentle rocking often decreases tone.

Position in space refers to changes in position of the body (e.g., upright, supine, and tipped back). These positions are registered through vestibular, proprioceptive, and tactile receptors that stimulate reflexive responses. Mature, functional responses include righting and equilibrium reactions. In children who have CNS dysfunction, reflex activity (i.e., involuntary, stereotypical movements in response to specific stimuli) often is primitive or pathological. A primitive reflex is one that normally occurs before the development of righting and equilibrium reactions and, therefore, under average everyday movement, should not recur after the first year of life. Such reflexes sometimes continue to happen in children who have CNS dysfunction and who have not developed normal postural reactions. A reflex is pathological when it occurs with greater persistence and when the child cannot willfully move out of the stereotypical pattern. An example of a primitive reflex influenced by the body's position in space is the tonic labyrinthine reflex, which is triggered by increased flexor tone in the prone position and extensor tone in the supine position. A pathological manifestation of this reflex may be a total extension pattern in the supine position, with the child unable to tuck his or her chin, close his or her jaw, or bring his or her hands together or up to his or her mouth.

Position of the head in relation to the body may affect reflex activity. Examples include asymmetrical tonic neck reflex and the symmetrical tonic neck reflex, each of which creates different movement patterns, depending on whether the neck is rotated, flexed, or extended. The asymmetrical tonic neck reflex interferes with midline activity, whereas the symmetrical tonic neck reflex interferes with freedom of arm movements and pelvic stability for sitting. In addition, changes in head position can produce stereotypical, whole-body reactions in the presence of neuromuscular dysfunction. For example, head extension in a hypertonic child can create a strong, total extension pattern with shoulder retraction, arched back, and extended hips. Conversely, when that child's neck is flexed passively, then the entire body relaxes.

Tactile stimulation includes light touch and deep pressure. Light touch often elicits phasic movements, which are undesirable in maintaining posture. Reflexes such as rooting and the Gallant are elicited by light touch and affect head or body position. The rooting reflex response takes the head out of the midline and may also elicit an asymmetrical tonic neck reflex, causing the entire body to be asymmetrical. The Gallant reflex causes trunk incurvation toward a source of touch on the lateral trunk, creating a temporary asymmetry of the spine.

The amount of stress or effort that an activity requires influences a child's movement and posture. An isolated movement that is difficult to execute may be accompanied by a total body reaction. For example, a child who easily is able to right his or her head when tipped forward 5 degrees may have more difficulty when his or her head is tipped forward 20 degrees. When the head is tipped forward 20 degrees, the child may respond with total body extension because of the effort needed to meet the increased demands on neck extension. Furthermore, strenuous activity or emotional stress also may exacerbate associated reactions. An associated reaction, such as tongue protrusion when a typical child concentrates on a fine motor task, may be more pronounced in a child who has neuromuscular difficulties. For example, when a child with neurological impairment engages in a writing task with the dominant arm, exaggerated mirror movements may occur in the other arm. In the extreme case, the associated reaction may result in the nondominant upper extremity retracting and flexing, accompanied by fisting of the hand. This asymmetrical posture would interfere with bilateral use of hands, such as holding down the paper as the child writes.

The temperature of the environment also may influence movement and posture. Cool temperatures can increase muscle tone. Neutral warmth that approximates body temperature (provided by warm clothing or ambient temperature) tends to reduce muscle tone.

Surface support refers to the surface on which a child is placed. Hard surfaces tend to be alerting and, therefore, may increase muscle tone. Hypertonic children may relax on well-cushioned but firm surfaces, whereas children who have lower tone may sink into the embrace of heavily upholstered surfaces and respond with more active postural control to a harder surface.

Frequent changes and high intensity of environmental stimulation often increase tone, whereas monotony and low levels of intensity have lulling effects and generally are associated with a reduction of muscle tone.

Affect also may influence posture and movement. Affect refers to the child's state of mind and his or her emotional responses to events that occur in the environment. Strong affectual responses increase tone, regardless of their positive or negative associations. The strong positive emotions associated with motivation, and particularly well-being, obviously should not be discouraged for the sake of modifying hypertonus.

The last major assumption related to the effects of neuromuscular dysfunction on postural reactions and function applies to Rood's concept of phasic and tonic muscles and their appropriate purposes (Stockmeyer, 1967). Tonic muscle groups are best suited to postural maintenance and are located more proximally. Physiologically, these muscle groups are better suited for sustained contractions. When these muscles are unable to perform their tasks adequately, the phasic muscles act as substitutes. Because the primary functions of phasic muscle groups are mobility and skill, they are ineffective in postural maintenance. For example, children who have CNS dysfunction may use their shoulders and arms to "hold themselves up" because of inefficient tonic muscle groups that cause poor postural tone. The result is fatigue and a lack of development in volitional skills for the extremities. Fatigue occurs because the phasic muscles are not well equipped for sustained contraction. Volitional skills do not develop because the extremities are used to maintain posture and are not free to engage in skilled activity

The fundamental goal of the biomechanical frame of reference for positioning children for functioning is to provide an artificial postural base from which the child can attend freely to his or her environment. An additional goal is to liberate the distal extremities so that the child can use them to interact with the environment. For one child, this may mean providing enough head control to make and maintain eye contact with a care provider or enough tone reduction to breathe deeply and easily. For another, it may mean providing sufficient support to enable the physical capacity to manipulate toys. This approach assumes that all children need consistent, effective postural responses for optimal manipulation of and interaction with their environments. When children are unable to do this effectively, therapists who use the biomechanical frame of reference for positioning children for functioning can help the child develop those postural responses or can provide external substitutions for them.

Factors that Interact with Postural Responses to Facilitate Participation in Occupation

Although the goal of the biomechanical frame of reference for positioning children for functioning is to enhance function through the use of artificial supports, success is dependent on attention to other factors that influence the development of motor control. These include, but are not restricted to, other body functions, environmental factors, and activities. The biomechanical approach cannot be applied in a vacuum; simply providing a good fit between supportive device and child will not adequately address functional goals. Here are some examples of situations where other factors must be addressed simultaneously:

- Introduction of positioning equipment is disruptive to the child's familiar routines, regardless of whether these routines facilitated, or were barriers to, participation.
- An adapted potty corrects posture, provides the child with a sense of safety, and reduces hypertonicity. However, the child has little success with bowel control because digestive functions are impaired since a diet with adequate fiber is difficult for him or her to manage orally.
- A student has better control during graphomotor tasks when positioned in a standing device, but feels apart from his or her friends who work and talk together at their desks.
- A baby has better oral control when supported in an adapted chair, but the mother wants to hold the baby in her arms when she feeds him or her.

Review of Assumptions

As discussed earlier, the biomechanical frame of reference for positioning children for functioning maintains the following six major assumptions:

1. The biomechanical frame of reference for positioning children for functioning contributes to independence by providing external supports to substitute for inadequate or abnormal postural reactions and therefore are as follows:

   It facilitates the development of some postural control by reducing the effects of gravity, or

   It provides a permanent support when potential to improve seems negligible.

2. Children learn to move effectively through sensory feedback, especially through the proprioceptive, vestibular, tactile, and visual systems. They repeat successful movements based on the sensory cues that the movements provide.

3. Normal motor development is predictable and sequential. The development of motor abilities depends on a stable base of support and on the righting and equilibrium reactions that allow a person to respond unconsciously to the forces of gravity.

   Posture depends on the body's response to gravity.

   Postural reactions develop sequentially. Each new skill is based on a previously developed skill.

4. Dysfunction or abnormalities of muscle, bone, or CNS may impair the development of normal postural reactions.

   Tone affects posture; tone is influenced by many internal and external factors, all of which can be modified.

   If normal postural reactions have not developed, the body compensates by using substitute movements, more effort, and more conscious attention. All of these things may interfere with function.

5. The manifestation of postural reactions is influenced not only by neurodevelopment but also by factors related to the child, environment, and task. These include, but are not limited to, other body functions; coping style; motivation; social, cultural, and physical environment; and the characteristics of the task in which the child is involved.

6. Occupational therapists must determine the level of postural dysfunction and the external factors that may affect performance. Treatment needs to provide substitutes for absent skills, yet still make demands on the child's existing capacity to function.

FUNCTION–DYSFUNCTION CONTINUA

There can be many causes of delays or dysfunction in a child's ability to interact with his or her environment. Only those things related to compromised postural reactions that interfere with skill development are appropriate targets for the biomechanical frame of reference. For example, the inability to use both hands at midline may be related to delayed sitting skills, which may result in retracted shoulders or the need

TABLE 15.1 Indicators of Function and Dysfunction for Range of Motion	
Full Passive Range of Motion	*Contractures and Deformities*
FUNCTION: Full range of motion	*DYSFUNCTION*: Limitations in range of motion or contractures
INDICATORS OF FUNCTION	**INDICATORS OF DYSFUNCTION**
Full, active range of motion	Functional limits of range of motion
	Fixed contractures

to always prop on one arm for support. Conversely, that same inability may be the result of perceptual processes such as poor bilateral integration or tactile defensiveness and may exist regardless of postural competence. On the one hand, lack of fine motor control in ocular, oral, or hand skills may be related to head and shoulder instability. Conversely, the problem may be specific to isolated distal muscles or it may come from a lack of organizational skills unrelated to posture. If postural reactions are delayed, weak, exaggerated, or performed by improper muscle groups, the biomechanical frame of reference for positioning children for functioning should be considered.

Indicators of Function and Dysfunction: Range of Motion

Range of motion is the ability to passively move a child's head and extremities through their full span of movement. Problems in this area are evident when a child has limitations in range of motion or contractures (Table 15.1).

Indicators of Function and Dysfunction: Head Control

In this continuum, function is represented by the child who can maintain his or her head in a righted position, when moving, and who can direct head movements as desired. This provides stability for ocular tasks such as eye control and visual fixation and for oral motor control and mobility for turning the head toward a source of stimulation. Dysfunction is represented by limited mobility or stability. This may occur primarily through inadequate muscular control or secondary to compensatory movements, such as stabilizing the head through use of shoulder elevation, which limits active range in the neck and shoulders (Table 15.2).

Indicators of Function and Dysfunction: Trunk Control

Function is represented by the child who demonstrates equilibrium reactions in the trunk as he or she reaches and interacts with the environment in an upright position. This child will also have full thoracic range for inspirations and expirations. With the biomechanical focus, respiration is only considered related to tone and position of the trunk. With less trunk control, dysfunction appears as (1) an inability to remain

TABLE 15.2 Indicators of Function and Dysfunction for Head Control	
Good Head Control	*Poor Head Control*
FUNCTION: Normal head control and mobility **INDICATORS OF FUNCTION** Head is righted and mobile in all planes	*DYSFUNCTION*: Poor head control and mobility **INDICATORS OF DYSFUNCTION** Child can maintain head in an upright position but loses head control when initiating a movement Child is unable to right head or control any head movements

upright once distal limb movements are initiated or (2) an inability to maintain any upright position at all. Abnormal muscle tone in the trunk can compromise respiratory capacity. Trunk deformities may occur from the force of gravity curving the trunk, asymmetrical muscle tone or muscle innervation, and consequently, from constant use of compensatory movements. Lateral or forward curvature of the spine (e.g., scoliosis and anterior kyphosis) reduces the thoracic space and may impair respiration with detriment to health, energy, and phonation (Table 15.3).

Indicators of Function and Dysfunction: Control of Arm Movements

The child who can reach in all planes, regardless of position, and who can maintain his or her hands where he or she would like them is at the functional end of the continuum. Dysfunction is represented by an inability to direct the hands because shoulders are involved in supporting the trunk (as a result of tone in the trunk being abnormal) or because arm movements against gravity are difficult to execute. Providing trunk support or changing the child's position in space can enhance function (Table 15.4).

TABLE 15.3 Indicators of Function and Dysfunction for Trunk Control	
Good Trunk Control	*Poor Trunk Control*
FUNCTION: Good trunk control **INDICATORS OF FUNCTION** Child's trunk is righted and stable in an upright position and is symmetrical when the child is seated or standing on a horizontal surface Child can take advantage of normal respiratory capacity	*DYSFUNCTION*: Poor trunk control **INDICATORS OF DYSFUNCTION** Child's trunk is righted but unstable when limb movements are initiated Child's trunk is not righted; child is unable to remain upright or remains upright with asymmetry Child's respiratory capacity is compromised by decreased size of thoracic cavity because of trunk and shoulder position Child's respiratory capacity is decreased because of abnormal muscle tone of the respiratory muscles, such as the intercostals

TABLE 15.4 Indicators of Function and Dysfunction for Control of Arm Movements	
Good Control of Arm Movements	***Poor Control of Arm Movements***
FUNCTION: Ability to reach in all planes **INDICATORS OF FUNCTION** Child can place, maintain, and control his or her hands where he or she pleases when in an upright position	*DYSFUNCTION*: Inability to reach in all planes **INDICATORS OF DYSFUNCTION** Child's arms are not liberated in an upright position; either they are needed for propping or shoulders are retracted to aid in upper trunk stability, bringing the hands back with them Child cannot move his or her arms in gravity resisted planes of movement and therefore, cannot place or maintain his or her hands where he or she wants them

Indicators of Function and Dysfunction: Mobility

The ability to move through space to attain a goal, explore an environment, or experience movement in many planes is at the functional end of the continuum. Mobility that is stressful or slow is dysfunctional because the child often may feel that the effort is not worth the goal or the child may be too fatigued to interact with the person or object once he or she attains his or her goal. Lack of mobility is also dysfunctional in that the child is deprived of essential sensory experiences, particularly vestibular and proprioceptive, which are provided by movement through space (Table 15.5).

Function and Dysfunction Continua Related to Participation in Life Activities

The goal of the biomechanical frame of reference for positioning children for functioning is to provide a secure postural base through positioning or with the assistance of external support. The previous section addresses specific components of motor development that provide a foundation for controlled movement. The following are examples of function–dysfunction continua that are specific to participation in life activities such as eating and accessing switches for technological aides.

TABLE 15.5 Indicators of Function and Dysfunction for Mobility	
Mobility	***Immobility***
FUNCTION: Mobility through space **INDICATORS OF FUNCTION** Child is mobile through space in all planes (walking; climbing in, out of, and over obstacles) Child can locomote in a horizontal position (crawling or creeping) on a flat surface	*DYSFUNCTION*: Slow, effortful mobility, or immobility **INDICATORS OF DYSFUNCTION** Child can only locomote by rolling Child cannot move his or her body through space

TABLE 15.6 Indicators of Function and Dysfunction for Eating	
Safe Eating	*Unsafe Eating*
FUNCTION: Safe, efficient eating **INDICATORS OF FUNCTION** Child can chew and swallow food successfully without aspirating	*DYSFUNCTION*: Difficulty with chewing and swallowing **INDICATORS OF DYSFUNCTION** Child is unable to grade jaw movements or control lips and tongue when eating Child frequently aspirates food

Indicators of Function and Dysfunction: Eating

The functional end of this continuum includes adequate oral motor control to ingest food safely in an average amount of time without choking. Although feeding difficulties may exist despite the development of postural control, the absence of good head and trunk control exacerbates oral motor dysfunction. Dysfunctional eating patterns (e.g., lack of jaw stability; poor tongue, cheek, and lip control; and disorganized swallowing) are affected by an unstable neck, compensatory movements in the shoulder girdle, impaired respiration, and abnormal tone associated with certain postures (Table 15.6).

Indicators of Function and Dysfunction: Toileting

Function in toileting includes the ability to sit independently on a toilet or commode and the ability to void. Dysfunction, with its concomitant lack of comfort and dignity, is represented by a lack of awareness or control of the voiding process or the inability to relax enough to void when sitting unsupported on a toilet. Awareness and control may be affected by abnormal tone, and postural control has a direct effect on the ability to relax when sitting independently (Table 15.7).

Indicators of Function and Dysfunction: Accessing Switch for Technological Aides

The child who can make and maintain contact with a switch, button, or joystick and release it at will is at the functional end of this continuum. The selection of switches

TABLE 15.7 Indicators of Function and Dysfunction for Toileting	
Continence	*Incontinence*
FUNCTION: Independence on toilet **INDICATORS OF FUNCTION** Child can empty bowel and bladder when seated on toilet	*DYSFUNCTION*: Inability to void in toilet **INDICATORS OF DYSFUNCTION** Child can only void intentionally when lying down Child cannot maintain sitting balance on a toilet Child can maintain sitting balance on a toilet but cannot direct the flow of urine into the bowl Child has no conscious bowel and bladder control

TABLE 15.8 Indicators of Function and Dysfunction for Accessing Switch for Technological Aides	
Switch Access	**Lack of Switch Access**
FUNCTION: Ability to independently use technological aides **INDICATORS OF FUNCTION** Child can approach, contact, and release switch with adequate speed and control using hand	*DYSFUNCTION*: Inability to independently use technological aides **INDICATORS OF DYSFUNCTION** Child cannot approach, switch, or maintain contact and control release Child cannot sustain approach or release sequence for duration of activity
Child can approach, contact, and release switch using body part other than hand	Child can approach, contact, and release switch with a body part, but the action impedes another function

to control augmentative communication devices and power wheelchairs, environmental controls, and other technological devices is extensive. The highest level of function consists of controlling the switch rapidly and efficiently without fatigue. Ideally, this would be accomplished through controlled arm and hand movements. However, movement in virtually any part of the body can be harnessed to drive a device. Switches may be controlled, for example, by inspiration/expiration or movements of head, neck, eyelids, shoulders, or feet. Function is decreased if, by harnessing one of these movements, another skill related to that movement is impaired (Table 15.8). For example, does a breath-driven device interfere with speech or create excessive drooling? Or does the child use a shoulder movement with significant postural asymmetry or with compensatory movements that eventually impair posture or mobility?

Each of these functions depends on the interaction of numerous factors. Cognition, perception, and behavior, as well as fine motor and organization abilities, contribute to these skills. Evaluation of the postural components necessary for function will determine whether and, specifically, which biomechanical assists are appropriate.

GUIDE TO EVALUATION

The purpose of the evaluation is to assess the postural components of a given dysfunction to plan intervention. This can be done by using the function–dysfunction continua.

Within the biomechanical frame of reference, the child's potential for change in the area of postural reactions is a major concern. This requires the use of professional judgment and may require ongoing assessment over a period of months. The child's potential for change is an important factor because it helps determine what type of postural aides should be used and how they will be most effective.

At times, the assessment of a child's needs within this frame of reference may be done by a therapist who has particular expertise in this area or through a clinic, as opposed to the therapist who is providing ongoing treatment. This is most likely to be considered when durable medical equipment, such as a wheelchair, is being considered. The therapist who treats the child should be actively involved in equipment decisions because of his or her long-term interaction with the child and understanding of the child's potential for change, both during the course of a day and over an extended period of time. This is particularly important for the child who needs the positioning device for the classroom. In these cases, the child's parents do not have the opportunity to observe their child's performance, needs, and responses in the context of the school, so the school-based therapist may be a critical resource during an off-site evaluation.

The assessment of the child begins by considering age, therapeutic history, physical status, prognosis, and environment because they all contribute to the child's potential for change. Age is an important consideration because of the plasticity of CNS. Therapeutic history is important because it indicates the types and focus of the child's previous contact with therapy and the child's responsiveness to intervention. Physical status indicates the child's general health, medication regime, and surgical history. Prognosis indicates the progression expected in relation to the child's diagnosis. The environment influences the child's potential for growth and motivation.

When a child is evaluated for positioning options, the therapist needs to observe carefully any sequence of specific elements of postural control. The outline in this section is intended to assist with this process.

• Can child move all body parts through full range against gravity?
• Can child right his or her head and is it mobile in all planes?
• Can child right his or her trunk and maintain stability?
• Can child place, maintain, and control position of his or her hands?
• Is the child mobile through space in all planes?
• Can child chew and swallow food successfully without aspirating?
• Can child void when seated on a toilet or potty?

It is important during this scrutiny to remember, however, that all elements of movement are interrelated, and that the therapist must step back and view the child's body as a whole. To take this further, it is imperative to apply the evaluation and intervention process to the child's life—the end goal is not that the child looks good from a postural perspective in the therapist's eye but that the child can do something that is important to him or her.

The assessment of the child should be done with the child involved in activities. This provides the therapist with an opportunity to analyze movement as it relates to posture and gravity. It is important to look at the child's ability to make rapid, unconscious postural changes within the context of an activity. References and charts are available to assist in this evaluation of the sequential development of motor skills (Bly, 1994; Fiorentino, 1981; Green, Mulcahy, & Pountney, 1995; Richardson, 1996). Concentration is on those central postural skills needed to support movement of the head and limbs to manipulate the environment. In addition, wheelchair seating assessment forms are found in textbooks (Barnes, 1991; Batavia, 1998; Bergen & Colangelo, 1985; Cook & Polgar, 2008; Rothstein, 2005). The long form covers the client information, environment of use, current position and equipment, mat evaluation, and measurements.

The following questions provide some guidelines for evaluating motor development in terms of functional posture, as derived from the function–dysfunction continua. In all cases, it is important to determine if dysfunctional movement is delayed (slow to develop) or pathological (influenced by abnormal tone or reflexes). Each of the following questions is directed toward the functional end of the continuum.

Can the Child Move All Body Parts through Full Range against Gravity?

This involves the assessment of the child's passive range of motion and the presence of fixed or dynamic contractures. Just as important as passive range of motion are the effects of movement and changes in position on functional range of motion. Is muscle tone high, low, or fluctuating? What kinds of stimuli increase pathological tone and, possibly, interfere with active range of motion? Does the effect of gravity prevent certain ranges of movement mechanically or physiologically, and can movement be enhanced by changing position to decrease the effects of gravity or by using gravity to assist movement? What movements or positions elicit reflexes that compromise full range?

If functional range is influenced by position, then the therapist needs to know how much of each day the child spends in different positions. A positioning log can be completed with the help of parents, care providers, and educators. How is the child fed, transported, toileted, and positioned for rest, recreation, and school? Which positions have been selected with function in mind, which can be modified to enhance movement, and which are selected to reduce stress on the family or care providers? In addition to the time spent in school chairs, high chairs, and wheelchairs, the child's time in backpacks, baby swings, car seats, and beanbag chairs and on the floor and bed should also be assessed. From the positioning log, the therapist can make modifications or suggestions to promote independent movement for the child and ease caregiving responsibilities for his or her family and school staff.

Can the Child Right His or Her Head and Is It Mobile in All Planes?

In the supine position, can the child maintain his or her head in midline, turn it to either side, and tuck his or her chin to observe people, body parts, and what may be in the child's hands? Is development delayed yet following a normal sequence, or is pathology present? Is difficulty with movement caused by low tone struggle against gravity, or is immobility caused by high tone? Is there increased extension in this position because of the influence of the tonic labyrinthine reflex? This may include neck hyperextension, an open jaw, retracted lips, or upward gaze. Does the rooting reflex cause the child to press one side of his or her face against the floor? Does the inability to maintain the head in midline elicit an asymmetric tonic neck reflex (ATNR)? When attempting to lift his or her head from the supine position, does the child use peripheral, phasic musculature (e.g., the sternocleidomastoids) to substitute for deep tonic work?

In the prone position, can the head be lifted to 90 degrees, or can it be turned freely to either side and be isolated from body movements so that the child does not flip over when he or she turns his or her head? Can the child raise and lower his or her head

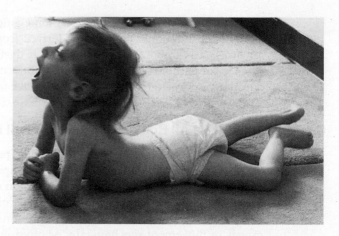

FIGURE 15.5 The child's head is thrown back for stability. Note the position of the mouth because of hyperextension.

with graded movements? Functionally, can the child turn his or her head to examine the world visually, and can the child control his or her mouth for age-appropriate speaking and swallowing in this position? If delay or pathology is present, is neck hyperextension necessary to keep the head upright (Figure 15.5)? If so, is it accompanied by extension throughout the body? Can the child close his or her mouth when the head is righted or is the jaw pulled into extension? Does the child simply collapse to lower his or her head?

In side lying, where the effects of gravity on the head are minimized, can the child look up and to the side without flipping into a prone or supine position? Can the child use lateral neck flexion against gravity to right his or her head or initiate movements of his or her body?

In the upright position (either sitting or supported standing), is the child's head aligned in space? Is it aligned with the child's body? It should be noted that the head may be righted but the neck may be flexed laterally or hyperextended to compensate for poor trunk position (e.g., in patients with scoliosis or kyphosis). If head control is poor, is shoulder elevation used to "nestle" the head for stability, thereby limiting neck mobility? Or, is the head generally thrown back or flopping forward? What is the controlled range of head movements? Can the child flex his or her neck forward 5 degrees and right it again but loses control if he or she flexes 10 degrees or more? If head control is inadequate, does tipping the trunk slightly forward or backward activate righting reactions or change muscle tone so that head stability is enhanced? If head control is minimal, how far back must the therapist tip the child's seat or stander until the child's head rests on a supporting back piece without flopping forward? If the therapist supports the head by tipping the seat back in space, is this a functional position for viewing the world and a safe position for swallowing?

Can the Child Right His or Her Trunk and Maintain Stability?

In this context, the trunk is seen not in terms of mobility but as a stable base of support for the head and arms (i.e., the primary parts of the body for seeking stimuli and manipulating the world). This is not meant to minimize the importance of the whole

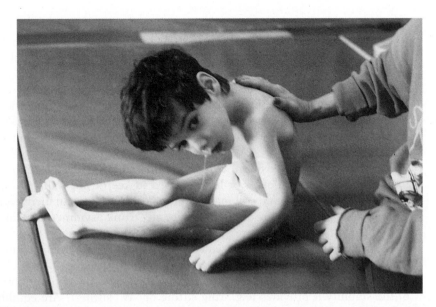

FIGURE 15.6 When placed in a sitting position, this child is unable to right his head or trunk. Protective extension is absent.

body in learning but to establish priorities for someone who is limited in functional movement. The therapist, therefore, looks at the trunk's capacity to stay upright in response to displacement (Hadders-Algra, Brogren, & Forssberg 1996, 1996a) and its ability to support the head and arms as they change position in relation to the trunk (Figure 15.6). The roles of the pelvis, legs, and feet are observed in conjunction with the trunk as part of the support basis for the body rather than in their roles of providing mobility through space.

A functional trunk also provides the base for good respiration; the rib cage is mobile and no fixed or functional contractures exist to reduce the thoracic space in which the lungs expand. For example, a fixed scoliosis may reduce the capacity of the lung on the flexed side (Nwaobi & Smith, 1986).

Although the ultimate goal is a trunk that works well in an upright position, the capacity of the lung is based on postural skills that have developed first in a horizontal position. Attention to this area is particularly important in a dynamic approach when goals include improving motor skills in a developmental continuum.

In the supine position, is the trunk free from the influences of abnormal tone or pathological reflexes? Is the back hyperextended or asymmetrical? Are the legs stuck in a frog-like position or extended and abducted? Can the trunk maintain the body's position when the head turns and the arms reach away from midline, or does the child inadvertently roll over during head/arm movement? Is the pelvis mobile enough to allow the child to play with his or her feet? Or is it tilted anterior as part of an extension pattern so that there is a space between the lumbar spine and the floor? If the child needs extra stability, can the child plant his or her feet on the floor?

In the prone position, is the child trapped by increased flexor tone or by the inability to extend against gravity? Is the pelvis flat on the floor or does hip flexion push the center of gravity toward the chest so that it is difficult to raise the chest off the floor? Likewise, do exaggerated hip abduction and external rotation tip the pelvis in the anterior direction? Do the arms help support the chest, or does the child need to use back hyperextension to raise the chest and reach out? When lifting the head and chest, is there associated hyperextension in the neck, lower back, and legs? When reaching upward, is there adequate abdominal activity to keep the child from rolling onto his or her back?

In the side lying position, can the child maintain the position without bracing himself or herself with arms or legs forward to keep from rolling? Can the child look and reach in all planes and still maintain the position? Does an increase in extensor tone create arching and flipping back? Are there any trunk asymmetries that are exaggerated when lying on one side (Figure 15.7)?

In an upright position (i.e., seated or standing at rest), is the trunk righted, stable, and symmetrical? Are adequate space and mobility evident in the chest for effective respiration? Can the child sit in various positions, or is the child limited to one because of the stability it provides (e.g., ring sitting or "W" sitting)? Are equilibrium reactions fully effective or only within a limited range of displacement? Are arms liberated; can the child reach in any plane without losing balance, or is activity in the shoulder girdle or arms necessary to maintain an upright trunk? For example, retracted shoulders may assist upper back extension, or there may be a need to prop on one or both arms. Can the

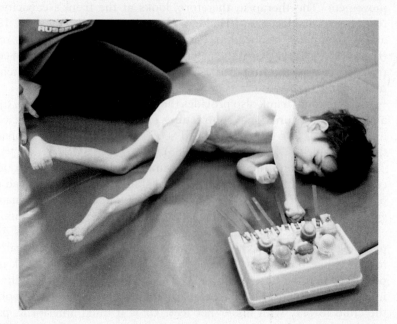

FIGURE 15.7 In an effort to maintain side lying, tone is increased. The lower extremities are not available for stabilization, and the hands are fisted.

trunk support the head and itself but not the weight of the arms? This can be determined if the child can sit erect only when resting, not when leaning, with his or her arms placed lightly on a tabletop.

How do the positions of the pelvis and legs affect the trunk? Is weight distributed equally to both sides of the pelvis? Is the pelvis relatively neutral or tilted in the anterior or posterior direction? Is the pelvis too far forward, requiring compensatory lumbar hyperextension or shoulder retraction to remain upright? Does a pelvis tilted toward the posterior create a rounded back, possibly with protracted shoulders and a hyperextended neck?

In the sitting position, does hip extension cause the child's back to press against the back of the chair, sliding him or her toward or off the front edge of the chair? Are the hips abducted in such a way that the child has no lateral stability, or abducted in such a way that he or she has little anterior stability? Can hips, knees, and ankles be maintained in a position that allows feet to be planted firmly on the floor? Does the child seem to be more functional in a standing or sitting position?

Can the Child Place, Maintain, and Control Position of His or Her Hands?

In this area, the therapist's concern is not fine motor skill but the ability to get the hands where they need to be, keep them there as long as necessary, and change their position through controlled movements of the shoulders and arms from a stable base. Improving function in this area may have secondary effects on fine motor skills in two ways. First, modification of muscle tone in the trunk and shoulders often improves tone in the extremities. Second, control of hand placement provides more opportunity for manipulation and the sensory experiences that contribute to fine motor control.

As with previous areas, the clinician must look at the quality of muscle tone. How can gravity impede or improve movement mechanically and physiologically? Mechanically, the concern is how gravity weighs limbs down in various positions. Physiologically, the concern is how it elicits righting or reflex activity in various positions. Also, what compensatory movements or associated reactions interfere with function?

In the supine position, can the child reach in all planes against gravity and maintain his or her hands away from his or her body without the need to stabilize by grasping an external object? For example, can the child reach up and touch a mobile or does the child need to hold onto it to keep his or her hand in that position in space? Can the child bring his or her hands to the midline or does gravity or the activity of an asymmetrical tonic neck reflex or tonic labyrinthine reflex prevent this? Can the child get his or her scapulae off the floor by protracting for an upward reach? Can the child look at and reach his or her tummy, knees, or toes, or must the child look up and initiate a symmetrical tonic neck reflex to reach down?

In the prone position, can the child lift his or her chest off the floor by using interaction of his or her flexors and protractors to bring arms forward as supports or with extensors to bring the child's head and back up so that his or her elbows are beneath the shoulders? In the absence of flexor activity, is the chest raised by back extensors with little or no weight bearing on the forearms? Can the child shift weight onto one arm to reach out with the other? Does the child collapse onto his or her chest when attempting to reach out, or compensate with neck and back hyperextension to keep from collapsing? Is shoulder stability adequate for sustained play in this position?

In the side lying position, is the upper arm fully mobile in the sagittal plane? Can the child reach up from the floor against gravity? Are shoulder movements isolated, or does the child need to initiate them with changes in the position of his or her head? Is the child's shoulder trapped in an internally rotated position by the effects of gravity in this position?

In an upright position, are the shoulders and arms free to move in all planes? Are there compensatory movements such as elevation, retraction, and external rotation or protraction and internal rotation to assist an ineffective head or trunk? Is the shoulder girdle mobile enough for full range but stable enough to maintain a position against gravity? Can the child use his or her arms only when supported by a tabletop? How does the position of the shoulder girdle affect mobility of the humeri and forearms? For example, protraction often is accompanied by internal rotation, adduction, extension, and pronation in children who have tone problems. How do the positions of the trunk and pelvis affect the position of the shoulders?

Is the Child Mobile through Space in All Planes?

In this area, the concern of the therapist who uses the biomechanical frame of reference for positioning children for functioning is not ambulation but mobility through space for two purposes: (1) Can the child move to attain a goal such as a toy, person, or food? (2) Can the child move to provide proprioceptive and vestibular input to enhance the development of body schema and spatial awareness? The clinician looks at how the child moves independently through space and if mechanical assistance would be beneficial.

Can the Child Get to a Desired Goal by Walking, Creeping, Crawling, or Rolling?

If so, does this process require pathological movements? Is the amount of time needed for the movement too extreme, or is the effort too exhausting? What alternatives for goal-oriented movement are realistic? Does the child have the potential to propel a wheelchair (either mechanical or powered), tricycle, or scooter board based on what the therapist knows about his or her functional range, postural reactions, and ability to maintain and control his or her hands? If the child has independent but not optimal locomotion, is the potential improvement gained through a piece of equipment worth the extra training required for the child, family, and care providers? Further, the therapist should explore with the child, family, and care providers their feeling about the use of this hardware and their ability to follow through with its use. Finally, the therapist should consider the expense of the equipment in relation to its need and the potential for reimbursement. If the child has no independent movement through space, which one of several methods is most appropriate for his or her physical and emotional growth and his or her life style? In addition to goal-directed movement through space, what kinds of passive movement through space can be provided? How can the child's position be modified so that he or she feels comfortable and secure?

Can the Child Chew and Swallow Food Successfully without Aspirating?

Feeding skills are assessed by the impact of posture on oral motor function. The assessment of hand placement and control, as discussed earlier, should yield similar information in relation to self-feeding skills. Although assessment of posture is critical to effective feeding intervention, it is only one part of a sophisticated evaluation of sensory, fine motor, cognitive, and behavioral skills that goes beyond the scope of this chapter.

Without describing an in-depth feeding evaluation, the following explanation gives examples of how posture and tone are incorporated into oral motor assessment. Are the trunk and neck stable to provide a base for movements and stability of the jaw? Can the head be maintained in a neutral or slightly flexed position? Is the neck extended so that the airway is open and aspiration of food is more likely, or is it flexed in such a way that swallowing is difficult? Is the trunk in an optimal position for respiration so that the coordination of swallowing and breathing is enhanced?

Does the presence of hypertonicity contribute to such oral reflexes as rooting or the bite reflex? Does it prevent isolated movements, such as separation of the tongue from the jaw? Are the tongue and lips retracted in association with extensor tone so that the tongue cannot come forward and the lips cannot come together?

Is gradation of oral movements affected? Does the jaw just open and snap shut when food is presented? Can support of the head and trunk or changes in body position in space modify high tone so that oral control is enhanced? How does gravity affect oral motor control in the presence of hypotonicity?

Does the child bite on the spoon because of ungraded jaw movements or because he or she is trying to keep his or her head from wobbling? Do the tongue and lips fall backward in a passively retracted position when the head is tipped back and forward when the neck is flexed? Can the child create enough lip pressure to keep food from falling out of his or her mouth? Is there enough activity in the cheeks to keep food from spilling over the teeth and pocketing in the cheeks? Does the child manage better in supported standing or reclined sitting positions? Does a change in position increase postural tone, or is extra support needed to accommodate for lack of tone?

Can the Child Void When Seated on a Toilet or Potty?

As with feeding, the biomechanical frame of reference is part of a complex evaluation of independent toileting. Information about the child's levels of cognition and sensory awareness is essential. Furthermore, it would be helpful for the therapist to know about the child's diet and behavior patterns.

The postural component addresses comfort, trunk stability, and the ability to relax hip extensors and abductors that otherwise may interfere mechanically with controlled elimination. The assessment is the same, then, as an evaluation of the child's capacity to sit in a stable, comfortable position with hips flexed and slightly abducted. In addition, the child should be assessed for the ability to direct the flow of urine into the toilet rather than onto the floor. This can be an issue with boys and girls alike and often is related to pelvic position.

An additional, extremely important component of the assessment is consideration of the family's or care provider's acceptance of any toileting aid or device in terms of size, management, and cosmesis.

Can the Child Access a Switch to Activate a Technological Device?

Again, the components of this task from a biomechanical frame of reference refer to the capacity to control the head, trunk, and arms. Regardless of their complexity, most devices can be driven by either an intermittent or sustained contact with a switch. However, the fewer demands on motor output when accessing a switch, the greater the cognitive/perceptual demands when using a complex device (such as augmentative communication or powered wheelchairs), where one action must be performed in a specific sequence. The process of selecting the best child/switch match is dependent on skilled team assessment of a multitude of performance components.

Physical components to be considered include the following:

- Does the child need additional postural supports while mastering the fine control necessary for this skill?
- Where in space can the switch be placed to maximize control? (This is referred to as the "sweet spot"). If using the hand, is the most successful placement for learning to activate the switch at midline or to the side? If using movement of another body part, in what position does switch activation require the least energy and minimize compensatory movements?
- Can the necessary movements for activation be performed against gravity, or does the switch need to be placed where movements are performed in a gravity-eliminated position?
- Can the child produce adequate force to depress the switch that is selected?
- Can the child release the switch in a timely manner?
- Does the child have various movements available to activate the device (e.g., keyboard, joystick) or must the child rely on one movement to activate a switch in a coded fashion?
- Is the child able to sustain the movement of a momentary switch (e.g., holding the joystick in a forward position to "drive" forward) or does the best switch/child match consist of a switch that is latched? It requires a contact to start it and stays on until a switch is activated to stop it.

Once the child's postural components have been assessed, the primary intervention plan addresses the need for and type of postural supports. However, the physical device cannot be effectively provided in a vacuum. For the biomechanical framework to support change, consideration of other factors must be built into the plan. The following questions can guide this process.

What Personal Factors Might Restrain or Support Use of the Equipment?

Personal style will influence how a child adapts to the use of postural supports. As liberating as it may ultimately be, the use of adapted positioning devices creates changes in routines, physical sensations, and habits and patterns of movement. The child's coping style and level of motivation will influence his or her ability to adapt to these changes. Other personal factors to consider are age and past experience with positioning devices. A young child may be less likely to tolerate the limitations of movement through space imposed by equipment than a student whose daily routines include longer periods of sitting in the classroom. It is important to note that any child may balk at new interventions if he or she has had similar but negative experiences in the past.

What Activities Will the Child Engage in When Positioned in the Device?

The appropriately selected activity will enhance the benefits of biomechanical intervention when it is selected in collaboration with the child and is set up in a way that makes reasonable demands on the motor skills that are being addressed. The positioning of the objects involved in the task is part of the therapeutic design. For example, if the goal of a prone lyer is to promote the development of weight shifting in the shoulders, an activity that requires the child to reach forward and upward with one arm (such as block constructions) is more demanding than one that can be accomplished with both forearms resting on the floor (such as coloring). The child's participation in choosing the activity will affect the extent to which he or she engages in it.

Will the Device Support Participation in Life and Social Engagement?

While addressing postural goals, is the equipment a barrier or support to the routines and interactions which the child would otherwise be engaged in? Can the child transition (or be assisted with transitions) between activity stations in the classroom in a timely fashion with his or her peers in the classroom when he or she is in a stander or seating unit? Should he or she be in a manual wheelchair during recess or is most of the action in the sandbox? Can he or she receive spontaneous hugs of comfort or glee, or does the lap tray, head support, and protraction wings make him or her physically inaccessible?

Will Physical, Cultural, and Social Environmental Factors Be Supports or Barriers to Effective Use of the Device, and Vice Versa?

How does the device fit into the space available in home or school? Is it cumbersome to move when the locus of activity changes? How does it look, does it have visual appeal, or does industrial construction hide the presence of the child within it? Do the parents feel that it liberates their child or does its presence exacerbate their sense of their child's differences and needs? Does the classroom teacher resent the time and space that it requires, or does he see the equipment as facilitating his student's participation in the classroom? The culture and goals of school programs vary widely in relation to the appropriateness and acceptance of supportive devices in the classroom. Some programs for physically challenged prioritize sensory and motor skills in their curricula. On the other end of the continuum, schools that practice full inclusion are more likely to emphasize social and academic participation, relegating the more intensive physical intervention to the home. The attitudes and priorities of families and systems play a significant role in how, if, and when the device is used, and how the child feels about using it.

POSTULATES REGARDING CHANGE

The biomechanical frame of reference for positioning children for functioning uses external devices to promote the child's functioning. On the basis of the evaluation data, the occupational therapist establishes functional goals for the child that may be developmental or task specific. For example, a developmental goal may be to provide the child with a device to facilitate weight bearing on the forearms in preparation for controlled mobility. A task-specific goal may be to provide the child with a switch plate to activate his or her communication device.

Postulates regarding change define relationships between concepts that structure the environment for change. These postulates help the therapist determine how and when to use adaptive equipment. In the biomechanical frame of reference, specific guidelines for the design, fabrication, and fitting of special devices are found in the "Application to Practice" section.

1. If practice time for a skill is increased, then the skill is developed more rapidly.

   During therapy sessions, the therapist often handles a child so that he or she is better able to perform a task. A great increase in therapeutic handling time generally is as impractical for the staff as it is intrusive for the child. Adapted equipment can help the child practice certain skills because equipment can simulate the therapist's hands, albeit in a static fashion, to enhance function.

   Regarding this postulate—that an increase in practice results in an increase in skill—the therapist must remember that there is a point of diminishing return. Judgment must be exercised in determining how often the child uses equipment and at what point its use restricts the child's participation in life. Without moderation, a good tool can become counterproductive.

2. If the therapist combines knowledge of the developmental progress of postural skills along with an awareness of the effects of gravity and sensory stimulation on normal and compensatory movement, then the therapist can determine appropriate positions to enhance a child's function.

   The therapist needs to determine at what point dysfunction occurs in the development of the child's postural skills and then how this dysfunction affects goal achievement. Another important consideration for the therapist is to explore which positioning options are most effective for a specific child.

3. If the therapist handles the child in various ways, the therapist can determine how best to enhance normal postural responses in any one position.

   Once the therapist determines an appropriate position, the therapist often finds that the child cannot maintain the position independently without using compensatory movements. Because compensatory movements result in significant secondary complications (permanent deformity that will ultimately decrease function), it is counterproductive to use these to enhance function. The therapist must identify the best way to help the child engage in functional activities and maintain as much normal postural activity as possible. This should be done by providing as much support as the child needs, but no more.

The process of determining an effective way to enhance a child's ability to tolerate an upright sitting position includes a combination of handling and manipulation of the child, an understanding of theoretical information, and trial and error. The understanding of theoretical information helps the therapist gain insight into what may be happening as a child moves or is moved; the therapist should not depend exclusively on that insight, however, to predict what will happen. Objective observation is essential so that the therapist sees and responds to what is happening, not what is expected to happen. This is the point at which trial and error become important: the therapist makes an adjustment in the child's position based on theoretical handling principles (e.g., proximal over distal handling) and then evaluates the child's response. If the response is not a desired one, the therapist continues to experiment and evaluate until the desired response is attained. Although the many principles for more aligned positioning are discussed in the "Application to Practice" section, no rules should be accepted without question.

What follows are postulates that may be helpful when handling a child to determine how to facilitate an effective position:

1. If the therapist first provides control centrally, then the distal parts of the body may be freed from the task of assisting the trunk or from the influence of associated reactions.

   For example, if a child cannot prop in the prone position, it may be because his or her body weight is shifted onto his or her chest. Before supporting him or her under the chest, the therapist should extend the child's hips fully by pressing down on his or her buttocks. With weight shifting back over the hips, the child may now be able to bear weight on the forearms.

2. If the therapist uses the effects of gravity to the child's benefit, then the therapist may reduce the need for more intrusive pieces of equipment.

   For example, a child positioned in a prone stander may exhibit poor head control. A prone stander provides full support to the child's ventral body surface, with a slightly forward tipping. When the child attempts to right his or her head, a full extension pattern appears so that his or her neck becomes hyperextended, his or her arms retract actively, and his or her back arches. A supine stander provides support to the child's dorsal surface with the body tipped back slightly. A supine stander should be considered for actual trial because with a supine stander, this child can use slight neck flexion to right his or her head and lean back against the head support when fatigued. This would eliminate the need for the additional head and back controls in the prone stander. A supine stander provides support to the child's dorsal surface with the body tipped back slightly.

3. If the therapist modifies the child's sensory environment, the therapist may enhance the positive effects of adapted equipment.

If the therapist observes how the child responds to factors (e.g., ambient noise and light, temperature, and the texture or firmness of a supporting surface), the therapist should make changes in the environment to compliment the postural device. For example, a child who responds to being placed on a cold plastic chair with a startle reaction and accompanying increase in extensor tone may exhibit more postural control with a lightly padded surface. A child who becomes lethargic in the presence of soft, slow music may maintain an upright position more easily with an increase in the volume and tempo of the music.

4. If the therapist can identify an effective position through handling, the therapist can attempt to simulate that handling by using an adapted device.

The therapist can attempt to "translate" a position from handling to a durable piece of equipment by recording exactly what support the therapist provides with his or her hands or body (e.g., minimal or moderate support) and at exactly which body location the supports contact the child's body. This record will provide a blueprint for constructing or ordering equipment. Although specifications for measuring are included in the following section, some general principles that apply to all positioning devices include the following:

- The surface of support units should be solid and stable so that it does not "give" or change with the child's movements. Flexible surfaces such as beanbags or sling seats on wheelchairs accommodate to the child's weight shifting, can result in instability, and as a result, can exacerbate asymmetries or compensatory postures.
- Ancillary supports, such as lateral trunk supports, leg abductors, or protraction blocks, should be assessed in a proximal to distal method and the least amount of support necessary to facilitate postural support should be used.
- Ancillary supports should be both small and thin enough so that they actually "fit" the child; however, at the same time they should be large enough to distribute pressure over the surface of the body part. In this way, the controlling support does not dig in and cause discomfort or, in some cases, active resistance. Whenever possible, blocks rather than straps should be used to control.

Too often, a child's wheelchair and seating system looks very similar to other children's systems with lateral support, hip guides, medial thigh supports, a headrest, a harness, and so on. In addition, too often there is a big wheelchair and seating system with a little person who is supposed to grow into it. The team involved in these decisions should consider how they would feel in an outfit and pair of shoes that are two sizes too large for their frame. For certain, their mobility would be compromised. This is exactly the same for the child in a large seating system he or she is supposed to grow into. There are advantages and disadvantages to every piece of equipment. The challenge is finding the best piece of equipment to meet each individual child's specific needs.

The positioning devices should be fitted to the child; the child should not be fitted to the device. It may be tempting to place a child in a piece of equipment, to see how it "fits." Once in the equipment, ill-fitting parts may be difficult to observe.

5. If the therapist considers the needs of the child's care providers, the therapist may provide equipment that is more likely to be used effectively.

Factors that influence care providers' attitudes include cosmesis, how much space the equipment takes up, how difficult it may be to place the child in and out of the equipment (McDonald, Surtees, & Wirz, 2003), how much assistance does the child need to use the device, how the device enhances or interferes with social interaction, and the cost of the device in relation to its effectiveness. For example, does the adapted commode fit in the bathroom at home? Or, does the chrome and plastic standing device look too industrial? If the equipment is offensive to those persons expected to use it, it is less likely to be used.

6. If the occupational therapist engages in team decision making, then the child is more likely to gain the benefits from using a particular piece of equipment.

Working with family members, physical therapists, speech pathologists, teachers, teaching assistants, physicians, and equipment vendors as a team provides more information about the child and makes the problem easier to solve. Each member of the team has a unique area of expertise and concern for the child. Accordingly, each team member provides distinctive input. All team members, including the family, should participate whenever appropriate in goal setting and problem solving. This is an effective way to address the complex factors such as cultural, social, and physical environment.

APPLICATION TO PRACTICE

Application to practice is divided into two sections. The first section discusses common positions in which central stability can be provided artificially. The second section deals with postural components or pieces of equipment as they relate to functional skills.

Central Stability

Intervention related to central stability covers the function and dysfunction continua of range of motion, head control, and trunk control. In these interventions, the therapist takes a primary role to determine the appropriate position and equipment. Any one position may be appropriate for various goals, depending on where supports are provided and how the equipment and, therefore, the child's body are oriented in space. Is the equipment perpendicular or parallel to the floor or tilted, and how does this affect the child? The following section provides an outline of what general goals may be approached in various positions, and how to fit equipment to the child. Each section contains a brief review of expected skill development in each position, along with the therapeutic advantages of the position.

Supine Position

The following is a list of functional skills that begin to develop in the supine position:

- Flexor activity develops head control: midline control and chin tuck
- Shoulder protraction and flexion against gravity
- Hands to midline

- Reduced demands on trunk; more effort can be given to head, oral, ocular, and shoulder control

Although not normally functional beyond infancy, practicing some movements in a restful supine position may be beneficial for a child who has severe physical impairments. Keeping in mind how gravity affects the child who has low tone and how reflex activity may increase hypertonicity in the supine position, the therapist may alleviate these effects by providing passive flexion. A pillow may be placed beneath the head and shoulders of a child so that it enhances neck flexion, supports the head laterally, and protracts the shoulders passively. A roll beneath the thighs can place the hips in a flexed position and yet allow the soles of the feet to be in contact with the floor. Positioning materials for the child to engage with is challenging in this position. Often it may simply provide an opportunity for the child to bring his or her hands to midline to explore the body. If the child is able to reach up against gravity, the activity must be suspended or supported above the child's body using an easel or rod. Oral motor control is taxed in this position, as it is more difficult to bring the tongue forward and lips together and to stabilize the jaw.

Prone Position

The following is a list of functional skills that begin to develop in the prone position:

- Head righting in a horizontal plane
- Interaction of dorsal extensors and ventral flexors for propping on forearms
- Shoulder stability during weight bearing (propping) and mobility on stability during weight shift
- Increased range of shoulder flexion is necessary when reaching from horizontal position
- Decreased effects of gravity on lateral asymmetries that occur with upright positioning
- Hands more likely to be in visual field by nature of shoulder position when propping

A wedge provides the basic support unit to enhance prone positioning for a child who cannot prop independently. The wedge should be wide enough so that it does not tip if the child starts to roll over. The length of the wedge is determined by the point of support at the chest and hips. The demand on the shoulder for weight bearing is influenced by the amount of contact of the wedge on the chest. Consequently, the lower the contact of the wedge on the chest the greater the demands on the shoulder girdle for weight bearing. However, for some individuals, if the front edge is too far back, the child may flex his or her trunk and curl over it. The front edge of the wedge, where it contacts the child's chest, may also affect respiration (Figure 15.8). This should be monitored carefully to ensure that weight bearing on the chest is not compromising respiration.

If a child tends to be kyphotic in the upright position but has a mobile, flexible spine, then the lumbar spine can be extended passively in prone. This can be accomplished by having the lower portion of the wedge end at the child's waist. Conversely, a lordotic child who lies in the prone position with an anterior tipped pelvis should be provided with a wedge that extends well beyond the hips so that the lumbar curve is not exaggerated. In addition, the pelvis can be stabilized further by strapping an "X" across the buttocks,

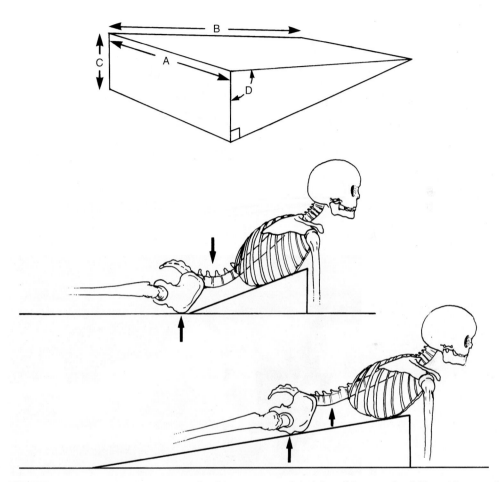

FIGURE 15.8 Measurements to consider for a prone wedge. (*A*) Width: unit should be wide enough so that it will not tip over if the child rolls over when strapped to it. (*B*) Length: contact of the front edge with the chest will determine how much shoulder stability is needed; the lower on the chest, the more the child is taxed. Lumbar curve and pelvic tilt are determined where the back edge ends in relation to the child's trunk or legs. (*C*) Height of the wedge will determine if weight is borne on forearms or extended arms. (*D*) Depending on which side of the wedge is chosen as the top surface, shoulders will be placed in either 90-degree flexion or a lesser degree of flexion.

each strap beginning at the iliac crest and crossing down to the opposite hip. This pelvic position, assisted by the straps, keeps the center of gravity at the hips. The straps also can prevent the child from pulling himself or herself forward over the front edge of the wedge. It should be noted that the use of a single strap often results in the strap sliding up to the lumbar area, causing an increase in lumbar extension and pelvic tilt (Figure 15.9).

The distance of the front edge of the wedge from the floor determines the demands placed on the shoulder girdle. A very low wedge provides support to the chest as the

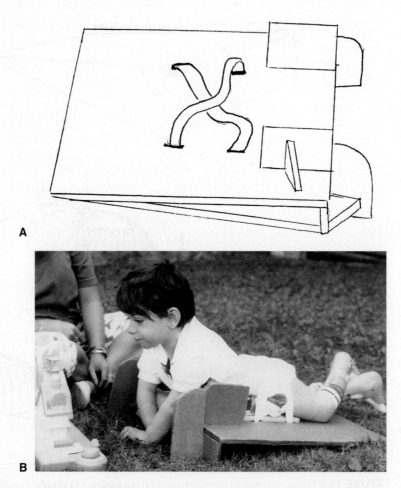

FIGURE 15.9 The prone lyer (**A**) provides hip control, lateral controls, and wings to prevent shoulder abduction and extension, keeping the arms forward of the shoulders (**B**).

child fatigues, but places high demands for weight bearing on the arms and allows more upper trunk mobility for weight shifting. A higher wedge that fully supports the chest but is low enough so that the forearms contact the floor reduces stress on the shoulders, provides proprioceptive feedback, and allows the less stable child to reach out without collapsing. A very high wedge may be used to eliminate demands on upper extremity weight bearing. In this position, a child's arms may dangle downward, in the same direction as the force of gravity. As the influence of gravity is minimized on the arms by the position, when the child makes a slight shoulder movement it results in a larger movement of his or her hands in his or her visual field. It is important to remember that the activity provided and the height of the activity relative to the child determine how the child uses his or her arms. For example, the child may play with small figures when weight bearing on both elbows but must weight shift to place rings on a stack pole.

When used in conjunction with hip straps, lateral supports to the trunk can help provide midline guidance and, if necessary, align the spine in the prone position. With some children, head raising in a prone position is accompanied by associated extensor patterns in the lower extremities, including hip adduction and ankle plantar flexion. This pattern can be modified by abducting the hips by placing an abductor between the knees, distributing pressure along the inner legs. It is important to remember that *too much abduction creates an anterior pelvic tilt.* A small roll beneath the ankle supports the instep so that the ankles are not stretched passively into plantar flexion.

Maintaining the head upright when in a horizontal position can be stressful. The therapist must carefully monitor the amount of time a child is in this position.

The child's options for social interaction in this position are limited. Other people need to be sitting or, preferably, lying, on the floor to engage with the child. While prone lying opposite the child maximizes interaction, this is a difficult position for many parents and teachers to maintain. The plan to provide a prone lyer needs to include appropriate activities and realistic expectations for parent–peer interaction when the child is in this position.

Side Lying Position

The following is a list of functional skills that develop in the side lying position:

- Lateral head righting (a component of neck stability in the upright position)
- Differentiation of two sides of the body (bottom side weight bearing, top side mobile)
- Hands easily placed in visual field
- Hypertonicity reduced; tonic labyrinthine reflexes inhibited
- Effects of gravity on shoulder flexion/extension reduced

The child who cannot maintain the side lying position independently will benefit from front or back supports to prevent inadvertent rolling (Figure 15.10). The back support can be a wall or a board perpendicular to the floor. The front support can be a block that contacts the trunk but allows movement of the shoulders and hips. This block is preferred to straps because it distributes pressure more evenly.

The child's head should be supported by a pillow or padded block that keeps the head and neck aligned laterally with the spine to prevent asymmetry and to facilitate lateral head righting. This also helps relieve pressure on the lower, weight-bearing shoulder. It is important to make sure that the pillow is wide enough so that the child's head does not fall when the child flexes his or her neck. If the child tends to extend his or her neck, slight padding can be attached to the back support behind the head to encourage a more neutral anterior/posterior neck position.

If the child tends to retract his or her shoulders, the therapist can use gravity to facilitate protraction by rolling him or her slightly forward. This can be done by angling the back support slightly forward. As the child's upper arm falls toward the floor, the shoulder tends to adduct horizontally and rotate internally. If this is not a desirable position, the top of the trunk support block can be used as an armrest. This does, however, eliminate functional hand use in this position.

The lower, weight-bearing leg generally is extended and the upside leg is flexed. If necessary, the weight-bearing leg can be extended by blocking the knee, distributing

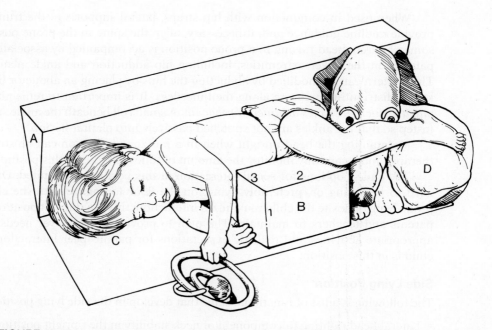

FIGURE 15.10 Possible components of a side lyer. (*A*) Wedged back tips child forward and assists in passive protraction. (*B*) Chest block/leg support: (*1*) Height determines the position of the upper hip (adduction/abduction; internal/external rotation). (*2*) Length determines if chest alone is supported or if hip, leg, and foot of upper leg are supported while lower leg is held in extension. (*3*) Depth is an issue only if the block also is used to maintain the position of the lower arm in shoulder flexion and elbow extension. (*C*) Surface is padded beneath this child's head, but no pillow is used because his head is proportionately large in relation to his body. A pillow would flex his neck laterally. (*D*) Stuffed animal acts as a leg block to extend the lower leg while supporting the upper leg in flexion. A longer chest block/leg support could have been used.

pressure along the thigh and skin. The child who has lower tone generally does not need this blocking at the lower knee because the leg will stay where you position it. In addition, the upside leg can be flexed easily, adducted, and rotated internally. This is important because the child who has low tone tends to position his or her hips in abduction and external rotation. When placing the child who shows extensor hypertonicity in side lying, his or her hips generally are positioned more appropriately in neutral abduction/adduction and neutral rotation. This is accomplished by supporting the higher knee, calf, ankle, and foot with a long block to position the hip properly and, simultaneously, to prevent the tibial torsion and ankle inversion/plantar flexion caused by lack of support to the foot.

It is important that the child be positioned in side lying on both sides equally in most cases. A side lyer can be provided with detachable parts so that the head and leg supports switch, allowing the child to be placed on either side. One exception is the child who has a functional scoliosis; generally the scoliosis is reduced when the "C" curve faces down and is exaggerated when the "C" faces up. A functional scoliosis is one that is completely flexible in supine. It is just the position that the body assumes for stabilization when positioned upright against gravity. The goal for side lying in a child with a functional scoliosis is to elongate the "shortened" side by lying on that side to facilitate elongation. Another consideration for determining on which side to place a child is to encourage specific arm/hand use: the upside arm is more liberated and most likely to be used.

The side lyer places the child in a very dependent position and limits the child's visual field because of restrictions on head movements. It offers excellent opportunities for the severely involved child to practice components of movement in a comfortable position with limited influence of abnormal tone. Those benefits must be weighed against restrictions to engagement with others and the environment when determining when and where the side lyer would be best used. For the less involved child who might benefit from the side lying position, temporary and softer supports such as foam blocks and pillows might be used so that the child might volitionally and independently roll out of the position.

Sitting Position

The following is a list of functional skills that begin to develop in the sitting position:

- Anterior/posterior and lateral stability of the neck and trunk
- Weight shift on hips; hips in a slight anterior tilt
- Arms liberated; shoulder position independent of trunk
- Shoulders girdle: provides stable base for arm movements

The biomechanical frame of reference for positioning children for functioning goal of providing external supports to increase alignment and postural stability for overall increased independent functioning is supported by numerous studies. Hulme et al. (1987) found that increased alignment led to increased head control, Howard et al. (2006) found that increased alignment led to improved femoral head position, and Heller, Forst, & Hengtler (1997) found that increased alignment via adaptive seating devices decreased scoliosis deformity. This increased postural alignment and support led to increased communication (Clarke & Redden, 1992), increased "mental performance" (Miedaner & Finuf, 1993), increased feeding, and increased ability to play (Vekerdy, 2007).

The child who is unable to sit independently basically needs stability in the pelvis and lower body to use the upper trunk, arms, and the head actively (Blair, Ballantyne, Horseman, & Chauvel, 1995; Colbert, Doyle, & Webb, 1986; Myhr et al., 1995) (Figure 15.11). This stability can be provided by the seating system to increase a child's social interaction and ability to participate in his or her activities of daily living (Clarke & Redden, 1992; Trefler et al., 1993). Compensatory movements often occur in response to an inadequate central base of support and controlled upper extremity movements are restricted (Boehme, 1998). The therapist must first correct or support any inadequacies in the base, especially at the pelvis (Reid & Rigby, 1996). This may decrease tone, compensatory movements, or associated reactions elicited by stress, giving the therapist a better idea of what, if any, corrections need to be made in the more mobile, upper parts of the body. It is important to provide the least amount of artificial supports necessary, providing flexibility for the development of dynamic movement (Brogren, Hadders-Algra, & Forssberg, 1996; Myhr et al., 1995). Various studies have hypothesized and supported

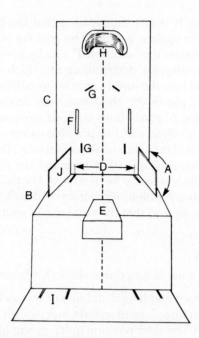

FIGURE 15.11 Possible components of an adapted chair: (*A*) Hip angle is commonly 90 degrees, open more if hamstrings are very tight; close angle slightly if it helps to reduce extensor hypertonus. (*B*) Seat depth should support thighs fully without digging into calf behind knee. (*C*) Seat height is determined by need for trunk and head support. (*D*) Hip straps generally come from seat bottom to hold bottom of pelvis back. Slots or attachments should be placed directly alongside the body to prevent lateral shifting of pelvis. (*E*) Abductor serves to keep legs centered; amount of abduction is determined once pelvis is secured in seating unit. Abductor starts at mid thigh, distributing pressure out to the front of the knees, beyond the front edge of the seat. (*F*) Lateral trunk supports are placed only as high as necessary to assist with trunk control. Lateral trunk supports should not interfere with humeral mobility because of height or thickness. (*G*) Slots or attachments for harness come in contact with shoulders without digging into the child's neck, and lower placement should be below the rib cage to allow for thoracic expansion during respiration. (*H*) Placement and angle of head support should be determined after hip and trunk controls are provided with decisions regarding tilt in space. (*I*) Foot straps may be needed if knee extension keeps feet from providing a base of support. (*J*) Hip guides may be necessary to keep pelvis centered and may help keep pelvic weight bearing symmetrical.

various seat positions for "optimal" posture in children with cerebral palsy. A slightly reclined posture is supported by Hadders-Algra et al. (1999) and McClenaghan, Thombs, & Milner (1992). An upright, erect posture for function is supported by Green & Nelham (1991) and (Nwaobi & Smith 1986, Nwaobi 1987). A straddle posture occasionally combined with a forward leaning of the trunk is advocated by Myhr & von Wendt (1991), Pope, Bowes, & Booth (1994), and Reid (1996). The "optimal" posture is one that allows a child to function as independently and efficiently as possible without significant compensatory movements. As a result, this will be different for different children depending on each individual's specific postural control and ability to use his or her extremities for function. It is also important to note that if compensatory postures are used for function, a home exercise program to elongate the "tightened" musculature is essential to minimize a child's risk of increased deformity and secondary complications.

Another way to modify tone to enhance the child's function is to consider the padding on the support unit. Sitting on a firmer support tends to increase arousal level. Adding medium density foam to create a softer support, which conforms to and supports the curves of the child's body, tends to reduce postural stress and hypertonicity.

The child's pelvis should be supported on a solid surface, padded if necessary, that extends to just behind the knees to support the thighs. Careful measurements must be taken when designing and ordering seating equipment. A seat that is too deep causes the edge to dig in behind the child's knees, pushing the legs and the bottom of the pelvis forward. A seat that is too shallow does not support the child's thighs, and the weight of his or her legs pulls his or her thighs downward and the bottom of his or her pelvis forward (Figure 15.12).

The back support should be no higher than necessary to discourage postural dependency. Some children do better with a back support that stops at the level of the pelvic crests or with no back support at all. If the goal is increased anterior shoulder movement, care should be taken to leave the scapula area clear for upward and downward rotation of the scapula with humeral movement. If a full back that also supports the head is being considered, attention should be given to the shape of the child's head. Young children and those with hydrocephalus often have large occipital regions. The high back support may push a large head forward, causing compensatory

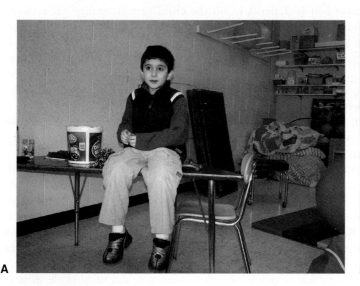
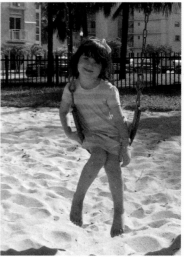

A   **B**

FIGURE 15.12 A solid surface (**A**) allows the hips to assume a relatively neutral position. The sling seat (**B**) forces the hips into adduction, asymmetry, and internal rotation.

curve in the neck. In such cases, a back support to shoulder height and a separate head support may be indicated to accommodate his or her head and allow for neutral cervical alignment.

The position of the child's pelvis also is controlled by the angle of seat to back (the angle of hip flexion) and the angle of the seating unit in space (amount that it tilts backward). These two factors should be explored simultaneously. The hip angle generally is most effective at 95 to 100 degrees. For individuals with increased extensor tone, increasing hip flexion or decreasing the angle of seat to back to 80 or 90 degrees may control or decrease severe extension hypertonicity. A child's tolerance for this position should be carefully evaluated. This may be a good position to attempt to increase strength in the trunk musculature via therapeutic activities. Once high tone is reduced, however, minimal postural tone may remain in the trunk. In another situation, when a child has very tight hamstrings, opening the hip angle slightly (5 to 10 degrees) to extend the hips may reduce the posterior pelvic tilt caused by the pull of his or her hamstrings. Opening the seat angle also can be effective with a low tone child. This can be accomplished by having the back perpendicular to the floor and using an anterior sloped seat. This position may facilitate increased proprioceptive input to the feet and consequently, postural alertness (Figure 15.13).

To secure the child's pelvis, a pelvic positioning belt is often used. Coming up from the point at which the seat meets the back of the chair, the belt is generally at a 60- to 90-degree angle to the hips and holds the pelvis in place. The belt itself should be appropriately sized and wide enough so that it does not dig into the child's flesh but narrow enough so that it places control only where desired and does further limit a child's movement and functional potential. Rather than coming from the outside edge of the seat, it should be attached alongside the hips to keep the child's pelvis centered. The angle and type of pelvic belt is dependent on the child's trunk and pelvic control, muscle tone, and positioning support needs. The various angles and types of belts can support the continuum of pelvic mobility to full pelvic stabilization.

For individuals with good trunk and pelvic control, a pelvic belt that is positioned below the anterior superior iliac spine (ASIS) and comes from the seat at a 90-degree angle, perpendicular to the floor, will adequately support the pelvis and will allow an anterior rotation in the pelvis for an individual to have forward reach.

If a child's pelvis can achieve a neutral alignment position but he or she cannot keep it there because of weakness, a pelvic belt that is positioned below the ASIS at a 60-degree angle to the seat is the general rule of thumb.

If a child has an anterior pelvic tilt tendency, the belt should be positioned directly over the ASIS and anchored on the back support parallel to the floor. This will hold back the top of the child's pelvis. This is helpful when an exaggerated anterior pelvic tilt exists but, in most cases, it is contraindicated because it does not allow for leaning forward to occur naturally with hip flexion. For a child *without* an anterior pelvic tilt tendency, it encourages a posterior pelvic tilt and a subsequent compensatory forward curve of the trunk (kyphosis) and therefore should be avoided.

If a child has a pelvic rotation or pelvic obliquity tendency due to muscle tone or muscle strength asymmetry, a more aggressive four-point, padded pelvic belt can be utilized to control the pelvis. The belt itself should be positioned directly over the ASIS

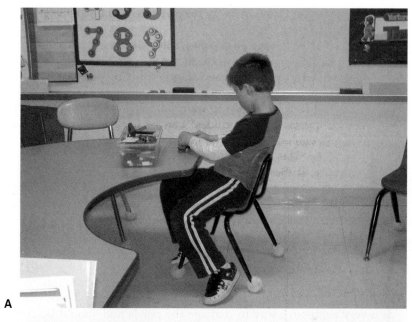

A

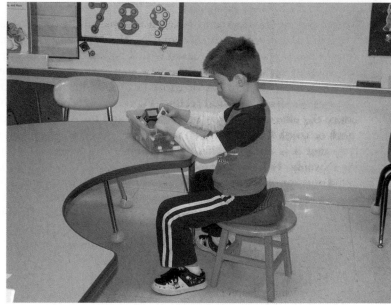

B

FIGURE 15.13 Tipping the pelvis forward (**A**), opening the hip angle, and removing the back support contributes to this student's postural competence (**B**).

and the secondary attachment straps can be anchored at 45-degree and 90-degree angles for optimal support.

With regard to pelvic positioning belts, size *does* matter. As noted in many pediatric seating systems, a too-wide strap placed at a 45-degree angle significantly limits pelvic mobility and can cause a posterior pelvic tilt by pulling the top of the child's pelvis backward.

If the child's pelvis tends to move laterally on the seat despite the seat belt, pelvic blocks also known as "hip guides" can be used for midline guidance and centering. These blocks can come from the seat cushion or the back support to nestle the child's pelvis in place. This is particularly important for a child who uses lateral trunk supports because, if the pelvis moves laterally while the trunk is positioned between the lateral trunk supports, a scoliotic position is created. In accordance with proximal to distal support principle, pelvic blocks should always be considered before lateral trunk supports are considered.

For some children with significant spasticity, an aggressive pelvic belt and hip guides is insufficient and a rigid pelvic stabilizer has been found helpful for anterior pelvic stabilization (Ryan, Snider-Riczker, & Rigby, 2005). Reid, Rigby, & Ryan (1999) found that caregivers and users preferred a rigid pelvic stabilizer over a pelvic belt and Rigby et al. (2002) found it increased a child's independence with bimanual tasks. This is a very aggressive way to manage the pelvis and should be considered only after all other options have been exhausted.

Depending on the degree to which it is done, tilting the seat unit slightly backward may increase or decrease postural demands. The stress and extensor tone that accompany an upright position can be decreased with a backward tilt. This provides the child with a back support on which he or she can lean intermittently. The same position may encourage activity in the neck or trunk flexors when the child comes forward into an upright position from a partial recline (Figure 15.14). When a reclining position is used to reduce the effects of gravity on the trunk and the child is incapable of flexing his or her neck or trunk forward into a righted position, it is important to support his or her head so that it is upright. This allows him or her to look forward rather than at the ceiling (Nwaobi, 1987). It is important to note that tilting back or reclining the seat back is a good position for increased stability. It is a good resting position for more sedentary activities such as watching television or being mobilized in a car/van. The slightly back position should not be used exclusively as it does not facilitate engagement in activity. For individuals who can tolerate more upright sitting, tilting the seating system to more upright position or unreclining the back is important for activity engagement and participation in dynamic activities such as feeding or writing.

The child's thighs contribute to his or her base of support. Too much abduction reduces anterior/posterior stability. Too much adduction reduces lateral stability and contributes to a pattern of extensor hypertonicity. Adductors are supports that run laterally along the child's thighs to reduce abduction. In general, the child's hips should be in neutral abduction/adduction. For some children, moderate hip abduction may be used to provide a wider base of support, to help reduce extensor tone in the hips, for orthopaedic stabilization reasons (Howard, et al., 2006; Manolikakis, 1992; Scrutton, 1991), or to facilitate an anterior pelvic tilt (Reid, 1996).

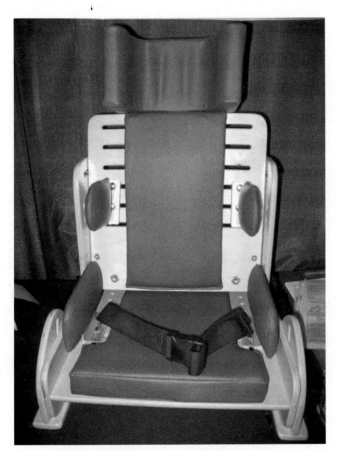

FIGURE 15.14 Another style of positioning chair with headrest and adjustable components.

A medial thigh support, also known as a "pommel," is a rhombus-shaped wedge that can be used to maintain the child's hips in abduction. When used, it should start at the middle of the child's thighs and extend to his or her knees, beyond the edge of the seat, to distribute pressure. A rhombus-shaped wedge also may be needed to keep the child's thighs symmetrical if one hip tends to abduct or to rotate externally while the other adducts or rotates internally (Figure 15.15). *This support is often misused and it is important to state that it should not be used to keep a child's hips back in the wheelchair.*

Care must be taken that the seat is not too high from the floor so that the child's feet can be placed firmly on the floor or on the foot support. Generally speaking, positioning the knees and ankles at a 90-degree angle is a good guideline for weight bearing for postural stability. If the seating unit is in a wheelchair, the seat height should be just high enough for 2 to 3 in. of footplate clearance from the ground. This will enable the child to better access the same tables and desks as his or her peers and will allow the child to come to the front edge of the seat and have his or her feet stabilized on the ground for an alternative, possible assisted, seating position. Foot orthotics should be considered to

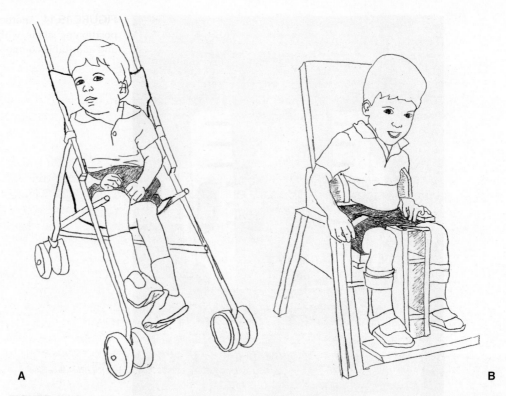

A **B**

FIGURE 15.15 Correction of this child's passive (**A**), rounded, and asymmetrical sitting posture requires appropriate seat depth, high back support, seat belt at 45 degrees, an abductor running from thighs to ankles, and lateral trunk support. In the adapted chair, the child's arms are free for play (**B**).

correct ankles that are unstable or pathologically positioned so that the child's feet can contribute to stability.

Once the child has been positioned so that his or her pelvis is aligned in a relatively neutral position, the therapist is better able to determine the positioning needs of the trunk, shoulders, and head. Lateral trunk supports provide lateral stability and increased postural alignment (Reid, 2002). They should be as thin as possible so that they do not interfere with upper extremity movement and function. They should be as shallow as possible and as low as possible if the child has fairly decent postural control and the potential to continue to gain postural control. Lateral supports should not be placed slightly away from the body to encourage the child to do more postural "work" because they will make contact with the sensitive area on the inside of the humerus and will cause the humerus to work in an abducted position which will compromise the movement pattern. A child may not be able to control his or her trunk and arms simultaneously. The higher the lateral supports, the more control they provide. Care should be taken to insure that the lateral supports are 1 to 2 in. below the axilla so that they are not suspending the child by the armpits. The two supports should be opposite each other, unless muscle control or tone in the trunk is asymmetrical. In that case, one support should be at the apex of the curve and the contralateral side should be higher to either "correct" or accommodate the scoliosis. Care should be taken that the supports are not so high that they press into the axilla where they may put pressure on the brachial plexus, nor so far apart that they hold the humeri in an abducted position. It is important to remember that improperly placed lateral supports interfere with shoulder mobility and hand use.

At times, a custom-molded seating system or a thoracic lumbar sacral orthosis is used to provide maximum trunk support to "correct" or support a child with a scoliosis or rotational scoliosis. Vekerdy (2007) found that the nonrigid custom-molded trunk support that was worn an average of several hours a day resulted in a significant change in posture of the trunk, extremities, head, chin and mouth. This increased alignment and trunk support also resulted in a change in the performance skills with increased eye-hand coordination, improvement in feeding, and improvement in ability to play. Shoham et al. (2004) noted a decrease in scoliosis on the contralateral side of the pelvic obliquity with orthosis use and Holms, Michael, & Solomonidis (2003) and Heller et al. (1997) found an improvement in posture for the duration of use of the support.

Lap trays or table surfaces can be designed to contribute to the child's more neutral shoulder and trunk positioning. It is important that they be provided only after optimal positioning has been attained through design of the seating or standing unit. With an improperly fitted basic unit, a child may use a lap tray to "hang" by his or her arms or to rest his or her head and upper trunk, rather than enhance arm position and function.

A lap tray should provide enough surface area to support the full length of the child's arms during all movements. Hands or fingers should not hang off the edge of the tray. If the tray trunk cutout is deep enough, the tray almost "wraps around" the child's trunk. The cutout should be large enough so that it does not dig into the child's chest or interfere with his or her breathing or slight weight shifts. It should be snug enough so that his or her arms do not slip between the trunk and the tray and become wedged. In general, it is preferable to provide a transparent tray for two reasons: (1) a child can see the rest of his or her body and (2) in a wheelchair, a child or care provider can see the floor through the tray to maneuver more easily through space.

The child's use of a lap tray can enhance arm and hand function by diminishing pathology in his or her shoulders. Although it cannot directly affect humeral rotation when supporting the humeri in slight forward flexion, this position modifies the pattern of external rotation, extension, and retraction. In addition, the humeri can be adducted horizontally, bringing the arms toward the midline, by using humeral "wings" also known as "protractor blocks." These are rectangular surfaces attached perpendicular to the lap tray. They push the humeri forward, preventing humeral extension and/or horizontal abduction. They also help to correct the position of humeri that are extended as part of a retraction/external rotation pattern. The humeral wings provide contact along the length of the humeri and should be high enough so that the child cannot lift his or her arms over them and get trapped behind them. The desired position for humeral wings can be determined by holding the child's humeri in slight flexion and running a pencil mark along the back of the elbows on the tray.

The child's use of a lap tray can contribute to trunk control by supporting his or her arms, thereby relieving the trunk of the weight of the arms. In this situation, the tray supports the arms, not the trunk. Position of a lap tray should be at or slightly above elbow height and be on height-adjustable armrests for optimal glenohumeral support. For children who habitually experience excessive trunk flexion, passive shoulder flexion that places the humeri in an almost horizontal position helps to elongate the thoracic spine as long as the child is not hanging by his or her arms on the tray.

It may be difficult for children who demonstrate inadequate shoulder flexion or tightness in shoulder extension to keep their elbows and forearms on the tray surface, because the arms are inclined to slide back from the tray edge and get trapped between the seat back and the back edge of the tray. Two possible solutions include the use of a "wrap-around" tray and the use of humeral wings. A more proximal approach to the problem of excessive shoulder retraction/extension would include the use of scapula wings, also known as "protraction wedges." These are small wedges placed on the seat back to bring the scapulae forward slightly. If the child retracts and pushes against the wedges, using a harness helps to maintain the trunk against the seat back, allowing the wedges to provide to the scapulae a gentle nudge forward.

Two issues prompt concern when using a lap tray on a seating or standing unit that tips back. First, if the lap tray is perpendicular to the back of the unit, it will be angled toward the child in an easel-like fashion when the unit is tilted back. The tilt of the lap tray can be controlled with adjustable hardware to keep it horizontal when the unit is tipped back. Second, by tipping the child slightly backward, gravity tends to push the humeri backward. It may be necessary to consider humeral wings that may not be otherwise needed when the child sits in a full, upright position.

The therapist may choose to tilt the lap tray like an easel if it helps correct trunk or head position. By resting his or her forearms on an easel surface, the child may use greater degrees of shoulder flexion. This may elongate the upper trunk, enhancing the upright position. Also, tilting the lap tray places visual stimuli closer to eye level. This may encourage the child to keep his or her head in a more upright position, rather than looking downward and initiating a flexion pattern in the neck and trunk when reading or drawing (Figure 15.16).

A lap tray should not be used exclusively. Its primary function is to support a child's arms and provide them with a surface to reach and access items when a standard table or desk is not available (e.g., in the park) and, when necessary, to support functional positioning of the arms for specific activities. As often as possible, it is important to remove the tray to allow the child to get close to others to interact more normally and close to tables and objects for manipulation and learning (e.g., books on bookshelves). Hopefully, the child's wheelchair seat height will be low enough to provide him or her with access to the same tables and desks as his or her peers. The issue of wheelchair height for small children presents a bit of a dilemma. If the lower height allows him or her to approach classroom tables and be at peer height when seated in the classroom, it will be too low for tables in the home and for matching height with peers when they are standing to work or play. In one environment or the other, the child would need to be transferred to another chair to be at the more appropriate level.

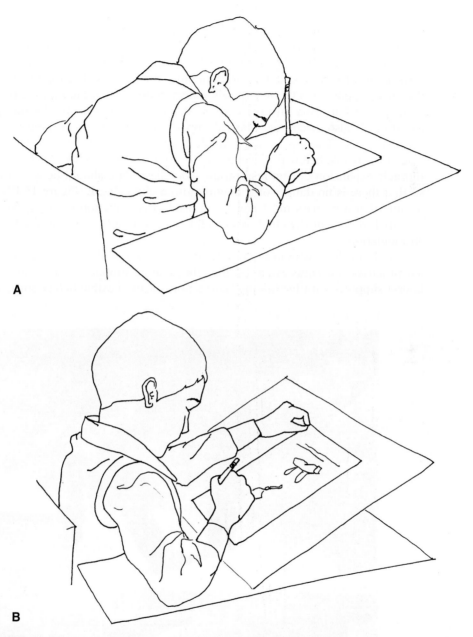

A

B

FIGURE 15.16 (**A**)., Flexion pattern, including overflow into hands, is created when this child looks down at his work. (**B**)., Angling the work surface changes the position of the head and modifies associated tone.

If a child's control of the trunk is so limited that he or she continually falls forward and cannot right himself or herself, a harness may be provided. This is an anterior trunk support that is traditionally made of a chest plate with four straps. Often, when a harness is used, the child's sitting unit is tipped slightly backward so that the child rests against the back and does not hang into the harness. The top two straps attach to the back support directly over the shoulders. Slots may be cut into the back for proper strap placement. This ensures a snug fit and, simultaneously, discourages shoulder elevation. It also discourages lateral upper trunk flexion by keeping the shoulders at the same level. The lower straps should attach to the back or through slots on either side of the trunk, below the level of the rib cage, so they are less likely to interfere with thoracic expansion during respiration. The chest plate should be at a mid chest level so that there is no danger of it digging into a child's neck (Figure 15.17). It is critical to note that a harness must always be used in conjunction with a pelvic belt. This is essential to prevent the child from sliding forward and down into the harness, risking strangulation.

For individuals with more complex positioning issues due to muscle strength or tone asymmetries, a harness can assist the other seating supports such as the hip guides and lateral supports with facilitating "correction" of the flexible deformities. This includes

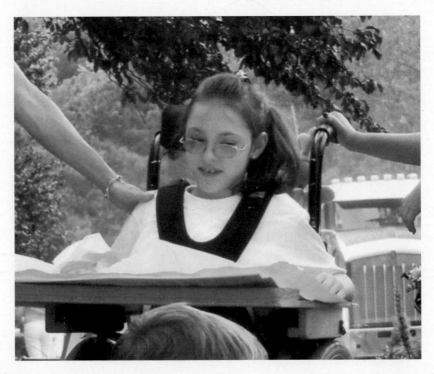

FIGURE 15.17 This harness prevents shoulder elevation and provides trunk support, contributing to postural symmetry and liberating hands.

"correction" of trunk lordosis, kyphosis, scoliosis, and a rotational scoliosis. There are various styles of harnesses along with strap length and direction modifications that can facilitate increased alignment. If the harness causes the shoulders to become retracted, protraction wedges can be used. Care should be taken that the sizes or positions of the wedges do not create rounding of the upper trunk. If retraction is mild and the scapulae are mobile, then the protraction wedge may be used without a harness.

Because of the complexity of the head, shoulder, and arm interaction, the therapist must be flexible and try several approaches to meet the child's needs. Supported alignment in the child's shoulders for more neutral positioning may provide more freedom of head movement or, conversely, may create a need for external head support. For example, by "correcting" a pattern of shoulder retraction and external rotation and straightening of the upper back, the child may no longer need compensatory neck extension to align his or her head with his or her body. Another child, with the same "corrections," however, may require a head support.

The first approach to improve inadequate head control or dysfunctional positioning of the head caused by tone problems is to correct total body position. Given enough external body support and reduction of physical stress, the child may be able to exercise control over his or her head on his or her own (Hulme et al., 1987). Alignment of the child's body with subsequent "normalization" of tone can reduce associated reactions and the need for compensatory movements in the neck. Conversely, it is important to remember that many pathological reflexes are elicited by head movement. In such cases, correction of head position can enhance body position. For example, slight flexion of a hyperextended neck may reduce extensor tone throughout the body, support midline head positioning, and may eliminate body asymmetry caused by the influence of an asymmetrical tonic neck reflex. That being said, these are small gentle positioning techniques. Aggressive head positioning should not be a primary goal of any child who exhibits head control.

Head position is the source of visual or auditory information and stimulation. There is a constant need to change head position continually throughout the day for function. Most children hyperextend their necks when seated in a chair to look at and speak with an adult who stands before or next to them. The position of the child in the environment or the stimulus in relation to the child must be considered when attempting to correct head position.

If a child has head control and a prominent ATNR that is used for function, such as to reach a water bottle on the table, then as long as the child can independently utilize this to access the water bottle and bring it to his or her mouth for drinking, restricting his or her head movement with an aggressive head support is not recommended. Conversely, if the child cannot control it and his or her limb movements are compromising environmental access with risk of injury upon entrance into a standard door then a more aggressive head support is recommended for safety. In addition, if these uncontrolled limb movements result in injury to others and intimidate others from socially interacting with the child, then a more aggressive head support is recommended for these times.

Aggressive head positioning is a goal for a child who has no head control when upright against gravity. Head supports have various posterior and lateral components to assist with this support. In addition, cervical collars are also utilized in conjunction with aggressive headrests for optimal support. Those children who have no head control may not be able to turn their heads even when supported by a headrest. The caregivers must attend to the child's position in the environment to assure that he or she has visual access to the important events.

The simplest support for the head may be a small posterior headrest. This provides a resting place but no lateral or anterior controls. In conjunction with a slight tip back of the unit, gravity assists in preventing passive, floppy forward flexion yet still encourages active neck flexion against slight resistance. The latter example may enhance active control of the head in some children. Another child may use an undesirable pattern of total flexion to right his or her head when tipped back. Care should be taken with head support because the headrest may provide a tactile cue that stimulates neck extension against the surface.

Another simple control consists of adding lateral support pads to the headrest. With all head supports, care should be taken that these supports do not interfere with the visual field or cover the ears. In addition, if the lateral contours of a head support touch the cheeks, a rooting reflex may result.

The suboccipital support is an attempt to simulate the shape of the therapist's hand where the therapist places his or her thumb and forefinger around the back of the child's neck with the occiput resting on the web space and the base of the temporal bones on thumb and fingertips. A suboccipital pad and neck collars contribute to head control with little interference to sensory receptors on the head and face. A suboccipital pad attaches to the seat back using a headrest hardware and cradles the base of the cranium. A child should be seated as upright as possible and the suboccipital pad should be placed at a height to support the base of the skull. A neck collar made of medium-density foam, cut in width to fit between the shoulders and the base of the skull snugly, supports and elongates the neck and can be used independent of the seating unit. To allow for slight neck flexion or jaw movements, the front of the neck collar should be connected in a yoke-like or V fashion.

If a child requires the support of a multicomponent headrest, the major headrest manufacturers offer a wide array of pad shapes, sizes, and contours to customize a head support for more aggressive contact. This aggressive support of the head and neck is important for a child who has no head control and is unable to prevent his or her head from falling forward, sideways, or backward when in an upright position. A slight backward tilt of the seating unit assists in keeping the head in contact with the support. When a child is tipped back more than 5 or 10 degrees for the sake of trunk control, however, it is necessary to right the head as much as possible by angling the head support or pushing it forward to flex the neck and align the head in space. The therapist must experiment with the child and caregivers to find the optimal relationship among head, trunk, and angle in space.

In extreme cases, a child may have a complete lack of head control. This child will also most likely have poor or absent trunk and lower extremity control. For this child, it is essential to first ensure that the trunk and pelvis are aggressively supported. Once that is accomplished, head support needs can be the primary focus. Along with the multicomponent headrest and/or cervical collar, a head strap or head cap (similar to a baseball cap appearance) can be utilized to adequately stabilize a child's head. Just as it is important to only utilize aggressive head supports after the trunk and pelvis are adequately stabilized, it is important to only use a head strap or head cap if the other components are insufficient to stabilize a child's head in the anterior direction.

Three notes of caution about more aggressive head and neck supports:

1. The lateral components of head support should not compromise circulation in the neck.
2. A full neck collar immobilizes the head and may interfere with jaw movements or swallowing.
3. A severe recline of the seating unit (up to 40 degrees tipped back) to provide head support limits the child's visual access to the environment, ability to interact with people in the environment, and can compromise swallowing.

In general, demands on active head control in the severely involved child should be minimized when the child is seated so that efforts can be directed toward intake of information, interaction with the environment, and fine motor skill or oral motor skill. The therapist should keep in mind that developing active components for head control may be addressed by using various positions and equipment such as standers, scooter boards, and prone wedges.

Case Study: Stephanie by Cheryl Cowart

Stephanie, a social, exuberant, 12-year-old child diagnosed with mixed athetosis/hypotonic cerebral palsy, attends a school in a children's rehabilitation hospital. She is beginning to desire the independence that most adolescents seek. Stephanie smiles and laughs often, and though she is unable to speak, she can communicate her needs and desires through facial expressions and eye gaze. She has the cognitive/perceptual and motor ability to access a communication device through single switch scanning (horizontal rows of commands are scanned on a timer, and after the user activates a switch to select a row, each command in the row is then scanned), though this process is very time consuming.

Stephanie presents with decreased central tone (hypotonic neck and trunk) and increased fluctuating peripheral extensor tone (Figure 15.18). This peripheral tone is usually precipitated by initiation of voluntary movement or by increased affect, such as when Stephanie is excited, frustrated, or startled. In unsupported sitting, Stephanie shows minimal equilibrium reactions and no functional protective reactions. Trunk control is poor and arms are not liberated. Owing to increased extensor tone, Stephanie sits with hip and knee extension, with a posterior pelvic tilt and compensatory kyphotic trunk. Fluctuating tone in her legs makes it impossible for her to maintain feet on the floor to contribute to a stable postural base. Stephanie can maintain her head in the midline to maintain visual contact with her environment, but she turns her head to the side to elicit an ATNR in order to initiate arm movements for reaching. She positions her reaching arm in elbow extension and shoulder abduction, while her nonreaching arm moves into shoulder abduction, scapular retraction, and elbow flexion. Stephanie is unable

FIGURE 15.18   Stephanie's lap tray positions her arms and allows full lateral visibility when driving her powered chair.

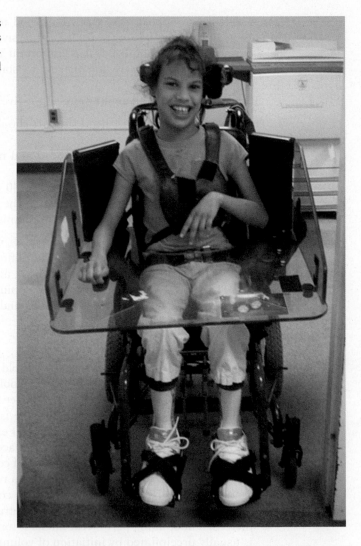

to accomplish graded volitional midrange arm movements or a functional grasp, though she can reach for, and briefly make contact with, a switch. Stephanie has no functional independent mobility through space in the same plane as her peers. She can roll and marine crawl for very short distances.

The biomechanical frame of reference for positioning children for functioning was used to increase Stephanie's occupational functioning in the areas of communication and mobility. A supportive seating system, including a solid seat and back, seatbelt, lateral trunk supports, hip guides, a chest harness, an anterior knee block (to maintain hips and thighs in a stable, symmetrical position), and sandal footplates with Velcro straps, was provided. This, with the addition of a lap tray for upper extremity support, enabled Stephanie to exercise sufficient postural and head control to drive a power wheelchair by using an airway surface liquid (ASL) proximity head array system. This is a semicircular headrest embedded with sensors that read relative head position rather than requiring physical contact. After training with an occupational therapist to improve graded head and upper extremity control, Stephanie gained enough left shoulder control to activate a reset switch (to restart the chair) located at the front of the lap tray, and enough head control to successfully maneuver her chair through busy school hallways. She uses head movements to access her communication device as well, because this is more efficient than harnessing an arm movement.

Despite this promising potential, Stephanie continued to require adult supervision with mobility in school. She was unable to safely move through doorways because her excitement when encountering a favorite teacher or friend increased her upper extremity tone; this resulted in shoulder abduction so that her arms caught against the doorframe. In addition, the head rotation pattern that Stephanie used to elicit an ATNR in order to initiate volitional arm movements precluded accurate use of the ASL sensors, and also resulted in decreased visual access to the space in which she needed to. Stephanie needed external controls for her arms so that she could maintain her head in midline to access switches. To promote Stephanie's increased safety and independence, a system was created to (1) contain Stephanie's arms within the parameters of the lap tray (without arm constraints), (2) allow full visibility for driving, (3) be sturdy enough to withstand Stephanie's severe tone fluctuations, (4) be manageable for family and caregivers, and (5) be adaptable in unforeseen circumstances. A lap tray unit was designed that included two detachable Plexiglas sides (anchored to the existing lap tray by two brackets and one manually removable screw) and bilateral padded protraction blocks to prevent Stephanie's elbows from lodging in the space between the seatback and the tray sides. To decrease the overall weight of the unit, the sides were sloped (starting at shoulder height at the seatback and descending to a height of 4 in. at the tray front). The present lap tray unit is adaptable when the seating system is "grown" as Stephanie gets taller (with minor adjustments), though a larger lap tray can be constructed using the same design in the years ahead. Although Stephanie was initially reticent to have a tray that looked "different" from other students', her hesitation was quickly overcome as she began enjoying her burgeoning school and community independence.

Supported Standing Position

The following is a list of functional skills that begin to develop in the supported standing position:

- Erect spine, liberated arms
- Neutral or slightly posterior pelvic tilt
- Hips extended with neutral rotation
- Knees stable but not locked in hyperextension
- Ankles in 90-degree flexion, neutral eversion/inversion

- Improved circulation and bone growth from upright weight bearing
- Increased alertness from upright position and extensor activity
- Decreased effects of flexor hypertonicity in the neck and trunk when weight bearing on extended hips and knees

The supported standing position should not be used for potential ambulators exclusively. This position not only provides increased opportunities of function for those children who are least likely to walk by enhancing circulation, growth, and alertness but also provides opportunities for head and arm control for children who have moderate to severe disabilities and is an alternative to long-term sitting (Manley & Gurtowski, 1985; Motloch & Brearley, 1983; Noronha, Bundy, & Groll, 1989).

The therapist first must decide which surface of the child's body is to be supported in standing. Providing support to the ventral surface of a child's body by using a "prone" stander at an 80- to 85-degree angle to the floor provides a close to normal standing position and requires slightly more extensor activity. If upright at 90 degrees, the prone stander tends to throw the child's body backward in space, and he or she may flex over the top edge of the stander to compensate. A supine stander provides full dorsal support for children who show very high or very low tone. For example, when slightly reclined in a supine stander, the very floppy child who has minimal head control is provided with total support. The child who has too much extensor tone and who throws his or her head, shoulders, and upper trunk back in a prone stander is encouraged to use flexion to right himself or herself intermittently in a slightly reclined supine stander.

Prone Stander

Through a series of trials and observations, the therapist can determine the optimal angle of a standing board to the floor. Postural demands and postural responses change as the stander is tipped farther forward or backward. In a prone stander, demands on head righting are less in an upright position than in a horizontal position (Figure 15.19). The child who cannot maintain a righted head in a full prone lying position may be successful in a prone stander at 75 degrees upright. In this case, with head control and tolerance in the prone position as the primary goal, the prone stander actually may be lowered as the child develops head control in increasingly higher horizontal positions.

The height of the stander determines how much support is provided to the trunk (and head in a supine position) and how much postural work must be done by the child. The therapist's goal is to challenge the postural system without causing fatigue or undesirable associated reactions that result from physical stress.

As with sitting, the pelvis should be positioned first. In the prone stander, crossed straps should stabilize the pelvis in the same way as in the prone position. If lateral shifting of the pelvis occurs, which would create a compensatory curve in the trunk, lateral pelvic blocks also known as "lateral hip guides" should be placed on either side of the pelvis. With hips in neutral, the knees should be directly below the hips. Occasionally, some hip abduction is desired. In either case, depending on the degree of abduction

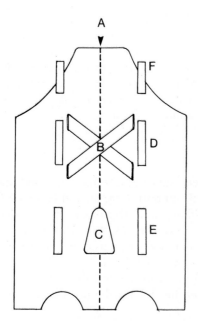

A

FIGURE 15.19 Possible components of a prone stander. (A) Height is determined by the child's need for ventral support, anywhere between the waist and sternoclavicular joint. When the support is cut high (as in this example), sides must be cut out to allow for shoulder mobility. (B) Hip straps come through slots right alongside the hips. They cross from the posterior crest of one side to the hip joint of the other side, placing pressure over the sacrum. (C) Abductor wedge keeps the legs aligned symmetrically and determines the amount of hip abduction. It runs above and below the knees but does not come in contact with the perineum. (D) Hip guides may be added for additional lateral stability, especially in the presence of a functional scoliosis. (E) Lateral leg guides prevent the external rotation/knee flexion pattern that often causes children with low tone to collapse in standing. (F) Lateral trunk supports may be necessary and should be placed as low as possible.

desired, a rectangular-shaped or trapezoid-shaped block should be placed between the knees. This spacer or abductor should extend above and below the knees to distribute pressure. Its primary purpose is to keep the legs aligned and symmetrical. If the child abducts and rotates his or her hips externally, knee flexion no longer is blocked by the surface of the stander because the knees will be facing laterally. Lateral supports at the level of the knees bring the hips into a more neutral abduction/adduction position and prevent collapse at the knees.

Padding in front of the knees on the prone stander is necessary to relieve pressure and prevent knee flexion. This should be done judiciously because too much padding can cause the knees to hyperextend. If the knees hyperextend regardless of padding, the joint can be flexed by slightly realigning the feet so that the ankle is slightly behind the knee. If a child wears foot orthoses, then the upper straps must be loosened because this position requires some ankle dorsiflexion.

Blocks placed laterally or medially to the child's feet or shoe holders can maintain the foot position if necessary. A nonskid surface could be just as effective. The integrity of the ankle and foot must be evaluated in standing. Although full discussion of this is beyond this chapter, ankle and foot orthoses must be provided for standing if pathology exists.

The need for and placement of lateral trunk supports can be determined once the lower body position is corrected and stable. The chest support or upper edge of the prone stander may end anywhere between the bottom of the sternum to just below the clavicle, depending on need. If the chest support is cut high, it should be narrow and contoured (something like the end of an ironing board) to free the shoulder girdle for movement.

As in the sitting position, height and angle of the lap tray contribute to facilitating postural control and alignment. A low lap tray may encourage weight bearing on extended arms. A child who has inadequate extension, however, may flex over the top of the chest support in an attempt to rest on the lap tray. In such cases, a lap tray at nipple level helps elongate the upper trunk and provide support for the arms as the child masters head control. The need for humeral wings on the lap tray should be assessed if retraction and extension are the dominant shoulder movements.

Supine Stander

In the supine stander, a pelvic strap is unnecessary because the chest and knee straps tend to encourage extension against the back support. Care should be taken to ensure that the chest strap does not dig into the axillary area. Hip blocks may be desirable to prevent lateral movement and any resultant asymmetries. As with the prone stander, abductor/spacer blocks or lateral adductors should be considered to align hips and legs. Padding should be placed behind the knees if there is any indication of hyper-extension at that joint. Ankle straps that come from behind the heel over the instep at a 45-degree angle or medial or lateral foot blocks may be needed to maintain foot placement.

A supine stander has a lap tray that supports the arms, provides a working surface, and encourages the child to use some active neck and upper trunk flexion to right his or her head and come forward to the working surface. Because the supine stander is tilted backward to some extent, protraction wedges on the stander or humeral wings on the lap tray may be necessary to assist the child in keeping his or her shoulders and arms forward against gravity. If head supports are needed, this is determined in the same way as for the partially reclined sitting position (Figure 15.20).

Functional Skills

The previous section discussed several common positions in which central stability is provided artificially to decrease pathological movement, encourage components of postural responses, and liberate the head and arms. Intervention in this section addresses the function–dysfunction continua that relate to hand control, mobility, feeding, and toileting, all of which involve more than postural responses. These functions also require cognition, perception, attention, motor planning, and fine motor skills. Postural control is a foundation for the development of these functions. The absence of postural control impedes the development of skills in these areas. The following sections describe postural components or equipment related to these functions.

Ability to Place, Maintain, and Control Hand Position

Although it is desirable to have shoulder and arm mobility in all planes, this is not always a realistic goal. If expectations must be graded or limited, then the most functional ranges of shoulder and arm movement are those that contribute to midline activity so

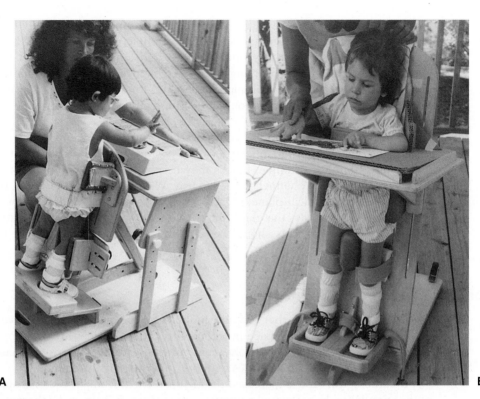

FIGURE 15.20 Two examples of standers: A., prone stander and B., supine stander.

that the child can bring objects toward his or her eyes, ears, and mouth for learning and survival. In this case, desirable ranges of volitional movement include neutral toward slight protraction; 30 degrees of external rotation toward full internal rotation; 0 to 90 degrees shoulder flexion, abduction, adduction, and horizontal adduction; and midranges of elbow flexion/extension and forearm rotation. The development of control in these ranges can be addressed in two ways: (1) by establishing skill in shoulder and elbow mobility and stability in developmental positions (enhancing the development of components of movement) and (2) by providing as much support as necessary to the body and proximal upper extremities to enable the child to perform a few distal isolated movements. (This improves distal function by providing proximal stability via external support to reduce the need for postural reactions.)

With a child who has moderate to severe disabilities, the therapist may choose to devise a specific pattern of movement related to one function. Examples of specific patterns of movement may be a hand-to-mouth pattern for feeding or a simple elbow movement to activate a switch. The first step is to provide an optimum base of support to modify tone, reduce demands on the rest of the body, and enhance attention to task. Side lying, sitting, prone standing, and supine standing are positions that should be considered. The second step is to determine how many arm movements the child can control and which ones need to be supported artificially by a table, lap tray, or other equipment components. For example, humeral wings, also known as "protraction blocks," on a tray minimize the child's ability to protract actively or to adduct horizontally when bringing his or her hand to his or her mouth. If the therapist raises the lap tray to axilla level, the child's movements are then limited to the horizontal plane, and demands for shoulder and elbow movements against gravity are eliminated.

In extreme cases, if a child has no control over arm movements (i.e., a child who has severe athetoid movements), one arm can be positioned so that movement is channeled in one direction. For example, blocks may be placed laterally and medially along the child's arm, creating a channel on the lap tray. With such an arrangement, the hand can move only in the vertical plane, regardless of extraneous shoulder, elbow, or forearm movements. In this way, the child may successfully depress a switch plate. Following a training period, supports should be withdrawn to assess potential for performance without aggressive supports.

Ability to Move through Space

There are various devices that facilitate mobility for the child who has a severe disability and cannot move through space independently. These devices are also appropriate for children who have less severe involvement but whose ability to perform a task efficiently or ability to participate in activities with his or her peers is impaired.

If pathological tone is increased through passive movement because of the intensity of the stimulation but affectual responses are positive, it is up to the therapist to provide a position in which unwanted overflow of tone can be controlled. For example, a child who hyperextends when swinging may be nestled in a flexed position within an inflatable tube placed on a platform swing.

Scooter boards may be effective in enhancing self-initiated movement in a child who has moderate to severe disabilities. They can also provide weight bearing, weight shifting, and rapid movement through space for the child who has a milder disability. The scooter board consists of an appropriately fitted prone wedge placed on highly responsive ball-bearing casters (Figure 15.21). Several modifications to the prone wedge can enhance its effectiveness. These include a chest wedge to provide the correct shoulder-to-floor distance and a narrower front wedge cut away to support only the chest and liberate the shoulder girdle (which is "ironing-board" shaped). The back edge of the wedge should end before the ankles so that the child's feet can hang freely over the end of the board. The child who has more severe disabilities may need an extension of the front edge of the wedge for intermittent head support. Directed, forward movement is not the goal in this case. The goal is movement for the experience of movement and interaction with the environment for physical (weight bearing, movement over stability), visual perceptual, sensory, and cognitive development. The child begins to initiate movement through space whenever his or her hands begin to bear weight through his or her arms. For the child who cannot roll or crawl, this may be his or her only opportunity to experience active movement through space.

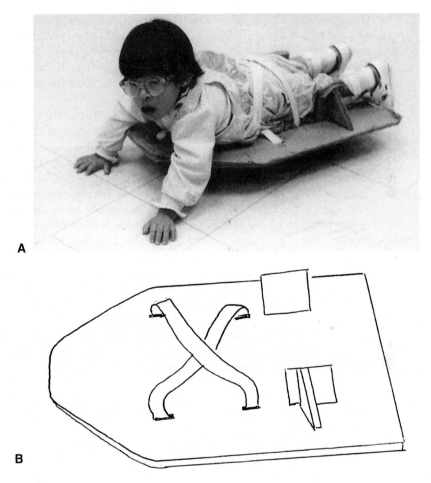

FIGURE 15.21 Scooter board (A, B) provides hip straps and abductors to prevent this low tone child from externally rotating her hips and dragging her legs on the floor.

Case Study: Max

Max is a typical 2-year-old boy who is the only child of working parents; their extended family lives a distance away. Max broke his right femur in his daycare program. After a brief stay in the hospital, he was sent home in a spica cast, which was to be removed, if healing occurred as expected, in 4 months. The hospital treated this as an orthopedic, not a developmental, issue. While in the cast, Max would not need physical therapy, so no rehabilitation referral was made.

Max's ability to engage in occupation as he knew it came to a screeching halt. Before the injury, he was physically active. He fed himself, assisted in dressing, took some interest in manipulative and imaginative toys, and spent most of his time running, climbing, playing with balls and trucks, and exploring physical space.

Once confined by the cast, Max cried with frustration a good deal of the time. His mother took a leave of absence to care for him. She spent hours entertaining him and carrying him around because he was almost inconsolable when left by himself. There was little support for her during the daytime because her family was not nearby and her closest friends were from work. Despite help in the evening from her husband, she was exhausted.

The plaster spica cast encompassed Max's trunk from the level of his nipples and continued to his legs, ending at the right toes and above the left knee. His hips were positioned in about 20 degrees of flexion and 90 degrees of abduction. There was a horizontal bar between Max's knees to support the cast and maintain the abducted position. The cast was very heavy. While Max retained his postural competencies, he could not exercise them because of mechanical restrictions imposed by the cast. He could not sit in a chair or lie on his stomach because of the position of his semiflexed hips. Mom carried Max, facing away from her, by supporting his buttocks on her hip and grasping the horizontal bar that was between his legs. When not being carried, Max was lying supine or propped precariously on the couch in a semisupine position. In neither position could he access toys for extended play, though he could briefly manipulate objects in space. He had no independent mobility. Max's mom requested an occupational therapy (OT) consult. Her plea for help was global—she had no specific request other than that life for Max and herself be more manageable.

The performance areas of occupation to be addressed by a biomechanical frame of reference for positioning children for functioning were play, self-care, and social participation: (1) independent mobility through space and (2) the ability to manipulate objects/toys for play and self-feeding. We would address the physical and social context, returning to Max the mom who was able to function as a supportive and competent parent.

Max had adequate neck, upper back, and arm control to propel a scooter board. However, when placed in prone his body was forced into a position similar to that of a newborn: his pelvis was higher than his chest because of the hip flexion imposed by the cast, weight was on his chest and face. Max did not have the endurance and excessive passive extension in neck and upper back to lift his head or move his arms in this position. However, by placing a pillow on the scooter board beneath his chest, Max's trunk was positioned horizontally so he was able to lift his head and his arms were liberated to propel the scooter board. When his mother sat on the floor, Max could also engage in object play with her, as the scooter board also provided a supported prone position for him.

Max could tolerate 15 minutes of play or movement in the scooter board before he fatigued. He needed opportunities for an upright position to spend the bulk of his time. When Max's trunk was held in an upright position he could not be placed on a horizontal surface due to the position of his legs. He could be propped upright with a beanbag beneath his legs; this conformed to and supported the contours of the cast but did not prevent him from falling to the side or backward, or sliding forward and down. Because of the weight of the cast, Max needed to be strapped into the upright position. A triple-thickness cardboard unit was constructed to contain the beanbag and to support Max's back. It had a floor, two sides, and a high back. Two slots were cut into the back at the level of Max's hips. However, because of the open angle of Max's hips, a traditional seatbelt would not hold him in place; the weight of his body would cause him to slide down through the belt. Rather, once Max was positioned in the chair, a strap was attached to one side of the horizontal bar, threaded through the slots, and then brought down to attach to the other side of the bar. Thus Max was suspended in his cast by the strap, the lower part of his body was supported by the beanbag, and his back was supported by the cardboard seat back. The unit was built to fit up to the coffee table in the living room, where Max was able to eat, socialize, and play.

Children who are nonambulatory or who walk slowly with crutches may be less taxed when using a tricycle. A tricycle also allows them to engage with peers in gross motor activity. Tricycles can be purchased with back supports, hip straps, abductors along the handlebar uprights, and footplates with straps (Fernandes, 2006) (Figure 15.22).

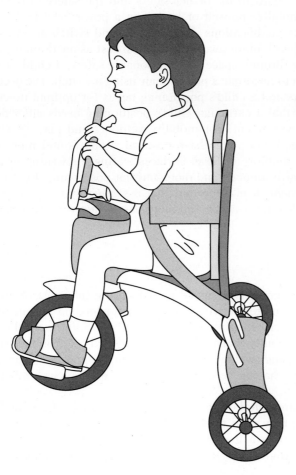

FIGURE 15.22 Adaptive tricycle provides back support, lateral trunk support, hip straps, abductors, foot straps, and horizontal bar to hold onto. Grasp on the original handle bar had encouraged shoulder elevation, internal rotation, elbow flexion, and ulnar deviation.

The therapist's role is to determine the tricycle measurements and provide appropriate supports for a particular child's sitting and mobility skills. Arm and hand positioning as well as lower extremity positioning should be assessed. The handlebars can be raised to encourage an upright trunk. Adapted vertical handgrips that place the forearm in a neutral rotation also encourage an erect trunk, provided there is forearm mobility. An appropriate seat height and abductor wedge can facilitate more neutral lower extremity alignment.

For individuals who do not have the mobility control to mobilize manual wheelchair functionally, a powered wheelchair can provide efficient and functional mobility. This is an important consideration for the nonambulator who finds a manual wheelchair painstakingly slow to propel and requiring excessive effort to move. To dispel a common myth, it is important to emphasize to the full team: parents, children, teachers, and other clinicians, that propelling a manual wheelchair is not a good exercise. The purpose of the wheelchair is mobility and if it is inefficient mobility, it is not assisting a child in participation. As long as a child demonstrates some understanding of awareness of space and judgment with regard to his or her safety and the safety of others, he or she has the potential to mobilize himself or herself in a power wheelchair. There is a wide range of electronics modifications and "joystick" and switch access devices to provide mobility to a child with more severe disabilities. Just as an 18-month-old child can direct his or her body through space with reasonable safety, a child of the same maturational age can learn to negotiate a power chair using a switch. The occupational therapist's role is to understand a child's positioning needs for optimal function. It is important to acknowledge that a particular child's positioning needs differ depending on the activity and the environment. For mobility outdoors and playing with his or her peers, a child may need more aggressive postural supports and more posterior positioning. However, for mobility on level surfaces, eating, or writing at a desk, a child may need less aggressive supports and more anterior positioning. Even for a child with more severe involvement, it is important that a seating system allows for easy modification to accommodate more active and more passive activities that make up an average child's day.

Ability to Feed

Positioning in a feeding program is designed to reduce the influence of low muscle or high muscle tone on oral motor activity. Positioning for feeding also involves minimizing situations that may trigger primitive reflexes and providing central stability to enhance controlled distal mobility (Larnet & Ekberg, 1995). This promotes skills such as sucking, biting, chewing, and swallowing. Vekerdy (2007) found significant improvement with feeding children having cerebral palsy using a thoracic lumbar support orthosis.

Tone can be modified through the choice of position and supports. A child who has very high or very low tone may need total support, such as that provided by reclined sitting or supine standing with a harness to provide shoulder control and thoracic support. A child who has slightly low tone may respond well to increased postural demands (e.g., a seat with low back support or a prone stander). In other cases, the best positioning device may be the therapist's body. The child who is positioned properly in an adult's lap benefits from physical warmth, touch, and social interaction, all of which may be the most effective therapy during his or her feeding.

For more involved individuals, head support may be needed to provide a stable base for jaw movements. A neutral or slightly flexed position of the neck contributes to controlled swallowing, reduces extensor hypertonicity, and prevents a child who has a disability from throwing his or her head back and "bird feeding." This is uncontrolled swallowing that uses gravity rather than musculature to get the food down. If the child has poor lip closure or lip pressure, keeping food in his or her mouth may be facilitated by a slight tipping back of his or her head. It is important that the neck not be extended. The appropriate position of the head can be accomplished by reclining the trunk partially and by bringing the head forward to an almost-righted position.

The head support should not contact the face to avoid a rooting reflex. Activation of the rooting reflex turns the child's head towards the source of food and also may initiate asymmetries because the turning of the head can produce asymmetrical tonic neck reflex activity.

Special attention should be paid to shoulder position during feeding. High tone in elevation, retraction, protraction, or humeral rotation can compromise swallowing and the coordination of swallowing with respiration.

Case Study: Paul

Paul is a 15-month-old boy who lives with his parents in a two-family home. His grandparents and extended family live next door. Paul receives home-based early intervention services. His speech therapist and OT requested a consult to evaluate for a seating device to support Paul at mealtime. Currently, mom feeds Paul as he sits on her lap.

Paul has full passive range of motion, but active movement of limbs is restricted by hypertonicity and poor postural stability. Head control is poor; he has difficulty righting his head. His neck is usually flexed forward and, in order to direct his gaze upward, he laterally flexes his neck, tipping his chin up. Lack of neck stability exacerbates poor oral motor control. Paul cannot sit independently and has no functional protective reactions. Given hip support, Paul sits with a kyphotic spine and can move his hands along the floor surface. His shoulders are held in elevation and retraction in the upright position so active range for reaching is limited. When supported at the trunk, he can bat at toys, occasionally making contact, but cannot maintain his arms in space without a surface beneath them. He can briefly sustain a gross grasp on a toy and bring it to his mouth. He cannot bring a bottle or direct a spoon to his mouth. While Paul can safely swallow soft food, the performance skills of biting, chewing, and swallowing are compromised. Mealtime is hard work for both Paul and his mom.

Meeting Paul's positioning needs for mealtime was relatively straightforward. An insert was constructed from triple-layer cardboard for his (previously unused) highchair. Paul's hips were positioned at 90 degrees of flexion and his pelvis was supported by a seatbelt at a 45-degree angle to his hips. The back of the insert was high enough to support his head. The insert was tipped back 5 degrees so that he would naturally rest his head against the seat back, avoiding his tendency to forward flex his neck. Lateral trunk and head supports were provided. The insert was elevated in the high chair so that the tray supported Paul's arms with his shoulders in 45 degrees of flexion; this support reduced the demands on his trunk and gave him a surface to support arm movements (Figure 15.23). Paul's mom was instructed to present food to him from an angle that encouraged him to slightly tuck his chin. Once the insert was properly fitted, Paul's direct service providers (OT and speech therapist) continued to address the activity demands, such as the properties of the tools used (type of spoon, plate, and cup), the sequence and timing of emerging hand-to-mouth skills, and the social demands of balancing the hard work of managing food with playful mealtime interaction between mom and Paul.

During the assessment, it became clear that Paul's engagement in occupation was restricted, inadvertently, not only by delayed performance skills, but also by habits, coping style, and cultural context. The biomechanical frame of reference, applied through a collaborative process with the family, could contribute to improved participation. When asked how Paul engaged himself when left unattended (i.e., how he moved independently and what toys/activities interested him), mom replied that he did not move on the floor because he was almost always being held by an adult, and that toys were always presented to him by another person. The advantage of having a loving and supportive extended family reduced the caregiving stressors that mom was subjected to, but unintentionally restricted Paul's development. There was tacit agreement in the family that Paul's role was that of a helpless infant who needed to be protected and made happy by more competent adults and children; there were minimal expectations for independence.

Paul's potential for developing motor skills necessary for play, self-care, and social participation was restricted by his lack of opportunity for independent movement. He needed time on the floor both to develop independent movement through space (rolling or crawling) and to develop shoulder stability/mobility in weight-bearing positions (prone) so that he could exercise more control of head and arm movements in an upright position. He also needed time in supported sitting to experiment with emerging manipulative skills and to engage in independent problem solving. Paul's distress in the prone position was disturbing to his family, so they rescued him to the comfort of their arms. The problem was addressed in two ways: (1) the prone position was made less stressful for Paul and (2) the relation between time in this position and Paul's success in self-feeding and play was explained to the family.

In this home, the presence of a prone lyer would have been offensive and unacceptable at this point in time. To introduce Paul to the prone position, he was given support with a small rolled towel. The ends of the towel were rolled inward to create lateral support to prevent him from rolling over into supine. Paul's first task was to tolerate this position and briefly right his head while socially engaged with a family member lying at his level (some family members needed their own rolled

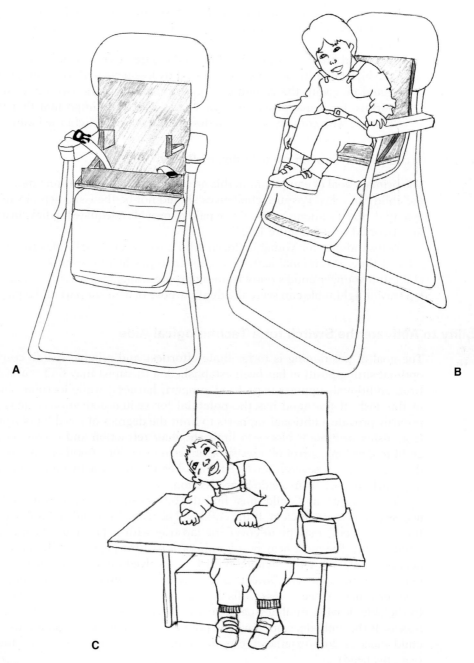

A

B

C

FIGURE 15.23 Paul's modified high chair contributes to oral motor control and emerging self-feeding skills (A and B). His adapted chair provides less support so that he can play with controlling lateral head and trunk movements (C).

up towels!). Again, the treating therapists, over time, addressed activity demands so that Paul could eventually play with toys in this position and develop crawling skills.

In addition, a cardboard chair and lap tray were provided. This was similar to the high chair insert but provided slightly less head and trunk support so that Paul could play with the demands of postural control. The lap tray provided a larger surface for age-appropriate toys. It was especially important that the chair was covered with contact paper of a design that would delight the family.

Ability to Void When Seated on a Toilet or Potty

The primary goal of equipment in this area is to provide support and modify tone so that the child can relax. Postural challenges should not be the issue here, instead comfort is essential. Special attention should be paid to provide adequate hip flexion and abduction in supported sitting (Figure 15.24).

Potty training for young children who have severe disabilities frequently requires a lot of time. Diversional activities are sometimes helpful to motivate and engage the child. If a younger child's potty training program includes diversional activities, then a lap tray or light table can serve the dual purpose of arm support and a play surface.

Ability to Activate the Switch for a Technological Aide

The goal of positioning is to facilitate effortless and reliable switch control. Once an optimal sitting position has been established, a therapist may find that a child benefits from additional supports (e.g., head support, harness) while learning the refinements of this task. If the hand has the potential for switch activation, it may help to temporarily provide additional supports to limit the degrees of freedom of arm movements (e.g., using protractor blocks to limit shoulder retraction and extension to enable the child to develop control of a wrist or finger movement). Another way to reduce motor demands when a severely involved child begins switch activation training may be to approach the task from a side lying position.

The therapist and child must find the best position in space for the switch, where access to it is most efficient. If the child will be using his hand, a graphic way to identify this "sweet spot" may be to cover the lap tray with paper and attach a marker to the child's hand. The most heavily colored portion of the paper usually represents the most accessible place for the switch. With less involved children, clinical observation can determine this spot. The "sweet spot" may be at midline for some children and to the side for others. Once access skills emerge, it is good to gradually move the switch off to the side, leaving midline space for the placement of other activities and table/desk access. If the child does not have the potential to use his or her hand, the therapist and child must explore together the options for a reliable movement in other body parts (e.g., the head).

Switches with a multitude of characteristics are available commercially (Weiss, 1990). If the child can control more than a single movement, he or she has potential to access more standard switches such as joysticks and keyboards. These tend to be more

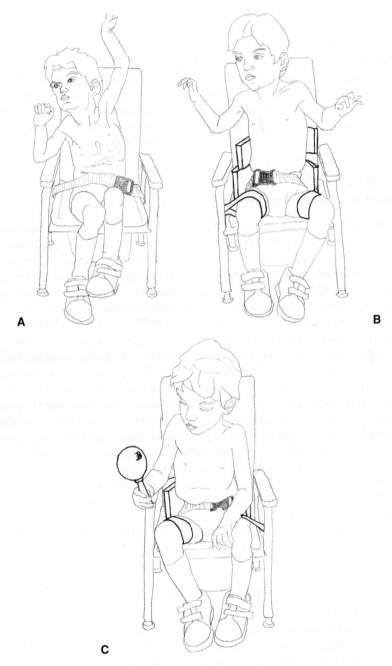

FIGURE 15.24 (**A**)., Child in commercially available adapted potty with seat belt. (**B**)., Child sitting with additional control facilitated by lateral trunk supports, hip guides, and abductor straps (*dark lines*). (**C**)., Relaxation is enhanced by the use of an activity.

efficient switch methods. If a child cannot efficiently operate a standard or modified joystick or keyboard, the therapist must find a match between the child's motor ability and the type of switch, in terms of force and speed needed, the distance traversed to activate/deactivate, and the cognitive/perceptual components to plan coded sequences of single movements (such as the attention and discrimination necessary to select one word from a vocabulary of hundreds on a communication device).

If the child has an adequate agonist musculature to activate a switch but inadequate antagonist to release it (or a similar scenario), the switch can be placed in a gravity eliminated position to facilitate the weaker movement. There is an array of hardware available to position switches to accomplish this.

Summary of Application to Practice

The last part of this chapter has addressed the more technical aspects of the biomechanical frame of reference for positioning children for functioning (i.e., the practical problems of translating a therapeutic intention into a piece of equipment). This process requires some mechanical skills and an ability to manipulate three-dimensional space mentally. Although it is only one component of treatment implementation, the actual prescription or design of equipment often makes the greater demands on the novice therapist. Frequent hazards involved in this process include that concentration becomes too focused on the product (i.e., adaptive device) and various other factors that enhance posture and function are overlooked. With this rapidly changing technology, it is easy to get caught up in particular devices and difficult to stay current on updated products and reimbursement trends. Long, Woolverton, Perry, & Thomas (2007) reported on a national survey of 272 pediatric therapists, who responded to questions about their training needs in assistive technology service delivery. These therapists identified a significant need for additional training in funding for assistive technology products, collaboration with families and other service providers, and accessing knowledgeable vendors. The novice therapist should be reminded that his or her role is to "know" the child and his or her positioning needs for function and articulate those specifications to a vendor. The vendor can then assist with his or her knowledge of the pros and cons of various products and product selection.

The following story illuminates some of the difficult decisions that a team needs to make in prioritizing goals and interventions when applying the biomechanical frame of reference.

Case Study: Ivan by Debra Fishers

Ivan is a 6-year-old kindergartener with cerebral palsy who attends school in a fully inclusive classroom. He has age-appropriate receptive language skills and impaired articulation and expressive language skills. He is beginning to use a communication device that produces synthesized speech. He rarely initiates interaction with his peers, but responds to their overtures. He enjoys being a part of their imaginative play and, when alone, prefers to explore the sensory aspects of toys and media. Engagement in construction and writing activities is restricted by fine motor impairments. However, he uses a keyboard to participate in classroom literacy activities.

Ivan has full passive range of motion but hypertonicity limits functional range of his arms and legs. He has fair head and trunk control with delayed protective and equilibrium reactions in sitting. When sitting unsupported, functional use of his arms is limited to the midranges, with no control of the forearm and wrist movements necessary to position hands and objects for optimal exploration. Without external trunk support, Ivan cannot use both hands simultaneously. He is unable to transfer from chair to floor, but can creep slowly and walk with effort using a walker.

As a student in an integrated classroom, Ivan's requirements for postural support serve a different purpose than they might in a clinical setting, or in a classroom for children with physical impairments, or at home. In a different setting, Ivan's motor development may take priority and equipment may be provided primarily to address motor skills. His "menu" of daily interventions might include a scooter board to support development of neck and upper back extension, stability and mobility of the shoulder girdle, and rapid independent movement through space; a prone lyer; a seating device to support him during floor activities (such as carpet time), consistent use of an adapted chair that supports optimal posture and hand control, and use of his walker within the classroom (Figure 15.25).

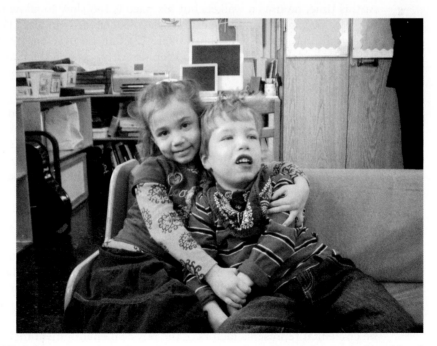

FIGURE 15.25 Ivan much prefers a hug to sitting in his adapted chair. (His friend has borrowed his seating wedge.)

However, in the culture of Ivan's classroom, full participation in academic tasks with his peers is a priority. The selection of appropriate equipment is made in collaboration with his teachers; their input is essential in determining a match between educational goals and Ivan's equipment. In this context, communication/interaction skills take priority over motor skills. It is essential that Ivan be available for all instruction, that he transition from one activity to another fluidly with his classmates, and that he not be physically isolated by his equipment. When he needs physical support, Ivan relies on the assistance of paraprofessionals rather than equipment. For use when keyboarding, Ivan uses a properly fitting chair with a seatbelt; that is the extent of adaptive positioning. In choosing this educational setting, Ivan's family recognizes that his routines at home will need to include more intensive attention to motor skills and more time for Ivan to practice independence with movement, including positioning equipment that supports these goals.

Prioritizing for a student with greater than average physical needs looks different in every classroom. Some classroom cultures emphasize the acceptance of differences, allotting time for physically challenged children to practice motor independence at the expense of total participation in the academic schedule. Others, such as Ivan's, emphasize full participation in the flow of classroom activities (both social and academic) as well as helping relationships over physical independence.

One area that has not yet been addressed for Ivan is his mobility at recess. At this time, he uses a walker, but his pace is too slow to allow him to be a part of active peer play. Future questions to consider for Ivan are: (1) Can he develop more skill and speed with the walker? (2) Can he develop the skill to propel a manual wheelchair fast enough to keep up with peers on the playground? (3) Can he develop the skill to control a powered wheelchair safely during play? This is a critical component of Ivan's development as yet unexplored.

The diagram in Figure 15.26 illustrates an approach to postural control that is more complete than a simple device to support the child. It should be viewed as a series of "excentric" rather than concentric circles with the supportive device in the center. The circles widen to demonstrate a more holistic approach to biomechanical intervention. As the circles grow from the center, the factors produce effects on posture and function that are less direct and specific but that are greater in scope.

The first, smallest circle represents the most direct approach: the child in the supportive device which is the "hardware" that taxes the therapist's mechanical and spatial skills. The next circle includes the physiological reactions that modulate posture (e.g., reactions to tactile cues provided by the equipment or reactions to changes in head or body position in space). The next circle represents effort—the amount of work the child must do to stay upright and interact with his or her environment. Too much effort may cause fatigue or frustration; too little effort may limit the potential for growth and change.

The circle that represents factors of the physical environment includes those things that influence levels of arousal, attention, and tone and indirectly enhance or disrupt

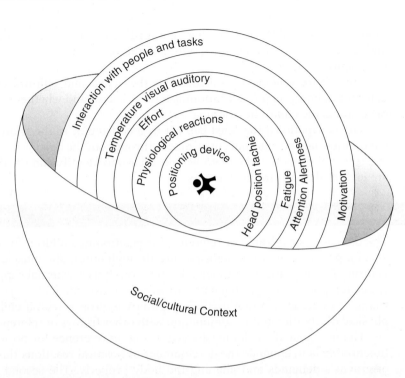

FIGURE 15.26 Diagram presenting an approach to postural control which is more complete than a device that merely supports the child.

postural reactions. Temperature can be changed to enhance posture by altering the heat in the room, adding or removing layers of clothing, or providing close physical contact between the child and another person. The position of visual cues may affect how the child holds his or her head, with resultant changes in tone and posture. The element of motion with visual stimulation can enhance attention or increase fatigue, depending on the child's head control and ocular motor skills. For example, practical implications include where the teacher stands or sits in relation to the child and whether the instructor moves about as he and she speaks. Another aspect of this circle is auditory stimulation. Background noise and changes in volume or tempo of voice or music enhance alertness, elicit dysfunctional startle responses, or cause a child to "shut down," depending on the person. These factors and many others in the physical environment have a subtle yet cumulative impact on posture and function and should be incorporated into the therapist's treatment plan.

The outermost circle encompasses opportunities for interaction with people and objects. Although this appears to be the least direct channel to modify posture and function, changes often include observable phenomena. For example, significant improvement in posture may be noted when a child is drawn into a song made up about himself or herself and his or her friends or when the child is given the opportunity to apply finger paint to his or her therapist's face. Interaction with people, animals, and materials and the associated senses of mastery and self-esteem represent goals and therapeutic tools.

This entire schema is embedded in the social and cultural environment, which determines how and if the positioning device is used and whether it ultimately supports or restrains the child's functioning.

The occupational therapist can act as a consultant to the team to help modify the child's internal and external environment throughout the day. As part of the biomechanical frame of reference, the therapist must learn to identify and use the many forces that are greater than the force of gravity.

Summary

The biomechanical frame of reference for positioning children for functioning is used when a person cannot maintain posture through automatic muscle activity because of neuromuscular or musculoskeletal dysfunction. It uses external supports or equipment, either temporarily or permanently, to substitute for the lack of postural control. The frame of reference is often used as a primary approach with a child exhibiting severe physical disabilities and in conjunction with other frames of reference.

The first goal of the biomechanical frame of reference for positioning children for functioning is to enhance the development of postural reactions through the reduction of gravity's demands and aligning the body properly. The second goal is to improve functional performance through the use of external supports, reducing the need for and demands in postural reactions and compensatory movements. An understanding of this frame of reference is dependent on a thorough understanding of the typical sequence of development. This frame of reference is the first approach. However, it is not used in a vacuum or at the expense of function. If function is possible using more pronounced asymmetrical postures and compensatory movements, that function should be permitted and encouraged for independent activity performance. That being said, the secondary sequelae (deformity and contractures) that are associated with a dominant asymmetry must be addressed through therapy and a home exercise program to minimize the potential for deformity and to promote symmetrical muscle length and postures.

Function–dysfunction continua include measures of central stability incorporating range of motion, head control, and trunk control and functional skills that incorporate control of head and arm movements, mobility, feeding, and toileting.

Application to practice involves the translation of therapeutic intentions into equipment that enhances posture and function. Through the use of "hardware," posture and central stability can be enhanced to enable the child to engage in functional activities and more actively participate in his or her home, school, and community environments. That is the goal of this intervention and this, in turn, will allow for continued development, functional gains, and participation.

ACKNOWLEDGMENTS

The authors wish to thank Cheryl Cowart for Stephanie's case study Debra Fishers for Ivan's case study and the Brunini family and Anthony Sicuranza for assistance in providing photographs. We also thank the clients at Kessler Institute for Rehabilitation for their cooperation and assistance with providing photographs for this chapter.

REFERENCES

Barnes, K. J. (1991). Modification of the physical environment. In C. Christiansen, & C. Baum (Eds). *Occupational Therapy: Overcoming Human Performance Deficits* (pp. 701–745). Thorofare, NJ: Slack Inc.

Batavia, M. (1998). *The Wheelchair Evaluation: A Practical Guide*. Boston, MA: Butterworth-Heinermann.

Bergen, A., & Colangelo, C. (1985). *Positioning the Client with Central Nervous System Deficits*. Valhalla, NY: Valhalla Rehabilitation Publications.

Blair, E., Ballantyne, J., Horseman, S., & Chauvel, P. (1995). A study of a dynamic proximal stability splint in the management of children with cerebral palsy. *Developmental Medicine and Child Neurology, 37*(6), 544–554.

Bly, L. (1994). *Motor Skill Acquisition in the First Year*. Tucson, AZ: Therapy Skill Builders.

Boehme, R. (1998). *Improving Upper Body Control*. Tucson, AZ: Therapy Skill Builders.

Brogren, E., Hadders-Algra, M., & Forssberg, H. (1996). Postural control in children with spastic diplegia: Muscle activity during perturbations in sitting. *Developmental Medicine and Child Neurology, 38*(5), 379–388.

Clarke, A. M., & Redden, J. F. (1992). Management of hip posture in cerebral palsy. *Journal of the Royal Society of Medicine, 85*(3), 150–151.

Colbert, A. P., Doyle, K. M., & Webb, W. E. (1986). DESEMO seats for young children with cerebral palsy. *Archives of Physical Medicine Rehabilitation, 67*(7), 484–486.

Cook, A. M., & Polgar, J. M. (2008). *Cook and Hussey's Assistive Technologies: Principles and Practice*. St. Louis, MO: Mosby, Elsevier Science.

Fernandes, T. (2006). Independent mobility for children with disabilities. *International Journal of Therapy and Rehabilitation, 13*(7), 329–333.

Fiorentino, M. (1981). *A Basis for Sensorimotor Development-Normal and Abnormal*. Springfield, IL: Charles C Thomas Publisher.

Green, E. M., Mulcahy, C. M., & Pountney, T. E. (1995). An investigation into the development of early postural control. *Developmental Medicine and Child Neurology, 37*(5), 437–448.

Green, E. M., & Nelham, R. L. (1991). Development of sitting ability, assessment of children with a motor handicap and prescription of appropriate seating systems. *Prosthetics and Orthotics International, 15*(3), 203–216.

Hadders-Algra, M., Brogren, E., & Forssberg, H. (1996). Training affects the development of postural adjustments in sitting infants. *Journal of Physiology, 493*(Pt 1), 289–298.

Hadders-Algra, M., Brogren, E., & Forssberg, H. (1996a). Ontogeny of postural adjustments during sitting in infancy: Variation, selection and modulation. *Journal of Physiology, 493*(Pt 1), 273–288.

Hadders-Algra, M., van der Fits, I. B., Stremmelaar, E. F., & Touwen, B. C. (1999). Development of postural adjustments during reaching in infants with CP. *Developmental Medicine and Child Neurology, 41*(11), 766–776.

Heller, K. D., Forst, R., & Hengtler, K. (1997). Scoliosis in Duchenne muscular dystrophy. *Prosthetic Orthotic International, 21*(3), 202–209.

Holms, K. J., Michael, S. M., & Solomonidis, S. E. (2003). Management of scoliosis with special seating for the non-ambulant spastic cerebral palsy population—a biomechanical study. *Clinical Biomechanics, 18*(6), 480–487.

Howard, S. B., Boyd, R. N., Reidt, S. M., Lanigan, A., Wolfe, R., Reddihough, D., & Graham, H. K. (2006). Hip displacement in cerebral palsy. _Journal of Bone Joint Surgery American, 88_(1), 121–129.

Hulme, J. B., Gallacher, K., Walsh, J., Niesen, S., & Waldron, D. (1987). Behavioral and postural changes observed with use of adaptive seating by clients with multiple handicaps. _Physical Therapy, 67_(7), 1060–1067.

Larnet, G., & Ekberg, O. (1995). Positioning improves the oral and pharyngeal swallowing function in children with cerebral palsy. _Acta Paediatric, 8_(6), 689–692.

Long, T. M., Woolverton, M., Perry, D. F., & Thomas, M. J. (2007). Training needs of pediatric occupational therapists in assistive technology. _American Journal of Occupational Therapy, 61_, 345–354.

Manley, M. T., & Gurtowski, E. (1985). The vertical wheeler: A device for ambulation in cerebral palsy. _Archives of Physical Medicine Rehabilitation, 66_(10), 717–720.

Manolikakis, G. (1992). Individual care of adduction contractures and threatening paralytic hip dislocations in cerebral palsy using sitting and lying expanding casts. _Orthopedic Technique, 43_, 810–815.

McClenaghan, B. A., Thombs, L., & Milner, M. (1992). Effects of seat surface inclination on postural stability and function of the upper extremities of children with cerebral palsy. _Developmental Medicine and Child Neurology, 34_(1), 40–48.

McDonald, R., Surtees, R., & Wirz, S. (2003). A comparison between parents' and therapists' views of their child's individual seating systems. _International Journal of Rehabilitation Research, 26_(3), 235–243.

Miedaner, J., & Finuf, I. (1993). Effects of adaptive positioning on psychological test scores for pre-school children with cerebral palsy. _Pediatric Physical Therapy, 5_(4), 177–182.

Motloch, W. M., & Brearley, M. N. (1983). Technical note—a patient propelled variable-inclination prone stander. _Prosthetic Orthotics International, 7_(3), 176–177.

Myhr, U., & von Wendt, L. (1991). Improvement of functional sitting position for children with cerebral palsy. _Developmental Medicine and Child Neurology, 33_(3), 246–256.

Myhr, U., von Wendt, L., Norrlin, S., & Randell, U. (1995). Five year follow-up of functional sitting position in children with cerebral palsy. _Developmental Medicine and Child Neurology, 37_(7), 587–596.

Noronha, J., Bundy, A., & Groll, J. (1989). The effect of positioning on the hand function of boys with cerebral palsy. _American Journal of Occupational Therapy, 43_, 504–512.

Nwaobi, O. M. (1987). Seating orientations and upper extremity function in children with cerebral palsy. _Physical Therapy, 67_(8), 1209–1212.

Nwaobi, O., & Smith, P. (1986). Effect of adaptive seating on pulmonary function of children with cerebral palsy. _Developmental Medicine and Child Neurology, 28_(3), 351–354.

Pope, P. M., Bowes, C. E., & Booth, E. (1994). Postural control in sitting. The SAM system: evaluation of use over three years. _Developmental Medicine and Child Neurology, 36_(3), 241–252.

Reid, D. J. (1996). The effects of the saddle seat on seated postural control and upper extremity movement in children with cerebral palsy. _Developmental Medicine and Child Neurology, 38_(9), 805–815.

Reid, D. T. (2002). Critical review of the research literature of seating interventions focusing on adults with mobility impairments. _Assistive Technology, 14_(2), 118–129.

Reid, D. T., & Rigby, P. (1996). Towards improving anterior pelvic stabilization devices for pediatric wheelchair users with cerebral palsy. _Canadian Journal of Rehabilitation, 9_, 147–158.

Reid, D. T., Rigby, P., & Ryan, S. (1999). Functional impact of a rigid pelvic stabilizer on children with cerebral palsy who use wheelchairs: Users' and caregivers' perceptions. _Journal of Pediatric Rehabilitation, 3_(3), 101–118.

Richardson, P. K. (1996). Use of standardized tests in pediatric practice. In J. Case-Smith, A. S. Allen, & P. N. Pratt (Eds). _Occupational Therapy for Children_ (pp. 200–224). St. Louis, MO: Mosby.

Rigby, P., Reid, D., Schoger, S., & Ryan, S. (2002). Effects of a wheelchair-mounted rigid pelvic stabilizer on caregiver assistance for children with cerebral palsy. _Assistive Technology, 13_(1), 2–11.

Rothstein, J. M. (2005). _The Rehabilitation Specialist's Handbook_. Philadelphia, PA: FA Davis Co.

Ryan, S., Snider-Riczker, P., & Rigby, P. (2005). Community-based performance of a pelvic stabilization device for children with cerebral palsy. _Assistive Technology, 17_(1), 37–46.

Scherzer, A., & Tscharnuter, I. (1982). _Early Diagnosis and Therapy in Cerebral Palsy_. New York: Marcel Dekker Inc.

Scherzer, A., & Tscharnuter, I. (1990). _Early Diagnosis and Therapy in Cerebral Palsy_ (2nd ed.). New York: Marcel Dekker Inc.

Scrutton, D. (1991). The causes of developmental deformity and their implication for seating. _Prosthetic Orthotic International, 15_(3), 199–202.

Shoham, Y., Meyer, S., Katz-Laurer, M. et al (2004). The influence of seat adjustment and a thoracic lumbar sacral orthosis on the distribution of body seat pressure in children with scoliosis and pelvic obliquity. *Disability Rehabilitation, 26,* 21–26.

Stockmeyer, S. (1967). An interpretation of the approach of Rood to the treatment of neuromuscular dysfunction. *American Journal of Physical Medicine, 46*(1), 900–956.

Trefler, E., Hobson, D., Taylor, S., Monahan, L., & Shaw, G. (1993). *Seating and Mobility for Persons with Disabilities.* Tucson, AZ: Therapy Skill Builders.

Vekerdy, Z. (2007). Management of seating posture of children with cerebral palsy by using thoracic-lumbar-sacral orthosis with non-rigid SIDO frame. *Disability and Rehabilitation, 29*(18), 1434–1441.

Weiss, P. L. (1990). Mechanical characteristics of micro-switches adapted for the physical disabled. *Journal of Biomedical Engineering, 12*(5), 398–402.

Issues When Applying Frames of Reference

CHAPTER 16

Frames of Reference in the Real World

JIM HINOJOSA • PAULA KRAMER

This chapter discusses the importance of appropriately using frames of reference in clinical practice. The first section focuses on understanding a frame of reference so that a therapist can articulate it clearly when treating a patient. In the second section, the art of practice with children—emphasizing therapeutic relationships—is covered.

ARTICULATING THE FRAME OF REFERENCE

When entry-level occupational therapists or occupational therapy students are asked to explain why they are doing a particular activity with a child, some common responses are "I'm not sure," "It was just intuition", "I know why, but I just can't put it into words," "I saw another therapist do it, and it worked well," or "I was taught this in school, and my instructor said it works well." It is uncomfortable oftentimes to respond quickly to such a complex question. As professionals, however, therapists must understand what they are doing and why they are doing it. They also need to be able to explain this rationale to patients, observers, other professionals, and especially parents.

In a recent clinical experience, for instance, an occupational therapy fieldwork student was asked to explain what she would do during a treatment session. She stated that she intended to play with the child because the child would benefit from all types of stimulation. This response indicated a lack of understanding about the child's individual needs and also a lack of clearly articulated goals. Furthermore, this suggests that the intervention was not thoroughly planned or probably not based in theory. Subsequently, any response or reaction from the child during this treatment situation could not be explained from a theoretical perspective.

In this example, the student's lack of understanding or inability to articulate a rationale for intervention may have resulted from a theoretical perspective that has not been clearly identified or understood. This student has predetermined that the child will benefit from any sensory stimulation but has not stated specific problem areas or expected responses from the child. But interventions cannot be viewed in such a simplistic way. They are step-by-step approaches geared toward addressing problem areas while providing a well-thought-out activity designed to bring about change. The appropriate structure for developing this organized, systematic approach to intervention is the frame of reference. The above-mentioned occupational therapy student may have had a clear idea of what her goals were, but without the structure of the frame of reference her intervention appears to have no theoretical basis for treatment. Furthermore, based on her intervention, she would have difficulty measuring change without this theoretical structure.

In another situation, an occupational therapy student was asked to explain why she placed a child (who had cerebral palsy) in a prone position on an adapted scooter board. She answered that it seemed like the right position. When the instructor asked for further clarification of what theoretical framework the student was using, the student was able to explain that this developmentally appropriate position facilitated the child's exploration of the environment. She said she was using the biomechanical frame of reference to allow the child to interact with and learn from his surrounding environment. Although her first response indicates her initial intuition, when pressed for details, the student was able to demonstrate a theoretical understanding of the intervention. What students and therapists often call intuition often is actually based on sound knowledge.

When occupational therapy students or therapists respond that their actions are based on intuition, they are not acknowledging their bases of learning. Sometimes, students and therapists do not appreciate what they have learned during their professional education, so they see their actions as being intuitive. For whatever reason, it is difficult to articulate a theoretical rationale for their actions when prompted. Identification of a frame of reference (which is grounded in theory) again allows a therapist to clearly cite his or her knowledge base and rationale for treatments.

Therapists can undermine their interventions by giving simplistic reasons for the work they do with children. Much of occupational therapy practice looks like play to a casual observer. When a therapist says that she is playing with a child to "provide stimulation," the response of the casual observer might be that anyone can play with a child and do the same thing. But when that therapist acknowledges that she is working from a theoretical base, she is able to show that play designed to provide specific stimulation is really a highly skilled and well-thought-out intervention plan designed to bring about targeted responses. The purpose of the frame of reference is to provide this blueprint for use in practice.

When therapists are asked what frame of reference they use most, some may respond, "I'm eclectic." In this case, the therapist has not identified from which of the various frames of reference her interventions are based. The therapist may not have a thoroughly constructed plan. She may not be using a frame of reference or may not have an understanding of the appropriate theoretical rationale necessary to bring about change. This therapist bases her interventions on various sources without synthesizing them into a focused frame of reference.

If a therapist randomly picks and chooses concepts, postulates, and techniques from many different approaches without concern for theoretical consistency, then specific outcomes cannot be anticipated. The base of a frame of reference is built upon theories that agree with each other and that present a unified, consistent approach to the change process. A frame of reference delineates what outcomes are to be expected from each specified intervention. The statement "I'm eclectic" lacks a theory-based intervention.

Just as a physician should not prescribe medication without knowing its possible consequences, a therapist should not use a procedure without understanding its potential effects. On the basis of a child's presenting problems, a therapist selects a frame of reference to specify changes or outcomes that she or he would like to promote. Techniques or procedures not derived from a frame of reference do not usually lead to an organized change that can be explained. At times, a misunderstood procedure can have consequences similar to a misused medication, such as when a neurophysiological technique like vestibular stimulation is used without a clear rationale for an expected response. To use vestibular stimulation without an understanding of the sensory integration frame of reference may result in an inappropriate behavioral response or a more severe central nervous system reaction.

Finally, because occupational therapy is concerned with and uses routine daily activities as the focus for interventions, it may appear to lack the scientific, empirical, and procedural bases used in other professions as "therapeutic." Because occupational therapy with children is activity oriented and often uses play, it is crucial that the therapeutic value of chosen activities is readily explainable. Therapists need to be able to explain that what they are doing is not just playing for the sake of fun, but focused activities for a purpose. Frames of reference provide the appropriate scientific and theoretical bases that explain the complexity of the activities used during the intervention process. What appears to be simple usually has complex theoretical underpinnings that are clarified for a therapist through the frame of reference, which brings the theories to a level at which they can be applied.

THE ART OF PRACTICE WITH CHILDREN

Earlier chapters in this book presented specific frames of reference that are important in current pediatric practice. Working with children effectively involves more than just knowing about and understanding frames of reference; it requires the ability to put them into practice effectively. Other occupational therapists have discussed and highlighted the "art of practice" in a global way as it applies to the entire profession (Crepeau, 1991; Gilfoyle, 1980; Mosey, 1981a,b; Peloquin, 1989, 1990, 2002). For example, Mosey presents the art of practice in a broad perspective as part of the philosophical origins of occupational therapy (Mosey, 1981a). The authors of this chapter intend to discuss it in a much more specific way as it relates to children and to the implementation of frames of reference.

Working with children presents interesting challenges that are different from those found while working with adults. Children are not miniature adults. They need to be approached in a way that is meaningful to them. But like adults, children have thoughts and feelings that must be taken into consideration, although they may not be able to express them.

The therapeutic relationship is an interactive process between therapist and child. The goal is to effectively assist the promotion of positive change within the child. It does not, however, necessarily involve an equal participation of therapist and child. It is the therapist's responsibility to establish the tone of the relationship. He or she guides the relationship, and, to some extent, manipulates it to the child's benefit. Initially, it is important to engage the child, get to know him or her, and involve him or her in the intervention process. The therapist often acts as a stimulator or cheerleader, a provoker of responses. At other times, the therapist must be more relaxed and give comfort.

For an occupational therapist, to fully engage a child in effective intervention is the essence of artful practice. Unlike most adults, children may not necessarily see therapy as beneficial. The art of occupational therapy involves captivating a child through toys, objects, games, or through the therapist's own actions so that the child becomes involved in the therapeutic process. This art is almost intangible and, therefore, difficult to describe. It is more than a skill; it is a mix of creativity, enthusiasm, an ability to choose objects based on a firm foundation of knowledge, and the use of the self in a way that engages a child so that a relationship can be developed and intervention can promote growth. The "trick" is to appreciate that the child must be dealt with as a whole person, not as component parts or as an aspect of an occupational performance area. This must be done with each child individually because each child is a unique human being.

The therapeutic relationship is important to the intervention process in any frame of reference. In some cases, it may be addressed specifically in the change process of the theoretical base. However, in many cases, it is not discussed at all. In specific frames of reference in which it is addressed, a particular type of relationship may exist that helps foster development. For example, in the sensory integrative frame of reference (as presented in Chapter 6) the therapist takes an active part in treatment and needs to playfully engage with a child. At the same time, he or she must allow the child to be self-directed to an extent in the treatment setting. In those situations in which the therapeutic relationship is not discussed, it is incumbent upon the therapist to formulate a relationship that promotes growth and change and is also consistent in that frame of reference. As discussed here, the art of practice relates broadly to all frames of reference.

Many characteristics color an effective therapeutic relationship. Perlman (1979) describes some of these characteristics as warmth, acceptance, caring/concern, and genuineness. Mosey (1981a) adds sympathy and empathy to this list. It often is difficult to describe a therapeutic relationship because its uniqueness depends on its special components—the therapist and the child. It is an emotional experience based on feelings and interactions. The relationship involves not only sympathy but also empathy. Sympathy occurs when people share common feelings that often involve commiseration. Empathy involves the projection of one's personality onto another in an effort to understand the feelings, emotions, and thoughts of the other. Often, especially with entry-level therapists, sympathy is a strong initial part of the therapeutic relationship. It is important, however, to move on to the point at which the therapist can be empathetic because it is empathy that assists her or him in being more effective during interactions with the child.

Unconditional acceptance is also an essential aspect of the relationship between therapist and child. The therapist accepts the child and his or her abilities as is. This precludes a judgmental attitude about the child and his or her lifestyle. Granted, the role of the therapist is to develop the strengths of children and to remediate or minimize their deficits. Therapists should not, though, base their abilities to care and interact on what the child is able to do or how he or she progresses. When children cannot do particular tasks or have experienced previous failures, they are less likely to try that activity again. The therapist needs to let the child know that the attempt to do something is more important than completing the entire activity itself, that making an attempt is more important than succeeding.

The manner in which an occupational therapist uses the legitimate tools of the profession is another part of the art of practice. As adapted by the therapist, the nonhuman environment becomes a component in practice. Some frames of reference delineate this therapeutic nonhuman environment. For example, the biomechanical frame of reference for positioning children for functioning (as presented in Chapter 15) describes the use of specific equipment to promote positive change as part of the nonhuman environment.

Other frames of reference do not address the specific environment, but may make implications about or give guidelines for effective types of environments. To use any frame of reference effectively as presented in this book, a therapist must create a safe therapeutic environment. To raise this legitimate tool to the level of art, the therapist must use understanding of the frame, along with creativity, to manipulate the environment so that it effectively engages the child and promotes improvement.

Time and experience are needed to develop the art of practice. It is not something that can be presumed of an entry-level therapist, although, like with painters or musicians, some therapists have an innate talent for it. The art of practice is not just skilled application of the frames of reference; rather, it is a combination of knowledge, self-confidence, self-understanding, self-acceptance, and awareness. It is hoped that new generations of entry-level therapists will become actively involved in exploring this process to become artful practitioners.

ALTERNATIVE APPLICATION OF FRAMES OF REFERENCE

Effective practice involves a therapist's ability to match a client with the most appropriate frame of reference within the context of his or her life. After a patient is referred to occupational therapy, the therapist does a preliminary screening. This helps determine the appropriate frame of reference to use, and thereby, the evaluation tools that should be used for the particular client. Sometimes, this can be one specific frame of reference, but at other times, one is not adequate enough to deal with the complexity of problems presented by the child or family. In this section, alternative ways that frames of reference can be applied are discussed, including the use of frames alone, in sequence, in parallel, and/or in combination. Additionally, the chapter discusses the development of new and unique frames of reference.

Single Frame of Reference

To be comfortable with and understand how to use frames of reference, the entry-level therapist must first work with one at a time. An important distinction should be made here: the therapist does not use only one frame of reference with all clients. For instance, with any given child, an entry-level therapist must first concentrate on the one frame of reference that fits that particular child's needs. With another child, that same therapist may need to use another frame of reference that is more suitable.

Entry-level therapists are often not fluent with theories relevant to pediatric practice. In the clinic, their primary concern is rightly how to help the child. This concern tends to focus them on what they are doing rather than on the reasons why—that is, whether the practice is (or is not) effective. To become truly competent, however, novice therapists must take time to familiarize themselves with all aspects of the frame of reference. To do this, they almost always have to start by using one frame with each client. As discussed in Chapter 1, the frame provides a blueprint for practice based on theoretical material.

When a therapist begins to use a frame of reference, he or she should first become comfortable with the entire frame by concentrating on its theoretical base. Once this is clearly understood, then the other sections of the frame (function–dysfunction continua, evaluation, postulates regarding change, and application to practice) are easier to grasp. The theoretical base, therefore, holds the key to understanding the important concepts for intervention. Assumptions are also stated in that section, and the significant relationships between concepts and postulates are presented and described. The function–dysfunction continua, evaluation, postulates regarding change, and application to practice all flow from the theoretical base.

By studying one frame of reference at a time, a therapist can become comfortable with the theoretical material and its transition into application. In understanding this material, the therapist develops the ability to use each function–dysfunction continuum systematically as a means to identify a child's strengths and limitations. On the basis of findings relative to the continua, the therapist then can determine what areas (if any) require intervention. Intervention is applied sequentially, using the postulates regarding change to practice, as illustrated in the application. At this point, the therapist creates an environment to bring about a desired response from the child. This empirical approach to intervention based on theory differentiates the skilled, competent professional from the highly technical practitioner. The skilled, competent professional bases the intervention on a firm theoretical base that allows for careful evaluation of the intervention process and its efficacy.

When one frame of reference is used properly (as outlined in this text) consistency in the intervention is ensured. Concepts and postulates as well as postulates regarding change agree, and consistency in that one segment flows from the other. As long as the therapist works with one frame, all actions agree and the theoretical principles and the application to intervention are congruent. This consistency could not be achieved if a therapist took only one concept or postulate from one section and then proceeded on to application. For example, in the Neuro-Developmental frame of reference, handling is a major concept. By itself, handling does not comprise the entire frame. If the therapist uses handling without the other therapeutic constructs from the theoretical base or the postulates regarding change, it is just a technique and not a sound way to apply the Neuro-Developmental Treatment frame of reference.

It is important to note that when only one frame of reference is used, it ensures that concepts and postulates and also postulates regarding change are all consistent and that the end result will be a more cogent intervention process. If, during the course of the intervention, the therapist notices that something is not working, then he or she can go back to the frame, the theoretical base, postulates regarding change, and the application to practice sections. These should provide some insight for modifying the plan for intervention.

Once a therapist becomes competent in using a frame of reference and has a thorough understanding of its application, he or she may tend to use it exclusively with all children. Unfortunately, this will deter the therapist from deciding on an individual basis which frame is most appropriate for each client. At times, such exclusivity could create a certain "tunnel vision"—that is, the therapist may come to believe that the one frame of reference is superior to all others. In this case, he or she may identify with that frame and begin to refer to himself or herself as a "neurodevelopmental therapist" or a "sensory integration therapist," for instance, instead of an occupational therapist. When this occurs, the therapist may be overlooking the individual needs of the child and instead be working from a strong belief dedicated to one specific frame of reference. The dangers of this are twofold: (1) a child may not receive intervention that meets his or her needs, and (2) therapists may not recognize the extent of their knowledge bases in terms of other frames of reference. This may preclude any chance of meeting the clients' needs.

Multiple Frames of Reference

In the real world, many children cannot have their needs met during an intervention with only one frame of reference. The problems children face often are more complex than those of "paper patients" (i.e., the classic textbook case). It would be easier if one frame of reference could address all the problems of a particular child, but in reality frames are limited by the scope of their theoretical bases. For example, in the sensory integrative frame of reference, activities of daily living (ADL) are not addressed comprehensively in the theoretical base. The theoretical base for sensory integration suggests that when a child has developed integrative abilities, he or she is then able to accomplish age-appropriate skills, which should allow for the performance of ADL. Although this may happen for some children, other children require additional direct intervention to bring them up to age-appropriate levels in these specific tasks. For this, an additional frame of reference must be used, perhaps one that addresses specific skill acquisition. Such an additional frame would have to focus on teaching the child specific skills to perform ADL successfully, such as the acquisitional frames of reference discussed in Chapter 14. In these situations, the occupational therapist must resort to using more than one frame of reference.

Constructing a relevant plan of intervention for a child with multiple problems often requires more than one frame of reference (Mosey, 1986). When a frame of reference is used in the purest sense (as each chapter in this book suggests) then it may deal with some of a child's most significant problems at the time, but it frequently is not adequate for the entire course of treatment. Whenever the therapist considers using combined or sequenced frames of reference, it is necessary to develop a basic understanding of what each one entails, as well as its unique approach to intervention.

Frames of Reference in Sequence

Frames of reference can be used in sequence—that is, one frame of reference is used primarily while another is employed for a separate and more discrete problem. For example, a child who has cerebral palsy may be treated first with the Neuro-Developmental frame of reference. After seeing the child for several months, the therapist might observe that the child also appears to be having visual perceptual problems. The therapist then evaluates the child based on the visual perception frame of reference. In this situation, the therapist decides to continue with the Neuro-Developmental Treatment frame but also decides to use the visual perception frame. Each frame of reference addresses different performance components and draws from different theories. Furthermore, each is based on different developmental perspectives as well as a belief that change occurs in different ways.

The study of these two frames of reference leads the therapist to understand that neither is congruent with the other in its approach to the change process. They are not in conflict, however, when applied separately. Conflict is when constructs or postulates do not agree because they are contradictory from a theoretical perspective. In this situation, each frame interprets the change process in a different way. Because of this, neither one will be compatible with the other should the therapist attempt to integrate them. The therapist will decide, therefore, to use these frames of reference in sequence, with the Neuro-Developmental Treatment frame as the basic approach. Each session will begin with the Neuro-Developmental Treatment frame, and toward the end of the time, switch to the visual perception frame.

Each aspect of the intervention is clearly delineated and grounded in the theoretical base for each frame of reference. This clear demarcation is evident in the environment that the therapist creates for change and also in the use of legitimate tools. During the Neuro-Developmental Treatment portion of the treatment session, the child and the therapist may be on a mat, with the therapist using rolls, balls, and/or therapeutic handling in play activities. During the visual perception portion of the treatment session, the child may sit at a table and participate in drawing activities. The techniques and activities of intervention from each frame of reference are not integrated. The therapist, though, is always aware of the frame of reference used at any given point in the session.

The characteristics of sequential intervention require that one frame of reference be designated as primary, followed by others in a set order that addresses discrete problems. Each frame of reference maintains its own integrity, and the therapeutic goals are separate. The intervention and the legitimate tools are distinctly tied to each unique theoretical base.

Frames of Reference in Parallel

Frames of reference can also be used in parallel. In this situation, two frames of reference are used at the same time to address similar or related problems from different perspectives. Each frame is used separately in different treatment sessions or even in separate intervention processes. Although they may not share the same theoretical perspectives, they do not conflict. Two frames of reference used often in parallel are the

Neuro-Developmental and biomechanical frames of reference. A therapist may treat a child who has cerebral palsy by first using the Neuro-Developmental Treatment frame of reference. She has selected this one to enhance the child's movement abilities and to assist him or her in developing as many normal patterns as possible. During the course of treatment, the therapist may reason that the child would benefit from using adaptive equipment. She then selects the biomechanical frame of reference to determine what equipment or devices might provide proper positioning for the child to improve motor skills.

The primary tool of the Neuro-Developmental frame of reference is therapeutic handling whereas the biomechanical frame relies on specific devices and therapeutic equipment to position the child. This is not meant to oversimplify either frame of reference. It is, rather, to point out that they do not conflict with one another, work toward similar goals, and, therefore, can be used well in parallel manner. In this case, the Neuro-Developmental frame of reference addresses a child's primary motor development, whereas the biomechanical frame of reference is used to address the child's static positioning needs. The Neuro-Developmental Treatment frame guides a therapist's regularly scheduled treatment sessions whereas the biomechanical frame of reference for positioning children for functioning provides proper seating equipment that positions a child throughout the day. Separately, each frame of reference addresses separate aspects of the child's motor performance. Jointly, the two facilitate intervention.

There is a relatively fine line between using frames of reference in sequence and using them in parallel. When using frames of reference in sequence, one frame of reference is primary, while the second (or third) frame of reference is more adjunctive. When using frames of reference in parallel, both are used at the same time, but relatively discretely, to address different areas. The two frames of reference are never integrated together.

Frames of Reference in Combination

Frames of reference can be used in combination in an integrative way. This can be done when the constructs of a theoretical base are consistent in that they agree about how change occurs. To use frames of reference in combination requires a skilled, experienced therapist who understands each frame. A therapist has to examine each one to determine whether its basic postulates are congruent with those of the other frames of reference. To use the postulates regarding change together, the basic concepts should be consistent in stating the same or similar things.

Two frames of reference that can easily be used in combination are the frames of reference for sensory integration and Neuro-Developmental treatment. Both are oriented developmentally and propose that specific skills and abilities are achieved in a specified sequence. When frames of reference are used in combination, the techniques of both are integrated during each intervention session. Chapter 15 discussed how the biomechanical frame of reference can be used frequently in combination with NDT.

The main characteristic of combined intervention is that two separate frames of reference can be integrated to best address the needs of a child as a whole. Both frames must be somewhat consistent with each other in terms of their underlying principles, and the therapeutic goals are integrated. The intervention is a blend that involves the combined use of various legitimate tools.

A skilled, competent therapist who combines two frames of reference over time may begin to view them as one. This is truly the use of two frames in combination. To make this into one "new" frame of reference, a therapist must reconstruct the theoretical base, carefully exploring the concepts, postulates, and assumptions from each to interweave them into a unified theoretical base that is internally consistent. From that point, the therapist must reformulate the entire frame of reference. This process is intense and generally requires postprofessional education and scholarship. The development of a new frame of reference provides new options for practice and contributes to the body of knowledge of the profession.

FORMULATION OF ORIGINAL FRAMES OF REFERENCE

The formulation of new and original frames of reference is an ongoing process in occupational therapy. As a dynamic profession, the endemic problems change continuously. This section focuses on the need for new frames of reference and serves as an overview of the process of developing new frames. Additional information can be found in discussions of applied scientific inquiry for occupational therapy (Mosey, 1989, 1992).

Over time, knowledge increases and technology advances. This creates change not only in society but also in the problems with which occupational therapists are concerned. One example is the technological strides made in neonatal intensive care that have resulted in the survival of more low–birth-weight babies. This new population, with its unique needs, requires specialized intervention. This has been handled in several ways. Some therapists have modified or reformulated traditional frames of reference around the specific problems of low–birth-weight infants. Other therapists have begun to evolve new frames of reference based on new theoretical information to work with this specific population. Each case requires advanced skills and knowledge.

As society changes, the profession of occupational therapy adapts, mandating the search for innovative approaches and solutions to problems. This situation requires that occupational therapists develop new frames of reference. Infants born addicted to cocaine or those born with human immunodeficiency virus (HIV) infections are examples of "new" client groups. Another reason that might stimulate the development of new frames of reference is the need to change or add legitimate tools or when the context or setting for therapy is changed.

A change in knowledge also precipitates the need for new frames of reference. This "new" knowledge may result from the refinement of theory, the development of new theories, or new research findings that modify the theoretical bases of old frames of reference. This may also occur when a therapist finds that specific postulates regarding change from a particular frame of reference no longer work, or when he or she is unable to find one that addresses a specific dysfunction.

The process of developing and articulating a frame of reference is complex. It requires a strong, scholarly knowledge base combined with advanced clinical reasoning skills. It follows the sequence discussed in Chapter 1, concentrating first on raw theoretical information which is then woven into a comprehensive and cohesive theoretical base. From this sound foundation, a therapist formulates the rest of the function–dysfunction continua, identifies behaviors indicative of function and dysfunction, specifies evaluation procedures and tools, writes postulates regarding change, and outlines an application for practice. Throughout this process, the therapist is concerned about the systematic ordering of concepts and constructs combined with internal consistency so that a clear design can be formed to link theory to practice. The development of new frames of reference is critical to the profession because these frames of reference expand the knowledge of the profession and provide additional tools for addressing problems found in society.

 ## Summary

With experience, therapists become more adept at identifying clients' problems and figuring out ways to deal with different deficits. The novice therapist begins understanding the intervention process by using a single frame of reference for the treatment of each client. After the therapist becomes comfortable with the theories that guide pediatric practice, he or she can then experiment with different ways of using various frames of reference, including sequential, parallel, and combined uses. The sophisticated, scholarly therapist eventually may move toward formulating a new frame of reference to guide intervention in new areas of practice.

REFERENCES

Crepeau, E. B. (1991). Achieving intersubjective understanding: Examples from an occupational therapy treatment session. *American Journal of Occupational Therapy, 45*, 1016–1025.

Gilfoyle, E. M. (1980). Caring: A philosophy for practice. *American Journal of Occupational Therapy, 34*, 517–521.

Mosey, A. C. (1981a). *Occupational Therapy: Configuration of a Profession*. New York: Raven Press.

Mosey, A. C. (1981b). Introduction: The art of practice. In B. Abreu (Ed). *Physical Disabilities Manual* (pp. 1–3). New York: Raven Press.

Mosey, A. C. (1986). *Psychosocial Components of Occupational Therapy*. New York: Raven Press.

Mosey, A. C. (1989). The proper focus of scientific inquiry in occupational therapy: Frames of reference (Editorial). *Occupational Therapy Journal of Research, 9*, 195–201.

Mosey, A. C. (1992). *Applied Scientific Inquiry in Health Professions: An Epistemological Orientation*. Rockville, MD: American Occupational Therapy Association.

Peloquin, S. M. (1989). Sustaining the art of practice in occupational therapy. *American Journal of Occupational Therapy, 43*, 219–226.

Peloquin, S. M. (1990). The patient-therapist relationship in occupational therapy: Understanding visions and images. *American Journal of Occupational Therapy, 44*(1), 13–21.

Peloquin, S. M. (2002). Reclaiming the vision of reaching for heart as well as hands. *American Journal of Occupational Therapy, 56*(5), 517–526.

Perlman, H. H. (1979). *Relationship: The Heart of Helping People*. Chicago, IL: The University of Chicago Press.

CHAPTER 17

Applying the Evidence-Based Practice Approach

TIEN-NI WANG • JIM HINOJOSA • PAULA KRAMER

Evidence-based practice (EBP) has been enthusiastically promoted in the last two decades. Therapists want to implement their practice with the support of evidence. EBP was originally developed in the area of medicine and is now part of nearly every healthcare discipline and professional education program. Currently, therapists must be concerned about the evidence they have to support their interventions. Therefore, it is critical to engage in research to support the efficacy of the frames of reference.

WHAT IS EVIDENCE-BASED PRACTICE?

EBP originated from the field of medicine and was initially referred to as "evidence-based medicine," which is the "conscientious, explicit, and judicious use of the current best evidence in making decisions about the care of individual patients" (Sackett et al., 1996). An expanded definition of evidence-based medicine/EBP came from Rosenberg & Donald (1995), who defined it as: "the process of systematically finding, appraising, and using contemporaneous research findings as the basis for clinical decisions. Evidence-based medicine/evidence-based practice asks questions, finds and appraises the relevant data, and harnesses the information for everyday clinical practice" (p. 1122). The two terms are often used interchangeably. Though, technically, evidence-based medicine refers only to the medical field, whereas EBP denotes other fields of healthcare (Law, 2002).

In evaluating clinical research, EBP involves the application of standardized criteria to grade the strength of relevant evidence. The evidence can be ranked from (at the most rigorous) highly variable, randomized, controlled trials published in a peer-reviewed professional journal to, at the other end, a trusted colleague's professional opinion or one's own experience. The terms "level of evidence" or "strength of evidence" refer to the system that classifies scientific studies in a hierarchy from highly valid to exhibiting serious flaws. Such a system can be used to judge and evaluate a level of evidence by reviewing research designs or derived and published data (Johnston, Sherer, & Whyte, 2006). According to this ranking system, systematic reviews or randomized controlled trials are always viewed as providing the highest level of evidence. The strength/level of evidence decreases in the following order: cohort studies, retrospective studies, opinions of respected authorities based on clinical experience, descriptive studies, and reports from expert committees (Humphris, 2005; Johnston, et al., 2006). The major purpose of rating the level of evidence is to assess the likelihood of bias related to a study's conclusions. Although it may not be difficult to understand the different forms or levels of evidence, it is far more important to know exactly what critical questions to ask and how to make critical judgments about evidence (Humphris, 2005).

Moreover, although a randomized, controlled trial is always viewed as the gold standard of design providing the strongest evidence, one should not assume that EBP is restricted only to randomized, controlled trial or meta-analyses. When no randomized, controlled trial has been conducted in the area of interest, other forms of evidence can be graded to provide answers to the questions being posed. As a result, the evidence-based approach should be the integration of external clinical evidence from systematic research with individual clinical expertise and patient values (Sackett et al., 1996).

A distinction should be made between how EBP is used in clinical practice and in research, although the two are often intermingled. The importance of viewing EBP as an ideology is related to the fact that medical clinical practice is not and cannot be static. Because EBP emphasizes the current and best evidence, knowledge about a particular treatment or intervention approach should be an ever-evolving process. The effectiveness of an intervention should be evaluated and reevaluated. Such evaluation can be done by using clinical judgment related to individual patients, but, more importantly, by conducting systematic investigations or clinical trials on groups of patients. An intervention should be used to treat a condition if it brings about positive effects or abandoned if the opposite is true. This is what Sackett et al. (2000) meant by calling EBP "a dynamic process." It begins when information is converted into an answerable question. Then you track down the best evidence to answer that question, appraising the evidence critically, applying the results in practice, evaluating the effectiveness and efficiency of the result, and then replicating the process continuously to find the best and most up-to-date evidence.

The Advantages of Applying Evidence-Based Practice

As a basis for practice, looking to research evidence began in the mid-20th century when Cochrane (1972) critiqued the effectiveness and efficiency of healthcare services. Evidence-based medicine first surfaced in clinical epidemiology; that is, researchers started examining existing research evidence protocols by providing systematic summaries on treatment effects (Cochrane, 1972). In the late 20th century, evidence-based approaches were embraced by many health and education fields including nursing, psychosocial health, education, and rehabilitation.

Since that time, EBP has increased in popularity and has spread from medicine to other health-related fields (Dawes et al., 2005). Unlike medicine, however, which used precise protocols or stringent standards to examine evidence, health-related professions such as nursing or allied health disciplines do not use the same standards to scrutinize treatment effectiveness. Although the concept of EBP is endorsed by all medical fields, it has been applied differently in other health-related professions, such as occupational therapy (Holm, 2000).

After the evidence-based approach came into use, many health-related disciplines have journeyed in its direction. Hence, regardless of which field (whether education, social services, government, or healthcare) one works in, you are likely to have encountered EBP. There are many benefits and advantages to implementing the EBP approach in clinical practice. First, EBP meets ethical criteria. If you or a loved one were diagnosed with a serious or fatal illness, would you not want to know the best treatment options based on evidence from high-quality studies? Would you wish your doctor, therapist, or social worker were an evidence-based practitioner? Using ethical considerations, it is a clinician's responsibility to provide services that avoid inflicting harm during the process of treatment. A clinician should treat patients as efficiently as possible to "do things better" and "do the right things" (Gray, 1997; Lopez et al., 2008; Tickle-Degnen, 2002). EBP is a conscientious, discriminative process of applying the best evidence when making decisions regarding client care (Christiansen, 2001; Lloyd-Smith, 1997). It can fulfill practitioners' ethical obligations to fully apply evaluation and research evidence in their professional practices.

Secondly, from patients and their families' points of view, the major benefit of EBP is receiving the best care efficiently. EBP is the conscientious and careful application of the current best evidence integrated with clinical expertise and patient values (Sackett et al., 2000). EBP can provide the most up-to-date and valid intervention. When these three elements are integrated, patients receive the best service. Moreover, nonclinicians or consumers can participate in and benefit from the EBP approach as well. They can actively participate in the process of decision making or obtain optimal choice by accessing related evidence (Dracup & Bryan-Brown, 2006; Rosenberg & Donald, 1995).

Third, for clinicians, the EBP approach can help them to make better clinical decisions. Clinical decision making is the end point of a process that includes clinical reasoning, problem solving, and awareness of patient and healthcare context (Maudsley, 2000). Sometimes, there is no clear correct answer during this process. Hence, the EBP approach can be helpful in clarifying some of the uncertainties in this decision-making process by using explicit knowledge obtained from research (Dawes et al., 2005; Singleton & Truglio-Londrigan, 2006). Furthermore, EBP can transform clinicians from passive readers of journal articles into active inquirers. In other words, reading evidence-based summaries can help clinicians develop new research and maintain up-to-date practice (Rosenberg & Donald, 1995). The EBP approach is one of the most useful tools for every clinician because it helps in conducting self-directed and life-long learning skills to solve clinical problems (Sackett et al., 2000).

Finally, EBP can help in the development of the profession. EBP represents a shift from making decisions based on opinion, tradition, or past experiences toward decisions based on scientific research and evidence (Melnyk, 2005; Sackett et al., 2000). Often, traditional sources are inadequate because they are out-of-date, wrong, ineffective, or too overwhelming in their volume. Thus, EBP can help each profession to integrate the latest and most valid evidence to improve overall practices and build professional knowledge. Furthermore, EBP can improve communication and understanding between people from different backgrounds, such as between researchers and clinicians, or between practitioners and consumers (Rosenberg & Donald, 1995). It is the conscientious use of the best available research in combination with clinicians' expertise and judgment and patients' preferences and values to arrive at the best decision that leads to positive, high-quality patient outcomes (Sackett et al., 1996). Also, EBP can provide a common framework for problem solving and clinical practice by constantly updating and integrating current evidence. It is very important to adopt an EBP approach so that evidence can help a profession to establish credibility and trustworthiness of practice.

The Disadvantages/Limitations of Applying Evidence-Based Practice

Although EBP is embraced by most professions, we should be aware of the challenges and potential disadvantages of using it as the only paradigm through which to judge the quality of service. Several challenging issues in applying the EBP approach in clinical practice will now be discussed.

First, the EBP approach is time consuming to learn and to practice. It requires sufficient time to properly set questions, find and appraise the evidence, and then act on that evidence (Rosenberg & Donald, 1995; Sackett et al., 2000). Busy clinicians may have limited amounts of time to master and apply these new skills. Many report insufficient time on the job to search for and read research (Dubouloz et al., 1999).

Limited resources are a second problem. Evidence is lacking to answer many of the questions that arise in clinical practice. For example, there is often insufficient literature or research, poor quality research (Rosenberg & Donald, 1995), inconsistent scientific evidence including inconclusive, inconsistent results from previous studies (Straus & McAlister, 2000), and limited number of people who can conveniently obtain the information (Pape, 2003).

Third, to implement EBP, clinicians need to develop new skills, including the abilities to perform systematic research and appraise literature (Pape, 2003; Rosenberg & Donald, 1995; Sackett et al., 2000; Straus & McAlister, 2000). As discussed above, the EBP approach is a dynamic process; it emphasizes systematically searching for and organizing relevant evidence, critically evaluating and appraising that evidence for currency and validity, and using the best evidence to enhance clinical practice. During this process, clinicians should know where and how to obtain information, recognize what information is needed to guide practice, understand and interpret the meaning of statistical knowledge, analyze the strengths and limitations of methodologies, and then analyze or synthesize these findings (Rosenberg & Donald, 1995; Sackett et al., 2000). Most clinicians, however, are not trained well in this approach and may not have adequate research skills. They may not be skillful in conducting literature reviews, may not be able to distinguish poor quality studies, or may not know how to apply evidence in practice. Also, some may not be motivated to learn these new skills in clinical practice (Straus & McAlister, 2000). Still others view the EBP approach as a threat to routine ways of analyzing choices and implementing clinical practice (Dubouloz, et al., 1999).

Finally, EBP suggests using the best available evidence. Randomized, controlled trials are always viewed as the best evidence or "gold standard" allowing researchers to control for the factors (both known and unknown) that may account for the outcome of an intervention. The best evidence is then brought together in meta-analysis and systematic reviews of randomized, controlled trials. There are, however, challenges involved in this assumption. First, the number of randomized, controlled trials is limited (Straus & McAlister, 2000), especially in health-related fields other than medicine. Also, producing randomized, controlled trials sometimes raises ethical concerns. Second, clinical trials are based mostly on highly homogenous samples. It is difficult, however, to apply evidence to the care of individual patients who are seldom homogeneous or may not even remotely resemble patients described in the clinical trails (Dracup & Bryan-Brown, 2006). Furthermore, should randomized, controlled trials always be viewed as the best evidence? Often, the best evidence can also be generated through other means. For example, according to the criteria for levels of evidence, studies using secondary data analysis and statistical analyses are not regarded as powerful for providing evidence on effectiveness. However, these methodologies can indeed answer important questions that may not be clear from randomized, controlled trials (Kessler, Gira, & Poertner, 2005). Also, qualitative studies may often be considered the lowest level of evidence, but they can provide a wealth of information concerning clients' perspectives. These are critical to understanding clients' thoughts, emotions, and experiences in planning interventions (Kessler, Gira, & Poertner, 2005).

Applying Evidence-Based Practice in Occupational Therapy

Occupational therapy (like most healthcare disciplines) is increasingly urged to ensure that practice and decision making is based on the most valid scientific evidence (Holm, 2000; Law & Baum, 1998). The Accreditation Standards for a Master's-Degree-Level Educational Program for the Occupational Therapist (AOTA, 2006) require that therapists be prepared to provide "evidence-based evaluations and interventions" (p. 652).

It is our responsibility as occupational therapists to use the best available evidence in clinical decision making as a fundamental element in ethical practice. In 2004, the International Conference on Evidence-Based Occupational Therapy (Bethesda, Maryland, July 11–14, 2004) was designed to facilitate efficient and effective EBP in the field, to enhance dissemination of research information for EBP, and to identify and address gaps in research (Coster, 2005).

According to Tickle-Degnen (1999), EBP is like a toolbox of methods which can help clinical reasoning, and, thus, it can integrate research evidence into the clinical reasoning process. The EBP approach can help a practitioner select the best assessments and intervention procedures (Tickle-Degnen, 1999). Take, for example, the sensory modulation deficit. The diagnosis and its intervention effectiveness used to be questioned. Now, with the emergence of scientific evidence regarding interventions for it, the treatment is more convincing and acceptable. In this way, EBP can help to apply treatment and clinical skills with a strong evidence base of effectiveness instead of relying only on previous experience of traditional practices.

While the main principles of EBP are relevant (i.e., the use of the current best evidence to make treatment decisions), the question remains whether occupational therapy should directly apply the process to practice? Some specific challenges and limitations are raised by this question. First, the domain and practice of occupational therapy is multifaceted, and potentially relevant literature may be found in various medical, educational, psychological, and other social science sources. Occupational therapy deals with various situations ranging from individual problems to issues involving whole communities or even society as a whole. As a result, there are many variables that should be considered which may make searching for evidence very complicated. Additionally, the trust relationship between a therapist and a patient plays a very important role in patient outcomes. A solid, trusting relationship can increase patient motivation and his or her satisfaction with an intervention. This, however, is often neglected in studies and is difficult to study.

Finally, is the best evidence for medicine (such as randomized, controlled trials) also the best evidence for occupational therapy? As a profession, we need to clearly understand what kind of evidence is needed before determining what is the "best" evidence. Another general problem is that often healthcare workers are slow or even passive about adopting clinical practices based on scientific findings. As practitioners in occupational therapy, some of our evidence resides within individual practitioners. For occupational therapists in clinical settings, practices are generally based on their own personal experience, their colleagues' or mentors' experience, or the voice of an expert. Some active practitioners, however, may update their practice based on scientific literature, but they usually skip the most important part—methodology. Instead, they only apply information from the introduction and discussion sections of relevant papers. They may uncritically accept the findings of a single published study. They may get information from the Internet without questioning the validity of the source. Or, they may take whatever the author says for granted and apply it directly into clinical practice without modification.

EFFICACY OF A FRAME OF REFERENCE

How does one establish the efficacy of a frame of reference? What research is most appropriate? Dr. Anne Cronin Mosey clearly outlines two forms of applied research that are unique to examining the adequacy of the frame of reference (Mosey, 1996). Applied research is distinctly different from basic scientific inquiry. It is important to note that basic scientific inquiry is not appropriate for examining frames of reference. First, the purpose of basic scientific inquiry is to develop and test theories. While a frame of reference is based on theories, the frame of reference itself is not a theory. It is a way to put a theory into practice. The theoretical base of the frame of reference is a collection of theoretical concepts, definitions, and postulates from one or more theories. It is not the whole theory. When performing applied research on a frame of reference, you are not examining the theories that contribute to the theoretical base. You are hoping to explore some aspect of the outcomes of intervention with the frame of reference and not the underlying theories. Therefore, any research that examines a frame of reference does not examine the specific theories that the theoretical base of the frame of reference is based on.

Accordingly, examination of the frame of reference requires the use of applied research. Applied research answers practical questions. For example, does something work, is something effective, or how effective is something? Applied research uses the same methods of science and research designs as basic research but asks questions about whether something is effective or useful, rather than questions about the theory itself. Applied researchers can examine frames of references from two perspectives. First, research can assess the efficacy of the entire frame of reference. In this case, the researcher assesses whether the frame of reference accurately resolves the problems. For example, if the frame of reference is to develop young children's handwriting skills, the application of the frame of reference should result in significant improvement in handwriting.

Secondly, a researcher can also examine component parts of the frame of reference to determine their adequacy. The term "adequacy" is used to indicate that it is related to the specific frame of reference and is the degree to which the section of the frame of reference being explored is satisfactory for the whole frame of reference. The two component parts of the frame of reference that can be examined for adequacy are the evaluation section (accuracy of problem identification) and the postulates regarding change (precision at resolving the problem).

Efficacy of the Entire Frame of Reference

A frame of reference may be examined from multiple perspectives. Common questions may examine the reliability, applicability, and specificity. It may also look at the outcome of intervention using the frame of reference. Does a child who is treated using this frame of reference demonstrate improvement in the expected areas of performance?

Reliability of a frame of reference examines the entire frame of reference or the application of the frame of reference by a therapist. For example, a researcher might examine whether the results or outcomes of the intervention are the same between two matched groups. Another researcher might examine whether individual clients have the same outcomes, when the same intervention is used. Another aspect of reliability is whether two or more therapists who use the frame of reference have the same results. In these studies, a researcher examines the consistency of the application of the frame across participants. Reliability would be the extent to which two or more therapists have the same outcomes. The focus on all these studies is the entire frame of reference.

Applicability of a frame of reference refers the extent to which the frame of reference can be applied to different individuals. It is similar to external validity of a quantitative study. There are two major concerns: First, are the outcomes important and applicable in terms of the client's life? Secondly, are the outcomes valued and significant to the client and/or his or her family? Third, are the outcomes significant to alter performance as viewed by external individuals, such as school personnel? Two research designs that can be useful to examine applicability are surveys and qualitative observational and interview designs.

Specificity examines when, how often, and how long a specific frame of reference should be used. In these studies, the researcher is concerned with examining the use of the frame of reference under various conditions. For example, is the frame of reference more effective when it is used twice a week as compared to once a week? Or, is the frame of reference effective for only a short period of time? For example, a researcher might be interested in knowing whether therapy to improve handwriting once a week for 6 months is more or less effective than intensive therapy every day for 1 hour for 3 weeks.

Efficacy of the Component Parts of a Frame of Reference

Examining the efficacy of the components parts of the frame of reference involves looking at the adequacy of both the evaluation section and postulates regarding change. Both these areas are discussed separately.

Adequacy of the Guide to Evaluation Section

This involves exploring the evaluation tools listed in the Guide to Evaluation section. These tools should be studied one at a time. Are they effective tools? Are they reliable and valid? Have these tools been adequately tested with the age range of children whom this frame of reference addresses?

The therapist also needs to determine if the tools recommended in the Guide to Evaluation section give a comprehensive picture of the child, and will allow the therapist to determine, plan an appropriate intervention, and then decide whether the intervention chosen will meet the needs of the child. Each tool or area of the guide to evaluation should be explored individually and then as a group. A review of the psychometric properties of the assessment tools (e.g., reliability and validity) would be a way to begin this evaluation. Quantitative methods using various experimental designs would also be appropriate for exploring this area.

Adequacy of the Postulates Regarding Change

When exploring the adequacy of the postulates regarding change, therapists can test the efficacy of one postulate at a time or a specific group of postulates regarding change. The therapist has to define a way to determine if a postulate can be effectively examined individually or not. It might be easier to explore postulates in groups, such as general postulates listed in the frame of reference or the sections into which the frame of reference divides them. One has to look at how the child responds to the intervention, whether progress has been made, and whether the progress made was as expected based on the theoretical base. Ultimately, you are looking at whether the postulates are addressing the issues that the frames of reference professes to address, and whether the child is showing changes in behavior or performance as outlined in the theoretical base. This can be done through both qualitative and quantitative methodologies, range from surveys and interviews to single case studies, and randomized controlled trials.

Summary

EBP is critical to the acceptance and growth of occupational therapy in general. It is essential that we research our frames of reference to determine their efficacy. This research should lead to modifications, either major or minor, of the frame of reference, so that ultimately we receive the expected outcome with our clients. Another alternative may be that research consistently demonstrated that the frame of reference does not yield the expected outcomes, even with modifications and therefore will no longer be used. The ongoing research of frames of reference in various formats presented in this chapter, with both qualitative and quantitative methods, is necessary for the continued growth of occupational therapy.

REFERENCES

American Occupational Therapy Association. (2006). The accreditation standards for a master's-degree-level educational program for the occupational therapist. *American Journal of Occupational Therapy, 61*(6), 652–661.

Christiansen, C. (2001). Ethical considerations related to evidence-based practice. *American Journal of Occupational Therapy, 55*, 345–349.

Cochrane, A. L. (1972). *Effectiveness and Efficiency: Random Reflections on Health Services*. Leeds: Nuffield Provincial Hospitals Trust.

Coster, W. (2005). International conference on evidence-based practice: A collaborative effort of the American Occupational Therapy Association, the American Occupational Therapy Foundation, and the Agency for Healthcare Research and Quality. *American Journal of Occupational Therapy, 59*(3), 356–358.

Lopez, A., Vanner, E. A., Cowan, A. M., Samuels, A. P., Shepherd, D. L. (2005). Sicily statement on evidence-based practice. *BMC Medical Education, 5*(1), 1–7.

Dracup, K., & Bryan-Brown, C. W. (2006). Evidence-based practice is wonderful… sort of. *American Journal of Critical Care, 15*(4), 356–359.

Dubouloz, C. J., Egan, M., Vallerand, J., & von Zweck, C. V. (1999). Occupational therapists' perceptions of evidence-based practice. *American Journal of Occupational Therapy, 53*, 445–453.

Gray, J. A. M. (1997). *Evidence-Based Healthcare: How to Make Health Policy and Management Decisions*. New York: Churchill Livingstone.

Holm, M. B. (2000). Our mandate for the new millennium: Evidence-based practice, 2000 Eleanor Clarke Slagle lecture. *American Journal of Occupational Therapy, 54*, 575–585.

Humphris, D. (2005). Types of evidence. In S. Hamer, & G. Collinson (Eds). *Achieving Evidence-Based Practice* (2nd ed., pp. 15–42). New York: Bailliere Tindall, Elsevier Science.

Johnston, M. V., Sherer, M., & Whyte, J. (2006). Applying evidence standards to rehabilitation research. *American Journal of Physical Medicine and Rehabilitation, 85*(4), 292–309.

Kessler, M. L., Gira, E., & Poertner, J. (2005). Moving best practice to evidence-based practice in child welfare. *The Journal of Contemporary Social Services, 86*(2), 244–250.

Law, M. (2002). Introduction to evidence-based practice. In M. Law (Ed). *Evidence-Based Rehabilitation: A Guide to Practice* (pp. 3–13). Thorofare, NJ: Slack Inc.

Law, M., & Baum, C. (1998). Evidence-based occupational therapy practice. *Canadian Journal of Occupational Therapy, 35*, 131–135.

Lloyd-Smith, W. (1997). Evidence-based practice and occupational therapy. *British Journal of Occupational Therapy, 60*, 474–478.

Lopez, A., Vanner, E. A., Cowan, A. M., Samuel, A. P., Shepherd, D. L., & Lopez, A., et al. (2008). Intervention planning facets—four facets of occupational therapy intervention planning: Economics, ethics, professional judgment, and evidence-based practice. *American Journal of Occupational Therapy, 62*(1), 87–96.

Maudsley, G. S. (2000). Science, critical thinking and competence for tomorrow's doctors. A review of terms and concepts. *Journal of Medical Education, 34*, 53–60.

Melnyk, B. M. (2005). *Evidence-Based Practice in Nursing and Healthcare: A Guide to Best Practice*. Philadelphia, PA: Lippincott Williams & Wilkins.

Mosey, A. C. (1996). *Applied Scientific Inquiry in the Health Professions: An Epistemological Orientation* (2nd ed.). Bethesda, MD: American Occupational Therapy Association.

Pape, T. M. (2003). Evidence-based nursing practice: To infinity and beyond. *The Journal of Continuing Education in Nursing, 34*(4), 154–161.

Rosenberg, W., & Donald, A. (1995). Evidence based medicine: An approach to clinical problem-solving. *British Medical Journal, 310*, 1122–1126.

Sackett, D. L., Rosenberg, W. M., Gray, J. A. M., Haynes, R. B., & Richardson, W. S. (1996). Evidence based medicine: What it is and what it isn't. *British Medical Journal, 312*, 71–72.

Sackett, D. L., Straus, S. E., Richardson, W. S., Rosenberg, W., & Haynes, R. B. (2000). *Evidence-Based Medicine: How to Practice and Teach EBM* (2nd ed.). New York: Churchill Livingstone.

Singleton, J. K., & Truglio-Londrigan, M. (2006). Is best practice in your practice? If you use this step-by-step guide to evidence-based practice, you'll say "yes!." *Nursing Spectrum (DC/Maryland/Virginia Edition), 16*(15), 28–29.

Straus, S. E., & McAlister, F. A. (2000). Evidence-based medicine: A commentary on common criticisms. *Canadian Medical Association Journal, 163*(7), 837–841.

Tickle-Degnen, L. (1999). Organizing, evaluating, and using evidence in occupational therapy practice. *American Journal of Occupational Therapy, 53*, 537–539.

Tickle-Degnen, L. (2002). Evidence-based practice forum—client-centered practice, therapeutic relationship, and the use of research evidence. *American Journal of Occupational Therapy, 56*, 470–474.

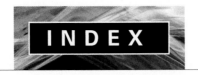

INDEX

Page numbers in *italics* refer to illustrations